Goodheart's Photoguide to Common Pediatric and Adult Skin Disorders

Diagnosis and Management

Goodheart's Photoguide to Common Pediatric and Adult Skin Disorders

Diagnosis and Management

FOURTH EDITION

Herbert P. Goodheart, MD
Associate Clinical Professor
Department of Dermatology
Icahn School of Medicine at Mount Sinai
New York, New York
Director of Dermatology
Elmhurst Hospital Center
Elmhurst, New York

Mercedes E. Gonzalez, MD
Assistant Clinical Professor
Department of Dermatology and Cutaneous Surgery
University of Miami Miller School of Medicine
and Department of Dermatology
Herbert Wertheim College of Medicine
Florida International University
Director, Pediatric Dermatology of Miami
Miami, FL

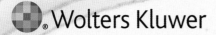

. Wolters Kluwer

Philadelphia • Baltimore • New York • London
Buenos Aires • Hong Kong • Sydney • Tokyo

Acquisitions Editor: Kel McGowan
Senior Product Development Editor: Kristina Oberle
Senior Production Project Manager: Alicia Jackson
Marketing Manager: Stephanie Kindlick
Design Coordinator: Steven Druding
Senior Manufacturing Coordinator: Beth Welsh
Prepress Vendor: Aptara, Inc.

9 8 7 6 5 4 3 2 1

Printed in China

978-1-45112-062-2

Library of Congress Cataloging-in-Publication Data
available upon request

LWW.com

Authors

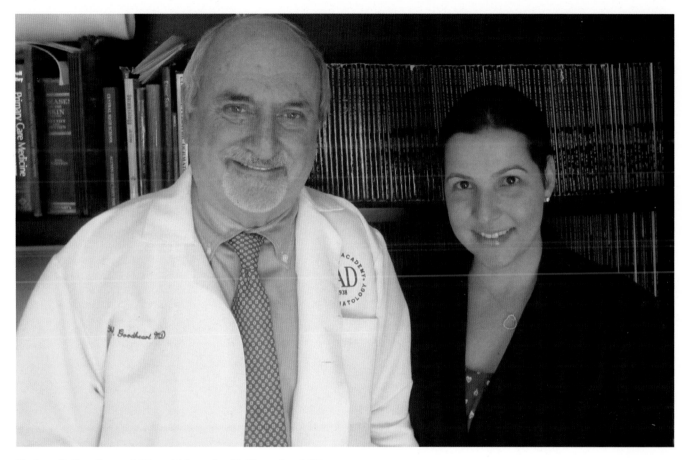

Herbert P. Goodheart, MD and Mercedes E. Gonzalez, MD

To our families, Karen and David, & Rogerio, Rogie and Maggie, who have provided immense support and encouragement throughout.

Herbert P. Goodheart, MD
Mercedes E. Gonzalez, MD

What the mind
does not know,
the eyes cannot see.
ANCIENT PROVERB

Foreword

As a second-year medical student, I recall studying cardiology one evening when my brother Andrew asked me to look at a rash that developed on his trunk. I did not have a clue as to how to make *any* dermatologic diagnosis. So, after Andrew accused my father of wasting tuition money on my evidently inadequate education, I thought it proper to register for a dermatology elective in my fourth year. I reasoned that, regardless of whatever field I would ultimately choose, I would inevitably be confronted with some cutaneous dilemmas. It was with tremendous fortune that I subsequently trained at the Albert Einstein College of Medicine in the Bronx, New York, under the tutelage of Michael Fisher, MD, the former head of the illustrious division of dermatology. It was during my training that I befriended the attending physician, Dr. Herb Goodheart. Herb always provided special insights, wisdom, and compassion in the evaluation of even the most rudimentary dermatologic disorders. He is a stellar teacher and dermatologist, who has compiled his years of perspicacity into this guide to dermatology.

As we begin the twenty-first century, the landscape of American medicine and dermatology is changing at an accelerating pace. Even though we can now comprehend many skin disorders at a molecular level and have advanced our therapeutic realm to include laser technology and immunobiology, the cornerstone of all dermatologic endeavors will always be careful clinical observation. As venues of practice shift toward a greater proportion of primary dermatologic care being delivered by nondermatologists, resources for these providers must be accessible, comprehensible, and practical.

Dr. Goodheart's guide to dermatology is divided into common disorders, the interrelationship between the skin and systemic diseases, basic and advanced dermatologic procedures, and a very useful appendix that provides patient handout material in both English and Spanish. Importantly, it combines features of an atlas with Herb's pithy perspectives, as though he is standing over your shoulder in the dermatology clinic. I am pleased to see that this fourth edition of Goodheart's has Dr. Mercedes E. Gonzalez contributing her considerable knowledge of pediatric dermatology and pediatrics. I am certain that such an addition will be an invaluable tool to help clinicians navigate through the various dermatologic disorders of all ages and will make it an invaluable resource for pediatricians as well as those in primary care.

Those who use this guide will come to appreciate many of the finer points and opinions that Drs. Goodheart and Gonzalez provide and even more so when becoming more facile with the discipline. Use this guide as a primer, an atlas, a consultant, and as a supplement to more in-depth dermatology texts and medical literature. Your dermatologic knowledge base will flourish, your appreciation of the field will blossom, and most importantly, your patients will benefit from your expertise.

Warren R. Heymann, MD
Head, Division of Dermatology
UMDNJ—Robert Wood Johnson School of
Medicine at Camden
Newark, New Jersey

Preface

Dr. Mercedes E. Gonzalez, board certified in pediatric dermatology, dermatology and pediatrics, has joined me in writing this expanded 4th edition, now retitled "Goodheart's Photoguide to Common Adult and Pediatric Skin Disorders: Diagnosis and Management."

Herbert P. Goodheart, MD

Our goal is to provide a comprehensive approach to the diagnosis and care of common skin disorders for patients of all ages. We have tried to make this the most practical resource for dermatologists, dermatology residents, medical students, residents in various areas of medicine, practicing physicians, physician assistants, nurse practitioners, and the general population i.e., anyone that encounters disorders of the skin.

Eleven new chapters: Birthmarks, Neonatal and Infantile Eruptions, Acne, Eczema, Superficial Bacterial Infections, Superficial Viral Infections, Viral & Bacterial Exanthems, Lumps, Bumps and Linear Eruptions, Hair and Nail Disorders, Cutaneous Manifestations of Systemic Disease and Neurocutaneous Syndromes have been added.

In addition to the new chapters on pediatric dermatology, the book has been further enlarged to encompass a wider assortment of cutaneous disorders. The book now includes presentations of disorders in racially and ethnically diverse populations and in the aging population, who are now presenting with a greater incidence of pre-cancers, basal cell and squamous cell carcinomas, melanoma, as well as rare skin cancers such as Merkel cell carcinoma.

The content has been updated to remain current and the formularies contain the latest in over-the-counter and prescription medications. We have also included many of the recent "biologics" that have become exciting tools for the targeted treatment of many immunologic and neoplastic disorders in dermatology.

Herbert P. Goodheart, MD and Mercedes E. Gonzalez, MD

Acknowledgments

We owe a great deal of gratitude to the team with which we worked who made the writing of this fourth edition a truly gratifying and enjoyable experience.

It began with Kristina Oberle and Rebecca Gaertner who had the foresight and determination to take on the project, followed by Kel McGowan who took over as acquisition editor and carried it over the finish line.

Other key players include:

Senior Production Project Manager: Alicia Jackson
Marketing Manager: Stephanie Kindlick
Design Coordinators: Steven Druding and Doug Smock
Senior Manufacturing Coordinator: Beth Welsh
Prepress Vendor: Aptara, Inc.
Project Manager: Harish Kumar

We are especially indebted to Kristina Oberle, our developmental editor, who kept track of a stream of disconnected material and buttoned up so many loose ends. Kristina's attention to detail and her availability to answer a multitude of questions has brought this complicated project to completion.

Thanks again to Peter Burk, Mary Ruth Buchness, and Ken Howe who were contributors to the first three editions.

This project never would have been realized without the initial foresight of Sonya Seigafuse who contributed to the second and third editions and was the catalyst for this fourth edition of our book.

Our art director, Larry Pezzato who focused on the illustrations and the processing of digital images, has been an essential contributor to this book, a book that depends on images.

Muchas gracias to Marcos and Rosa Sastre, who supplied the Spanish translations on some of the new handouts.

For this fourth edition, my appreciation also goes to Ashit Mahar and Ben Barankin for their excellent clinical photographs and to Ross Levy, whose advice about wound healing has been a great addition; his hands and surgical skills are featured more than once in this book.

Thanks go to the "brain trust" of many colleagues at Derm-Chat/Derm-Rx, who kept us up-to-date on the latest diagnostic and therapeutic issues in dermatology. Art Huntley who founded and Haines Ely carried on with this valuable online resource. Also thanks to Pam Basuk who has taken on the mantle. To the heavy posters—Joe Eastern, Jerry Bock, Diane Thaler, Pat Condry, Kevin Smith, Linda Spencer, Steve Stone, Gail Drayton, Steve Emmet, Ashit Mahwar, Otto Bastos, Bob Rudolph, Sahar Ghannam, Larry Finkel, Bill Danby, Lynn Margesson, Sate Hamza, Noah Scheinfeld, Steve Feldman, Bernie Recht, Barry Ginsberg, Bill Smith, Pierre Jaffe, Omid Zargari, Becky Bushong, Thomas Vaughn, Ed Zabawski, Jerry Litt, JoBohanon-Grant, Ben Treen, Rhett Drugge, Catelin Popescu, Lennie Rosmarin, Jo Herzog, Peter Panagotacos, Nejib Doss Koushik Lahiri, Emily Altman, Chuck Fishman, Susan Bushelman, Orin Goldblum, Robin Berger, Maida Burrow, Stu Kittay, Diane Davidson, Chuck Miller, Norm Guzick, Walter Wood, Sandeep Gupta, Alice Do, and many, many others who are too numerous to mention. You have been our "online classmates and teachers." We thank you all.

Dr. Gonzalez would like to acknowledge her mentors in pediatric dermatology whose tutelage, guidance, and pearls of wisdom aided in the writing of the pediatric section. Specifically, Julie V. Schaffer, Seth J. Orlow, Harper Price, Helen T. Shin, Lawrence Schachner, Maria C. Garzon, and Miguel R. Sanchez have been important mentors.

We are immensely pleased with the superb job our publisher Wolters Kluwer Health has done in producing this edition.

Contents

The following patient handouts can be found in the companion eBook edition:

Acne

Acne: How to Apply Duac Gel, BenzaClin Gel, and Benzamycin Gel

Acne: How to Apply Topical Retinoids

Alopecia Areata

Athlete's Foot (Tinea Pedis)

Atopic Dermatitis

Atypical Nevus (Mole)

Basal Cell Carcinoma

Bleach Baths

Burow's Solution

Contact Dermatitis

Cysts

Dry Skin (Xerosis)

Fungal Nails (Onychomycosis)

Genital Warts

Granuloma Annulare

Hair Loss (Androgenic Alopecia)

Hand Eczema

Head Lice

Herpes Simplex

Herpes Zoster (Shingles)

Hives (Urticaria)

Keratosis Pilaris (Rough Bumpy Skin)

Lichen Planus

Lyme Disease

Lyme Disease: Prevention

Malignant Melanoma

Melasma

Molluscum Contagiosum

Pityriasis Rosea

Poison Ivy and Poison Oak (Rhus Dermatitis)

Pseudofolliculitis Barbae (Razor Bumps)

Psoriasis

Rosacea

Scabies

Scalp Psoriasis: Scale Removal

Seborrheic Dermatitis of the Face

Seborrheic Dermatitis of the Scalp and Dandruff

Seborrheic Keratosis

Short-Term Cortisone Therapy

Skin Tags

Soak and Smear Instruction Sheet

Solar Keratosis (Actinic Keratosis)

Squamous Cell Carcinoma

Sun Protection Advice

Tinea Capitis

Tinea Cruris (Jock Itch)

Tinea Versicolor

Vitiligo

Warts

Illustrated Glossary of Basic Skin Lesions

Topical Therapy

Illustrated Glossary of Basic Skin Lesions

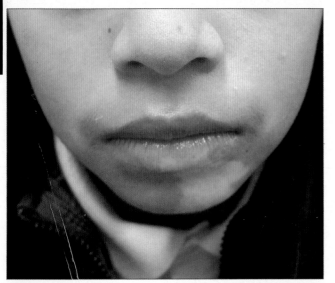

Macule. Freckles (ephelides).

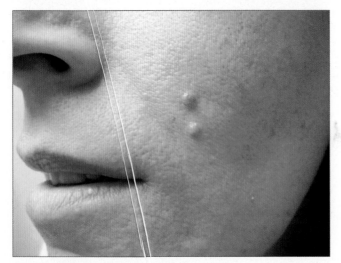

Patch. Vitiligo.

PRIMARY LESIONS

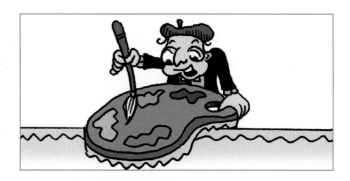

Macules are small, flat, nonpalpable skin lesions (you cannot feel macules, if you close your eyes, they "disappear"). They occur in various colors, shapes, and sizes.

Examples: tattoos, flat nevi, postinflammatory hyperpigmentation, postinflammatory hypopigmentation, erythema, purpura, and freckles.

Patches are large macules. There is some confusion regarding patches; some dermatologists refer to a patch as a large macule, whereas others refer to patches as macules with overlying fine scale (e.g., the scaly patches seen in pityriasis rosea and tinea versicolor).

Examples: melasma and vitiligo.

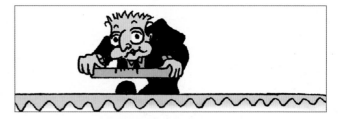

Papules are small, solid elevations with no visible fluid. Papules can vary in shape, color, and size from pinhead-sized up to 1 cm in diameter. They may be flat-topped (planar), umbilicated (e.g., molluscum contagiosum), yellowish (e.g., xanthoma), or brown/black (e.g., dermal nevus).

Examples: molluscum contagiosum, warts, and palpable nevi (moles).

Note: *"Maculopapule" is a contradiction in terms, and the use of this term should be abandoned. An eruption may be described as being macular and papular, rather than "maculopapular." Preferably, the term, "morbilliform" (measles-like) should be used.*

Papule. Melanocytic nevi (moles).

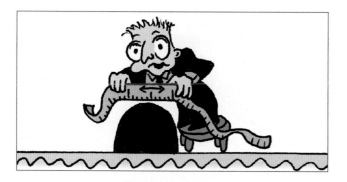

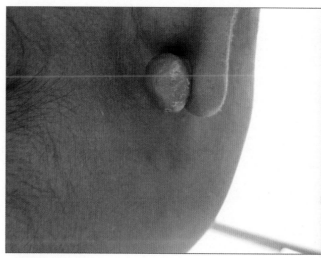

Nodules are firm, solid palpable lesions that are generally greater than 1 cm in diameter. They may be seen as elevated lesions or, if deeper, can be palpated without any elevation of the skin (subcutaneous nodules such as cysts and lipomas).

Examples: erythema nodosum, lipoma, pyogenic granuloma, rheumatoid nodules, basal cell carcinoma, squamous cell carcinoma, and keloids.

Nodule. Keloid.

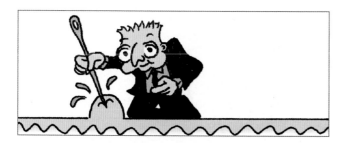

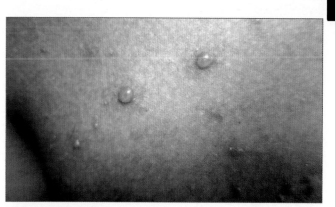

Vesicles (small blisters) are clear, fluid-filled lesions generally 1 cm or less in diameter.

Examples: herpes simplex, acute vesicular tinea pedis, and early chickenpox.

Vesicle. Chickenpox.

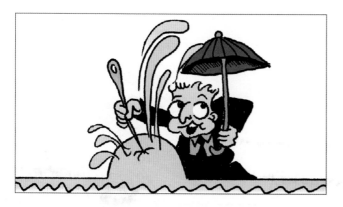

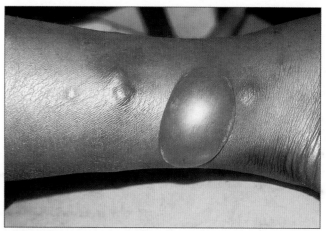

Bullae (large blisters) are clear, fluid-filled lesions generally 1 cm or more in diameter.

Examples: second-degree burns, herpes zoster, and insect bite reactions.

Bulla. Bullous insect bite reaction.

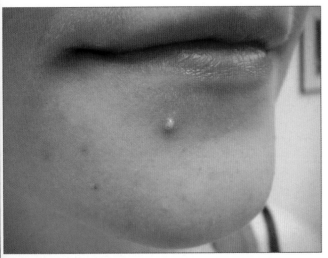

Pustule. Acne pustule.

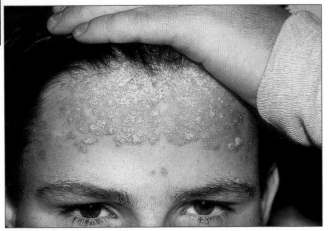

Plaque. Psoriasis vulgaris.

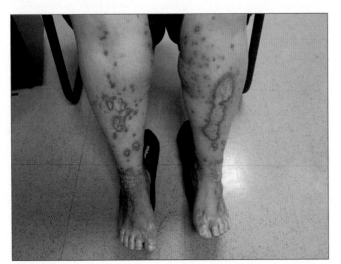

Atrophic plaque. Multiple atrophic plaques of lichen planus.

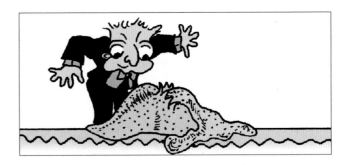

Pustules are raised, circumscribed, superficial lesions that contain purulent, cloudy material.

Examples: evolving chickenpox, folliculitis, and pustular acne.

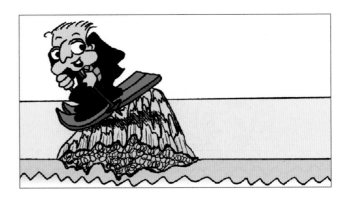

Plaques are well-circumscribed, elevated, or depressed (*atrophic*), plateau-like lesions that are usually >1 cm. They may arise from papules that coalesce or they may arise *de novo.* Crust and scale are commonly present.

Examples: chronic eczematous dermatitis and psoriasis.

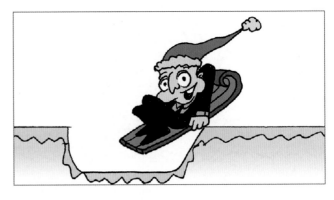

Atrophic plaques result from a thinning process that is associated with a decreased number of cutaneous cells, often with a loss of normal skin markings. Dermal atrophy may result in a depression of the skin.

Examples: discoid lupus erythematosus, morphea (localized scleroderma), atrophy caused by intralesional cortisone injections, and atrophic lichen planus.

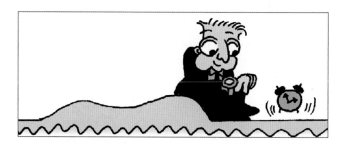

Wheals are raised, flesh-colored or erythematous papules or plaques that are transient. They last less than 24 hours, and later reappear with a different shape, size, and location.

Examples: urticaria (hives) and angioedema.

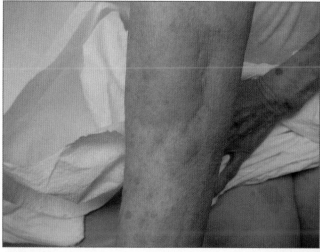

Wheal. Urticaria.

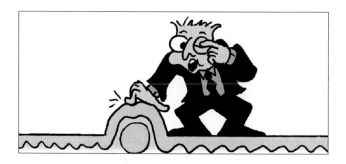

Cysts are walled-off, ballotable lesions containing fluid or semisolid material. (They feel like an eyeball when palpated.)

Examples: pilar and epidermoid cysts.

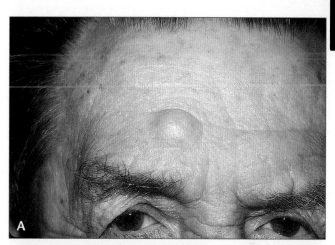

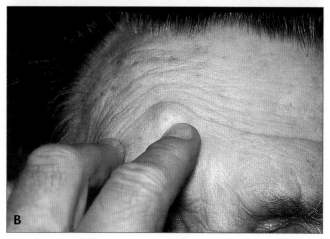

Cyst. Epidermoid cyst.

SECONDARY (MODIFIED) LESIONS

Secondary features on primary lesions may evolve naturally or develop as a result of patient manipulation.

Scale. Dandruff.

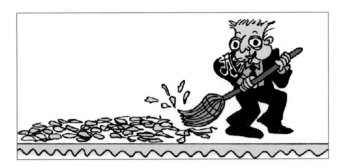

Scales (desquamation) comprise the outer layer of epidermis that normally desquamates or sheds imperceptibly on a daily basis. In many dermatologic conditions, when this shedding becomes visible, it is then considered to be abnormal. Visible scale is the result of increased production of corneocytes or delayed desquamation.

Examples of conditions that commonly produce scale are psoriasis, dandruff, xerosis, and ichthyosis.

Crust. Bullous impetigo with "honey-colored" crusts.

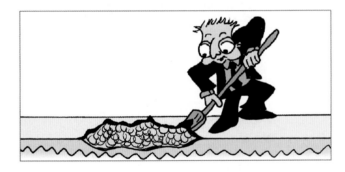

Crusts (scabs) are formed from blood, serum, or other dried exudate. "Honey-colored crusts" *(impetiginization)* are often a sign of superficial bacterial infection.

Examples: excoriated or infected insect bites and evolving lesions of bullous impetigo.

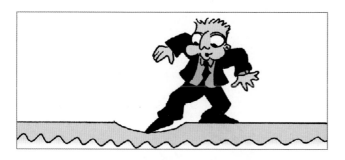

Erosions are shallow losses of tissue involving only the epidermis ("topsoil"). They often result from blisters and pustules and usually heal without scarring.

Examples: secondary lesions of herpes simplex, herpes zoster, and aphthous stomatitis.

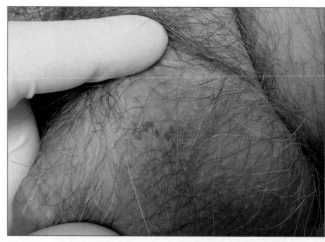

Erosion. Grouped erosions of resolving herpes simplex.

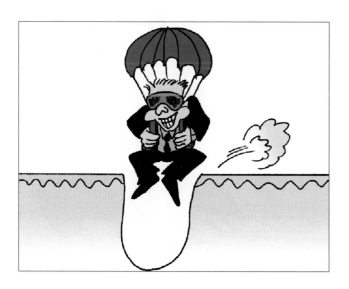

Ulcers are defects deeper than erosions. Ulcers involve complete loss of the epidermis as well as the dermis or deeper layers. They usually heal with scarring.

Examples: pyoderma gangrenosum, venous stasis ulcers, and vasculitis.

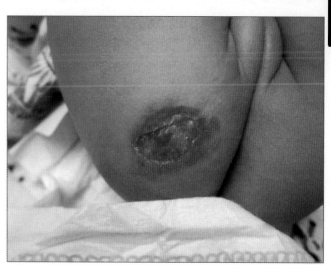

Ulcer. Ulcerated infantile hemangioma.

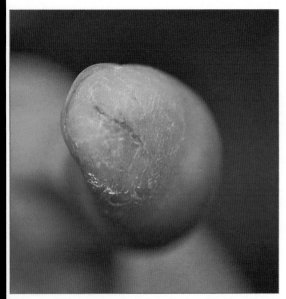

Fissure. Hand eczema.

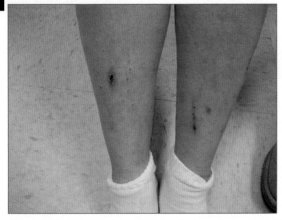

Excoriation. Punctate and linear lesions from scratching.

Fissures are small, linear ulcers or cracks in the skin. They are often painful.

Examples of conditions in which fissures may be seen: angular stomatitis (perlèche), eczema of the lips, and eczematous dermatitis of the fingers.

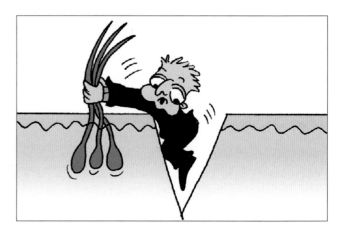

Excoriations are linear or punctate erosions or excavations induced by scratching, picking, or digging.

Examples: insect bites, cat scratches, and self-induced lesions.

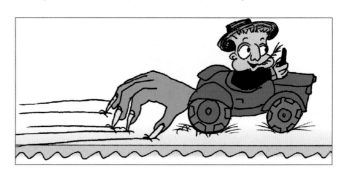

REACTION PATTERNS, SHAPES, AND CONFIGURATIONS

Diseased skin has a limited number of clinical manifestations. Many skin disorders tend to occur in characteristic shapes, distributions, arrangements, and reaction patterns that often serve as diagnostic clues.

REACTION PATTERNS

The convention of describing skin disorders in terms of certain reaction patterns is inexact and there is often a great deal of overlap. For example, the blistering acute eruption of poison ivy can be described as both a vesicobullous as well as an acute eczematous reaction pattern. However, using these patterns to describe individual skin lesions or eruptions often helps greatly in formulating a differential diagnosis.

A **papulosquamous reaction pattern** refers to an eruption in which the primary lesions consist of macules, papules, or plaques with scale. Thus, a papulosquamous reaction pattern suggests a differential diagnosis that includes psoriasis, tinea corporis, tinea versicolor, lichen planus, parapsoriasis, mycosis fungoides, and pityriasis rosea.

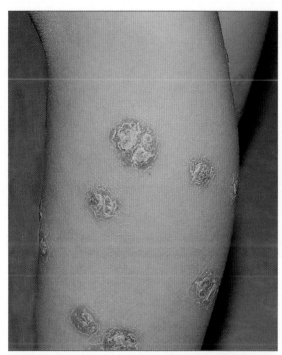

Papulosquamous reaction pattern. Psoriasis.

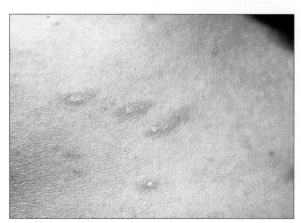

Papulosquamous reaction pattern. Pityriasis rosea.

Eczematous reaction patterns are a little more difficult than papulosquamous patterns to describe (see Chapters 4 and 13), because they often have various presentations and, at times, may be impossible to distinguish from papulosquamous patterns.

- **Acute and subacute eczema.** Examples include erythematous "juicy" papules or plaques and/or weeping vesicobullous lesions. A classic example is poison ivy.

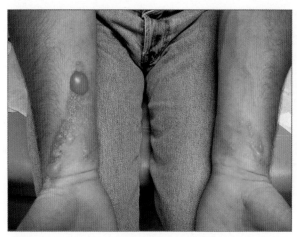

Acute eczematous reaction pattern. Poison ivy. Note "honey-colored" *(impetiginized)* vesicobullous fluid.

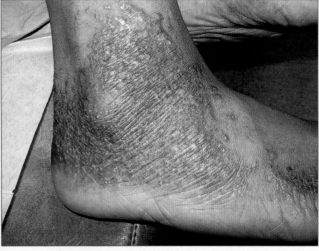

Chronic eczematous reaction pattern. Atopic dermatitis with lichenification.

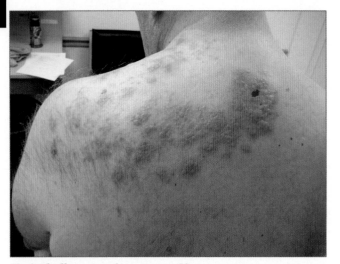

Vesicobullous reaction pattern. Herpes zoster.

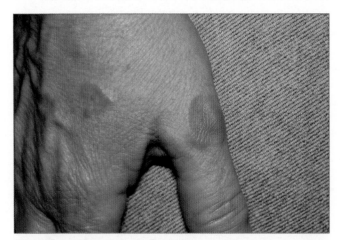

Dermal reaction pattern. Granuloma annulare.

- **Chronic eczema.** The hallmark lesion of chronic eczematous dermatitis is *lichenification,* which is caused by repeated scratching and/or rubbing. Typical examples are long-standing atopic dermatitis and lichen simplex chronicus.

The **vesicobullous reaction pattern** consists of fluid-filled blisters.

Examples: second-degree burns, primary bullous disorders, varicella, herpes simplex and herpes zoster infections.

In a **dermal reaction pattern** the lesions or eruptions are confined to the dermis. There is generally an absence of scale or changes in the epidermis.

Examples: cutaneous sarcoidosis, depositional processes involving uric acid (gouty tophi), or lipids (eruptive xanthomas) and granuloma annulare.

A **subcutaneous reaction pattern** is characterized by lesions or eruptions that are confined to subcutaneous tissue. There may or may not be an elevation of the skin and in general there is an absence of scale or epidermal change.

Examples: erythema nodosum and lipomas.

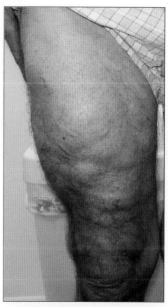

Subcutaneous reaction pattern. Multiple lipomas.

A **vascular reaction pattern** refers to erythema or edema resulting from changes in the vasculature, such as vasodilatation, purpura, or vasculitis.

Examples: first-degree burns, viral exanthem, urticaria, erythema multiforme, vasculitis, and drug rashes.

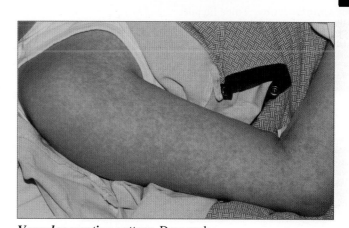

Vascular reaction pattern. Drug rash.

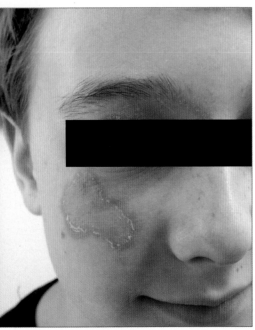

Annular lesion. Tinea faciale.

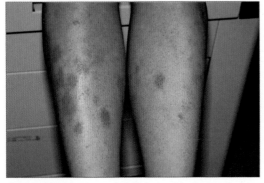

Nummular lesions. Coin-shaped lesions of nummular eczema.

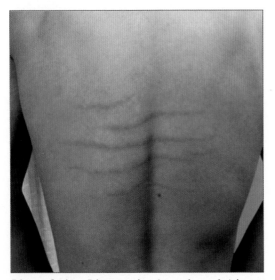

Linear lesion. Linear striae (stretch marks) in a teenager.

SHAPE OF LESIONS

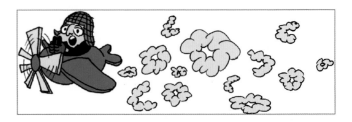

Annular and **arciform** are terms used to describe lesions that are ring-shaped or semiannular.

Examples: urticaria, granuloma annulare, and tinea corporis ("ringworm").

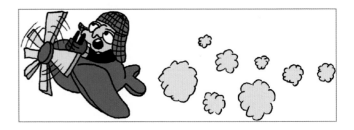

Nummular is a term that describes coin-shaped lesions.

Examples: discoid lupus erythematosus, psoriasis, and nummular eczema.

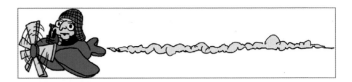

Linear lesions may result from exogenous agents, inflammatory eruptions, excoriations, congenital growths, and striae (stretch marks).

Examples: lesions of poison ivy and dermatographism.

CONFIGURATION OF LESIONS

The arrangement (configuration) of lesions is the interrelationship of multiple lesions.

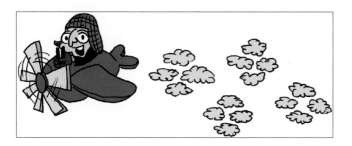

Grouped (clustered) lesions are noted in "herpetiform" and "zosteriform" vesicles or bullae.

Examples: insect bite reactions, herpes simplex and herpes zoster.

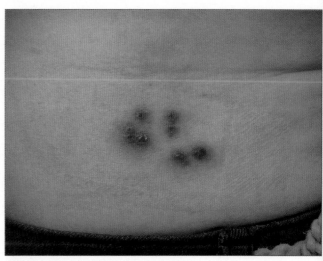

Grouped lesions. Grouped vesicles.

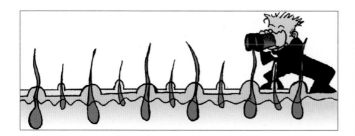

Follicular arrangement of lesions involves hair follicles. Lesions are often papular or pustular, at times with a visible central emerging hair. Lesions are spaced at fairly equal distances in a gridlike pattern.

Examples: keratosis pilaris and folliculitis.

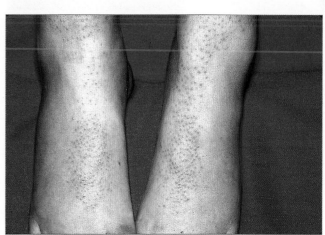

Follicular lesions. Follicular eczema. Note the gridlike pattern of tiny papules.

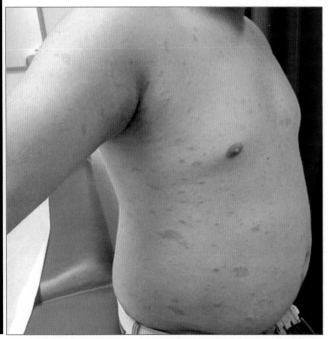

Lines of cleavage. Pityriasis rosea.

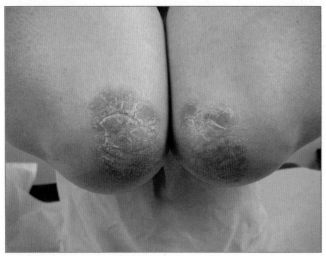

Bilateral symmetry. Psoriasis.

DISTRIBUTION OF LESIONS

Observing the overall distribution of skin lesions can be helpful for establishing the correct diagnosis. Lesions may be generalized (e.g., extensive exfoliative erythroderma and drug rash) or focal (e.g., a nodule of basal cell carcinoma and melanoma). They may follow the lines of cleavage (aka Langer's skin tension lines; e.g., pityriasis rosea), be dermatomal (area of skin innervated by a single spinal nerve; e.g., herpes zoster), follow the lines of Blaschko (which reflect patterns of the skin's embryonic development; e.g., epidermal nevi), or have characteristic bilateral symmetry (e.g., psoriasis, vitiligo).

OVERVIEW

Topical therapy, the mainstay of dermatologic treatment, has traditionally been the bailiwick of dermatologists. Thus, it is no surprise that an understanding of the appropriate use and abuse of these agents has been either neglected or misunderstood by other health care professionals. The following is an attempt to provide a practical overview of topical therapy. The primary focus is on the use of topical steroids; other topical agents such as antibiotics and antifungals will be discussed in other sections of the book. Topical antibiotics used for acne are listed in Chapter 12 and topical antibiotics used for other cutaneous infections such as impetigo are described in Chapters 5 and 16.

BASICS

- Topical therapy is generally safer than systemic therapy.
- Creams are generally more popular with patients than ointments because they are less greasy and messy; however, they are usually less potent and more drying.
- In addition, to their enhanced potency, ointments are more moisturizing than creams, gels, and foams.
- Gels and foams are greaseless; they spread more easily and are very practical for treating acne and for application to hairy areas of the body.
- The amount of a topical preparation applied does not affect its penetration or potency. The thicker the application, the greater the wastage—only the thin layer that is in intimate contact with the skin is absorbed; the remainder is rubbed off. **More is not always better!**
- Once- or twice-daily applications are usually sufficient for most preparations.

VEHICLES

- The active drug is combined with a vehicle, or base. Vehicles vary in their ability to "deliver" to the target site in the skin.
- The rate of penetration and absorption of a topical medication into the skin depends on how occlusive its vehicle is and on how readily the vehicle releases the active chemical.
- A vehicle should be cosmetically acceptable and nonsensitizing.

A CREAM, AN OINTMENT, A GEL, OR A LOTION?

- Creams are oil in water preparations; their water content makes them more drying than ointments.
- Generally, ointments are more potent, more lubricating, less irritating, and less sensitizing than are creams or lotions.
- Lotions, gels, aerosols, foams, and solutions are useful on hairy areas.

WET DRESSINGS

- There is some validity to the old adage: "If it's dry, wet it; if it's wet, dry it."
- Wet dressings help dry wounds, and aid in their debridement by removing debris (e.g., serum, crusts). They also have a nonspecific antifungal and antibacterial effect, especially when chemicals such as aluminum sulfate, silver nitrate, acetic acid (vinegar is dilute acetic acid), and potassium permanganate are added.
- For example, the application of **Burow solution** (aluminum sulfate and calcium acetate) helps dry out weeping and oozing lesions such as from poison ivy, tinea pedis, herpes simplex, and herpes zoster.

 SEE PATIENT HANDOUT "BUROW SOLUTION" IN THE COMPANION eBOOK EDITION.

TOPICAL STEROIDS

See Tables I.1 and I.2.

BASICS

- Topical steroids are used to treat the vast majority of inflammatory dermatoses. They are the cornerstone of therapy in dermatology, and, when used properly, are quite safe.
- The unwanted side effects of topical steroids are directly related to their potencies.
- Whenever possible, a low-potency steroid should be used for the shortest possible time. Conversely, one should avoid using a preparation that is not potent enough to treat a particular condition.
- For severe dermatoses, a very potent steroid may be used to initiate therapy ("strong, but not long"), and a less potent preparation may be used afterward for maintenance ("downward titration").
- **Hydration** of the stratum corneum increases penetration, which, in turn, increases efficacy and potency (Fig. I.1A,B).
- **Occlusion**, which involves placing medications under occlusive dressings, produces increased hydration of the stratum corneum (the "reservoir effect").
- **Tachyphylaxis** (tolerance) occurs when the medication loses its efficacy with continued use. It is most often seen in the treatment of psoriasis.
- To help minimize tachyphylaxis, a high-potency preparation is applied until a dermatosis clears and then a lower-potency topical steroid is prescribed for intermittent flares.

MECHANISM OF ACTION

- Topical steroids have two basic mechanisms of action: anti-inflammatory and antimitotic.
- Anti-inflammatory properties are of particular importance when they are used to treat eczematous and other primarily inflammatory conditions.
- Antimitotic properties of topical steroids help to reduce the buildup of scale.

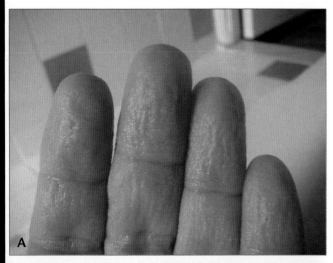

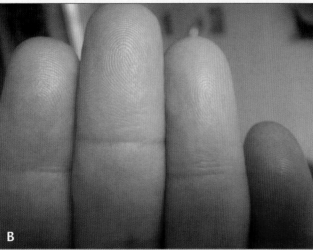

I.1   **A:** *Hydration.* These fingers have been immersed in water for a prolonged period to increase the penetration of a topical drug. **B:** *Hydration.* Five minutes later. The skin resumes its presoaking appearance.

POTENCIES

- Fluorinated topical steroids are generally more potent than other topical steroids. For example, triamcinolone acetonide, which contains a fluoride ion, is 100 times more potent than nonfluorinated hydrocortisone.
- When treating children and elderly patients, clinicians should take extra measures to avoid the use of potent or superpotent fluorinated compounds, when possible.
- Only nonfluorinated, mild topical steroids should be applied to the face and, ideally, only for short periods of time, to avoid atrophy and steroid-induced rosacea. However, this rule can be broken. For example, for the treatment of severe acute contact dermatitis of the face, a superpotent topical steroid used briefly may be preferable to a mild, ineffective topical steroid or a systemic steroid.
- Thin eyelid skin requires the least potent preparations for the shortest periods of time.

- The intertriginous (skin touching skin) areas similarly respond to lower potencies because the apposition of skin surfaces acts like an occlusive dressing. The axillae and inguinal creases are particularly prone to higher absorption and resultant steroid atrophy.

DELIVERY (PERCUTANEOUS PENETRATION)

- Topical steroids and other topical preparations are ineffective unless they are absorbed into the skin. Percutaneous penetration can be manipulated by hydrating the skin, by using occlusive dressings, and by changing the vehicle (e.g., to an ointment).
- The ability to penetrate varies by anatomic site as follows:

> Mucous membranes > Scrotum > Eyelids > Face > Torso > Extremities > Palms and soles

Because the stratum corneum serves as a "reservoir"—a storehouse of medication—it continues to release a topical steroid into the skin after application. Consequently, once-daily application is often sufficient to manage many inflammatory dermatoses. The following are methods of increasing topical medication penetration:

- **Soaking.** Soaking an affected area in water before the application of a topical agent allows that water to hydrate the stratum corneum and thus allow a topical steroid to penetrate more deeply into inflammatory foci.

   If there is no bathtub at home or the patient cannot use a bathtub, a prolonged lukewarm shower, followed by the application of the prescribed ointment underneath a wet towel can serve the same purpose.

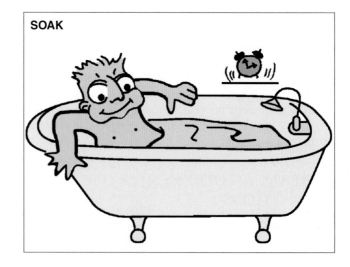

- **Smearing.** After soaking, the application ("smearing") of a topical steroid (particularly an ointment-based preparation) to wet skin traps the absorbed water, which cannot easily evaporate through such a greasy, occlusive barrier.

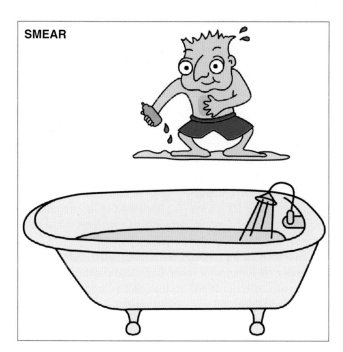

SMEAR

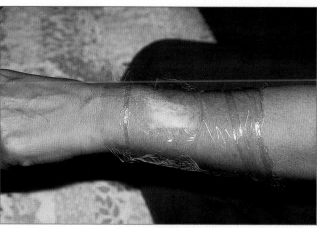

I.2 *Occlusion.* A topical steroid cream has been applied, and a "nonbreathing" polyethylene wrap is used to cover it.

POTENTIAL SIDE EFFECTS

- **Skin atrophy.** Epidermal atrophy is a local reaction demonstrated by shiny, thinned skin and telangiectasias. It generally reverses when topical steroids are discontinued.
- **Striae** (linear atrophic scars) may occur after repeated use of a potent topical steroid in one area. These permanent scars are seen most often in intertriginous areas, such as the axillae and groin, where the skin is generally thin, moist, and naturally occluded.
- **Acneform/rosacea-like eruptions** of the face (Fig. I.3). Lesions resembling acne vulgaris, rosacea, and perioral dermatitis may result from the regular use of topical fluorinated steroids on the face. These eruptions manifest as persistent

- **Soak and smear for cutaneous infections.** Dilute bleach baths have become a very popular and safe adjunctive treatment for many skin infections. Patients can be reassured that it is the same as what is done when swimming pools are chlorinated to kill bacteria.
- During the "soak and smear" (described above) household bleach can be used as follows:
  - For adults: 1 cup of common liquid bleach such as Clorox Bleach mixed in with a full bathtub.
  - For children: ¼ to ½ cup in a half full bathtub; for small infants: 1 to 2 caps full in a gallon jug.
  - If there is no bathtub at home or the patient cannot use a bathtub, 2 caps full of bleach can be mixed in a spray bottle with water and sprayed onto the skin while showering.
- **Occlusion.** A "nonbreathing" polyethylene wrap such as **Saran Wrap** or **Handi-Wrap**, held in place by tape, a bandage, a sock, or an elastic bandage, can provide occlusion to an area where topical steroids have been applied (Fig. I.2). The wrap may be left on while the patient sleeps or worn for several hours while the patient is awake. Specific areas may be occluded as follows:
  - A plastic shower cap can be used when the scalp is treated with a topical steroid.
  - **Cordran tape**, a preparation that is impregnated with the steroid flurandrenolide, is helpful for occlusive therapy when relatively small areas are treated.
  - Rubber or vinyl gloves or finger cots may be used for the hands and fingers.
  - Small plastic bags (e.g., **Ziploc bags**) may be used for the feet.
  - Occlusive garments ("sauna suits") can be worn when extensive areas are involved.

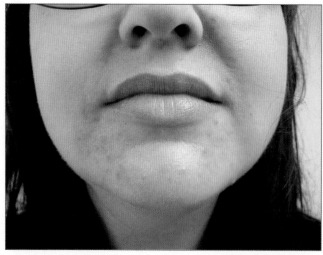

I.3 *Perioral dermatitis resembling rosacea and peroral dermatitis.* This reaction was caused by long-term use of a potent topical fluorinated steroid.

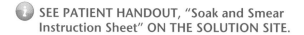

SEE PATIENT HANDOUT, "Soak and Smear Instruction Sheet" ON THE SOLUTION SITE.

erythema, papules, pustules, and telangiectasia. The condition often flares once the steroid is withdrawn ("rebound rosacea").

- **Tinea incognito,** a superficial fungal infection. This condition may be misdiagnosed because its clinical signs may be obscured by the use of topical steroids, which reduce inflammation and itching without killing the fungus.

Less common side effects include the following:

- **Hypersensitivity reactions.** Allergic contact dermatitis to the steroid molecule may occur and may easily be overlooked. The hypersensitivity can be evoked by the steroid, the vehicle, or both, and it is often not suspected clinically. A clue to its presence is a lack of the expected anti-inflammatory effect of the topical steroid.
- **Purpura.** This condition may be noted after prolonged topical steroid use, particularly in elderly patients.
- **Other local effects.** These include hypopigmentation, excess facial hair growth, and delayed wound healing.
- **Systemic absorption** may result from extensive use, often with occlusion, of potent topical steroids. In the rare event that there is hypothalamic–pituitary–adrenal axis suppression, it is quickly reversible upon discontinuation. Infants, particularly those born prematurely, have a greater risk of systemic absorption because of their increased body surface compared to body mass as well as their less efficient cutaneous permeability barriers.

HELPFUL HINTS

- Large, economical amounts of triamcinolone cream and ointment may be purchased in 454-g (1-lb) jars.
- Become familiar with only one or two agents from each potency class; that should be enough to treat most skin conditions that are responsive to topical steroids.
- Prolonged application of combination topical antifungal/corticosteroid preparations such as **Lotrisone** and **Mycolog II** that contain potent topical steroids can result in striae, particularly when used in skinfold sites.

TOPICAL IMMUNOMODULATORS (CALCINEURIN INHIBITORS)

BASICS

- Tacrolimus (**Protopic**) ointment and Pimecrolimus (**Elidel**) cream are nonsteroidal, anti-inflammatory agents that are widely utilized in dermatology.
- Tacrolimus 0.1% ointment is indicated for the treatment of moderate-to-severe atopic dermatitis in adults (>16 years) and the 0.03% ointment is approved for use for moderate-to-severe AD in patients ≥2 years of age.
- Pimecrolimus 1% cream is indicated for the treatment of mild-to-moderate atopic dermatitis in patients >2 years of age.
- Both Protopic and Elidel have been used "off-label" as effective treatments for other dermatoses such as seborrheic dermatitis, discoid lupus erythematosus, and psoriasis and are especially useful as "steroid sparing agents" in areas at high risk for skin thinning (atrophy) such as the face, eyelids, groin, and axillae.

MECHANISM OF ACTION

- Tacrolimus and pimecrolimus inhibit calcineurin preventing T-cell cytokine release and inflammation.

POTENTIAL SIDE EFFECTS

- Skin irritation (burning, stinging, or a warm sensation) can occur and is more likely to happen with Protopic.

SAFETY

- Protopic and Elidel include black box warning labels stating that the long-term safety has not been established and that there is a potential for future lymphoma or malignancy. The theoretical risk was based on data from virus-infected lab monkeys who were treated with 26 to 47 times the maximum recommended dosage of oral tacrolimus.
- Several task forces from the American Academy of Dermatology, American College of Allergy, Asthma and Immunology, and the National Eczema Foundation have found no evidence of an increased level of risk from the use of these agents and are working to remove this label.
- There has been no evidence of systemic immunosuppression or an increased risk for malignancy in clinical studies or post-marketing surveillance of either medication.
- Nonetheless, Protopic and Elidel are best used intermittently in rotation with topical steroids and it is important to discuss the black box warning with patients.

POINTS TO REMEMBER

- Intertriginous areas such as the axillae and inguinal creases are physically occluded, so less potent preparations should be used to avoid atrophy.
- When treating children and the elderly, avoid the use of potent fluorinated compounds, when possible.
- Soaking and occlusion increase penetration and potency; they also can make a low-potency agent as strong—in efficacy and side effects—as a mid- to high-potency agent.
- How much cream, ointment, or lotion should one apply? Application should be thin, not thick—a little works as well as a lot.
- Higher-potency steroids bring more rapid clearing and limit the overall exposure to the preparation. In contrast, prolonged application of low-potency agents takes much longer to produce comparable effects.

Table I.1 TOPICAL STEROIDS ("THE SHORT LIST")[a]

CLASS/POTENCY	GENERIC NAME	BRAND NAMES
Class I: Superpotent	Clobetasol propionate 0.05% cream/gel/ointment/ foam, lotion	Temovate, Olux foam, Clobex lotion, spray, Cormax scalp solution
	Diflorasone diacetate 0.05% ointment	Psorcon
	Halobetasol propionate 0.05% cream/ointment	Ultravate
	Fluocinonide 0.1% cream	Vanos
	Flurandrenolide	Cordran tape (small roll, large roll)
Class II: Very high potency	Desoximetasone 0.25%, cream/ointment, 0.05% gel	Topicort
	Fluocinonide 0.05% cream/ointment/solution/gel	Lidex
	Mometasone 0.01% ointment	Elocon
Class III: High potency	Fluticasone 0.005% ointment	Cutivate
	Triamcinolone acetonide 0.1% ointment	Kenalog
Class IV: Medium-high potency	Fluocinolone acetonide 0.025% ointment	Synalar
	Hydrocortisone valerate 0.2% ointment	Westcort
	Fluticasone 0.05% cream	Cutivate
	Triamcinolone acetonide 0.1% cream	Kenalog
Class V: Medium potency	Hydrocortisone valerate 0.2% cream	Westcort
	Hydrocortisone butyrate 0.01% ointment/cream/lotion	Locoid
Class VI: Low potency	Desonide 0.05% gel/cream/ointment	DesOwen
	Alclometasone dipropionate 0.05% ointment/cream	Aclovate
	Fluocinolone acetonide 0.01% cream/solution	Synalar
Class VII: Very low potency	Hydrocortisone 0.5%, 1.0%, 2.5% cream/ointment/ lotion[b]	Hytone, Cortizone 10, Cortaid, and many other over-the-counter brands

The agents listed should provide more than enough treatment options for the conditions discussed in this book.

[a]Most preparations are available in tubes of 15, 30, or 60 g; lotions and solutions are available in bottles of 20 to 60 mL.

[b]Prescription 2.5% hydrocortisone is hardly more potent than 1% hydrocortisone.

Table I.2 CLASSIFICATION, STRENGTH, AND VEHICLE OF SOME COMMONLY USED TOPICAL CORTICOSTEROIDS ("THE LONG LIST")

GENERIC NAME	BRAND NAME(S)
Class I: Superpotent	
Betamethasone dipropionate 0.05% gel/ointment/lotion	**Diprolene**
Clobetasol propionate 0.05% cream/ointment/gel/lotion/foam	**Temovate, Olux foam, Clobex lotion, spray, Cormax scalp solution**
Diflorasone diacetate 0.05% ointment/lotion/gel	**Psorcon**
Halobetasol propionate 0.05% cream/ointment	**Ultravate**
Flurandrenolide	**Cordran tape**
Fluocinonide 0.1% cream	**Vanos**
Class II: Very high potency	
Amcinonide 0.1% ointment	**Cyclocort**
Betamethasone dipropionate 0.05% ointment	**Diprosone**
Desoximetasone 0.05% cream/ointment; 0.25% gel	**Topicort**
Diflorasone diacetate 0.05% cream	**Psorcon**
Betamethasone dipropionate 0.05% cream	**Diprolene AF**
Fluocinonide 0.05% cream/ointment/gel	**Lidex**
Halcinonide 0.1% cream/ointment/solution	**Halog**
Mometasone furoate 0.1% ointment	**Elocon**
Class III: High potency	
Amcinonide 0.1% cream/lotion	**Cyclocort**
Betamethasone dipropionate 0.05% cream/lotion	**Diprosone**
Betamethasone valerate 0.1% ointment	**Valisone**
Diflorasone diacetate 0.05% cream	**Florone, Maxiflor**
Fluticasone propionate 0.005% ointment	**Cutivate**
Triamcinolone acetate 0.1% ointment; 0.5% cream	**Aristocort A**
Class IV: Medium-high potency	
Betamethasone valerate 0.12% foam	**Luxiq Foam**
Desoximetasone 0.05% cream	**Topicort LP**
Fluocinolone acetonide 0.2% cream	**Synalar-HP**
Fluocinolone acetonide 0.025% ointment	**Synalar**
Hydrocortisone valerate 0.2% ointment	**Westcort**
Mometasone furoate 0.1% cream	**Elocon**
Triamcinolone acetonide 0.1% ointment	**Kenalog, Aristocort**
Hydrocortisone probutate 0.1%	**Pandel**
Class V: Medium potency	
Betamethasone valerate 0.1% cream/lotion	**Valisone**
Desonide 0.05% ointment	**DesOwen, Tridesilon**
Fluticasone propionate 0.1% cream	**Cutivate**
Fluocinolone acetonide 0.025% cream	**Synalar, Synemol**
Flurandrenolide 0.05% cream	**Cordran SP**
Hydrocortisone butyrate 0.1% cream/ointment/solution	**Locoid**
Hydrocortisone valerate 0.2% cream	**Westcort**
Prednicarbate 0.1%	**Dermatop-E**
Triamcinolone acetonide 0.1% cream/lotion	**Kenalog**
Triamcinolone acetonide 0.025% cream	**Aristocort**
Class VI: Low potency	
Alclometasone dipropionate 0.05% cream/ointment	**Aclovate**
Betamethasone 17-valerate 0.1% lotion	**Valisone**
Desonide 0.05% cream/lotion	**DesOwen**
Desonide 0.05% am	**Tridesilon**
Fluocinolone acetonide 0.01% cream/solution	**Synalar**
Fluocinolone acetonide 0.01%	**Capex shampoo, Derma-Smoothe**
Mometasone furoate 0.1% cream/ointment	**Elocon**
Class VII: Very low potency	
Hydrocortisone 0.5%, 1.0%, 2.5% cream/ointment/lotion	**Hytone, Cortaid, Cortizone-10, Cortizone 5 Creme**

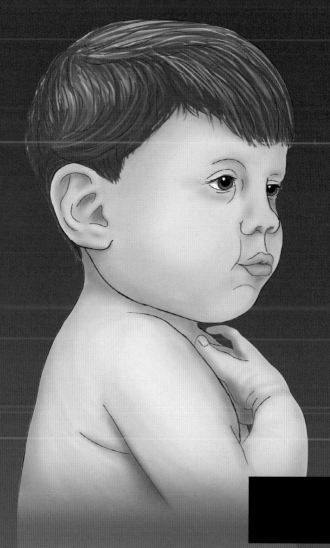

PART ONE

Common Pediatric Skin Conditions: Diagnosis and Management

Birthmarks

OVERVIEW

Birthmarks are visible skin lesions present at birth or shortly thereafter, that can be frightening to parents. Birthmarks can be red, blue, brown-black, or white; flat or raised; hairy or warty and occur as a single or multiple lesions or distributed over a segment of the body. Fortunately, regardless of color or shape, the vast majority of congenital skin lesions or "birthmarks" are a benign, isolated finding and parents can be reassured.

Occasionally, a birthmark may be a sign of an associated congenital defect or an underlying syndrome. The location and morphology of a birthmark can help determine the risk of an association and direct the appropriate workup.

It is important to quickly differentiate a worrisome birthmark from an insignificant lesion and reassure parents as soon as possible. However, even benign and medically insignificant birthmarks can be of great cosmetic significance and require treatment. This chapter will discuss the most common birthmarks, their potential associations and the necessary workup and management.

IN THIS CHAPTER...

➤ **APLASIA CUTIS CONGENITA**

➤ **NEVUS SEBACEOUS**

➤ **NEVUS SIMPLEX**

➤ **PORT-WINE STAIN**

  • Sturge–Weber syndrome
  • Klippel–Trenaunay syndrome

➤ **INFANTILE HEMANGIOMA**

➤ **CAFÉ AU LAIT SPOTS**

➤ **DERMAL MELANOCYTOSIS**

➤ **CONGENITAL MELANOCYTIC NEVUS**

➤ **EPIDERMAL NEVUS**

➤ **NEVUS DEPIGMENTOSUS**

Aplasia Cutis Congenita

BASICS

- Aplasia cutis congenita (ACC) refers to a congenital defect that results in a localized area of absent skin at birth and is most commonly seen on the scalp (Fig. 1.1).
- Usually there is absence of the epidermis and dermis in the affected area but occasionally subcutaneous tissues, bone, and dura can also be missing.

PATHOGENESIS

- The exact cause of ACC is unknown and most cases are sporadic.
- Proposed theories include genetic factors, birth trauma, teratogens, and intrauterine infection.
- A popular hypothesis suggests that ACC is the result of compromised vasculature of the placenta.

CLINICAL MANIFESTATIONS

- Most often ACC presents on the scalp as a single, localized area of smooth alopecia in close proximity to the hair whorl.
- Less commonly, ACC presents as multiple areas of alopecia on the scalp or can be found on the face, trunk, or extremities (Fig. 1.2).
- ACC can have a variable appearance at birth including a well-formed hairless scar, ulceration with a granulating base, a superficial erosion, or a translucent, glistening membrane ("membranous aplasia cutis"—uncommon variant) (Fig. 1.3).
- Lesions are usually sharply demarcated, oval, circular, or stellate, and measure 1 to 3 cm in diameter.

*This consists of a hand-held magnifier that allows inspection of skin lesions unobstructed by skin surface reflections.

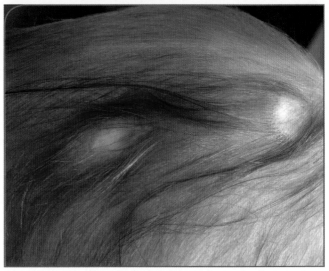

1.2 *Aplasia cutis congenita.* Two lesions of aplasia cutis congenita on the scalp, both with a surrounding "hair collar sign" which can signal an underlying neural tube defect. (Figure courtesy of Seth J. Orlow, MD, PhD.)

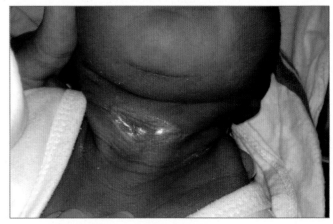

1.3 *Aplasia cutis congenita.* Membranous aplasia cutis on the anterior neck.

- ACC is an isolated defect in the majority of cases, but it can be associated with other developmental anomalies or a feature of a variety of syndromes.
- A ring of long, dark hair around membranous aplasia cutis (the hair collar sign) is thought to herald an underlying neural tube defect (see Fig. 1.2).

DIAGNOSIS

- Diagnosis is clinical.

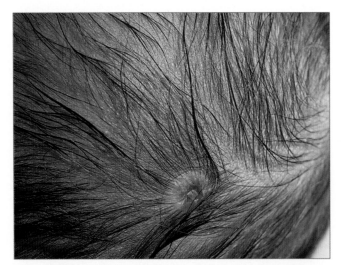

1.1 *Aplasia cutis congenita.* Typical presentation of aplasia cutis congenita: a small well-demarcated healing ulceration on the vertex scalp of a neonate. (From Burkhart CN, Morrell DS. *Visual Dx Essential Pediatric Dermatology.* Philadelphia, PA: Lippincott Williams & Wilkins, 2010.)

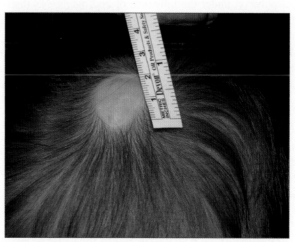

 DIFFERENTIAL DIAGNOSIS

Birth-related Skin Injury from Forceps or Scalp Electrodes
- *Birth history will reveal use of instruments.*

Nevus Sebaceous
- *Pink, yellow, pebbly surface often visible on close inspection.*

Erosion from Herpes Simplex Virus (HSV) Infection
- *History of exposure to HSV.*

 POINT TO REMEMBER

- A collar of thick hair surrounding ACC ("hair collar sign") should prompt neuroimaging to rule out an underlying neurologic anomaly.

 HELPFUL HINT

- Lesions of ACC remain devoid of hair and ultimately appear scar-like.

 MANAGEMENT

- Prognosis is excellent and most lesions heal completely in the first weeks to months of life.
- A complete physical examination should be performed to rule out other congenital defects.
- Conservative wound care with antibiotic ointments and nonstick dressings will help heal most small defects quickly.
- Lesions heal with scarring and alopecia (Fig. 1.4).
- Most scars become relatively inconspicuous and require no correction but large and/or obvious scars can be treated with plastic surgical reconstruction in the future.
- If lesion appears large, deep, or stellate or if located in the midline, a radiologic evaluation to assess for an underlying defect is necessary.

1.4 *Aplasia cutis congenita.* Aplasia cutis congenita persists as a well-healed scar that lacks hair follicles (alopecia). (Figure courtesy of Seth J. Orlow, MD, PhD.)

Nevus Sebaceous

BASICS

- Nevus sebaceous (NS) is a common congenital hamartoma (benign tumor) composed of malformed sebaceous glands (large and not associated with follicular units), apocrine glands, and follicular units that typically present on the scalp.

CLINICAL MANIFESTATIONS

- NS can occur anywhere on the body, but >97% of lesions occur on the head or neck, most often on the scalp.
- NS initially presents as a solitary, well-circumscribed, oval or linear, hairless, pink or yellow-orange/tan, finely papulated plaque (Fig. 1.5).
- Occasionally, NS can be thicker or have papillomatous projections, simulating a wart; or present as a large pedunculated lesion at birth (Fig. 1.6).
- After infancy, lesions flatten and grow proportionately with child.
- At puberty, under the influence of androgens, NS thicken, become darker yellow or brown, more papular or verrucous, and can be friable or pruritic (Fig. 1.7).
- Warty growths, representing secondary adnexal neoplasms, may develop within an NS during adolescence or later.

PATHOGENESIS

- NS represents at defect in cutaneous embryologic development; its exact etiology is unknown.
- NS occurs sporadically.

DIAGNOSIS

- Diagnosis is clinical.
- Dermatoscopy showing bright yellow dots, and an absence of hair follicles can help make the definitive diagnosis, before the characteristic features become apparent.

This consists of a hand-held magnifier that allows inspection of skin lesions unobstructed by skin surface reflections.

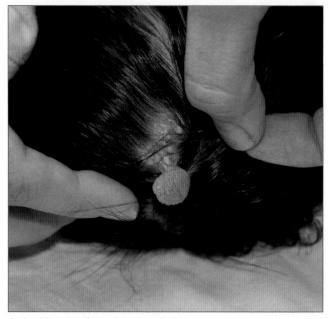

1.6 *Nevus sebaceous.* Atypical large, verrucous, pedunculated nevus sebaceous on the scalp of a neonate.

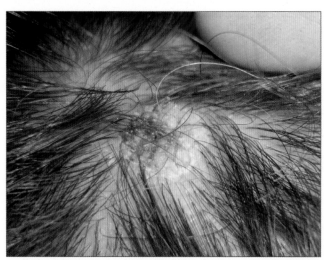

1.7 *Nevus sebaceous.* Nevus sebaceous showing the typical verrucous changes that occur at puberty.

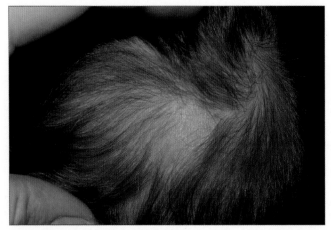

1.5 *Nevus sebaceous.* Typical yellow-tan color, oval shape, and finely papulated appearance of a nevus sebaceous.

DIFFERENTIAL DIAGNOSIS

Aplasia Cutis Congenita
- *Close inspection will reveal a lack of yellow dots.*

Congenital Triangular Alopecia (see Chapter 9)
- *Skin-colored, flat, lancet-shaped, alopecic patch that remains stable over time.*

Other Congenital Hamartomas (i.e., Epidermal Nevus)
- *Close inspection will reveal a lack of yellow dots.*
- *Hyperpigmented velvety surface.*

 ### MANAGEMENT

- A complete physical examination should be performed to rule out other congenital defects and determine extent of NS.
- Complete surgical removal remains the treatment of choice for NS given the concern for warty proliferation, permanent alopecia, and the development of secondary tumors at puberty.
- More recent investigations have shown that the risk of developing a malignant neoplasm within an NS is quite low.
- Recommendations for timing of excision vary. Advantages of removing the lesions in infancy are greater laxity of tissues, smaller size of lesion, and removal of any cosmetic impact on a developing child; the main disadvantage to early removal is the need for general anesthesia.
- Most often, a NS is removed in late childhood, prior to the onset of puberty, when the patient is able to cooperate with excision under local anesthesia and the lesion has not yet thickened under the influence of androgens.
- In cases of an extensive or widespread NS, a thorough medical history and physical examination should be performed with special attention to the ocular, neurologic, and musculoskeletal systems. Radiologic evaluation and further workup should be symptom-directed.
- Various ablative treatments including cryotherapy and electrodessication have been used to treat NS, but these do not remove risk of neoplasia and can still leave areas of alopecia.

Nevus Simplex (aka Salmon Patch)

BASICS

- Nevus simplex is now the preferred term for the most common vascular birthmark of infancy formerly known as the salmon patch.
- A nevus simplex is evident at birth as a pink-red vascular patch in characteristic locations on the face or on the occipital scalp.

CLINICAL MANIFESTATIONS

- A nevus simplex presents as an ill-defined, flat, dull pink or red, blanchable patch most commonly on the posterior scalp (aka "stork bite"), glabella (aka "angel's kiss"), forehead, upper eyelids, nose, and/or upper lip (Figs. 1.8 and 1.9).
- Less often, a nevus simplex can have a more extensive, widespread distribution.
- Lesions become deeper red with crying and physical exertion.
- Complete resolution within the first 2 years of life is expected for >95% of lesions on the face.
- Occipital lesions tend to persist for longer, some indefinitely.

PATHOGENESIS

- Etiology is unknown.
- Many experts believe it to be a form of persistent fetal circulation rather than a true vascular malformation.

DIAGNOSIS

- Diagnosis is clinical.

 DIFFERENTIAL DIAGNOSIS

Port-Wine Stain
- *Well demarcated and darker pink in color.*
- *Persistent and darkens over time.*

Early Hemangioma
- *Not present at birth.*
- *Rapid volumetric growth in the first few weeks of life.*

 MANAGEMENT

- No treatment is necessary as the vast majority of lesions on the face fade completely.
- More extensive lesions and occipital lesions can persist beyond the first year of life.
- Pulsed dye laser (PDL) is effective for persistent lesions.

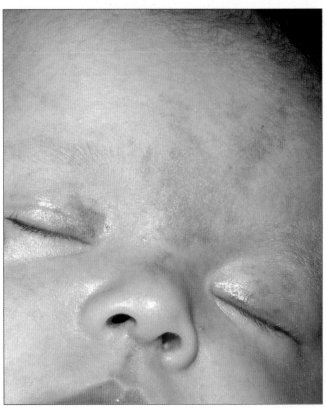

1.8 *Nevus Simplex.* Nevus simplex in a V-shape on the central forehead and on upper eyelids of a neonate. Lesions become more apparent with crying or straining.

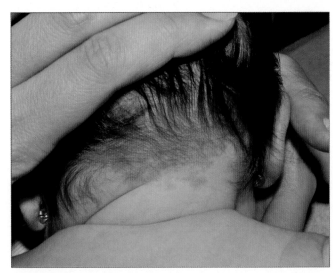

1.9 *Nevus Simplex.* Nevus simplex on the posterior scalp.

 HELPFUL HINTS

- Nevus simplex are common, occurring in 30% to 40% of newborns.
- Nevus simplex should be distinguished from a port-wine stain (PWS) early on so parents can be reassured of their eventual resolution and lack of associated findings.

Port-Wine Stain (Nevus Flammeus)

BASICS

- A PWS is a congenital capillary malformation that typically presents as a deep pink to reddish-purple discoloration of the skin on the head and/or neck.
- Most of the time a PWS is an isolated lesion but it can be seen as part of a variety of syndromes.

PATHOGENESIS

- The pathogenesis is unknown.

CLINICAL MANIFESTATIONS

- A PWS presents at birth as a flat, well-demarcated, pink to dark red ("port-wine" color) blanchable patch most commonly noted on the face (Fig. 1.10).
- PWSs are usually unilateral, but can be bilateral.
- Lesions darken progressively and can become thickened over time. Some develop secondary proliferative nodules on their surface.
- A PWS present in certain locations can be a clue to an associated syndrome (see Table 1.1 for a list). Two of the most common syndromes will be discussed below.

DIAGNOSIS

- The diagnosis is made clinically.
- Workup for an underlying syndrome association is based on the location of the PWS.

DIFFERENTIAL DIAGNOSIS

Early Infantile Hemangioma
- *Rapid proliferation will begin at 3 to 6 weeks of age.*
- *Complete involution is expected.*

Nevus Simplex
- *Ill-defined vascular patch usually located on central face or occipital scalp.*
- *Lightens over time, and complete involution is expected.*

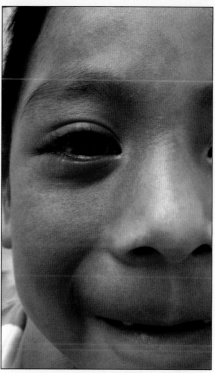

1.10 *Port-wine stain.* Port-wine stain in the typical location on the face. Note the sharp midline demarcation.

Table 1.1 LOCATION OF PWS AND ASSOCIATED SYNDROME	
LOCATION	**SYNDROME**
Face, in V1 (+/– V2 and V3) distribution	Sturge–Weber syndrome
Extremity, geographic shape	Klippel–Trenaunay syndrome
Face and limbs (multiple small lesions, surrounded by white halo)	Parkes Weber syndrome
Dermatomal capillary malformation on the back	Cobb syndrome
Midforehead, glabella, and upper eyelids	Beckwith–Wiedemann syndrome

MANAGEMENT

- A complete physical examination should be performed to determine location and extent of PWS and if there are any other congenital defects.
- If a PWS in a high-risk location (see Table 1.1) is identified, appropriate workup and referrals should be made.
- Once a potential syndrome association has been ruled out, the PWS can be approached as a cosmetic issue.
- The decision of whether and when to treat a PWS depends on its size, location, and the age of the child. Parents should be educated as to their natural history of persistence and gradual darkening and thickening over time. The potential psychosocial impact of the lesion (especially facial PWS) on the developing child should also be considered.
- The treatment of choice is the PDL (585 to 595 nm) which targets oxyhemoglobin and destroys dermal blood vessels without damage to the epidermis.
- Early and frequent treatment (every 2 to 4 weeks) of a PWS with the PDL can lead to significant and sometimes complete clearance.
- The number of treatments needed to achieve clearance varies from >6 to 12. Parents will often stop treatments once cosmetically acceptable lightening has occurred.
- Laser treatments can be performed in an outpatient setting with or without topical anesthesia or under general anesthesia, depending on the age of the patient and the location and extent of the PWS.
- For PWS resistant to PDL, combination with other vascular lasers (i.e., potassium-titanyl-phosphate (KTP) or Nd:YAG) can often achieve excellent results.

HELPFUL HINT

- The early initiation of PDL treatment can lead to complete clearance in infancy.

STURGE–WEBER SYNDROME

BASICS

- Sturge–Weber syndrome (SWS) is the association of: (1) a PWS on the face in the distribution of the first trigeminal nerve (V1) with or without involvement in the V2 and/or V3 distribution (see Fig. 1.10), (2) ipsilateral leptomeningeal vascular malformation, and (3) ipsilateral glaucoma.
- The risk of SWS is determined by the distribution of the PWS—all patients with SWS have all or part of their PWS in the V1 distribution.
- The overall incidence of SWS in patients with a PWS appearing in the V1 and V2 distribution is 8%, and the risk increases if multiple segments are involved or if the PWS is bilateral.

CLINICAL MANIFESTATIONS

- Seizures are the most common neurologic manifestations of SWS and usually present in infancy.
- Glaucoma is the most common eye finding and can occur anytime from infancy through adulthood.
- Children with SWS can also suffer from headaches, strokes, focal deficits, or have cognitive or behavioral impairments.

DIAGNOSIS

- All patients with a PWS in the V1 distribution should have baseline and at least yearly complete ophthalmologic examinations to determine presence of ocular involvement.
- Although a CT scan may be better at picking up the typical cortical calcifications ("tram-track" calcifications), an MRI with gadolinium is the test of choice and first-line study for identifying the presence of intracerebral vascular anomalies.

MANAGEMENT

- Management of patients with SWS is multidisciplinary. Patients should be followed by dermatology, pediatric neurology, and pediatric ophthalmology.
- Seizures are usually treated with medications but occasionally require surgical intervention.
- PDL may be used to treat the cutaneous PWS once seizures have been controlled.
- Close ophthalmologic follow-up is required for early detection and treatment of glaucoma.

HELPFUL HINT

- Referral to support foundations such as the Sturge–Weber Foundation (www.sturge-weber.com) is often beneficial to families of affected children.

KLIPPEL–TRENAUNAY SYNDROME

BASICS

- Klippel–Trenaunay Syndrome (KTS) is the triad of: (1) a PWS located on an extremity, (2) underlying typical varicose veins, venous or lymphatic malformations (VMs or LMs), and (3) progressive hypertrophy of the underlying soft tissues and/or bone.
- The diagnosis of KTS requires two out of the three features listed above.

CLINICAL MANIFESTATIONS

- The PWS associated with KTS are typically those that are "geographic" in shape which means that the borders are sharply demarcated resembling the outlines of countries on a map (Fig. 1.11) rather than those that are blotchy with smudgy borders (Fig. 1.12).
- Prominent superficial veins or varicosities as well as soft tissue overgrowth will develop with age. Occasionally, bony overgrowth of the affected limb also occurs.
- KTS may lead to localized intravascular coagulopathy and thromboses that result in pain and an increased risk of skin ulcers and pulmonary embolism.
- Limb length discrepancy can lead to scoliosis and hip asymmetry.

DIAGNOSIS

- Infants at high risk for KTS should be followed closely for evidence of venous and lymphatic malformations and limb length discrepancy. Limb lengths can be evaluated clinically early on; later they can be assessed radiographically.
- A color Doppler ultrasound of the affected extremity can determine the composition and extent of the underlying vascular malformation. Occasionally an MRI and MRA are needed.
- A coagulation profile should be checked periodically to determine the presence of intravascular coagulopathy.

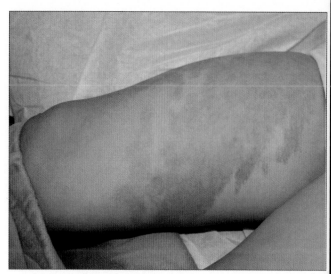

1.12 *Port-wine stain.* Blotchy port-wine stain on the leg.

 MANAGEMENT

- The management of KTS is aimed at prevention of and surveillance for the known potential complications.
- A multidisciplinary team involving dermatology, orthopedic and vascular surgery, and hematology is often required.
- Compression therapy with stockings, elastic bandages or massage will reduce pain and limb engorgement in most patients with KTS.
- The PWS and the cutaneous vascular blebs can be treated with laser therapy.

 HELPFUL HINT

- Referral to the Klippel–Trenaunay Support Group (http://www.kt-foundation.org/) is often beneficial for patients and families.

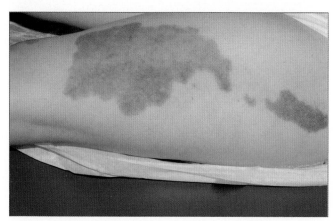

1.11 *Port-wine stain.* Well-demarcated "geographic" port-wine stain on the thigh. These lesions have a higher-risk KTS (Figure courtesy of Seth J. Orlow, MD, PhD.)

Infantile Hemangioma

BASICS

- The infantile hemangioma (IH) is the most common tumor of infancy, present in 5% to 10% of all infants.
- IHs are more common in female infants and low–birth-weight newborns.

PATHOGENESIS

- The exact etiology and pathogenesis of IH is unknown but is an area of vigorous investigation that has been accelerated by the development of an IH mouse model.
- IH is neoplasm of benign endothelial-like cells that possess the markers GLUT-1, Lewis Y antigen, Fc®RII, and merosin and stem cells, and pericytes.
- The etiology is unknown, but popular theories include a placental embolus, a somatic mutation in a gene-mediating endothelial cell proliferation, or origination from an endothelial progenitor cell (CD34+, CD133+).

CLINICAL MANIFESTATIONS

- IHs are not present at birth.
- They present in the first few weeks of life with a precursor lesion that can appear as a bluish bruise-like patch, telangiectasias with a rim of pallor, or a red flat stain.
- IHs have a characteristic natural history consisting of three phases:
  1. The ***rapid proliferation phase***: 3 weeks until 6 to 7 months of age; IHs experience rapid volumetric growth and appear red, firm and have a rubbery texture (Fig. 1.13).

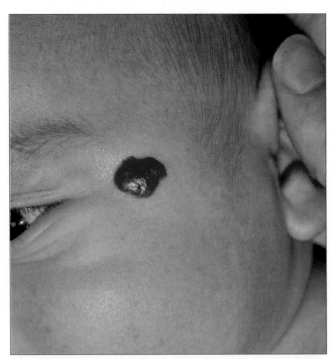

1.13   *Infantile hemangioma.* The bright red color and firm rubbery appearance are typical of an infantile hemangioma in the growth phase.

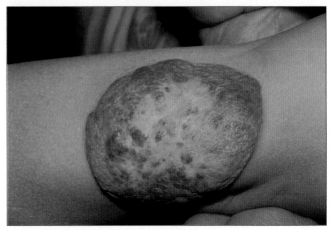

1.14   *Involuting infantile hemangioma.* Red color is breaking apart and texture is soft and spongy. The hemangioma is being replaced with fibrofatty tissue.

  2. The ***plateau (or late proliferative) phase***: variable length, usually 7 to 12 months of age; IHs have a slower rate of growth and color changes to a dull red to gray and begins to break apart and lesions feel soft or spongy.
  3. The ***involution phase***: usually starts at 1 year of age and is a gradual process that can last for years; the color continues to fade, some lesions involute completely while others leave fibrofatty residua (Fig. 1.14).
- IH can be superficial (Fig. 1.15), deep or mixed (superficial and deep) (Fig. 1.16).
- Lesions with a deep component will grow for about month longer than superficial IH.
- More recent studies show that most IH growth is complete by 5 months of age and that involution ends at median age 3 years.
- Ulceration is the most common complication and is heralded by a gray-white color during the proliferative phase (Fig. 1.17).

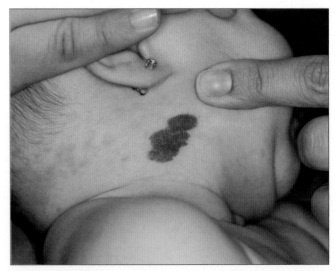

1.15   *Infantile hemangioma.* A superficial infantile hemangioma is a thin, flat bright red plaque. Also note nevus simplex or "stork bite" on posterior scalp.

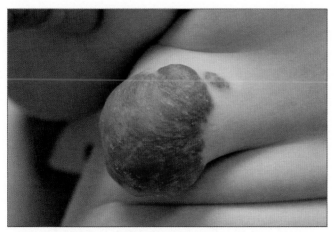

1.16 Infantile hemangioma. Mixed infantile hemangioma has both a superficial component and a deep component that often extends beyond superficial component. (Figure courtesy of Lawrence Schachner, M.D.)

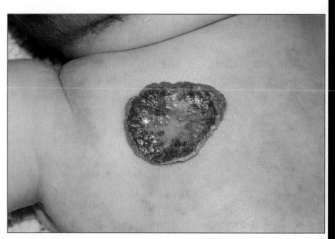

1.17 An ulcerated infantile hemangioma. Ulceration is the most common complication of IH and occurs during the growth phase.

- IHs in certain locations and of certain morphologies are at higher risk for development of complications and/or associated systemic involvement (see Table 1.2, for a list of high-risk IHs and intervention required). For example, IHs in the perineum are at highest risk for early ulceration, IHs in the central face can lead to permanent cosmetic disfigurement, and large segmental IHs (configuration corresponding to a recognizable and/or significant portion of a developmental segment) on the face should prompt workup for PHACES syndrome.
- Early recognition of high-risk IH will allow for more timely intervention.

DIAGNOSIS

- Diagnosis is clinically based on the typical morphology and characteristic growth pattern.

 DIFFERENTIAL DIAGNOSIS

Congenital Hemangiomas
- **Rapidly involuting congenital hemangioma (RICH)**— *present at birth, undergoes rapid spontaneous involution in the first year of life. Negative for GLUT-1.*
- **Noninvoluting congenital hemangioma (NICH)**— *present at birth, remains stable in size, does not involute. Negative for GLUT-1.*

Vascular Malformations (Capillary, Mixed Capillary-Venous or Venous-Arterial)
- *Vascular malformations are present at birth and grow proportionately with child over time.*

Table 1.2 HIGH-RISK INFANTILE HEMANGIOMAS LOCATION AND REQUIRED INTERVENTION

ANATOMIC LOCATION/ MORPHOLOGY	RISK	INTERVENTION
Perineal, axilla, neck, perioral	Ulceration, disfigurement, feeding difficulties (perioral)	Close monitoring, identify premonitory gray-white color, treat early (i.e., <8 weeks)
Nasal tip, ear, large facial (esp. deep component)	Permanent scarring, disfigurement	Identify risk and treat early (i.e., <8 wks)
Periorbital and retrobulbar	Ocular axis occlusion, astigmatism, amblyopia, tear duct occlusion	Identify risk and treat early (i.e., <8 wks), baseline ophtho evaluation
Facial, large (>5 cm), segmental	PHACES syndrome (posterior fossa malformations, hemangiomas, arterial anomalies, cardiac defects, eye abnormalities, sternal clefting)	MRI/MRA head and neck Echocardiogram Ophtho evaluation Systemic treatment
Segmental overlying lumbosacral spine	LUMBAR syndrome (lower body hemangioma, urogenital abnormalities, myelopathy, bony, and anorectal deformities)	MRI with contrast of spine <3 mo can use ultrasound as initial screen +/−Systemic treatment
Segmental "beard area" central neck	Airway hemangioma	Imaging Systemic treatment
Multiple hemangiomas (>5)	Visceral involvement (esp. liver and GI tract) "Multiple cutaneous hemangiomas with or without systemic hemangiomas"	Liver ultrasound, systemic treatment if liver IH present

MANAGEMENT

- The vast majority of IHs will proliferate and involve with minimal consequence. In these cases, active non-intervention is the treatment of choice and consists of education on the natural history of IH, close monitoring (with or without the use of photography), and reassurance.
- It is important to recognize IHs that are at high risk for complications (i.e., ulceration, cosmetic disfigurement, and interference with vital functions) or associated anomalies and intervene quickly with treatment (see below) and proper workup (see Table 1.2).
- For IH requiring treatment, the options include topical, local, or systemic therapy.

Topical Treatments

- **Timolol 0.5% gel-forming solution** is a nonselective beta-blocker that is highly effective for ulcerated and superficial hemangiomas.
- Timolol 0.5% gel-forming solution is dosed as one drop twice daily on the IH for at least 3 months for best response.
- **Imiquimod 5% cream** has shown some efficacy in treatment of small superficial IH.
- **PDL therapy** (585 to 595 nm) is useful for early superficial lesions, ulcerating lesions (accelerates healing and decreases pain), and the residual erythema and telangiectasias left behind once IH has involuted.
- **Fractionated CO_2** or **Fraxel Lasers**—useful for treatment of the residual scarring and telangiectasias.
- Mid to superpotent topical corticosteroids (**triamcinolone 0.1% ointment or clobetasol 0.05% ointment**) applied twice daily to IH can also halt growth and hasten involution.

Intralesional Therapy

- Intralesional triamcinolone (**Kenalog**), 5 to 10 mg/cc, can stabilize growth and decrease the size of IH.
- This treatment is most useful for early localized IH on the lip and nasal tip.
- Injections should be initiated early and repeated every 3 to 4 weeks for maximal benefit.

Systemic Treatments

- Systemic therapy is reserved for larger IH with more aggressive growth characteristics that pose a high threat to a vital function, for cosmetic disfigurement, or for those IH not responding to local therapy.

Propranolol

- The nonselective beta-blocker, propranolol, has become the first-line treatment for IH requiring systemic therapy, given its greater efficacy and better side effect profile compared to systemic corticosteroids.
- Consensus guidelines on the use of propranolol for IH recommend a baseline cardiopulmonary evaluation prior to initiating propranolol and inpatient initiation if patient is <8 weeks old, or has inadequate social support or comorbidities.
- **Hemangeol** (propranolol hydrochloride 4.28 mg/mL) is a new infant friendly, paraben- and alcohol-free formulation of propranolol that is FDA approved and indicated for the treatment of IHs.

Dosing

- Optimal dosing is based on weight with goal therapeutic dose of 2 to 3 mg/kg/day divided and given three times daily with a minimum of 6 hours between doses.
- Multiple dosing regimens are used; one commonly used method is:
  - Start at 0.33 mg/kg/dose, three times per day, for 3 to 7 days then,
  - Increase to 0.5 mg/kg/dose, three times per day, for 3 to 7 days then,
  - Increase to *goal* of 0.66 mg/kg/dose three times per day.
- Recommended dose of **hemangeol** based on the results of a large multicenter randomized trial is 3.4 mg/kg/day divided twice daily for 6 months.
- HR and BP should be checked between 1 and 3 hours after initial dose, and after the first dose of a dose increase of >0.5 mg/kg/day.
- Propranolol is usually continued through the growth phase of the IH and then tapered off.

Side Effects

- Sleep disturbance, intermittent acrocyanosis, gastrointestinal symptoms, and respiratory symptoms.
- Serious side effects are rare and include hypotension, bradycardia, and hypoglycemia.
- Propranolol should be given during the day with a feeding shortly after administration.
- Parents should be educated on the symptoms of hypoglycemia and instructed to ensure regular feeding times, avoid prolonged fasts, and discontinue propranolol during times of decreased oral intake.

continued on page 35

MANAGEMENT *Continued*

Atenolol

- Atenolol, a selective β1 receptor antagonist, has demonstrated similar efficacy for problematic infantile hemangiomas.
- Commonly used dose is 1 mg/kg/day.

Systemic Corticosteroids

- Oral corticosteroids (**prednisone or prednisolone**) are used to treat IH requiring systemic treatment when there is a contraindication to the use of propranolol.

Dosing

- Range is 2 to 4 mg/kg/day divided twice daily.
- Treatment is continued until IH growth has stopped and then tapered slowly to avoid rebound growth and adrenal suppression.

Side Effects

- Weight gain, increased irritability, stomach upset, hypertension, and immunosuppression.

- **Interferon α2a or 2b** and **Vincristine** are systemic treatments occasionally used in the treatment of refractory IH requiring treatment.

Treatments for Ulceration

- Topical **timolol 0.5% gel-forming solution**, one drop twice daily, can hasten healing.
- Local wound care with topical antibiotic ointments and nonstick dressings, or becaplermin gel.
- Pain management with acetaminophen or topical lidocaine gel or cream.
- **PDL therapy** has been shown to accelerate healing and decrease pain.

Surgery

- Excisional surgery is sometimes necessary in cases of airway hemangiomas and certain facial lesions.

 POINTS TO REMEMBER

- Most IHs require no treatment; active nonintervention is all that is needed.
- Recognize high-risk hemangiomas and treat early.
- Consider a cardiac evaluation in patients who are using topical timolol for ulcerated IH.

 HELPFUL HINTS

- IH may resemble PWSs early on, but close monitoring in the first month of life will demonstrate the characteristic growth pattern of an IH.
- Propranolol is now considered first line for IH that require systemic treatment.
- Prior to propranolol initiation for IH, patients should have a baseline cardiopulmonary evaluation.

Café au Lait Spots

BIRTHMARKS

BASICS

- Café au lait spots or café au lait macules are light brown flat lesions on the skin that are noted at birth in up to 1/3 of newborns.
- Most of the time, children will have less than three café au lait spots as an isolated finding. The presence of more than five café au lait or a single, large unilateral café au lait may be indicative of an underlying genetic syndrome.

PATHOLOGY

- Histologically, there is increased basal cell layer melanin and giant melanosomes.

CLINICAL MANIFESTATIONS

- Lesions present as light brown, evenly pigmented, round or oval, flat macules or patches that can vary in size from small to very large (Fig. 1.18).
- Café au lait spots are more common in children with darker skin color.
- May occur anywhere on the body and most children have one to three lesions.
- Lesions persist and remain stable over a lifetime.
- Six or more café au lait spots should prompt consideration for neurofibromatosis (NF) (see Chapter 11). The café au lait spots associated with NF are usually oval with smooth, sharply demarcated borders ("typical" café au lait; Fig. 1.19).
- Atypical café au lait spots are larger, have irregular or "smudgy" borders and nonhomogeneous pigment and are less likely to be associated with NF1 (Fig. 1.20; Chapter X).
- Large, geographic café au lait spots especially those on the abdomen may be a marker of McCune–Albright syndrome.

DIAGNOSIS

- Based on clinical recognition.

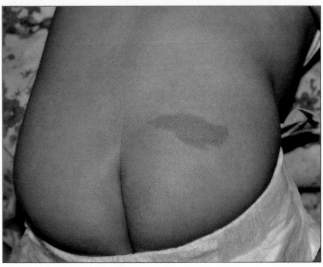

1.18 *Café au lait macule.* Large café au lait spot on buttock of infant.

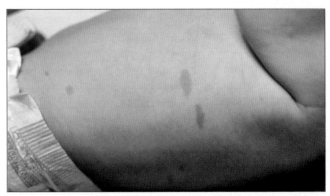

1.19 *Café au lait macule.* The café au lait macules seen in neurofibromatosis typically have smooth borders.

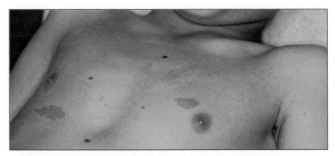

1.20 *Café au lait macule.* Two café au lait macules on chest showing smudgy irregular borders.

DIFFERENTIAL DIAGNOSIS

Congenital Melanocytic Nevus
- *Darker brown in color, may be raised.*
- *Thickens and changes color over time.*

Congenital Nevus Spilus (see below)
- *May initially look identical to a café au lait; over time smaller foci of darker brown nevi will develop within the lighter brown background patch.*

Epidermal Nevus (see below)
- *May initially be flat and light brown but over time become raised and can become warty.*
- *Typically present in a Blaschkolinear pattern.*

Becker Nevus
- *An ill-defined hyperpigmented patch that can resemble a café au lait (Fig. 1.21).*
- *Presents during adolescence; typically unilateral and on the chest.*

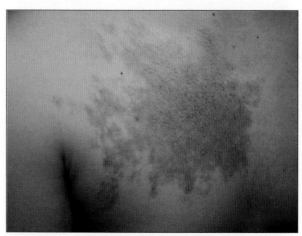

1.21 *Becker Nevus.* Becker nevus in the typical location on the chest can mimic a large café au lait spot.

 MANAGEMENT

- Patients with café au lait spots noted at birth should have a complete skin examination to determine number of café au lait and the presence of other congenital defects.
- No specific treatment is necessary.
- Laser therapy, including the Er:YAG, or the Q-switched Nd:YAG, Q-switched alexandrite or ruby, for lightening or removal of café au lait has produced variable results. Most studies show ~50% of patients experience total clearance but there is a high relapse rate.
- Parents should be reassured of their benign and static nature.

Dermal Melanocytosis (aka Mongolian Spot(s))

BASICS

- Mongolian spots are very common bluish-gray stains that are typically seen on the lower back of darker skinned newborns (Fig. 1.22).
- Lesions occur in >90% of African-American neonates, 60% to 70% of Asian and Hispanic neonates but are only seen in <10% of Caucasian babies.

PATHOGENESIS

- The cause is unknown, but represents a collection of spindle-shaped melanocytes located deep in the dermis.

CLINICAL MANIFESTATIONS

- Presents at birth as a flat, deep brown to slate gray or blue-black, ill-defined large flat (macular) lesions.
- There can be single or multiple lesions that often coalesce into larger lesions.
- The borders are usually irregular and occasionally indistinct.
- Most commonly located on the lumbosacral areas and buttocks; occasionally seen on the lower limbs, back, flanks, and shoulders.
- Sometimes can be widespread and extensive (Fig. 1.23).
- Lesions tend to fade during first 2 to 3 years of life.
- Occasionally, persist into adulthood.

DIAGNOSIS

- The diagnosis is clinical.

 DIFFERENTIAL DIAGNOSIS

Congenital Melanocytic Nevus
- *Usually are smaller and well demarcated.*
- *Color is homogeneous light or dark brown and some are raised and have excess hair.*

Blue Nevus
- *Dark blue macule or papule, occasionally present at birth and is usually small (<1 cm) and located on an extremity.*

Nevus of Ito or Ota
- *Speckled blue-black lesion that progresses over time in a characteristic location.*
- *Nevus of Ito is located over the shoulder and Nevus of Ota is usually periorbital.*

Bruising
- *Occasionally Mongolian spots may be mistaken for bruises. Bruises will fade within 1 to 2 weeks.*

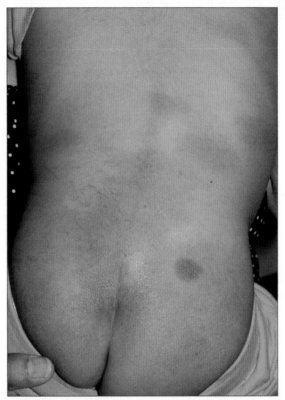

1.22 *Dermal Melanocytosis.* Mongolian spot in the characteristic location on the lower back of an infant.

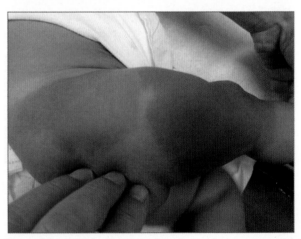

1.23 *Dermal Melanocytosis.* Mongolian spots on the thigh.

🔧 **MANAGEMENT**

- A complete physical examination should be performed to determine extent of the lesion and to determine the presence of other skin lesions.
- Parents should be reassured that these lesions are benign and that spontaneous, complete resolution without sequelae is expected.
- Blue-black pigment–specific lasers can be used for lesions that persist into adulthood and are of cosmetic significance.

Congenital Melanocytic Nevus

BASICS

- Nevi that are present at birth or develop within the first 2 years of life are considered congenital melanocytic nevi (CMN).
- Small or medium CMN are common and occur in 1% to 3% of neonates.

PATHOLOGY

- As opposed to acquired nevi that present later in life, CMN show melanocytes extending deeper into the dermis and tend to surround hair follicles and nerves. Melanocytes are also found singly lined up in between collagen bundles.

CLINICAL MANIFESTATIONS

- CMN present as tan to light or dark brown/black, flat or raised macules or papules of varying size.
- CMN are classified according to their predicted final adult size as small, medium, or large.
  - **Small CMN** have a final size of <1.5 cm in largest diameter.
  - **Medium CMN** have a final size of 1.5 to 19.9 cm in greatest diameter (Fig. 1.24).
  - **Large (or giant) CMN** have a predicted adult size of ≥20 cm (equivalent to ≥9 cm on the head of an infant or ≥6 cm on the body of an infant) (Fig. 1.25).
- Large CMN have an estimated incidence of 1 in 20,000 and are associated with an increased risk of melanoma and neurocutaneous melanosis.
- Lesions enlarge in proportion to the child's growth.
- Over time CMN can become darker or lighter in color, develop a mottled pigmentation, increase in thickness, and even spontaneously regress. Surface changes such as hypertrichosis, verrucous changes, and proliferative nodules can also occur (Fig. 1.26).

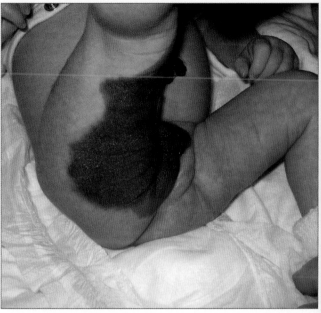

1.25 *Congenital Melanocytic Nevus.* Giant congenital melanocytic nevus on the thigh of a neonate. Giant CMN have an increased risk of developing melanoma.

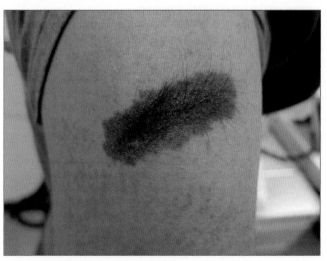

1.26 *Congenital Melanocytic Nevus.* Medium congenital melanocytic nevus demonstrating hypertrichosis.

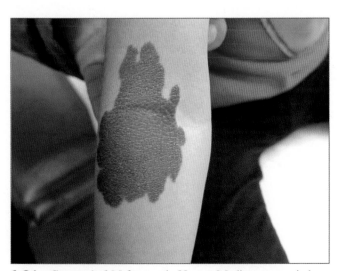

1.24 *Congenital Melanocytic Nevus.* Medium congenital melanocytic nevus are 1.5 to 19.9 cm.

CLINICAL VARIANT

- **Speckled lentiginous nevus or nevus spilus** (Fig. 1.27) is a subtype of CMN that initially presents as a variably sized (usually 1 to 4 cm) tan patch, resembling a café au lait spot, that over time develops superimposed darker pigmented macules and papules, representing nevi.
- The risk of melanoma development within nevus spilus is thought to be proportional to the size of the lesion and suspicious changes within lesions should be evaluated histologically.

ASSOCIATED RISKS

- The risk for the development of melanoma in CMN is not exactly known and is the subject of much debate and investigation but is believed to correlate with the size of the CMN.
- Currently the risk of melanoma in small and medium CMN is thought to be <1% over a lifetime and almost always occur after puberty.
- For large CMN, the risk of melanoma is approximately 5% to 10% over a lifetime and commonly occurs in childhood.
- Melanoma can present as a focal area of change within the nevus or as a proliferative nodule.
- Patients with large CMN who also have numerous smaller ("satellite") nevi (Fig. 1.28.) or those with multiple medium-sized nevi are at increased risk for the development of neurocutaneous melanosis, which is the proliferation of melanocytes within the leptomeninges.

DIFFERENTIAL DIAGNOSIS

Dermal Melanocytosis (aka Mongolian Spot)
- *Ill-defined irregular borders, fades over time.*

Café au Lait Spots
- *Remain lightly pigmented and stable over time.*

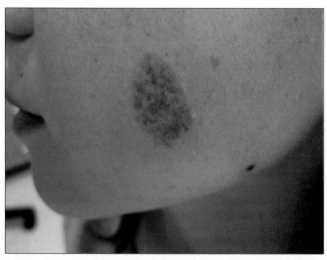

1.27 *Nevus spilus.* Typical presentation of a nevus spilus as a tan patch with superimposed darker brown macules within.

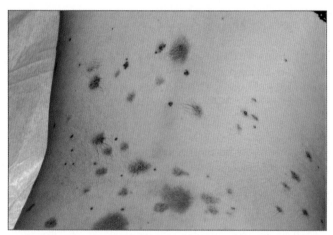

1.28 *Satellite Nevi.* Numerous satellite nevi can be associated with neurocutaneous melanosis.

MANAGEMENT

- A complete skin examination should be performed and the CMN should be measured and categorized as small, medium, or large.
- Parents should be counseled about the risk for the future development of melanoma.
- In general, prophylactic removal of small and medium CMN is not recommended if there are no concerning features and no obstacles to monitoring.
- Small and medium CMN can be managed on a case-by-case basis taking into account whether there are worrisome clinical features, cosmetic or parental concerns, and the ease of monitoring lesion given its location.
- Most of the time regular clinical monitoring is all that is needed.
- Surgical excision can be performed especially for cosmetically disfiguring lesions to avoid the potential psychosocial impact of the lesion on the developing child.
- Patients with large CMN, especially those on the posterior axis or those with smaller satellite nevi, and patients with multiple medium CMN should be screened for neurocutaneous melanosis with an MRI of the brain and spine ideally before 4 to 6 months of age.

- For large CMN, early and complete surgical excision is often recommended and desired by parents. However, decision to perform surgical removal should be individualized taking into account the risks of the procedure versus the benefits of surgical removal.
- Staged excision with tissue expansion can be performed by specialized surgeons and is often initiated between 6 and 9 months of age when the risk of anesthesia decreases.
- While surgical excision will improve cosmetic appearance, it does not completely eliminate the risk for melanoma because it is usually impossible to remove every nevus cell due to their deep extension into the fat, fascia, and muscle.
- In some large CMN, surgical removal is not feasible and other methods such as curettage, dermabrasion, or resurfacing lasers can have a cosmetic benefit.
- Regardless of intervention, large CMN should be closely followed with periodic skin examinations, dermoscopic evaluation, photographic documentation, and palpation.

HELPFUL HINTS

- The risk of melanoma in small and medium CMN is estimated to be <1% over a lifetime.
- Patients with large CMN and their families may benefit from organizations such as Nevus Outreach, Inc. (www.nevus.org), which offers annual family conferences, educational information, and a social support network.

POINTS TO REMEMBER

- Parents should be counseled on how to recognize concerning features in nevi and bring to the attention of the physician any focal changes in color, border, or surface appearance of the nevus.
- When examining large CMN it is important to palpate the lesions to detect for presence of firm nodules as melanoma can arise deep.
- Risk of neurocutaneous melanosis is greater if more than 20 satellite nevi are present or if large CMN is >40 cm.

Epidermal Nevus

BIRTHMARKS

BASICS

- The term epidermal nevus (EN) is applied to a variety of congenital hamartomas that are composed of cells derived from the embryonic ectoderm.
- Epidermal nevi are categorized based on the predominant ectodermal cell type present. For example, an NS is a type of EN, so named because sebaceous glands predominate (see earlier in this chapter).
- Keratinocytic epidermal nevi (composed mostly of keratinocytes) are the most common type of EN and are the type that is discussed here.

PATHOGENESIS

- Epidermal nevi reflect cutaneous mosaicism and are thought to result from a somatic mutation in a single ectodermal cell that then gives rise to a clone of genetically identical cells (see below).

CLINICAL MANIFESTATIONS

- The clinical appearance of EN is variable.
- EN are often seen as a variably sized linear plaque(s) along the lines of Blaschko which represent the embryonic migration of skin cells.
- EN can be skin-colored to pink or hyperpigmented and flat or slightly raised (Fig. 1.29).
- EN are typically localized but can be widespread (Fig. 1.30).
- EN can be present at birth or appear in infancy or early childhood.
- Initially lesions are flat or slightly raised and over time, some lesions thicken and can become warty.
- EN are usually an isolated finding but occasionally, especially large and extensive EN, can be associated with an underlying syndrome or extracutaneous defect.

DIAGNOSIS

- Diagnosis is usually made clinically.
- A skin biopsy may occasionally be necessary to determine subtype of EN or to differentiate an EN from an inflammatory skin condition such as psoriasis.

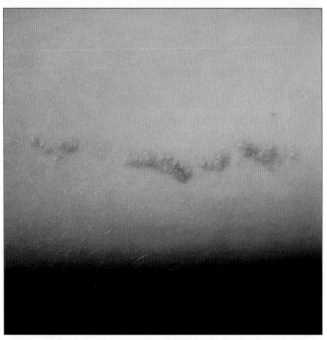

1.29 *Epidermal Nevus.* Localized epidermal nevus on the leg. (Figure courtesy of Lawrence Schachner, M.D.)

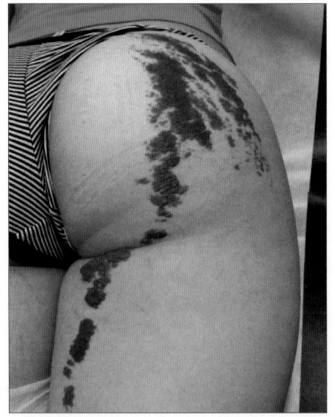

1.30 *Epidermal Nevus.* Extensive hyperpigmented verrucous epidermal nevus on the posterior thigh of a teenage girl.

DIFFERENTIAL DIAGNOSIS

Hyperpigmented Pigmentary Mosaicism (aka Segmental Pigmentation Disorder; see Fig. 1.34)

- *Linear and whorled hyperpigmented streaks present at birth and remain stable and flat over time.*

Psoriasis

- *Occasionally psoriasis may present in a linear or segmental distribution and can be mistaken for an EN.*
- *Psoriasis will be pink-red with overlying silvery white scale and responds to topical steroids.*

Lichen Striatus

- *Long, linear plaque composed of flat-topped papules commonly seen on the extremities in children.*
- *Not present at birth and spontaneously resolve over months to years.*

Verruca Vulgaris

- *Can occasionally present as a small linear plaque resembling a verrucous EN.*
- *Not present at birth, black dots will be visible after paring lesion.*

 MANAGEMENT

- Patients with large or extensive EN require a thorough medical and family history and physical evaluation with particular attention to the neurologic, ocular, and cardiovascular systems. A symptom-directed workup should be performed as necessary.
- Most EN lack associated defects and are only of cosmetic concern.
- Because most EN thicken and become warty over time, many patients request complete removal or destruction.
- Method of treatment depends on size and location of the lesion. Surgical excision will provide the most definitive result for most small, localized lesions.
- Larger lesions are often treated with a combination of superficial destructive and surgical methods.
- Superficial destructive methods such as cryotherapy, electrodessication, and laser ablation have variable results and are often followed by recurrence.
- Ablative CO_2 laser therapy and Fraxel laser are effective in removing EN.
- Topical therapies such as topical retinoids, 5-fluorouracil and topical corticosteroids can improve the appearance of the EN in some cases.

Nevus Depigmentosus

BASICS

- A nevus depigmentosus (ND) is a common, well-circumscribed hypopigmented patch that can be seen at birth or becomes apparent later infancy or early childhood as the surrounding skin pigmentation increases.
- Although the name implies absence of pigment, ND are usually hypopigmented and have reduced pigment but not a total lack of pigment.
- ND are usually an isolated finding.

PATHOGENESIS

- ND are thought to result from a defect in melanin transfer to keratinocytes.
- Histology shows a decrease in amount of melanin.

CLINICAL MANIFESTATIONS

- Presents as a solitary, hypopigmented (flat) macule or patch with well-defined irregular borders (Fig. 1.31).
- ND can occur anywhere on the skin but are typically seen on the trunk and grow proportionately with child.
- Persists lifelong, remains unchanged.
- Occasionally, can present as multiple lesions or as a linear and/or segmental lesion (Fig. 1.32).
- When more extensive, the term **pigmentary mosaicism** or **segmental pigmentation disorder** is applied.
- If multiple small lesions are present, ND must be distinguished from an ash leaf macule that is associated with the neurocutaneous genetic disorder, tuberous sclerosis (see Chapter 11).

CLINICAL VARIANTS

- Hypopigmentation at birth sometimes presents in a more widespread, patterned distribution such as block-like or a checkerboard pattern; or as streaks and swirls along the lines of Blaschko (Fig. 1.33).
- This type of patterned pigmentation was previously termed hypomelanosis of Ito but now **pigmentary mosaicism** or **segmental pigmentation disorder** are the preferred terms.
- Alternatively, there can be patterned *hyper*pigmentation on the skin at birth or developing shortly thereafter (also called **linear and whorled nevoid hypermelanosis**) (Fig. 1.34).
- Although programmed in utero, sometimes these birthmarks do not become apparent until the first few years of life when pigmentation increases.
- Parents are often frightened because the pigment alteration can be extensive.
- Cells within the hypo- or hyperpigmented area of skin reflect genetic mosaicism whereby a clone of cells were programmed during embryologic development to make more or less pigment.
- Associated systemic findings usually of the neurologic, musculoskeletal, or cardiac system are found in a minority

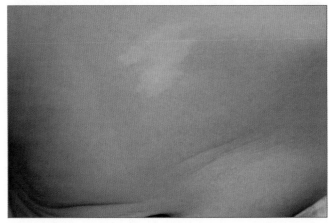

1.31 *Nevus depigmentosus.* Localized nevus depigmentosus on trunk.

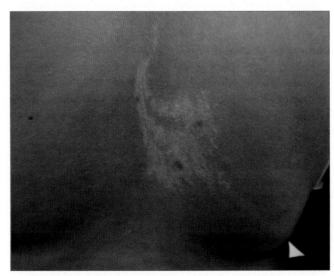

1.32 *Nevus depigmentosus.* Segmental nevus depigmentosus.

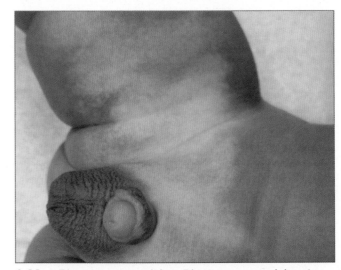

1.33 *Pigmentary mosaicism.* Pigmentary mosaicism (or segmental pigmentation disorder) presenting as block-like hypopigmentation present since birth.

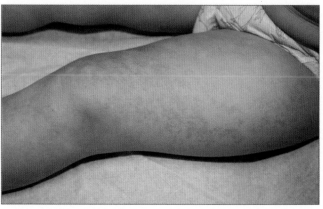

1.34 *Pigmentary mosaicism.* Pigmentary mosaicism presenting as streaky hyperpigmentation on the leg.

of patients with pigment alterations along Blaschko lines and workup should be symptom-directed.
• In the vast majority of patients this patterned hypo- or hyperpigmentation is merely a cosmetic issue.

DIAGNOSIS

• Diagnosis is based on clinical recognition.
• Examination with a Wood lamp may be helpful.

 DIFFERENTIAL DIAGNOSIS

Vitiligo
• *Rarely present at birth.*
• *Depigmented patch, will appear chalk white under Wood light.*

Ash-leaf Macule
• *Hypopigmented oval or leaf-shaped macules and patches; usually multiple are present.*
• *Other clinical features of tuberous sclerosis may be present.*

Pityriasis Alba (P. alba) or Postinflammatory Hypopigmentation (PIH)
• *In older children, P. alba may be confused for ND.*
• *P. alba or PIH presents as ill-defined areas of hypopigmentation on the face or arms often associated with background xerosis or atopic dermatitis.*

 MANAGEMENT

• Patients with ND should have a complete physical examination to determine extent of lesion and presence of other skin findings.
• ND are benign and nonprogressive and parents can be reassured.
• Specific treatment is not necessary.
• For lesions in cosmetically sensitive areas or for those who desire treatment, autologous skin grafting and transfer with melanocyte-rich suspensions have been successful in some cases.
• There are also reports of improvement with excimer laser (308 nm) treatments.
• Cosmetic cover-up is also an effective albeit temporary treatment.

 HELPFUL HINT

• When in doubt the use of a Wood lamp will help distinguish an ND which will appear milky white, from vitiligo which will appear chalk white.

 POINTS TO REMEMBER

• Large and patterned areas of hypo- or hyperpigmentation (aka pigmentary mosaicism) is a relatively common birthmark that sometimes does not become apparent until later in infancy and is usually only a cosmetic issue.
• Although the name implies lack of pigment, ND are hypopigmented.

Neonatal and Infantile Eruptions

OVERVIEW

There are numerous skin eruptions that characteristically occur during the neonatal period and in infancy. Most of these are transient physiologic phenomena or benign, self-limited eruptions that are unique to newborns and infants and often bother parents much more than they do the babies. Less often, a skin rash on a neonate or infant can represent an infection, a genetic skin disease, or a systemic condition. It is important to recognize the clinical morphology and distribution of the common, benign eruptions so that they can be quickly distinguished from more significant conditions that may require further workup and treatment.

When in doubt, simple, reliable tests such as a potassium hydroxide stain (KOH), Gram stain, and cultures can help to rule out an infectious etiology. A skin biopsy is rarely indicated. Many of the conditions described in this chapter can have widespread, extensive presentations but are generally asymptomatic. Treatment, when necessary, is aimed at the alleviation of symptoms and the prevention or treatment of infection. In addition, the level of parental anxiety should be assessed and addressed.

IN THIS CHAPTER...

> **CUTIS MARMORATA**

> **SEBACEOUS GLAND HYPERPLASIA**

> **TRANSIENT NEONATAL PUSTULAR MELANOSIS**

> **ERYTHEMA TOXICUM NEONATORUM**

> **SUCKING BLISTERS**

> **MILIA**

> **MILIARIA**

> **NEONATAL LUPUS ERYTHEMATOSUS**

> **SEBORRHEIC DERMATITIS**

> **DIAPER DERMATITIS**

> **ACROPUSTULOSIS OF INFANCY**

> **EOSINOPHILIC PUSTULAR FOLLICULITIS OF INFANCY**

> **ACUTE HEMORRHAGIC EDEMA OF INFANCY**

BASICS

- Cutis marmorata is a physiologic response of the dermal capillaries to cooler ambient temperatures that is commonly seen in newborns.

PATHOGENESIS

- Cool ambient temperatures cause vasodilatation of capillaries.

CLINICAL MANIFESTATIONS

- Symmetric, blanchable, reticulated deep red to violaceous patches usually located on the extremities; less often on the trunk (Fig. 2.1).
- Lesions typically resolve with rewarming.
- Cutis marmorata may persist for several weeks to months but usually completely resolves with no sequelae.
- In patients with Down syndrome or hypothyroidism, cutis marmorata may persist for a longer time.

DIAGNOSIS

- Diagnosis is based on clinical recognition and evidence of resolution with rewarming.

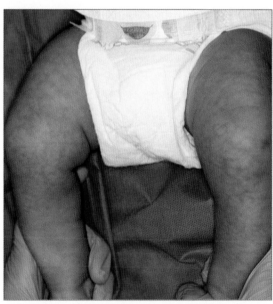

2.1   Cutis marmorata. Symmetric, blanchable, reticulated deep red to violaceous patches on the lower extremities; these will improve with rewarming.

HELPFUL HINTS

- If diagnosis is in doubt, attempt to rewarm patient by swaddling to see if skin lesions disappear.
- Physiologic cutis marmorata is blanchable and improves with warming.

DIFFERENTIAL DIAGNOSIS

Cutis Marmorata Telangiectatica Congenita (CMTC)

- *Persistent deep red or violaceous reticulated patches on an extremity that does not resolve with rewarming and does not blanch.*
- *CMTC can be seen in association with several genetic syndromes including Adams–Oliver syndrome or can be associated with underlying hypoplasia of the affected extremity (Fig. 2.2).*

Reticulated Port-Wine Stain

- *Will not disappear with rewarming.*
- *Progressively darkens over time.*

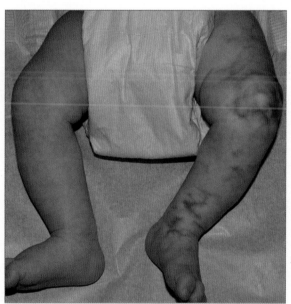

 2.2   Cutis marmorata telangiectatica congenita. Irregular, linear, violaceous reticulated, and atrophic patches that do not resolve with rewarming on the left lower extremity. By contrast, note physiologic cutis marmorata on the right lower extremity.

MANAGEMENT

- The most important first step in management is to distinguish physiologic cutis marmorata from CMTC or a vascular malformation.
- Physiologic cutis marmorata is a benign condition of no medical significance and will resolve spontaneously. Parents can be reassured.
- To prevent lesions, parents should keep infants warm.

BASICS

- Common transient condition seen in most newborns.

PATHOGENESIS

- Result of maternal androgens that stimulate sebaceous glands.

CLINICAL MANIFESTATIONS

- Yellow-white to skin-colored, monomorphic tiny macules to slightly elevated papules on the nose, cheeks, and upper lips of full-term infants (Fig. 2.3).

DIAGNOSIS

- Diagnosis is based on clinical recognition.

DIFFERENTIAL DIAGNOSIS

Milia (see later in this chapter)
- *Discrete, white, firm, tiny papules usually seen scattered on the face of a newborn.*

Neonatal Cephalic Pustulosis (Neonatal Acne)
- *Variably sized pink papules and pustules typically found on the cheeks, chin, and forehead.*

MANAGEMENT

- Reassure parents this is a benign eruption.
- Spontaneous resolution occurs within the first few months of life.

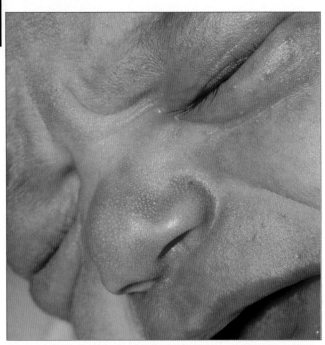

2.3   *Sebaceous gland hyperplasia.* Yellow-white monomorphic tiny macules and elevated papules on the nose in this full-term infant.

Transient Neonatal Pustular Melanosis

BASICS

- Transient neonatal pustular melanosis (TNPM) is a benign, self-limiting condition that affects 5% of black and <1% of white neonates.

PATHOGENESIS

- The etiology is unknown.

CLINICAL MANIFESTATIONS

- Lesions are typically evident at birth and evolve through three phases:
  - **Phase 1:** Flaccid vesiculopustules with minimal to no erythema, last 24 to 48 hours (Fig. 2.4).
  - **Phase 2:** Collarettes of scale (representing ruptured vesicles) (Fig. 2.5).
  - **Phase 3:** Hyperpigmented macules, resolve over weeks to months (Fig. 2.6).
- Phases 1 and 2 can happen in utero and baby is born with only brown "freckle-like" macules, or baby can be born with a combination of pustules, collarettes of scale, and hyperpigmented macules.
- Any site can be affected but lesions have a predilection for forehead, chin, neck, lower back, and diaper area.
- Rarely, may be seen on the scalp, palms, and soles.

DIAGNOSIS

- Diagnosis is based on clinical recognition.
- A Wright stain of pustule fluid will demonstrate neutrophils and solidify the diagnosis.
- KOH, Gram stain, and Tzanck smear will be negative.

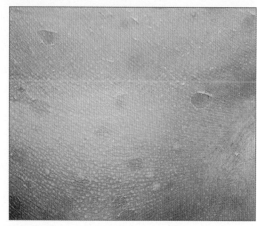

2.5 *Transient neonatal pustular melanosis.* Phase 2: Collarettes of scale from ruptured pustules as well as residual pustules.

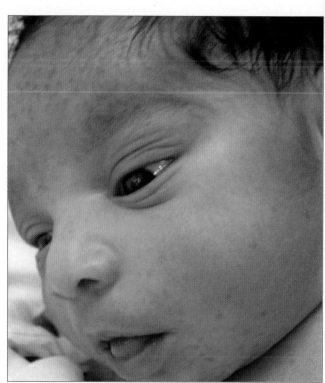

2.6 *Transient neonatal pustular melanosis.* Phase 3 of TNPM, hyperpigmented macules on the forehead and chin of this newborn. Phases 1 and 2 may have occurred in utero.

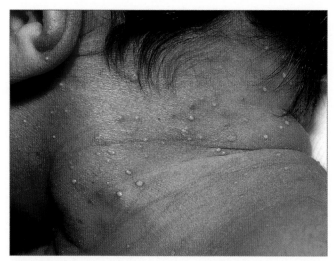

2.4 *Transient neonatal pustular melanosis.* Phase 1: Thin roofed pustules on a dark-skinned neonate. (From Burkhart CN, Morrell DS. *Visual Dx Essential Pediatric Dermatology.* Philadelphia, PA: Lippincott Williams & Wilkins; 2010.)

DIFFERENTIAL DIAGNOSIS

Bullous Impetigo
- *Superficial flaccid pustules and bullae typically found in the diaper area, axillae, or sites of wounds (circumcision or umbilical cord).*
- *Gram stain will reveal gram-positive cocci.*

Erythema Toxicum Neonatorum (see below)
- *Pustules on a blotchy erythematous base, usually not present at birth.*

Congenital Candidiasis
- *Tiny pustules or collarettes of scale on an erythematous base.*
- *When present at birth is usually widespread and often present on palms and soles.*
- *KOH of pustule contents will reveal pseudohyphae and budding yeast.*

Café au Lait Spots
- *Variably sized well-demarcated tan patches that present at birth as 1 to 3 discrete lesions.*
- *Persist unchanged over time.*

 MANAGEMENT

- TNPM should be distinguished from a congenital skin infection.
- Reassure parents of complete spontaneous resolution within the first weeks of life.
- Hyperpigmented macules may take several months to fade completely.

 POINT TO REMEMBER

- In TNPM, a Wright stain of pustule fluid will show many neutrophils but a Gram stain will be negative for bacterial organisms.

Erythema Toxicum Neonatorum

BASICS

- Erythema toxicum neonatorum (ETN, also known as toxic erythema of the newborn) is a common idiopathic, self-limiting eruption in otherwise healthy full-term newborns.

PATHOGENESIS

- The exact cause is unknown.

CLINICAL MANIFESTATIONS

- ETN is usually not present at birth and normally develops on the third or fourth day of life. There are rare reports of its appearance anywhere from the first day of life through 2 weeks of age.
- Lesions typically begin as ill-defined pink macules or edematous papules of variable size, that later develop ~1- to 3-mm yellow to pale pink papules or pustules at the center.
- Lesions are typically discrete and scattered and occur on the face, trunk, and extremities (Fig. 2.7).
- The palms and soles are typically spared.
- Rarely, the erythema may become confluent and widespread (Fig. 2.8).
- Exacerbations and remissions can occur in the first 2 weeks of life.
- The eruption usually self-resolves without sequelae over several days.

DIAGNOSIS

- Diagnosis is based on clinical recognition.
- A Wright or Giemsa stain of pustule contents will reveal numerous eosinophils.

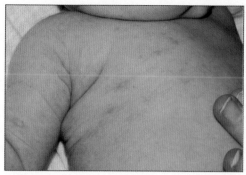

2.7 *Erythema toxicum neonatorum.* Ill-defined pink wheals with central pale yellow edematous papule scattered on the trunk.

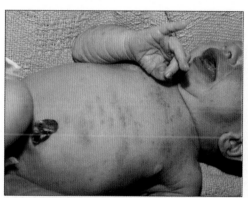

2.8 *Erythema toxicum neonatorum.* Areas of confluent erythema and several overlying papulopustules on the trunk. (From Burkhart CN, Morrell DS. *Visual Dx Essential Pediatric Dermatology.* Philadelphia, PA: Lippincott Williams & Wilkins; 2010.)

MANAGEMENT

- It is important to first rule out an infectious etiology.
- Parents can be reassured that this is a common, benign, asymptomatic, and self-limited condition.

HELPFUL HINT

- ETN affects up to 50% of full-term babies; it is rare in premature infants.

POINT TO REMEMBER

- A Wright stain of pustule contents will show numerous eosinophils, but a Gram stain will be negative for bacterial organisms and a KOH will be negative for yeast.

DIFFERENTIAL DIAGNOSIS

Transient Neonatal Pustular Melanosis (see above)

- *Present at birth as flaccid vesiculopustules that rupture easily leaving behind a collarette of scale and a hyperpigmented macule.*

Miliaria (see later in this chapter)

- *Occurs in first weeks of life secondary to heat and occlusion from excessive swaddling.*
- *Presents as small pink to red papules, vesicles, or papulovesicles with an erythematous rim commonly grouped on the trunk.*

Congenital Candidiasis

- *Tiny pustules or collarettes of scale on an erythematous base.*
- *When present at birth is usually widespread and often present on palms and soles.*
- *KOH of pustule contents will reveal pseudohyphae and budding yeast.*

Sucking Blisters

BASICS

• Blisters or erosions seen on the extremities in newborns due to vigorous sucking in utero.

CLINICAL MANIFESTATIONS

• Presents as a single, oval shaped, superficial vesicle or bullae or as an erosion with a collarette of scale (Fig. 2.9).
• Usually seen on the dorsal hands or fingers or forearms but can also be found on the lips.

DIAGNOSIS

• Diagnosis is based on clinical recognition.

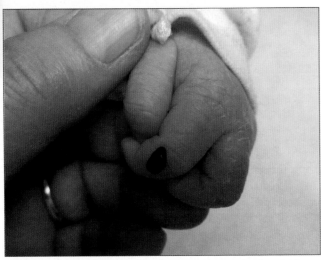

2.9 *Sucking blister.* Sucking blister on the finger of this newborn can be hemorrhagic, as seen in this picture.

 DIFFERENTIAL DIAGNOSIS

Bullous Impetigo
• *Superficial flaccid vesicles or bullae that rupture easily. Little to no surrounding redness.*
• *Typically multiple lesions and located in intertriginous areas such as the diaper area and axillae.*

Epidermolysis Bullosa
• *Genetic skin condition that presents with variable amounts of skin blistering and erosions at birth.*
• *New blisters will form easily at sites of trauma or friction.*

Neonatal Herpes Infection
• *Grouped vesicles on an erythematous base may be on any cutaneous surface and involve the mucosa; when ruptured, lesions appear as punched out erosions.*
• *Tzanck smear of vesicle base will show multinucleated giant cells. HSV culture or DFA will be positive for HSV1 or 2.*

 MANAGEMENT

• The most important first step in management is ruling out an infectious etiology or genetic skin condition.
• Sucking blisters heal completely without scarring within 2 weeks.
• Petrolatum ointment can be applied to lesion twice daily to hasten resolution.

Milia (See also Chapter 30)

BASICS

- Milia are tiny epidermal cysts that are commonly seen on the face of newborns.

PATHOGENESIS

- Lesions represent trapped keratin (the main structural protein in skin) just underneath the epidermis.

CLINICAL MANIFESTATIONS

- Appear as pinpoint (~1- to 2-mm) white or yellow superficial papules typically located on the cheeks, nose, chin, or forehead (Fig. 2.10).
- They may occur singly but more often present as multiple lesions or grouped.
- Occur in 40% to 50% of newborns, and self-resolve within the first month of life.
- Milia can also be seen in older children and adolescents on the face especially around the eyes or on the scrotum following trauma to the skin usually from scratching or rubbing (Fig. 2.11).

DIAGNOSIS

- Diagnosis is based on clinical recognition.

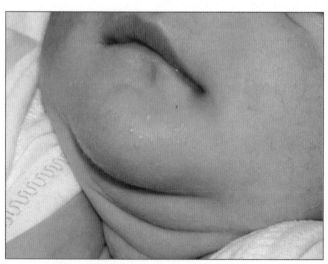

2.10   *Milia.* Superficial, pinpoint white papules are common on the face of newborns.

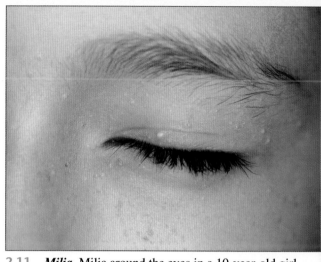

2.11   *Milia.* Milia around the eyes in a 10-year-old girl.

 DIFFERENTIAL DIAGNOSIS

Sebaceous Hyperplasia (see above)
- *Yellow-white monomorphic, tiny papules typically grouped on the nose of a newborn.*

Miliaria (see below)
- *Pinpoint vesicles and pustules with surrounding erythema grouped over trunk and occluded areas of skin.*

 MANAGEMENT

- No treatment is necessary as most milia on newborns resolve spontaneously without scarring in the first few months of life.
- Persistent milia or for milia in older children that are bothersome, lesions can be extracted manually by nicking the top of the lesion (with a lancet or an 11 blade) and manually removing contents, or using a comedone extractor to drain.
- Topical retinoids such as **tretinoin 0.025% cream** has also been used to help clear persistent milia.

NEONATAL AND INFANTILE ERUPTIONS

Miliaria

BASICS

- Miliaria is a relatively common vesicular eruption seen in the first few weeks of life and can occur in all newborns given the right conditions.

PATHOGENESIS

- Miliaria is the result of keratin plugging of the relatively immature neonatal eccrine sweat ducts with resultant trapping of sweat in the skin.
- When the trapped sweat triggers a localized inflammatory response, miliaria rubra is seen.
- Common triggers include excessive swaddling, heat, fever, and occlusive dressings.

CLINICAL MANIFESTATIONS

- Miliaria crystallina presents as pinpoint, 1 to 2 mm, clear to white superficial vesicles (Fig. 2.12).
- Miliaria rubra (also called "prickly heat") presents as grouped, small pink to red papules, vesicles or papulovesicles with a surrounding rim of erythema (Fig. 2.13).
- Miliaria rubra is most commonly seen in occluded areas of the body such as the body folds and the back.
- Palms and soles are never involved.

DIAGNOSIS

- Diagnosis is based on clinical recognition.
- A KOH preparation, Gram stain, and/or Tzanck smear can be helpful to rule out infectious causes of vesicles and pustules.

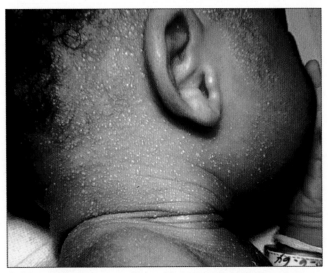

2.12   *Miliaria crystallina.* Closely grouped tiny clear vesicles.

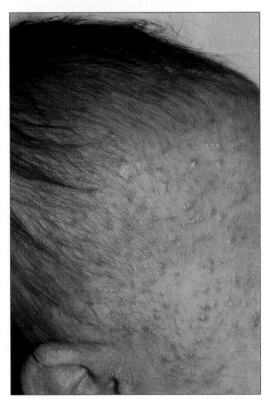

2.13   *Miliaria rubra.* This eruption is also called prickly heat or heat rash and typically presents as numerous small erythematous nonfollicular papules on the lateral face, neck, and upper trunk in young infants.

DIFFERENTIAL DIAGNOSIS

Congenital or Infantile Candidiasis
- *Tiny pustules or collarettes of scale on an erythematous base.*
- *When present at birth is usually widespread and often present on palms and soles.*
- *KOH of pustule contents will reveal pseudohyphae and budding yeast.*

Neonatal Herpes Infection
- *Grouped vesicles on an erythematous base.*
- *There is usually a history of maternal HSV infection and Tzanck smear will show multinucleated giant cells.*

Erythema Toxicum Neonatorum (see above)
- *Common eruption papules or pustules on erythematous wheal usually in haphazard distribution.*
- *Resolves completely within 2 weeks.*

Folliculitis
- *Perifollicular pustules with surrounding erythema.*

MANAGEMENT

- After an infectious etiology has been ruled out, parents can be reassured that this is a benign eruption.
- Spontaneous resolution with cooling usually occurs.
- Counsel on avoidance excessive heat, humidity, and swaddling.
- Avoid excessive use of thick (ointment based) emollients in hot, humid climates or in cold climates especially when bundling baby.
- Use of loose fitting cotton clothing, cooler baths, and air conditioning can be helpful in the prevention of outbreaks.

 HELPFUL HINT

- Perform a KOH, Gram stain, or Tzanck smear to rule out more serious causes of vesicles or pustules on a newborn's skin.

Neonatal Lupus Erythematosus

BASICS

- Neonatal lupus erythematosus (NLE) is a rare autoimmune syndrome that affects 2% to 4% of infants born of mothers who are anti-Ro (SSA), anti-La (SSB), and/or anti-RNP antibody positive.
- Most mothers do not show any signs or symptoms of connective tissue disease at the time of birth of the affected infant; however, Sjögren syndrome, systemic lupus erythematosus, or undifferentiated autoimmune syndrome does ultimately develop in some of these women.

PATHOGENESIS

- NLE is an autoimmune condition caused by the passage of maternal antibodies to the neonate in utero.

CLINICAL MANIFESTATIONS

- NLE has a varied clinical presentation that includes a characteristic skin rash with or without systemic abnormalities and congenital complete heart block.
- Most commonly, NLE manifests as a skin rash on the face (especially on forehead and periorbital), scalp, and extensor extremities, although lesions can occur anywhere.
- The spectrum of skin findings includes annular erythematous, flat or edematous lesions with or without scale, variably sized erythematous patches, periorbital erythema ("owl's sign" or "raccoon eyes"), scaly atrophic macules and patches, or telangiectasias (Figs. 2.14 and 2.15).
- Lesions can be present at birth or be delayed up to 20 weeks after birth, and have a mean age of onset of 6 weeks.
- Skin lesions can be precipitated or worsened by sun exposure.
- Thrombocytopenia or, less often, other hematologic abnormalities may be present. Liver dysfunction (elevated transaminases, cholestasis, or hyperbilirubinemia) occurs in 10% to 25% of infants with NLE and is usually transient.
- Complete congenital heart block, the most serious potential manifestation of NLE, occurs in 2% to 4% of patients and is usually apparent at birth. First- and second-degree heart blocks, cardiomyopathy, or myocarditis have also been reported in up to 10% to 20% of patients.
- There are isolated reports of neurologic abnormalities in children with NLE.

DIAGNOSIS

- NLE should be suspected in infants with the typical appearance and distribution of the skin lesions.
- Positive anti-Ro, anti-La, or anti-U1RNP antibodies in the infant and mother will confirm the diagnosis.
- Patients with positive antibodies require a thorough physical examination, complete blood count, liver function test, and a cardiac evaluation to determine the full extent of the syndrome.

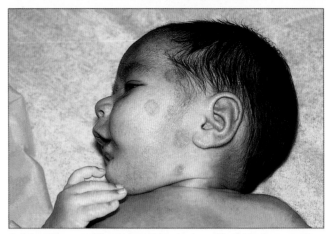

2.14 *Neonatal lupus erythematosus.* These scaly, annular erythematous plaques appeared shortly after birth and were mistaken for "ringworm." This infant's mother had anti-Ro antibodies.

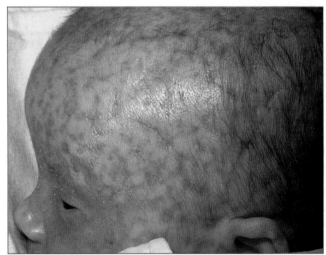

2.15 *Neonatal lupus erythematosus.* Atrophic plaques with telangiectasias on the face and scalp is another clinical presentation of NLE. (From Burkhart CN, Morrell DS. *Visual Dx Essential Pediatric Dermatology.* Philadelphia: Lippincott Williams & Wilkins, 2010.)

DIFFERENTIAL DIAGNOSIS

Urticaria
- *Pink, edematous, migratory, annular plaques that resolve within 24 hours.*

Tinea Corporis
- *Red, annular scaly plaques with advancing edge of scale.*
- *KOH will be positive.*

Infantile Seborrheic Dermatitis (see below)
- *Ill-defined eczematous pink plaques with greasy yellow scale on face and scalp.*
- *Occasionally brown adherent scale on scalp.*
- *Responds quickly to low-potency topical steroids and/ or topical antifungals.*

MANAGEMENT

- Skin lesions usually self-resolve by 6 to 12 months of age, concurrent with the clearance of maternal antibodies, and heal without sequelae.
- Occasionally residual atrophy and telangiectasias persist.
- Hematologic and hepatic complications also typically resolve when antibodies are cleared.
- Skin lesions are treated with meticulous photoprotection, emollients, and low- to mid-potency topical steroids (**desonide 0.05% ointment** or **fluocinolone 0.025% ointment**).
- Systemic abnormalities may require oral or IV corticosteroids or intravenous immunoglobulin.
- Cardiac complications require management by a pediatric cardiologist. Complete heart block is irreversible and often requires pacemaker insertion.
- Mothers of infants with NLE should be counseled that the risk of NLE in a subsequent child increases to 20%; consequently, they should have appropriate prenatal monitoring in subsequent pregnancies.

HELPFUL HINTS

- Periorbital erythema in a neonate should always prompt consideration of NLE.
- Studies show that infants with NLE have a similar risk as nonaffected siblings for the development of future autoimmune disease.

POINTS TO REMEMBER

- NLE presents with a characteristic skin eruption on photo-exposed areas at birth or shortly thereafter.
- Positive anti-Ro, anti-La, and/or anti-U1RNP antibodies in maternal and infant serum will confirm the diagnosis of NLE.

Seborrheic Dermatitis

BASICS

- Infantile seborrheic dermatitis also called *cradle cap* (when located on scalp (Fig. 2.16) in neonates and infants) is an eczematous eruption that develops in areas of high sebaceous gland activity.

CLINICAL MANIFESTATIONS

- Pink patches and plaques with greasy yellow scale classically occurring on the scalp, face (especially eyebrows and nasolabial folds), ears (posterior and ear canals), and skin folds (neck, axillae, groin, arm, and thigh folds).
- Tends to resolve around 3 to 4 months of age when levels of hormones subside.
- Its pathogenesis, differential diagnosis, and management are discussed in detail in Chapter 4.

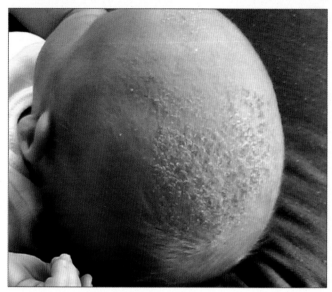

2.16 *Seborrheic dermatitis.* Thick greasy yellow scale can become stuck on or matted on the scalp and is often referred to as cradle cap.

Diaper Dermatitis

BASICS

- Diaper dermatitis, also called diaper rash, encompasses several different dermatoses that can occur on the skin underneath the diaper in infants.
- Primary irritant diaper dermatitis, the most common form of diaper rash, and its management is presented below; other causes of diaper rash are presented in Table 2.1.

(IRRITANT) DIAPER DERMATITIS

- The most common form of diaper rash is a primary irritant contact dermatitis, a type of eczematous dermatitis triggered by urine, feces, moisture, and occlusion (also discussed in Chapter 4).
- It can first present as early as the first few weeks of life, has a peak incidence at 9 to 12 months, but can occur any time when diapers are worn.

PATHOGENESIS

- Diaper dermatitis is the result of overhydration of the skin due to urine and sweat produced by the occlusive diaper that leads to increased permeability of the skin to irritants.
- Irritant triggers include friction, or rubbing of skin on skin, soaps, antibacterial and cleansing substances found in baby wipes and topical diaper ointments, urine, and proteolytic enzymes in stool.
- Urine increases the skin's pH which intensifies the activities of fecal proteases and lipases.
- When friction is the primary cause of the dermatitis, the term "chafing dermatitis" or "frictional dermatitis" is used.
- Irritant diaper dermatitis may also be exaggerated by the presence of atopic dermatitis, seborrheic dermatitis, or a secondary infection by *Candida albicans*.

CLINICAL MANIFESTATIONS

- Diaper dermatitis presents as erythematous, shiny, moist patches on the convex surfaces of the buttocks, the vulva, perineal area, proximal thighs, and lower abdomen.
- Eczematous plaques on the labia appear shiny and wrinkly (Fig. 2.17).
- Lesions typically spare the body folds (intertriginous creases) because such areas do not come into direct contact with the diaper.
- With neglect, erosions or ulcerations may develop.

DIAGNOSIS

- The diagnosis is made clinically.
- When irritant diaper dermatitis is not improving with adequate treatment, it is important to consider other less common causes of diaper dermatitis. The clinical features, diagnosis, and treatment of these are presented in Table 2.1.

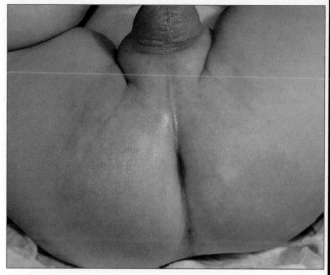

2.17 *(Irritant contact) diaper dermatitis.* Shiny, wrinkly eczematous plaques on convex surfaces of skin.

 MANAGEMENT

The two components to the management of irritant diaper dermatitis are ***treatment*** of the active dermatitis and ***prevention*** of recurrence.

SPECIFIC TREATMENT MEASURES

- Avoid wipes when an eczematous eruption is present as the skin barrier is compromised.
- Wash the affected area with a nonsoap cleanser (**Cetaphil cleanser**) or gentle soap and a soft, moistened paper towel or soft cloth.
- If the eruption is mild, use a low-potency steroid such as **hydrocortisone 2.5% cream** or **ointment** twice daily to affected areas and apply a generous coating of a petrolatum (**Aquaphor or Vaseline**) or a zinc oxide–based ointment (**Balmex, Triple paste, or A&D ointment**) over the topical steroid to the affected areas of skin at each diaper change.
- Stronger topical steroids such as **desonide 0.05%** (class 6), **hydrocortisone valerate 0.02%** cream (class 5), or ointment (class 4) may be used for brief periods when necessary.
- **Potent topical steroids, particularly fluorinated preparations such as those contained in Lotrisone, are to be avoided in the diaper area.**
- If there is no improvement after several days and the presence of *C. albicans* is suspected, a topical antifungal preparation such as **Triple Paste AF** or **Vusion ointment** (0.25% miconazole combined with 15% zinc oxide) should be used.

PREVENTION

- Keep skin of diaper area clean and dry.
- Change diapers promptly after voiding or soiling.

Table 2.1 DIFFERENTIAL DIAGNOSIS OF DIAPER DERMATITIS

	BASICS	CLINICAL MANIFESTATIONS	DIAGNOSIS AND TREATMENT
Infections **Candidal diaper dermatitis** (Fig. 2.18)	Candidal infection of skin, common May be triggered by recent systemic antibiotic use, diarrhea, and oral thrush. In chronic, recurrent cases candida may be present in patient's GI tract	Bright "beefy" red, well-demarcated scaly patches, collarette of scale at edge, and characteristic satellite papulopustules Unlike irritant diaper dermatitis, the inguinal fold is usually affected Can also be seen in oral mucosa and other intertriginous areas	A KOH will be positive and show pseudo-hyphae and budding yeast Topical anti-candida treatments including **miconazole 2% cream, nystatin cream,** or **ketoconazole 2% cream.** In resistant cases oral therapy with **nystatin** or **fluconazole** is required

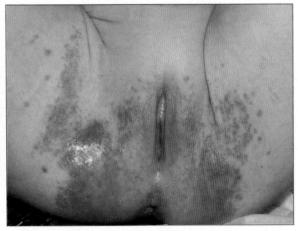

2.18 *Candidal diaper dermatitis.* Beefy red erythema and satellite papules and pustules are characteristic of a yeast-induced diaper rash. (From Edwards L, Lynch PJ. *Genital Dermatology Atlas*, 2nd ed. Philadelphia, PA: Lippincott Williams & Wilkins; 2011.)

Bullous impetigo (Fig. 2.19)	Infection with a toxin producing strain of *Staphylococcus aureus* that separates the upper layers of the epidermis Moisture and warmth can promote bacterial growth; sometimes umbilicus is colonized with the *S. aureus*	*Early:* small vesicles that enlarge to 1–2-cm superficial bullae *Late:* larger flaccid bullae, rupture easily leaving a collarette of scale, no thick crust, and usually no surrounding erythema Favors diaper area in newborns but also seen periumbilical, face, trunk, and body folds	Gram stain: gram-positive cocci in clusters; bacterial culture + *S. aureus* Treat with topical antibiotics (**mupirocin 2% ointment** or **fusidic acid cream or ointment**); oral antibiotics are used if there are systemic findings or not improving with topicals (**cephalexin**)

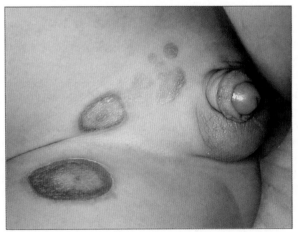

2.19 *Bullous impetigo.* Shiny erosions with peripheral scaly representing remnants of the blister roof. In infants, bullous impetigo typically presents in the diaper area. (From Burkhart CN, Morrell DS. *Visual Dx Essential Pediatric Dermatology*. Philadelphia, PA: Lippincott Williams & Wilkins; 2010.)

Table 2.1 DIFFERENTIAL DIAGNOSIS OF DIAPER DERMATITIS *(Continued)*

	BASICS	CLINICAL MANIFESTATIONS	DIAGNOSIS AND TREATMENT
Inflammatory conditions **Seborrheic dermatitis**	Results from increased activity of sebaceous glands secondary to elevated hormone levels in early infancy	Salmon-colored scaly plaques with greasy yellow scale Usually involves the inguinal folds and convex surfaces. Occasionally fissuring is seen No satellite lesions Typically eruption will also be present in other body folds, face, and/or scalp	Diagnosis is based on clinical recognition Responds quickly to low-potency topical corticosteroid (**hydrocortisone 2.5% ointment**) and/or topical antifungals (**ketoconazole 2% cream**). Spontaneous clearance
Psoriasis (Fig. 2.20)	Psoriasis is overall rare in infancy; however, diaper dermatitis with dissemination is the most common presentation of psoriasis in children <2 yrs. A positive family history of psoriasis may be present	Sharply demarcated confluent erythematous plaques, involve inguinal folds, typical scale of psoriasis may be lacking due to moisture in the diaper area Typical psoriasis lesions may be present elsewhere	Psoriasis will take longer to clear than seborrheic dermatitis and will require a more potent topical corticosteroid (**hydrocortisone valerate 0.2% or desonide 0.05% ointment**)

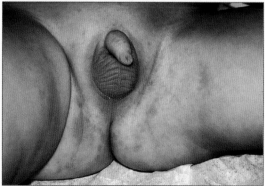

2.20   *Psoriasis in diaper area.* Sharply demarcated confluent erythema in the diaper area including the inguinal folds. Typical psoriatic plaques can be seen on the trunk, periumbilical skin, and the legs.

Atopic dermatitis (Fig. 2.21)	Uncommonly seen in the diaper area, typically in the inguinal creases	Appears similar to irritant dermatitis (shiny, wrinkled eczematous plaques) but is more chronic and resistant to treatment Is intensely itchy. Usually typical eczematous plaques are present elsewhere on body	Topical corticosteroids, frequent diaper changes, application of thick barrier ointment with each diaper change. Avoidance of harsh soaps and overuse of wipes

2.21   *Atopic dermatitis in diaper area.* Eczematous eruption in inguinal creases are evident in this infant.

(continued)

Table 2.1 DIFFERENTIAL DIAGNOSIS OF DIAPER DERMATITIS (*Continued*)

	BASICS	CLINICAL MANIFESTATIONS	DIAGNOSIS AND TREATMENT
Jacquet dermatitis (Fig. 2.22)	Represents the severe end of the spectrum of irritant diaper dermatitis	A severe erosive eruption, well-demarcated papules, nodules, and punched-out ulcerations, typically on the perianal skin	Management is similar to irritant dermatitis, frequent changes, application of thick barrier ointment with each diaper change, low threshold for antimicrobial treatment if not improving

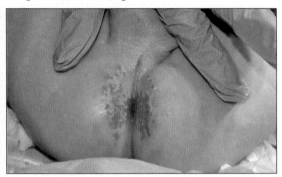

2.22 *Jacquet erosive diaper dermatitis.* This eruption is typically seen on the perianal skin and is thought to represent the severe end of the irritant contact diaper dermatitis spectrum.

Other			
Langerhans cell histiocytosis (Fig. 2.23)	Rare disease characterized by infiltration of Langerhans cells into various organs of the body	In infants, typically presents as a seborrheic dermatitis-like eruption admixed with petechial and purpuric papules some with red-brown crusting. Fails to respond to treatment Lesions can also be seen on the scalp and trunk Can involve skin only or skin + other organ systems	A skin biopsy can confirm the diagnosis in suspected cases Treatment depends on extent of extracutaneous involvement

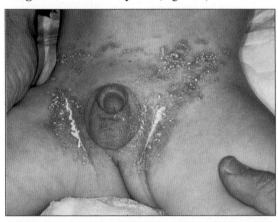

2.23 *Langerhan cell histiocytosis in diaper area.* In this infant, lesions are present in the diaper area. These findings can be differentiated from candidiasis, atopic dermatitis, and seborrheic dermatitis by their more infiltrated morphology and unresponsiveness to treatment for these conditions. (From Edwards L, Lynch PJ. *Genital Dermatology Atlas*, 2nd ed. Philadelphia, PA: Lippincott Williams & Wilkins; 2011.)

Table 2.1 DIFFERENTIAL DIAGNOSIS OF DIAPER DERMATITIS *(Continued)*

	BASICS	CLINICAL MANIFESTATIONS	DIAGNOSIS AND TREATMENT
Acrodermatitis enteropathica (Fig. 2.24A,B) 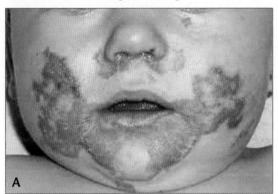 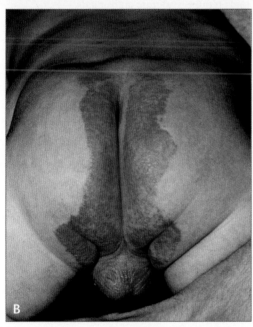	Rare condition caused by zinc deficiency that usually results from an inherited inability to absorb zinc; less often is acquired due to low levels of zinc in diet (or in maternal milk) or malabsorption from intestinal disease	Well-demarcated scaly plaques in the perineal skin and inguinal folds. Occasionally erosions, vesicles, and bullae. Older lesions become thick with drier scale. Typically, lesions are also present around the mouth and on hands and feet. Usually there is associated diarrhea and alopecia	Diagnosis is confirmed by detection of plasma zinc levels of <50 ug/mL and a low alkaline phosphatase Responds quickly to zinc supplementation

2.24 **A** and **B:** *Acrodermatitis enteropathica.* Severe desquamative eruptions are seen the perioral and diaper areas. (**B:** From Edwards L, Lynch PJ. *Genital Dermatology Atlas*, 2nd ed. Philadelphia, PA: Lippincott Williams & Wilkins; 2011.)

- Minimize friction—dry the skin by patting (not rubbing). Remember friction is one of the causes of irritant diaper dermatitis.
- Absorb moisture—use of disposable diapers with super absorbent gelling materials holds moisture in and keeps it away from the skin.
- Use gentle, soap-free cleansers such as **Cetaphil nonsoap gentle cleanser**.
- Apply a skin protectant/barrier cream to the skin at each diaper change. Recommended creams: **Aquaphor, Triple paste**, or **Desitin**.

POINTS TO REMEMBER

- Irritation (ICD) is the most common cause of an eruption in the diaper area in infants.
- Aim for prevention by changing diapers frequently, using superabsorbent disposable diapers and coating the skin with a barrier ointment.
- Avoid the use of high-potency topical steroids in the diaper area.
- Consider referral to a dermatologist, particularly in persistent, unresponsive cases.
- The term diaper rash is commonly used as a diagnosis but in fact there are many distinct dermatoses that can result in an eruption in the diaper area.

HELPFUL HINT

- Optimal management of diaper dermatitis relies on an early and accurate determination of the cause. Oftentimes more than one factor is playing a role.

POINTS TO REMEMBER

- If a case of seborrheic dermatitis in the diaper area is not improving with treatment—consider a skin biopsy to rule out Langerhan cell histiocytosis.
- Patients with recurrent candidal diaper dermatitis may be carriers of candida in their GI tract and a course of oral antifungals may be required.
- Infants with yeast infection of the skin and systemic symptoms require systemic antifungals.

Acropustulosis of Infancy

BASICS

- Acropustulosis of infancy (also called *infantile acropustulosis*) is an itchy, pustular eruption characterized by recurrent crops of vesiculopustules on the palms and soles and is more common in African-American children.
- Acropustulosis of infancy (AI) remits spontaneously.

PATHOGENESIS

- AI is idiopathic.
- Sometimes reported to be precipitated by a scabies infestation.

CLINICAL MANIFESTATIONS

- Lesions begin as pink papules that evolve into slightly larger tense pustules that spontaneously rupture leaving behind a collarette of thin scale (Fig. 2.25).
- Lesions appear in crops, predominantly on the palms and soles but can also be seen on the dorsal and lateral aspects of the hands, wrists, and feet and last for 1 to 2 weeks.
- Flares occur every couple of weeks to every couple of months.
- Occasionally the legs, forearms, and scalp are also involved.
- Lesions are intensely itchy.
- Over time, flares become less frequent and less severe.
- The condition eventually burns out within 2 to 3 years but it can remain uncomfortable until then.

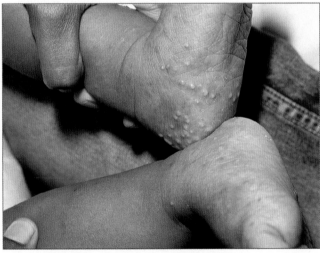

2.25 *Infantile acropustulosis.* Pruritic vesiculopustules on the sole recur in crops. (From Burkhart CN, Morrell DS. *Visual Dx Essential Pediatric Dermatology*. Philadelphia, PA: Lippincott Williams & Wilkins; 2010.)

DIAGNOSIS

- Diagnosis is based on recognition of the characteristic clinical course and appearance of lesions and the ruling out of scabies.
- A smear of pustule contents will show numerous neutrophils and some eosinophils.
- A Gram stain, KOH, and Tzanck smear will be negative for organisms.

 DIFFERENTIAL DIAGNOSIS

Scabies Infestation
- *Can mimic AI, and some clinicians advocate empiric treatment for scabies if clinical suspicion is present.*
- *Household contacts may also be itchy or have similar lesions.*
- *Sometimes, mite, eggs, or feces are seen on a scabies prep.*

Dyshidrotic Eczema
- *Small skin-colored papules and vesicles on palms and soles, usually on sides of fingers, rare in infancy.*

Transient Neonatal Pustular Melanosis (see earlier in this chapter)
- *Present at birth as flaccid vesiculopustules that rupture easily leaving behind a collarette of scale and a hyperpigmented macule.*
- *Resolves spontaneously in first few weeks of life.*

Impetigo
- *Honey-colored crusted papules and plaques.*
- *Gram stain and culture will show evidence of bacteria.*

 MANAGEMENT

- AI eventually self-resolves but can take several years.
- Itch can be severe and lead to irritability, inability to sleep, excoriations, and secondary infection.
- Pruritus usually requires the use of mid- to high-potency topical corticosteroids (**mometasone 0.1% ointment** or **clobetasol 0.05% ointment**) twice daily during flares.
- Antihistamines such as **cetirizine** can also be helpful. Sedating antihistamines can help induce sleep.
- Dapsone has been used in recalcitrant and highly symptomatic cases.

 POINT TO REMEMBER

- AI is usually intensely itchy and often requires potent to superpotent topical steroids as well as an antihistamine.

Eosinophilic Pustular Folliculitis of Infancy

BASICS

- Eosinophilic pustular folliculitis (EPF) of infancy presents as recurrent, grouped itchy papulopustules most often on the scalp.
- EPF of infancy has unique characteristics that distinguish it from the adult and HIV related forms.

PATHOGENESIS

- Unclear but thought to represent a reaction pattern to an antigenic trigger.
- A biopsy shows eosinophils around the hair follicle.

CLINICAL MANIFESTATIONS

- Lesions appear as recurrent crops of papules and papulopustules on an erythematous base located primarily on the scalp but the hands, feet, and trunk can also be affected (Fig. 2.26).
- EPF can be intensely itchy.
- Lesions evolve into yellow, crusted papules over 7 to 10 days and then heal without scarring but may leave residual hyperpigmentation.
- New crops will appear every 2 to 8 weeks.
- EPF typically presents in early infancy and eventually "burns out" between 6 to 36 months of age.

DIAGNOSIS

- Diagnosis is based on recognition of the characteristic location, clinical course, and appearance of lesions.
- Pustules in EPF are sterile; a Gram stain, KOH, and Tzanck smear will be negative for organisms.
- A Wright stain of pustule contents will show abundant eosinophils.

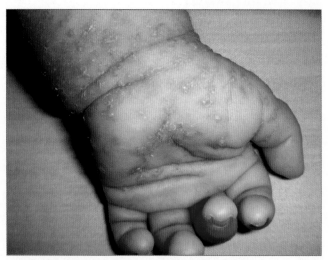

2.26 *Eosinophilic pustular folliculitis.* These very itchy lesions can easily be mistaken for a scabies infestation.

 DIFFERENTIAL DIAGNOSIS

Infantile Acropustulosis
- *Can mimic EPF of infancy; AI primarily occurs on hands and feet.*
- *Lesions last longer and resolve with collarettes of scale.*

Scabies Infestation or Insect Bites
- *Widespread, intensely, itchy papules.*
- *Household contacts may also be itchy or have similar lesions.*
- *Sometimes, mite, eggs, or feces are seen on a scabies prep.*

Bacterial Folliculitis
- *Follicular pustules on an erythematous base may be scattered on scalp and elsewhere on body.*
- *Gram stain and culture will reveal bacteria.*
- *Does not recur in crops.*

 MANAGEMENT

- EPF of infancy will self-resolve by 3 years of age in most patients.
- Treatment is symptomatic.
- Itch during flares can be severe and usually requires mid- to high-potency topical corticosteroids (**mometasone 0.1% ointment** or **clobetasol 0.05% ointment**).
- The antihistamine **cetirizine** can also be helpful for its eosinophil antimigration effect. Sedating antihistamines can help induce sleep in patients unable to sleep because of the itch.
- Dapsone and oral antibiotics (**erythromycin** and **cephalexin**) have been used with variable success in recalcitrant and highly symptomatic cases.

 POINTS TO REMEMBER

- EPF of infancy is a benign self-limited eruption that usually resolves by 3 years of age.
- It is important to clearly distinguish EPF of infancy as a distinct entity from the adult-onset and the HIV-associated types to prevent unnecessary parental anxiety from internet searches.

Acute Hemorrhagic Edema of Infancy (aka Finkelstein Disease)

BASICS

- A self-limited, leukocytoclastic vasculitis that presents as large urticarial plaques, fever, and edema in children between the ages of 4 months to 3 years.
- Although the clinical presentation can be alarming, the condition has a benign clinical course.

PATHOGENESIS

- Presumed to be an immune complex-mediated vasculitis.
- Onset is preceded by a recent respiratory infection, a medication, or an immunization in three out of four cases.

CLINICAL MANIFESTATIONS

- Acute onset of large, urticarial or annular, targetoid, purpuric plaques found primarily on face, ears, and extremities (Fig. 2.27).
- The trunk is relatively spared.
- Tender edema on face (especially eyelids and ears) and/or extremities is common (Fig. 2.28).
- Occasional petechiae, purpura, or necrotic lesions.
- Fever is usually low grade and involvement of kidneys, joints, and gastrointestinal tract is rare.

DIAGNOSIS

- Diagnosis is based on clinical recognition and the natural history of the condition.
- A skin biopsy will reveal a leukocytoclastic vasculitis. Direct immunofluorescence is negative for IgA deposition in the majority of cases.

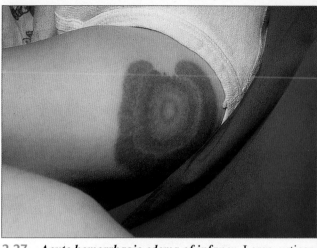

2.27 *Acute hemorrhagic edema of infancy.* Large, urticarial or annular, targetoid, purpuric plaques on the lateral thigh.

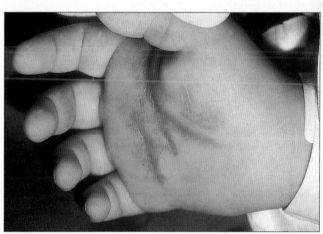

2.28 *Acute hemorrhagic edema of infancy.* Tender edema and erythema of the palm.

 DIFFERENTIAL DIAGNOSIS

Urticaria

- *Pink, edematous, migratory, annular plaques that resolve within 24 hours.*
- *Can be itchy but is nontender.*

 MANAGEMENT

- Acute hemorrhagic edema of infancy spontaneously resolves without sequelae within 1 to 3 weeks.
- No treatment is generally necessary.
- Treatment is supportive and includes treatment for pain and fever.

3 Acne

OVERVIEW

Acne is a common skin condition that will affect most people at some point in their lives. It is most commonly seen in adolescence as part of several visible signs of the hormonal surge that occurs with the onset of puberty. Less well known is its presentation during the neonatal period, infancy, and childhood, which can lead to significant parental distress.

Neonatal acne is a benign eruption that self-resolves without sequelae often requiring no treatment whereas infantile acne often requires treatment. Childhood acne is rare and should prompt investigation for causes of hyperandrogenism. Periorificial dermatitis, a rosacea-like condition, has a typical appearance and distribution and responds well to topical or systemic treatments. These forms of acne will be detailed in this chapter. Chapter 12 discusses the presentation and treatment of common adolescent acne, also called acne vulgaris.

IN THIS CHAPTER...

➤ **NEONATAL CEPHALIC PUSTULOSIS (NEONATAL ACNE)**

➤ **INFANTILE ACNE**

➤ **CHILDHOOD ACNE**

➤ **PERIOROFICIAL DERMATITIS**

➤ **ADOLESCENT ACNE (AKA ACNE VULGARIS)**

Neonatal Cephalic Pustulosis (Neonatal Acne)

BASICS

- Neonatal acne is now referred to as neonatal cephalic pustulosis to distinguish it from infantile and adolescent acne.
- Neonatal cephalic pustulosis is a benign self-limiting condition that is estimated to occur in 25% of neonates.

PATHOGENESIS

- Recent data suggest the papules and pustules in this condition may be the result of an inflammatory response to *Malassezia* spp.
- Increased rates of sebum secretion during the neonatal period are also thought to play a role.

CLINICAL MANIFESTATIONS

- Presents at 2 to 3 weeks of age as discrete erythematous papules and pustules on the cheeks, or, less often, on the forehead, chin, scalp, and chest (Figs. 3.1 and 3.2).
- Unlike infantile and adolescent acne there are no comedones and the course is self-limiting.
- Eruption is asymptomatic.
- Resolves spontaneously in weeks to months.

DIAGNOSIS

- Diagnosis is usually made clinically.
- A Giemsa stain may show yeast forms, neutrophils, and other inflammatory cells.
- When in doubt a Gram stain can rule out bacterial folliculitis and a KOH can rule out candidiasis.

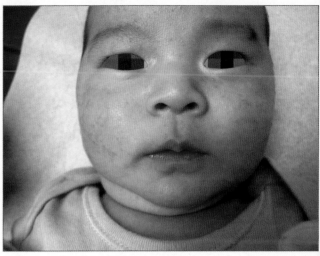

3.2 *Neonatal cephalic pustulosis.* Typical appearance of neonatal cephalic pustulosis. Note subtle erythematous papules and absence of comedones.

 DIFFERENTIAL DIAGNOSIS

Miliaria Rubra
- *Lesions can be indistinguishable from neonatal cephalic pustulosis, but will be located in body folds and areas subject to heat and occlusion.*

Erythema Toxicum Neonatorum
- *Lesions are more widespread and scattered in distribution over trunk and face.*
- *Lesions often associated with a pink edematous wheal.*

Candidiasis
- *Tiny pustules on erythematous base in a more widespread distribution.*
- *Lesions easily rupture leaving collarettes of scale.*

 MANAGEMENT

- No treatment is required as the condition self-resolves by 3 to 6 months of age.
- Parents should be instructed to gently wash the newborn's face twice daily with a mild soap and water.
- In severe cases, the application of topical imidazoles such as **ketoconazole 2% cream** or **econazole 1% cream** twice daily can lead to improvement.
- Topical **hydrocortisone 1% cream** can be helpful if lesions are very red.
- Application of oils or ointments may exacerbate condition.

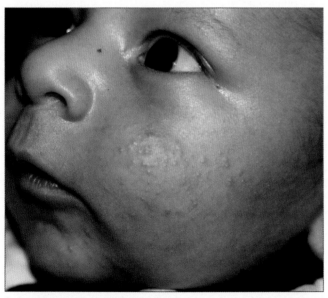

3.1 *Neonatal cephalic pustulosis.* Erythematous papulopustules on the cheeks resolved completely at 4 months of age in this infant.

 HELPFUL HINT

- Neonatal cephalic pustulosis lacks comedones.

Infantile Acne

BASICS

- Infantile acne is an uncommon condition that is the result of the intrinsic hormonal imbalances that can occur during infancy.
- Seen more often in boys and first appears between 2 to 6 months of age.

PATHOGENESIS

- Infantile acne results from increased androgens and sebum excretion in susceptible infants.
- All babies have elevated adrenal androgens in early infancy due to a transiently enlarged adrenal gland. In infant boys, the testes also produce luteinizing hormone (LH) and testosterone and levels can rise equal to those seen in puberty.
- Both sources of androgens markedly diminish by 1 year of age and remain low for most of childhood.

CLINICAL MANIFESTATIONS

- Infantile acne appears strikingly similar to typical acne vulgaris that is seen in adolescence with an admixture of acneiform papules, pustules, open and closed comedones, and cysts (Fig. 3.3).
- Lesions are typically located on the cheeks but can also be seen on the forehead, chin, and back.
- Cysts, draining sinuses, and deep nodules with potential for scarring occasionally occur.
- Onset is between 3 to 6 months and subsides at around 1 to 2 years of age commiserate with the normalization of androgen levels.
- Rarely persists through adolescence.

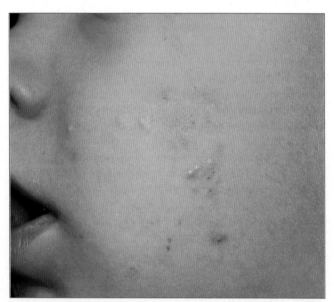

3.3 *Infantile acne.* In this 8-month-old boy there is an admixture of acneiform papules, pustules, open and closed comedones, and occasional cysts.

DIAGNOSIS

- Diagnosis is made clinically usually after other conditions are ruled out.

DIFFERENTIAL DIAGNOSIS

Miliaria Rubra
- *Small pustules on an erythematous base, usually located on occluded areas.*

Bacterial Folliculitis
- *Follicularly based pustules, clears completely with proper treatment.*
- *Gram stain will show gram-positive cocci, culture will grow organism.*

Periorificial Dermatitis
- *Acneiform papules and pustules around mouth, nose, and periorbital skin.*
- *Exacerbated or triggered by the use of topical or inhaled steroids.*

Pomade Acne
- *Occlusive ointments or oils applied to the skin can trigger an acneiform eruption resembling infantile acne.*

MANAGEMENT

- Patients with infantile acne should have a complete physical examination with particular attention to other signs of androgen excess, that is, clitoromegaly, hirsutism, or pubic hair. If signs of androgen excess are present, referral to a pediatric endocrinologist is warranted.
- Most cases resolve by 1 to 2 years of age, even without treatment. In rare cases, the condition can persist until 4 to 5 years old and even through adolescence.
- First-line treatments are similar to those used for adolescent acne and include topical **tretinoin 0.025% cream or benzoyl peroxide** with or without a topical antibiotic, such as Benzaclin (**benzoyl peroxide 5% and clindamycin 1%**).
- In severe cases, especially when there is scarring potential, oral antibiotics or isotretinoin may be required.
- Antibiotic choices for acne at this age include **erythromycin** and **trimethoprim/sulfamethoxazole**.

HELPFUL HINTS

- Severe cases of infantile acne may be a marker for severe disease in adolescence.
- Avoid use of tetracycline, doxycycline, or minocycline below the age of 8 years.

POINTS TO REMEMBER

	NEONATAL CEPHALIC PUSTULOSIS	INFANTILE ACNE
Onset	2–3 wks of age	3–6 mo
Clinical	Inflammatory lesions, no comedones	Comedones ++, papules, pustules, cysts
Etiology	*Malassezia* spp. or increased neonatal sebum secretion rates	Elevated levels of LH and testosterone Boys > girls
Duration	Weeks to months	1–2 yrs; rarely persists through adolescence
Treatment	Imidazoles (e.g., topical ketoconazole (Nizoral) 2% cream), benzoyl peroxide	Topical tretinoin, benzoyl peroxide, oral antibiotics, isotretinoin if severe

Childhood Acne

BASICS

- Acne during childhood (i.e., between 1 and 7 years) is rare and is primarily seen in two scenarios:
  1. Persistent infantile acne
  2. Hyperandrogenism

PATHOGENESIS

- Adrenal androgens are normally quiescent throughout childhood, rising at around 7 to 8 years of age during adrenarche.
- The appearance of acne prior to this age should raise concerns for hyperandrogenism that can be secondary to premature adrenarche, congenital adrenal hyperplasia (CAH), central precocious puberty, gonadal or adrenal tumors, or Cushing syndrome.

CLINICAL MANIFESTATIONS

- Presents similarly to infantile and adolescent acne with open and closed comedones, inflammatory papules, and pustules usually located on the face (Fig. 3.4).
- Cysts and nodules may also appear.

DIAGNOSIS

- Diagnosis is based on clinical recognition.

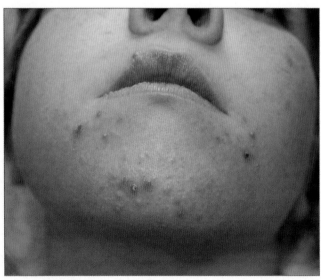

3.4 **Childhood acne.** Acne in children 1 to 7 years can represent persistent infantile acne or be the result of hyperandrogenism. (Figure courtesy of Lawrence A. Schachner, MD.)

 DIFFERENTIAL DIAGNOSIS

Periorificial Dermatitis (see below)
- *Acneiform papules and pustules around mouth, nose, and periorbital skin.*
- *History of topical or inhaled steroid use.*

Keratosis Pilaris of Cheeks
- *Pinpoint, keratotic, perifollicular papules on bilateral cheeks.*
- *Lesions and background skin become red with exertion and sweating.*
- *Seen more often in atopics.*

Milia
- *Discrete, white, superficial keratin cysts typically located around the eyes and upper cheeks.*

 MANAGEMENT

- Initial assessment should include a thorough history and physical examination, including height, weight, and tanner staging. Particular attention should be given to other signs of androgen excess (see Chapter 20) including body odor, axillary hair, pubic hair, etc.
- If an abnormality is detected, prompt referral to a pediatric endocrinologist is indicated.
- Treatment for acne lesions, is similar to treatment of acne vulgaris and includes topical retinoids (i.e., **tretinoin 0.05% cream**) and topical antibiotics (**benzoyl peroxide** and **clindamycin or erythromycin**). Systemic agents are reserved for more severe and recalcitrant cases (see Chapter 12 for formulary and treatment of acne).

 POINT TO REMEMBER

- Acne with onset during childhood is rare and should prompt a workup for hyperandrogenemia.

BASICS

- Periorificial dermatitis, also called periorificial dermatitis, is an idiopathic acneiform eruption that typically occurs in children.

PATHOGENESIS

- The etiology is not known but patients report a preceding use of topical, inhaled, or systemic corticosteroids.
- Given the histologic similarities to rosacea, some consider periorificial dermatitis a childhood form of rosacea.

CLINICAL MANIFESTATIONS

- Grouped, acneiform, tiny erythematous papules and pustules distributed in the perioral, periocular, and intranasal areas (Fig. 3.5A).
- In girls, similar lesions on the vulvar skin can be seen (Fig. 3.5B).
- Resolving papules and pustules may be replaced by redness or red desquamative scale.
- Eruption can be subtle and localized to one small area of the face or be extensive (Figs. 3.6–3.8).
- Some patients complain of associated itching or burning especially if creams or hot water is applied to the eruption.

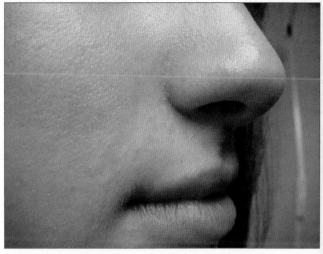

3.6 *Periorificial dermatitis.* Eruption can subtle and localized to perinasal skin.

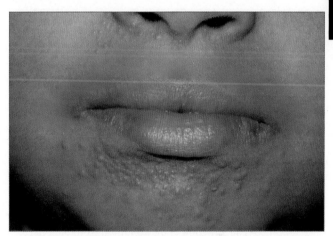

3.7 *Periorificial dermatitis.* Characteristic presentation with grouped erythematous papules and pustules around the nose and mouth.

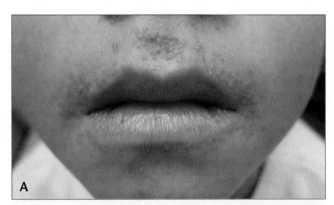

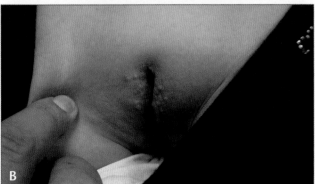

3.5 *Periorificial dermatitis.* **A:** Grouped erythematous papules and tiny pustules in a young girl. **B:** Lesions were also present on the labia majora.

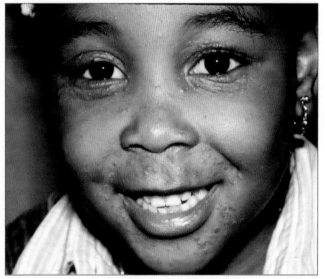

3.8 *Periorificial dermatitis.* Extensive presentation on the face, lesions are present on perioral and periorbital skin.

DIAGNOSIS

- Clinical recognition of typical appearance and distribution of lesions.

DIFFERENTIAL DIAGNOSIS

Acne
- *Rare in childhood when periorificial dermatitis typically appears.*
- *Lesions are more scattered on cheeks and forehead.*

Irritant Dermatitis
- *Ill-defined pink eczematous plaques.*
- *History of an irritant may be elicited.*

MANAGEMENT

- The condition is usually self-limiting but it can take months to years to resolve.
- If triggered by use of topical or inhaled corticosteroids, discontinuation of use can lead to improvement in condition.
- Topical antibiotics are first line for mild localized cases. **Metrocream 1%,** or **erythromycin 2% gel** applied twice daily can lead to resolution in mild cases.
- **Protopic 0.03% ointment** or **Elidel 1% cream** have also been successfully used but there are occasional reports of exacerbation of the condition from their use.
- Oral antibiotics such as **erythromycin, azithromycin, or tetracyclines** in patients >8 years old are used for extensive and recalcitrant cases. Antibiotics should be used for at least 6 weeks and then gradually tapered to avoid rebound flares.

HELPFUL HINT

- Periorificial dermatitis tends not to recur once successfully treated.

POINT TO REMEMBER

- In girls with extensive presentations, the vulvar region may also be involved.

BASICS

- Acne can be the first sign of normal adrenal maturation and the onset of puberty, sometimes appearing before pubic hair, breast buds, and testicular enlargement. Such preadolescent acne usually begins as comedones on the forehead and central face (Figs. 3.9 and 3.10).
- Acne is one of the most common reasons a teenager or preteen will visit a dermatologist.

- The etiology, pathogenies, and treatment of acne vulgaris (aka common acne) or adolescent acne is discussed in detail in Chapter 12.
- In this section, salient tips for successful acne treatment in adolescents and preadolescents will be discussed.

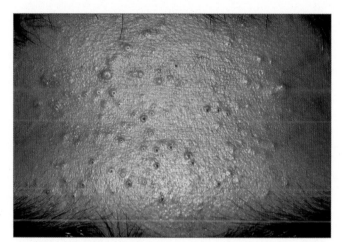

3.9 *Preadolescent acne.* Early acne often appears as open and closed comedones on the central face.

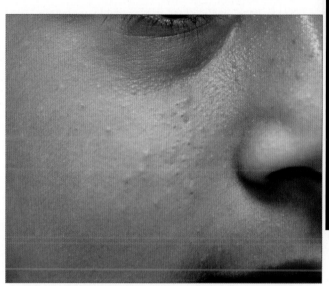

3.10 *Preadolescent acne.* Open and closed comedones, some slightly erythematous on the medial cheek, and prominent sebaceous glands on the nose in an 11-year-old girl.

 HELPFUL HINTS FOR ACNE IN ADOLESCENTS

- Reassure your teenage patient that over 90% of people of their age also have acne and that there are many excellent treatments available that can induce a **sustained remission**.
- Tell your patient that there is no, one best treatment for acne, there are many—the key is to **find** the **right combination** that will work for the patient's particular type of acne and skin type and will easily be incorporated into the patient's routine.
- Assess **level of motivation**, is it the patient who is bothered by the acne or is it a family member? Key questions to ask: Is the patient very self-conscious about their acne? Are they withdrawing from activities?
- Use the **least aggressive** and **simplest** regimen that will lead to prolonged remission.
- Teens will be more likely to stop using a treatment if they see that a particular treatment is not working, if the regimen is too complicated, or if they are experiencing side effects.
- For preadolescents (8 to 11 years) showing prominent sebaceous glands and early comedones suggest getting into the habit of washing their face twice daily with a mild acne wash such as **Neutrogena Acne** wash with salicylic acid 2%.

- For acne with a significant comedonal component always incorporate a topical retinoid such as adapalene (mildest), tretinoin, or tazarotene (strongest). For patients with dry or sensitive skin use a cream or lotion and avoid gels.
- **Anticipate side effects** and discuss them openly:
  - All acne treatments can dry out the skin, reassure patients that this is expected and will improve with continued use. The following suggestions can help counteract dryness: apply only a small amount of medication (pea size amount is enough for the entire face); decrease frequency of use to every other day; use a noncomedogenic moisturizer daily or twice daily on top of the topical acne medication.
  - Temporary redness immediately after application of acne medication can occur.
  - Topical acne treatments will make the skin burn more easily when exposed to the sun. Patients should use adequate sun protection when going out in the sun.
  - If prolonged burning or stinging occurs, stop using the medication.
- Counsel of avoidance of picking and squeezing pimples and over scrubbing.
- Provide **clear, simple written instructions** and hand out to patient at every visit.

HELPFUL HINTS

- Remember to ask your patient how much they are bothered by their acne. If it is primarily mom who cares, then it is less likely that the acne medication will be used.
- Some acne medications are available in pumps, a pump allows for easy one-step medication dispensing.
- Placing acne treatments in strategic locations such as night treatment on the nightstand and morning treatments near the toothbrush may make it easier for patients to remember to apply their medication.
- Place acne washes in the shower.

POINT TO REMEMBER

- Topical antibiotics should not be used as monotherapy for acne as this can lead to the development of bacterial resistance.

CHAPTER 4

Eczema in Infants and Children

OVERVIEW

Eczema is the most common inflammatory skin condition in both children and adults and is one of the chief reasons children visit a dermatologist. Eczema can present in various clinical forms and can be confusing for patients and their nondermatologic healthcare providers. The word *eczema* was coined by the Ancient Greeks to mean "a boiling out or over" and accurately describes both the microscopic and clinical appearances of acute eczema in which the epidermal keratinocytes are swollen and "boil over" creating epidermal vesicles. Currently, the term eczema is more widely applied to a heterogeneous group of inflammatory skin eruptions that share clinical (pruritus, erythema, and scale) and histologic (spongiosis) hallmarks.

Terminologic confusion may also arise if the word *dermatitis*—a more generalized, often vague designation that refers to inflammation of skin—is used synonymously with eczema or is coupled with it. In general, it is acceptable to use *eczema* and *dermatitis* interchangeably. *Eczematous dermatitis,* therefore, is somewhat redundant, although some might argue that the term is more inclusive than either word alone.

In this chapter, atopic dermatitis and irritant contact dermatitis, forms of eczema that commonly occur in children, will be discussed. Allergic contact dermatitis, nummular dermatitis (aka nummular eczema) and asteatotic eczema are other forms of eczema more often seen in adults and are discussed in Chapter 13.

HISTOPATHOLOGY

On a microscopic level, an acute eczematous epidermis contains intercellular and intracellular fluids and appears sponge-like (spongiosis). Vasodilatation of the dermis also occurs. These histologic abnormalities correspond to the clinical features of acute eczema: edema, erythema, vesicles, and bullae (e.g., as seen in poison ivy dermatitis; see Chapter 13).

In subacute or chronic eczema, the epidermis thickens (acanthosis) and retains nuclei (parakeratosis), and there is an abundant inflammatory cell infiltrate in the dermis. These changes account for the scale and lichenification of chronic eczema (e.g., chronic lichenified AD; see Fig. 4.1).

IN THIS CHAPTER...

➤ **ATOPIC DERMATITIS (*Infantile, Childhood, Adolescent phases*)**

➤ **KERATOSIS PILARIS**

➤ **ICHTHYOSIS VULGARIS**

➤ **PITYRIASIS ALBA**

➤ **SEBORRHEIC DERMATITIS**

➤ **IRRITANT CONTACT DERMATITIS**

- Diaper dermatitis
- Lip lickers dermatitis
- Juvenile plantar dermatosis

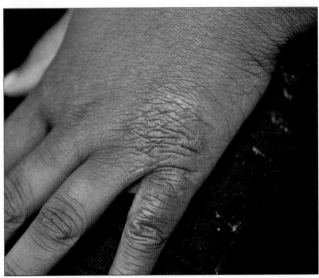

4.1 *Chronic atopic dermatitis.* Hyperpigmented lichenified plaque typical of chronic eczema.

77

Atopic Dermatitis

BASICS

- Atopic dermatitis (AD) is the most common form of eczema in children and is estimated to affect 15% to 20% of children worldwide, with increasing prevalence in some countries.
- "Atopic dermatitis" is a more precise term to describe the form of eczema that has a highly characteristic, age-specific distribution pattern and is associated with other atopic disorders such as asthma and allergic rhinitis.
- Clinical hallmarks of AD include pruritus, an unpredictable course of flares and remissions, early onset, and an age-specific morphology and distribution of lesions.
- Symptoms begin during infancy (usually after 2 months) in more than half of patients; and the onset is before 5 years of age in 90% of patients.
- AD is typically the first manifestation of the atopic triad and precedes the development of asthma and allergic rhinoconjunctivitis. The progression from atopic dermatitis in infancy, to asthma in childhood, and allergic rhinoconjunctivitis in late childhood/early adolescence is known as the "atopic march." It is estimated the 50% to 80% of children with AD will develop another atopic disease.
- AD has a substantial adverse impact on the quality of life of affected children and their families and the societal economic burden is high.
- AD tends to improve with age. Forty percent of children clear by 3 years of age and up to 70% clear by puberty.

PATHOGENESIS

- Atopic dermatitis results from intrinsic defects in the epidermal barrier, alterations in cutaneous innate and adaptive immunity and environmental triggers. The complex interplay among these factors is the subject of vigorous investigation.
- The traditional "inside-out" theory, which suggests that AD is primarily an immunologic disease, has now been complemented by the "outside-in" theory, which considers the barrier defect as primary.
- Barrier defects in AD include mutations in filaggrin (*FLG*), decreased epidermal lipid content (ceramides), and increased transepidermal water loss. This barrier dysfunction explains the dry skin and vulnerability to skin infections typical of AD.
- Immunologic abnormalities in AD include decreased levels of epidermal antimicrobial peptides (beta-defensins and cathelicidins), and a T-helper 2 (Th2) type response to penetrating antigens (microbial, aeroallergens, etc.), which promotes eosinophilia and IgE production. A T-helper type 1 response is noted only later, in chronic AD.

CLINICAL MANIFESTATIONS

- Patients invariably complain or demonstrate the presence of pruritus.
- AD is a chronic condition often with an unpredictable course of flares and remissions.

Table 4.1	CLINICAL CLUES TO THE DIAGNOSIS OF ATOPIC DERMATITIS

Xerosis, generalized
Excoriations (Fig. 4.14)
Hyperlinear palms (Fig. 4.15)
Dennie-Morgan folds (Fig. 4.16)
Allergic shiners (Fig. 4.17)
Circumoral pallor

- The different phases of AD are not always clearly distinct and any or all manifestations (i.e., acute, subacute, or chronic; see Chapter 13) of atopic dermatitis may exist in a single patient.
- The background skin is usually dry and rough to the touch.
- Other clinical clues are often present; see Table 4.1.

DESCRIPTION OF LESIONS

INFANTILE PHASE

- In infancy, AD usually presents after 2 months of age with intense itching or irritability.
- Skin lesions present with varying amounts of ill-defined, erythematous, edematous, papules and plaques on the cheeks, forehead, and scalp, as well as on the extensor extremities (Fig. 4.2). The eruption can also become more generalized.
- The face and/or scalp is involved in almost all affected infants (Figs. 4.3 and 4.4).
- There is often a history of seborrheic dermatitis or "cradle cap" and features of AD become prominent after the seborrheic dermatitis subsides.
- Infants indicate itching by rubbing their scalp and head on crib bedding, by pinching, scratching, or tapping of affected and unaffected areas of skin.
- Characteristically infantile AD spares the more moist "fold" areas such as the inguinal folds,
- diaper area, nasolabial folds, and axillae.

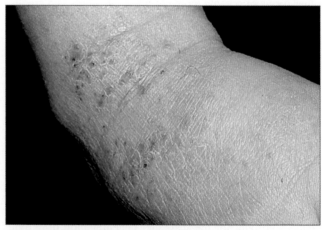

4.2 *Infantile atopic dermatitis.* Note erythema, crusts, scale, and mild lichenification on the dorsal foot of this infant.

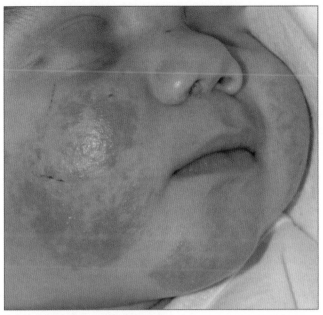

4.3 *Infantile atopic dermatitis.* Acute eczematous plaques on the cheeks of an infant.

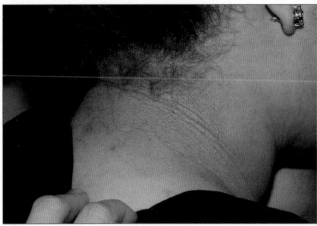

4.5 *Childhood atopic dermatitis.* Eczematous plaques on the nape of the neck in a 4-year-old girl with atopic dermatitis.

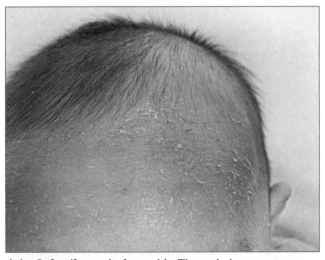

4.4 *Infantile atopic dermatitis.* The scalp is a common area of involvement in babies.

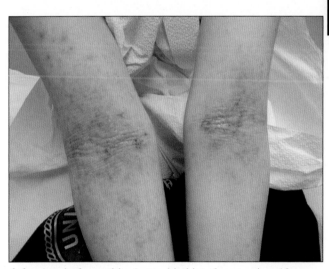

4.6 *Atopic dermatitis.* Antecubital involvement in a 10-year-old child.

CHILDHOOD PHASE

- The childhood phase of AD follows the infantile phase beginning at around 2 years of age and continues through puberty.
- Lesions localize to the flexural aspects of the elbows and knees (antecubital and popliteal fossae), the wrists, ankles, and posterior neck in a symmetric distribution (Figs. 4.5 and 4.6).
- Facial eczema typically presents on the periorbital skin and the lips.
- Lesions in childhood AD tend to be more well circumscribed, dry, and scaly.
- Repeated rubbing and scratching results in *lichenification* (Fig. 4.7).

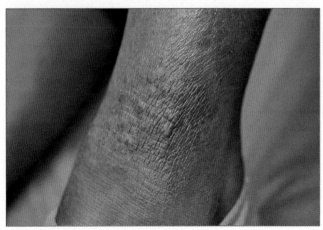

4.7 *Atopic dermatitis.* Lichenification is apparent from repeated rubbing and scratching.

Chapter 4 • Eczema in Infants and Children **79**

- Pruritus may make it difficult for children to sit still in school and negatively affects attention.
- In darker skin types, follicular prominence, or a "goosebump" feel to the skin, especially notable on the trunk, can be a presentation of AD.
- Lymphadenopathy can be severe especially in cases of long standing and untreated AD.

ADOLESCENT PHASE

- Predominant areas of involvement continue to be the flexural surfaces; in addition, the dorsal aspect of the hands and feet are also commonly affected.
- Lesions may also appear in other extensor locations such as the shins, ankles, feet (Fig. 4.8), and the nape of the neck. Sometimes lesions limited to the lips (atopic cheilitis; Fig. 4.9), eyelids (Fig. 4.10), vulvar or scrotal areas, or hands, which may be the only features of atopic dermatitis that persist into adolescence or adulthood.
- Lichenification is often seen.
- In adolescence, the morphology of eczematous lesions may change to follicularly based papules (e.g., follicular eczema; Fig. 4.11) or deep seeded vesicles on the hands (e.g., dyshidrotic eczema; Fig. 4.12).
- Nail dystrophy can occur in atopic dermatitis and represents involvement of the proximal nail fold and the underlying nail matrix (root).
- Postinflammatory pigmentary changes are also more apparent during the adolescent phase.

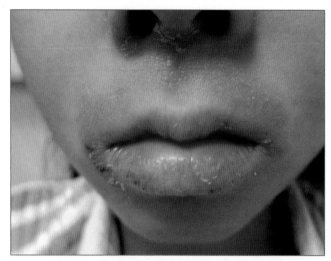

4.9 *Atopic cheilitis (atopic dermatitis of the lips).* Note the lichenification and the ill-defined outline of the vermilion border of the upper lip.

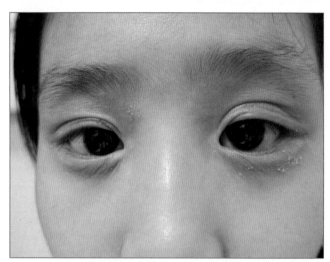

4.10 *Atopic dermatitis.* AD of the eyelids may be all that persists into adolescence.

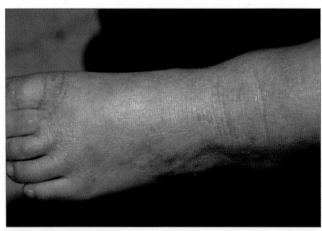

4.8 *Atopic dermatitis.* Severe subacute and chronic AD on the feet of this adolescent boy. Note linear hemorrhagic crusts from scratching.

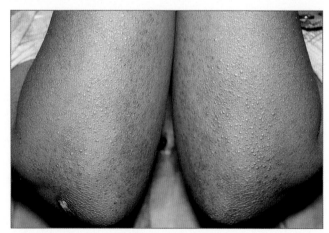

4.11 *Atopic dermatitis, follicular eczema.* Atopic dermatitis of the hair follicles. Note the grid-like pattern of tiny (1 mm) follicular papules. This is a common presentation in African-American patients.

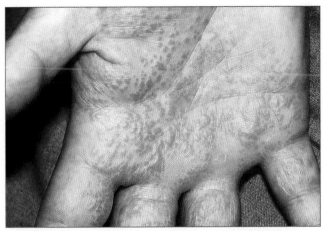

4.12 *Dyshidrotic eczema.* Deep-seeded vesicles on the palms or sides of fingers is the characteristic distribution of dyshidrotic eczema (see Fig. 13.28).

CLINICAL SEQUELAE AND POSSIBLE COMPLICATIONS

* Pruritus may interfere with sleep and school performance.
* Scratching and rubbing can result in lichenification and increase the sensation of itch resulting in the "itch-scratch cycle."
* *Staphylococcus aureus* is prevalent on AD skin and can be cultured from lesional skin in >80% of patients and clinically unaffected skin in 30% to 50% of AD patients.
* Secondary skin infection is the most common complication seen in AD. *S. aureus* and *Streptococcus pyogenes* are the most frequent culprits.
* The secretion of toxins (superantigens) by *S. aureus* may trigger flares.
* Secondary infection with herpes simplex virus may result in eczema herpeticum (**Kaposi varicelliform eruption**) (Fig. 4.13), which more commonly occurs in childhood.

DIAGNOSIS

* Diagnosis of atopic dermatitis is made clinically.
* Besides pruritus, other important clinical features include xerosis and other atopic stigmata (see Table 4.1); eczematous skin lesions in the typical age-specific distribution (i.e., face and extensor surfaces in infants and a flexural distribution in childhood); a chronic, unpredictable, and relapsing course; an early age at onset (usually <2 years of age); and/or a first degree relative with asthma or allergic rhinitis.

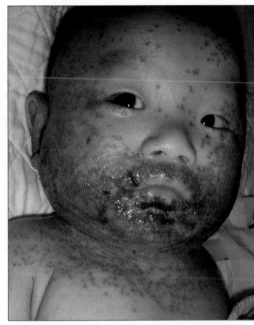

4.13 *Eczema herpeticum.* Punched out crusted vesicles in areas of atopic dermatitis.

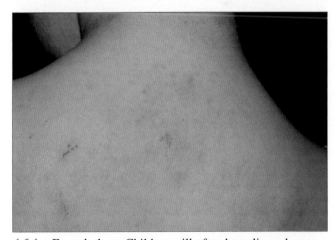

4.14 *Excoriations.* Children will often have linear brown crusts in areas of skin that are easily reachable due to scratching.

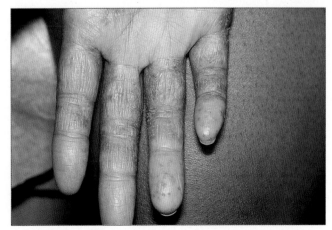

4.15 *Hyperlinear palms.* Lichenification and hyperlinearity are evident in this girl who has chronic hand eczema.

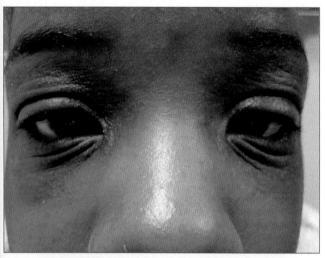

4.16 *Dennie-Morgan folds.* These comprise a characteristic double fold that extends from the inner to the outer canthus of the lower eyelid.

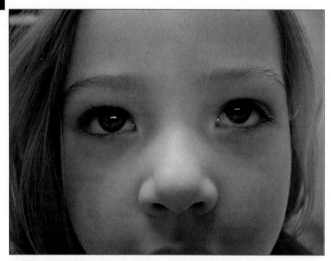

4.17 *Allergic shiners.* This term refers to a darkened, violaceous, or tan coloring in the periorbital area. Along with Dennie-Morgan folds, this dark coloring may be an instant clue to the diagnosis of atopic dermatitis.

DIFFERENTIAL DIAGNOSIS

- The diagnosis of atopic dermatitis is generally not difficult, especially in patients with an atopic history.

Contact Dermatitis (see later in this chapter)
- *Determine whether the patient was exposed to an allergen or irritant.*
- *The location of the lesions is limited to the area of contact with allergen; the morphology of the lesion may suggest an external cause.*

Psoriasis (see Chapter 14)
- *Lesions generally appear on extensor locations—the elbows, knees, and other large joints—rather than on flexor creases.*
- *Patients may have a positive family history of psoriasis.*
- *Usually, psoriasis is less pruritic than eczema.*
- *Psoriatic lesions tend to be clearly demarcated from normal surrounding skin, and the scale of psoriasis is adherent and silvery. However, psoriasis may at times be clinically indistinguishable from atopic dermatitis.*

Scabies (see Chapter 20)
- *A history of exposure is important in diagnosing scabies.*
- *Symptoms are present in other household members.*
- *Characteristic distribution (e.g., in the webs between the fingers and on the flexor wrists) can mimic that of eczema.*
- *A positive scabies scraping is diagnostic of scabies.*

Seborrheic Dermatitis
- *In infants, it may be difficult to distinguish atopic dermatitis from seborrheic dermatitis and at times both conditions overlap.*
- *Seborrheic dermatitis presents earlier in infancy (1 to 3 weeks of life) and characteristically affects the skin folds, as opposed to infantile atopic dermatitis that affects the extensor surfaces.*
- *The scale is greasier and has a yellow-brown color to it.*

MANAGEMENT

General Principles

- **Treat flares** promptly with the appropriate strength topical corticosteroid until complete clearance, that is, the skin is no longer rough, red, or itchy.
- A **daily maintenance** routine is required both during periods of active flares and when disease is quiescent.
- **Identification and avoidance of** known and possible **triggers** such as extremes of temperature, outdoor and indoor allergens (i.e., dust mites, grass pollens, animal dander, molds), and irritants (i.e., sweat, harsh soaps and detergents, bubble baths, fragrances, rough synthetic fabrics, etc.).
- **Communication** and education about AD is paramount. The use of a **Written Action Plan** (see Companion eBook) and close follow-up can help ensure adherence.

Treatment

Topical Therapy (see Chapter 13 and "Introduction: Topical Therapy")

- Topically applied corticosteroids to areas of active dermatitis is the mainstay of AD therapy.
- Maintenance therapy with daily gentle skin care and use of moisturizers must be a part of the treatment for all patients with AD.

Face and Body Folds

- For the face and intertriginous regions (axillae and inguinal creases—areas that are "naturally" occluded), treatment should be initiated with a low-potency (class 6 or 7) ointment, such as hydrocortisone 2.5% ointment or desonide 0.05% ointment.
- **Protopic ointment, 0.03% or 0.1%** (tacrolimus) and **Elidel 1% cream** (pimecrolimus) are nonsteroidal immunomodulators that have been shown to reduce the symptoms of AD and are used as an alternative to topical steroids or as part of maintenance therapy, particularly when the eruption involves the face or intertriginous areas, such as the axillae and groin, where the long-term use of high-potency steroids is limited.
- Protopic is considered to be equivalent to a class 5 topical steroid. Protopic 0.1% is approved for the treatment of atopic dermatitis in patients >16 years and older and the 0.03% concentration is approved for patients older than 2 years.
- Elidel 1% cream is considered to be equipotent to a class 6 topical steroid.

For information regarding the long-term safety of these agents, see "Introduction: Topical Therapy."

Body (Trunk, Arms, Legs, Scalp)

- For nonintertriginous areas, treatment can be initiated with a mid-strength (class 3 or 4) cream or ointment such as mometasone 0.1% ointment (**Elocon**) or fluticasone 0.05% cream or 0.005% ointment (**Cutivate**).

- For thicker lesions, initial therapy may be with a more potent topical steroid (class 2 or 3), such as fluocinonide 0.05% cream (**Lidex**) ointment.
- Long-standing, lichenified eczematous lesions on the body or lesions on the hands and feet may require a superpotent agent such as **clobetasol 0.05%** ointment.

Topical agents should be used until the dermatitis has cleared completely, that is, the skin is no longer rough, red, or itchy. It can be helpful to find an area on the child's skin that is free of dermatitis to show the patient and parent what clear means. Skin that is clear of dermatitis can still be hypo- or hyperpigmented.

Adjunctive Therapies to Consider During AD Flares

- Wet wraps and the "soak and smear" technique are useful adjuncts for the treatment of acute severe disease, especially when lichenified and/or localized to the upper and lower extremities.
- **Wet wrap treatment** involves the application of a topical corticosteroid to the areas of active dermatitis over which a double layer, first moist then dry, of close-fitting cotton bandages are applied. Any type of close fitting cotton garment can be used (i.e., elastic tubular cotton bandage [**Tubifast**], old cotton bed sheets or t-shirts cut into wrappable strips). The cotton wraps can be left in place 3 to 24 hours with longer applications being more effective. Wet wrap treatment is effective when used for an average of 7 days.
- **Soak and smear** involves soaking in a bath or shower for 10 to 20 minutes followed by *immediate* application of the topical medication while the skin is still damp. This technique allows for moisture trapping and better penetration of the medication into the skin.
- For the child with frequent flares, especially those with a history of staphylococcal infection, **"Bleach baths"** with **sodium hypochlorite (Clorox)** (1/4 cup of household bleach in a half full bath tub or ½ cup in a full bath tub) twice weekly can be beneficial as part of the maintenance plan for atopic dermatitis.
- Oral first generation H_1 antihistamines such as diphenhydramine (**Benadryl**) and hydroxyzine (**Atarax**) probably do not reduce itching, but they are sometimes useful as inducers of sleep, a positive side effect for many patients.
- If outdoor or indoor allergens are identified as a potential exacerbating factor, daily nonsedating antihistamines such as loratidine (**Claritin**) or cetirizine (**Zyrtec**) can be beneficial.

Daily Maintenance Therapy

Gentle Bathing Tips

- Despite popular belief, patients with AD, especially children, should bathe daily.

continued on page 84

MANAGEMENT *Continued*

- The benefits include removal of excess dirt, potential irritants and allergens and surface microbes; hydrating the skin and allowing for better delivery of corticosteroids and moisturizers.
- Baths should be short (no longer than 10 minutes) and with tepid water.
- Use mild, moisturizing soaps such as **Dove (sensitive skin beauty bar)** or nonsoap cleansers such as Cetaphil Gentle cleanser.
- After bathing, pat (do not rub) the skin dry; and then *immediately* (within 3 minutes) apply topical corticosteroid to areas of active dermatitis first, then apply moisturizer to all skin including over topical steroid.
- Moisturizers should be fragrance-free creams or ointments and contain ceramides.
- Suggested ointments: **Vaseline Petroleum Jelly, Aquaphor**
- Suggested creams: **CeraVe cream, Eucerin Daily Repair Creme, Cetaphil Cream**
- **Atopiclair, MimyX**, and **Epiceram and Eletone** are newer, multiple-ingredient nonsteroidal barrier repair creams that are available via prescription.

Other Therapeutic Measures

- For patients with secondary staphylococcal infection, oral antistaphylococcal therapy with **cephalexin** (or other agent) is required. Bacterial cultures should always be performed before starting an oral antibiotic.
- If infection with methicillin-resistant *S. aureus* (**MRSA**) is detected or suspected, therapy with **clindamycin,** **doxycycline** (if patient is older than 8 years), or **trimethoprim-sulfamethoxazole** is required.
- For patients with secondary herpes simplex infection (Kaposi varicelliform eruption), oral antiviral therapy and, possibly, hospitalization may be required. A viral culture taken from the base of a fresh vesicle should be sent before initiating antiviral therapy.
- When the child continues to have severe disease such that the condition is causing significant disruption in the child's and/or family's life, more aggressive systemic therapy is warranted.
- Before resorting to systemic therapy, "soak and smear" and/or wet wraps with potent topical corticosteroids should be attempted. (See above and "Introduction: Topical Therapy.")
- Systemic steroids should not be used for the treatment of flares of AD because of the unfavorable risk to benefit profile and the severe rebound flares of disease that often occurs upon tapering.
- Phototherapy with narrowband ultraviolet B rays and, less commonly, ultraviolet A rays, is often very effective for widespread skin involvement.
- Systemic immunosuppressive agents such as **cyclosporine, mycophenolate mofetil,** or azathioprine is sometimes necessary in patients with severe generalized atopic dermatitis that is refractory to topical and adjunctive therapies.

 SEE PATIENT HANDOUTS, "Atopic Dermatitis," "Written Action Plan," "Soak and Smear Instruction Sheet," and "Bleach Baths" IN THE COMPANION eBOOK EDITION.

HELPFUL HINTS

- Patients and their parents, caregivers, and teachers should be educated about the manifestations and management of atopic dermatitis at each visit.
- When topical steroids are applied immediately after bathing, their penetration and potency are increased.
- The "gooiest" and cheapest moisturizer is petrolatum.
- The National Eczema Association can be contacted at:
  415-499-3474 or 800-818-7546
  4460 Redwood Highway, Suite 16-D, San Rafael, CA 94903-1953
  info@nationaleczema.org or
  http://www.nationaleczema.org

POINTS TO REMEMBER

- Topical steroids should be applied only to areas of active disease (inflamed, rough, red skin) and not for postinflammatory hyper- or hypopigmentation.
- The application of an appropriately chosen topical steroid (more potent for thicker lesions and less potent for thinner lesions) can clear even the most severe dermatitis.
- "Stronger" is often preferable to "longer" in the use of topical steroids, because long-term application is more often associated with cutaneous side effects (i.e., striae, telangiectasias, atrophy, acne).
- Low-potency topical steroids or topical calcineurin inhibitors are recommended for use on the face and in skin folds, such as the perineal area and underarms.

 SEE PATIENT HANDOUT "Atopic Dermatitis" IN THE COMPANION eBOOK EDITION.

COMMON MYTHS ABOUT ATOPIC DERMATITIS

Myth: Soy formulas improve eczema in infants.
Fact: Food allergies contribute to flares of atopic dermatitis in less than 10% of patients. Thus, changing a formula from cow's milk protein to soy protein usually does not affect eczema. Urticaria (hives) is the usual skin manifestation of a food allergy.

Myth: Infants and children who have atopic dermatitis should be bathed infrequently.
Fact: The advantages of bathing (removal of scale, surface bacteria, etc.) far outweigh its disadvantages (see following) and potential drying effect of water on the skin.

Myth: Laundry detergents are a common cause of eczema.
Fact: This is very rarely the case. Most detergents are rinsed out, with very little soap remaining to trigger a flare of atopic dermatitis.

Myth: Potent topical steroids should not be used on infants or young children.
Fact: Topical steroids, when used properly, are quite safe. Choosing a topical steroid of adequate potency (even if potent or superpotent) to clear eczema completely will result in less overall use than the use of a mild topical steroid for a longer period of time. Not using topical steroids of adequate potency can lead to undertreatment, which can interfere with the child's and family's daily activities.

ASSOCIATED CONDITIONS

Patients with atopic dermatitis often exhibit one or more associated conditions that are listed in Table 4.2. These disorders are often found in patients with an atopic history. However, on occasion, they manifest in patients without an atopic predisposition.

Table 4.2 CONDITIONS ASSOCIATED WITH ATOPIC DERMATITIS

Keratosis pilaris
Ichthyosis vulgaris
Pityriasis alba

Keratosis Pilaris

BASICS

- Keratosis pilaris (KP), often referred to as "chicken-skin" because of its rough texture, is a common, benign eruption that frequently occurs in patients with atopic dermatitis but can also occur as an isolated condition.
- KP presents as an eruption of grouped, follicular, keratotic papules resulting in a sandpaper-like feel and is most commonly found on the lateral arms.
- KP runs in families, and most of the time an affected child has a parent or sibling with keratosis pilaris.

CLINICAL MANIFESTATIONS

- Each lesion of KP is characterized by a plug of hyperkeratosis at the hair follicle orifice with a surrounding halo of perifollicular erythema.
- Lesions are similar in size and can be red or skin-colored with a white keratotic plug.
- KP appears in preadolescent children on the lateral aspects of the cheeks (Fig. 4.18), the upper and lateral thighs, posterolateral arms, dorsal forearms, and/or the buttocks.
- In adolescents and adults, KP is most often found on the deltoid and posterolateral upper arms (Fig. 4.19). Less often, the eruption can extend on to the upper back and the lateral thighs.
- The cause of KP is unknown.
- KP is rarely symptomatic. Although some patients are bothered by the rough feeling and the appearance of the eruption, the condition is mostly of cosmetic significance.

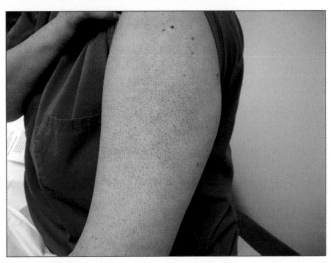

4.19 **Keratosis pilaris.** This teenager has tiny, rough-textured, red, follicular papules on his lateral upper arms.

 DIFFERENTIAL DIAGNOSIS

Acne
- *Lesions are variably sized, papules, pustules, and comedones.*
- *"T-zone" (forehead, nose, chin) distribution of lesions.*
- *Occurs in infancy, adolescence, and adulthood.*

Folliculitis
- *Lesions have more prominent erythema and a pustular, rather than keratotic, core.*

Perioral Dermatitis
- *Lesions are localized to the skin around the mouth and nose, rather than the lateral cheeks as in KP.*
- *Lesions look like acne and are exacerbated by topical steroids.*

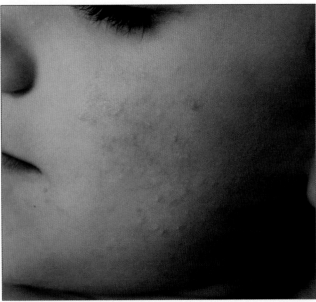

4.18 **Keratosis pilaris.** This preadolescent boy has keratotic, acne-like, perifollicular papules on his cheeks.

MANAGEMENT

- There is no cure for KP but treatment with salicylic acid or alpha-hydroxy acid (lactic acid or glycolic acid) containing emollients can help exfoliate the excess skin and result in a smoother feel to the skin.
- Lactic acid, available as 12% ammonium lactate cream or lotion such as is in **AmLactin Cream** or **Lac-Hydrin Cream**, is often a good place to start. The cream should be applied twice daily. If no improvement is noted after 6 weeks of use, an alternative, such as **Acqua Glycolic Cream** (glycolic acid) or **Cerave SA** (salicylic acid) can be tried.
- Emollients containing variable amounts of urea (10% to 40%), a keratolytic agent, can also help smoothen affected skin. Products containing urea include **Umecta** (40% urea), **Eucerin Repair Lotion** (10% urea), and **Keralac Lotion** (35% urea). Skin irritation is more likely to occur with preparations that contain higher percentages of urea.
- **Tretinoin** 0.05% or 0.1% cream and **Pulsed Dye Laser** have also been used to treat KP with positive results.
- Loofas and exfoliating scrubs that contain "microbeads" should not be used excessively, but once or twice a week may be beneficial.
- Treatment of KP in children who also have AD is more challenging as moisturizers that contain alpha-hydroxy acids can be irritating to their skin, so treatment is often discouraged unless of significant cosmetic importance.

Ichthyosis Vulgaris

BASICS

- Ichthyosis vulgaris (IV) is the most common type of hereditary ichthyosis and is seen in 10% to 30% of patients with atopic dermatitis.
- IV is now known to be due to mutations in profilaggrin, the precursor of filaggrin, a protein that is important for the maintenance of an intact skin barrier.
- IV is inherited in a semidominant manner, meaning that clinical manifestations are seen with a mutation on one allele.

CLINICAL MANIFESTATIONS

- IV is usually discovered in childhood and typically presents as fish-like, dry scale on the dorsal aspects of the legs (Fig. 4.20). Fine dry scale can also be seen on other areas.
- Characteristically, the flexor creases are spared in this condition (Fig. 4.21) and thickening of the skin of the palms and soles with hyperlinearity is typical.

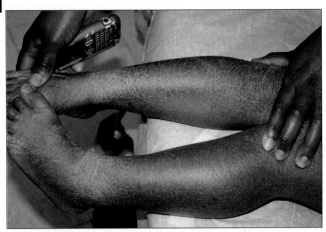

4.20 *Ichthyosis vulgaris.* Typical fish-like, dry scale on the dorsal aspects of the legs.

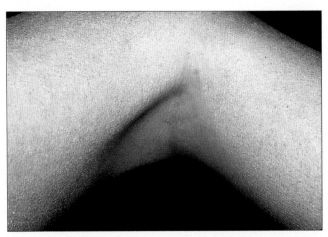

4.21 *Ichthyosis vulgaris.* Lesions resemble fish scales. Note the characteristic sparing of the popliteal creases.

- Patients with IV are more likely to have keratosis pilaris and also more likely to have an atopic condition—atopic dermatitis, asthma, and/or allergic rhinitis.
- Examination and questioning of an affected child's parent will often reveal dry skin and hyperlinear palms.
- The condition generally improves with age.

 DIFFERENTIAL DIAGNOSIS

Other Hereditary Ichthyoses
- *Flexural surfaces are involved in other congenital ichthyoses and are spared in ichthyosis vulgaris and X-linked ichthyosis (Fig. 4.21).*

Xerosis
- *Ichthyosis vulgaris is often confused for generalized xerosis or dryness of the skin. Dry skin has fine white scaling, and an ashy color but no fish-like scale as in IV.*

 MANAGEMENT

- There is no cure for icthyosis vulgaris. Treatment consists of emollients.
- Similar to the treatment for KP, emollients containing urea, salicylic acid, or alpha-hydroxy acids such as **Lac-Hydrin Cream, Umecta** (40% urea), **Eucerin Repair Lotion** (10% urea), and **Keralac Lotion** (35% urea) can help remove scale and result in a smoother look and feel to the skin. Higher percentages of urea may be more effective but are also more likely to be irritating.
- Topical retinoids such as tretinoin or tazarotene are helpful for some patients.
- In patients with concomitant AD, alpha-hydroxy acid and urea containing emollients can be irritating.

BASICS

- Pityriasis alba (P. alba) is a nonspecific, mild dermatitis characterized by hypopigmented macules and patches on the face and occasionally, on the arms.
- It is believed that this mild dermatitis interrupts the transfer of pigment from melanocytes to keratinocytes and thus the affected area appears lighter in color.
- P. alba frequently occurs in children with atopic dermatitis.

CLINICAL MANIFESTATIONS

- P. alba is often discovered in the summer, when sun exposure results in darkening of the normal skin and thus, increased contrast between normal and affected skin.
- Typically, P. alba presents as variably sized, ill-defined hypopigmented or light pink macules and patches with overlying fine white scaling on the face (Fig. 4.22).
- The cheeks are most characteristically involved, but P. alba can also be seen on the chest and arms (Fig. 4.23).
- P. alba is most often seen in children and adolescents with darkly pigmented skin.

DIFFERENTIAL DIAGNOSIS

Tinea Versicolor
- *Lesions of TV have an edge of scale and often have a pink-orange hue.*
- *Lesions are more well demarcated and are often more widespread on chest, back, and neck.*

Vitiligo
- *Lesions of vitiligo are more well demarcated and lack scale.*
- *Lesions appear chalk-white (signifying depigmentation) under a Wood lamp.*

Nevus Depigmentosus
- *Usually a solitary lesion, present from birth, unchanged, and more well demarcated than P. alba.*

MANAGEMENT

- In general, no treatment is necessary as pigment returns to normal over several months. Occasionally, repigmentation can take years.
- Treatment with a low-potency topical steroid such as **desonide 0.05% ointment** or a topical calcineurin inhibitor such as **Protopic 0.03% ointment** or **Elidel 1% cream** twice a day for a few weeks can clear the scale and allow for repigmentation to occur.
- Once scaling has resolved, frequent use of moisturizers and protection from sun exposure can help lessen the contrast between the hypopigmented area and the surrounding skin.

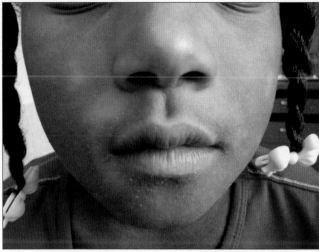

4.22 *Pityriasis alba.* Ill-defined hypopigmented slightly scaly plaques on the cheeks are characteristic of P. alba.

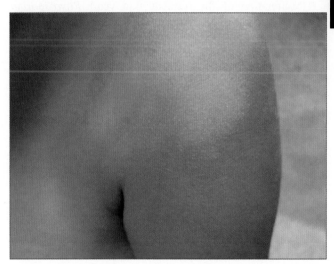

4.23 *Pityriasis alba.* P. alba can also be seen on the chest and arms.

BASICS

- Seborrheic dermatitis (SD) is a type of eczematous dermatitis that presents in the "seborrheic" areas of the body, that is, those regions of the body that have the greatest concentration of sebaceous glands and include the scalp, face, presternal region, interscapular area, umbilicus, and body folds (intertriginous areas).
- In the pediatric population, seborrheic dermatitis is seen in infancy and in adolescence.

PATHOGENESIS

- The cause of seborrheic dermatitis is not known.
- Currently, the following factors are believed to have an etiologic role:
  - Increased levels of androgens present in the first year of life and during puberty
  - High sebum production in response to increased androgens
  - Proliferation of the resident skin yeast *Pityrosporum ovale* (*Malassezia ovalis*) and/or *Malassezia furfur,* which thrive in areas of high sebum
  - Altered composition of skin surface lipids: high triglycerides and cholesterol with decreased squalene and free fatty acids

CLINICAL MANIFESTATIONS

INFANCY

- In infancy, SD typically appears at 3 to 4 weeks of life (range 1 to 10 weeks), with yellowish-brown, greasy adherent scales on the vertex and anterior scalp and is often called "cradle cap" (Fig. 4.24).
- SD can then progress to an erythematous scaly eruption involving the entire scalp.
- In infants, the scalp is almost always involved. Other areas of the body are variably involved.
- On the face, infantile SD appears as pink-orange greasy patches with varying amounts of overlying scale.
- On the body, well-demarcated pink to salmon-colored, shiny patches with greasy scale are seen on the retroauricular folds, trunk, and in the body folds including the axillae and inguinal folds (Fig. 4.25).
- Unlike atopic dermatitis, pruritus is usually slight or absent.
- Some infants with SD progress into atopic dermatitis.

ADOLESCENCE

- In adolescence, SD usually appears on the scalp and as erythema and scaling and is often called "dandruff." The face and body can also be affected.
- In severe cases, scaling can be thick and adherent and mimic psoriasis and is termed "sebopsoriasis" (see Chapter 14).

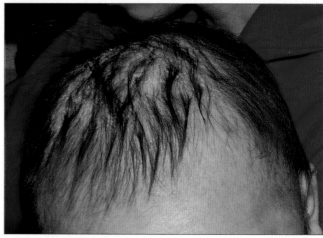

4.24   *Seborrheic dermatitis.* Yellowish greasy adherent scales on the scalp is often called "cradle cap" in infants.

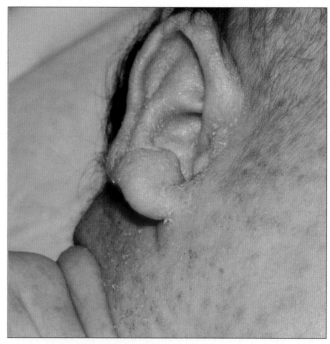

4.25   *Seborrheic dermatitis.* Typical greasy yellow scaling can be seen in and around the ears in infants.

- On the body, lesions typically appear on the face specifically the forehead, eyebrows, eyelashes, cheeks, beard, and nasolabial folds (Fig. 4.26) as variable amounts of erythema and greasy scaling. In the body folds (i.e., retroauricular folds, inframammary areas, axillae, inguinal creases, intragluteal crease, perianal area, and umbilicus) or in the presternal skin, lesions of SD appear as well demarcated pink-orange greasy patches with or without an overlying whitish scale.
- The eruption of SD tends to be bilaterally symmetric.
- SD is seen more commonly seen in boys.

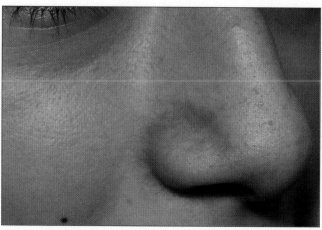

4.26 *Seborrheic dermatitis.* In adolescents, occurs on the face and chest.

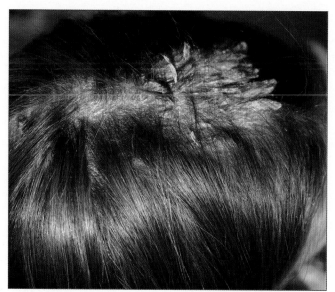

4.27 *Pityriasis amiantacea.* Long-standing untreated seborrheic dermatitis of the scalp can lead thick plate-like scales firmly adherent to the scalp.

CLINICAL SEQUELAE

- On the scalp, there may be itching and scratching which can lead to significant scale that is often noticeable on clothing.
- Occasionally, secondary candidal or bacterial infection can occur in SD and the neck fold and the inguinal folds are most susceptible.
- When infection is suspected, bacterial culture should be sent and topical anticandidal and/or antibacterial agents should be initiated. Topical agents are generally sufficient to clear an infection; however, occasionally systemic antibiotics are necessary.
- Pityriasis amiantacea (also called tinea amiantacea although it is not a fungal infection), a condition of thick plate-like scales firmly adherent to the scalp and hair (Fig. 4.27), can develop in untreated SD of the scalp.

 DIFFERENTIAL DIAGNOSIS

The differential diagnosis of SD varies depending on the age, and the location of the lesions.

Infants
Atopic Dermatitis
- *AD presents later in infancy (2 to 3 months).*
- *In AD, lesions are ill-defined, with dry scale and are very itchy.*
- *Occluded "fold" areas of the body are usually spared in AD whereas, seborrheic dermatitis which typically involves folds.*

Psoriasis
- *Infantile psoriasis often starts in the diaper area and can be difficult to distinguish from infantile seborrheic dermatitis.*
- *Typical psoriatic lesions—well-demarcated bright pink red patches and plaques with overlying silvery white scale—may be present elsewhere.*

Irritant Contact Dermatitis
- *Skin within the body folds is spared.*
- *Shiny pink patches in areas of contact with the irritant, that is, convex surfaces of labia and buttocks in diaper dermatitis.*

Candidiasis
- *Tends to occur in body folds but patches are brighter, more "beefy" red.*
- *Pinpoint satellite pustules and a typical odor may be present.*
- *KOH and fungal culture will be positive for Candida species.*

Adolescents
Psoriasis
- *Scalp psoriasis can be difficult to distinguish from SD.*
- *Well-demarcated plaques with silvery white scale.*
- *Psoriatic plaques and nail pits may be present elsewhere.*

Eczematous Dermatitis Such as Atopic Dermatitis
- *Eczematous lesions elsewhere on the body.*
- *Atopic history.*
- *Marked pruritus.*

Tinea Capitis
- *Scale is drier.*
- *Broken hairs may be present.*
- *Occipital lymphadenopathy sometimes present.*

MANAGEMENT

Infants

- SD in infants usually self resolves by 8 to 12 months of age.
- No treatment is required; in extensive cases treatment can be used to alleviate symptoms.

Scalp

- Frequent shampooing with a regular gentle baby shampoo usually suffices.
- Removal of scales can be facilitated by massaging the affected area of scalp with baby oil or mineral oil.
- Antifungal shampoos such as ketoconazole 2% are effective but should only be used as a last resort as they are drying and can irritate the eyes.
- When redness is present the use of a low-potency topical steroid in a lotion, solution, or oil base such as **hydrocortisone 2.5%** or **desonide 0.05%** applied twice daily is effective.

Face and Body Folds

- Either a low-potency topical steroid (class 5 to 7): **hydrocortisone 2.5%** or **desonide 0.05%** or topical antifungal agent: **ketoconazole 2%** cream or **econazole 1%** cream can clear SD when applied once to twice daily.

Adolescents

- Treatment of SD in adolescents is similar to treatment in adults and is discussed in detail in Chapter 13.
- Briefly, treatment of scalp SD involves frequent shampooing (at least four to five times per week) with shampoos that contain **tar, salicylic acid, selenium sulfide, zinc pyrithione, or antifungal agents (i.e., ketoconazole)**. Alternative use of different preparations on a regular basis is recommended as part of a treatment regimen. Suggested shampoos include **Sebulex, Selsun blue, T-sal, T-gel, Head & Shoulders,** and **DHS Zinc.**
- These antiseborrheic shampoos can also be used as body washes for SD on the body.
- For associated erythema and/or pruritus, medium- to high-potency (class 1 to 3) topical steroid lotions, gels, oils, or foams (**clobetasol 0.05%** gel/lotion/solution/foam, **fluocinonide 0.05% gel, fluocinolone 0.025% solution** or **betamethasone valerate foam 0.12%** [**Luxiq foam**]) applied twice daily are effective. Foams, solutions, and gels are less oily than ointments or creams.
- For SD on the face or in the body folds, a mild steroid (class 5 to 7) or a topical calcineurin inhibitor (i.e., **Elidel cream**) used twice daily can clear the redness, then an antifungal agent such as econazole 1% cream or ketoconazole 2% cream should be used on a daily basis as maintenance.

HELPFUL HINTS

- Infantile seborrheic dermatitis presents in the first few weeks of life, affects skin folds, and subsides by 3 to 4 months of age; whereas atopic dermatitis presents later, at around 3 months of age, and affects the extensor surfaces and spares the folds.
- SD of the scalp is generally not seen in preadolescent children; therefore, excessive use of shampoos should *not* be encouraged in this age group. The child may actually have atopic dermatitis, which is only aggravated by frequent shampooing.
- The application of topical antifungals may work as well or better than topical steroids in many cases.
- **Protopic ointment** (tacrolimus) 0.1% and **Elidel cream** (pimecrolimus) 1% may also be effective in the treatment of facial and intertriginous SD.

POINTS TO REMEMBER

- Infantile SD is often asymptomatic and self-resolves.
- Low-potency topical steroids or topical antifungal agents can help reduce redness and scaling in infantile SD.
- In adolescents, antiseborrheic shampoos should be used in combination with intermittent use of topical steroids.

SEE PATIENT HANDOUT "Scalp Psoriasis: Scale Removal" IN THE COMPANION eBOOK EDITION.

- Contact dermatitis is an inflammatory, eczematous eruption caused by contact with an external agent.
- In *irritant contact dermatitis* (ICD) an external agent produces an eczematous eruption by direct irritation of the skin. The eruption can occur in anyone who is exposed to the agent and is confined to the area of exposure. In contrast, *allergic contact dermatitis* (ACD) requires prior sensitization and there is no reaction on first exposure.
- Although allergic contact dermatitis can be seen with increased frequency in patients with atopic dermatitis, ICD is overall more common in children, including children with atopic dermatitis. See Tables 4.3 and 4.4 for a list of the most common contact allergens and irritants in children. Allergic contact dermatitis is discussed in detail in Chapter 13.

Table 4.3 MOST COMMON CONTACT ALLERGENS IN CHILDREN

ALLERGEN	SOURCE
Nickel	Jewelry, snaps, buckles, metal buttons, eyeglasses
Cobalt	Buttons, snaps, jewelry, often a contaminant in nickel products
Neomycin	First aid and antibiotic containing ointments and creams
Balsam of Peru	Included in perfumes, toothpaste, flavoring agents, skin lotions
Fragrance mix	Foods, cosmetics, perfumes, insecticides, dental products, etc.
Thimerosal	Used as a preservative in local antiseptics, vaccines, and skin creams
Formaldehyde	A preservative found in paper products, dry cleaning solvents, paints, cosmetic products, wrinkle-resistant clothes
Chromate	Found in tanned leather products such as shoes, paints, and cement
Thiuram	Elastic in waistbands, socks, and shoe insoles
Lanolin	Emollients (such as Aquaphor), lip balms, and soaps
Paraphenylene-diamine	Hair dyes, black henna tattoos

Table 4.4 TOP 10 SOURCES OF IRRITANT CONTACT DERMATITIS IN CHILDREN

Hand soaps
Bubble baths
Detergents
Cleaning products
Certain foods (especially citrus and tomato-based foods)
Saliva
Urine
Stool
Friction

- The severity of an ICD varies and is dependent on the duration of exposure, the concentration of the irritating substance, and the condition of the skin at the time of exposure. In addition, sweating, maceration, and occlusion can all potentiate a substance's irritating effect.
- Diaper dermatitis, lip licker's dermatitis, and juvenile plantar dermatosis are forms of ICD that are commonly seen in infants and children and will be discussed here.

(IRRITANT) DIAPER DERMATITIS

BASICS

- The most common form of diaper rash is a primary irritant dermatitis (Fig. 4.28), a type of eczematous dermatitis triggered by urine, feces, moisture, and occlusion (discussed in detail in Chapter 2).
- Diaper dermatitis can first present as early as the first few weeks of life, has a peak incidence at 9 to 12 months, but can occur any time when diapers are worn.
- Patients who have atopic dermatitis are more likely to develop ICD as a result of their inherent skin sensitivity and defective barrier function.

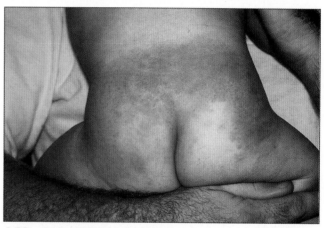

4.28 *Irritant diaper dermatitis.* The eruption conforms to the shape of the diaper.

LIP LICKERS DERMATITIS

BASICS

- Lip lickers dermatitis is an eczematous eruption on the lips and perioral skin that is caused by irritation from saliva due to an, often unconscious, licking habit.

CLINICAL MANIFESTATIONS

- Lip lickers dermatitis presents with dry, scaly lips and pink or hyperpigmented (in darker skin types) thin, scaly plaques, in a semicircular geometric shape on the upper and lower cutaneous portion of the lips (Fig. 4.29).
- The distribution of the dermatitis reflects the licking motion.

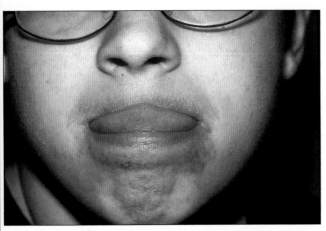

4.29 *Lip Licker's dermatitis.* The erythema and scaling are secondary to this child's habit of licking her lips.

- The skin immediately adjacent to the mucosal lip is often spared.
- The lips are dry and cracked. Sometimes fissures are present.

DIAGNOSIS

- The diagnosis is made from the clinical examination and by eliciting a history of lip licking.

DIFFERENTIAL DIAGNOSIS

Allergic Cheilitis (Allergic Contact Dermatitis of the Lips)
- *Eczematous eruption is limited to the mucosal lips and the adjacent skin. Usually due to cosmetics, personal hygiene products or foods.*

Atopic Cheilitis (Atopic Dermatitis of the Lips)
- *Eruption on mucosal lips—lips appear dry, pink and fissured.*
- *Often there is other stigmata of atopic dermatitis, that is, circumoral pallor, Dennie-Morgan folds. Evidence of atopic dermatitis elsewhere on skin.*

MANAGEMENT

- A low-potency (class 6 or 7) topical steroid such as **hydrocortisone 2.5% ointment** or **desonide 0.05% ointment** applied twice daily to the affected area can help clear the dermatitis.
- A skin protectant or barrier ointment applied to the lips two to six times per day can help keep the lips moist and protect the skin from contact with saliva.
- It is important to also attempt to stop the licking habit to prevent recurrence.

JUVENILE PLANTAR DERMATOSIS
BASICS

- Juvenile plantar dermatosis (JPD) is a common dermatosis of childhood seen on the plantar aspects of the soles and toes.
- JPD is also called "sweaty sock dermatitis," because it is triggered by sweat and friction and often worsens in the winter months when warm socks and closed shoes are worn.

CLINICAL MANIFESTATIONS

- JPD presents as a smooth, red, shiny well-demarcated patches with desquamative scaling on the balls of the feet and the toe pads. The eruption is often symmetric (Figs. 4.30 and 4.31).
- Fissures may be present, which are often painful.
- The interdigital web spaces are spared but the palms and finger pads may have similar lesions.
- Usually asymptomatic, but occasionally can be itchy.
- The eruption can wax and wane for some time but is a self-limiting condition.

DIAGNOSIS

- The diagnosis is made clinically.

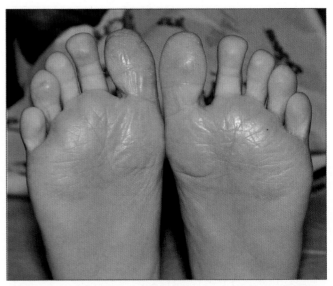

4.30 *Juvenile plantar dermatosis.* Smooth, shiny pink well-demarcated patches symmetrically distributed on the balls of the feet and the toe pads.

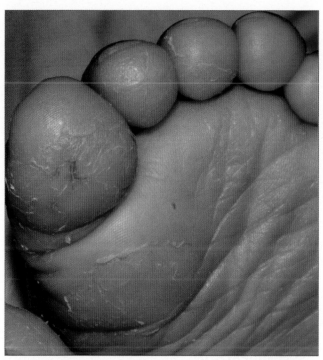

Tinea Pedis

- *Usually involves the interdigital spaces especially in between fourth and fifth toes.*
- *KOH will be positive.*

Palmoplantar Psoriasis

- *Plaques of psoriasis are more brightly pink and scale is drier and thicker.*

Shoe Allergic Contact Dermatitis

- *Allergic contact dermatitis secondary to shoe components is usually seen on the dorsum of the foot.*
- *ACD presents as a well-demarcated eczematous plaque in the area of skin where the shoe has contacted the skin.*

4.31 *Juvenile plantar dermatosis.* Fissures occasionally develop.

MANAGEMENT

- Take measures to decrease sweating:
  - Use **Zeasorb powder** on feet and in shoes before wearing shoes, or
  - Apply **aluminum chloride (hexahydrate)** containing preparations **(Hydrosal or Certain Dri)** to the skin of the feet prior to wearing shoes, and
  - Avoid impermeable socks and shoes, instead wear thin all cotton socks and shoes made with breathable materials
- Change socks frequently if wet to avoid overhydration of skin.
- Ointments and/or acid-based emollients or keratolytics should be applied twice daily to help protect the skin and prevent irritation by sweat.
- A medium to high potency (class 1 to 3) topical steroid such as **mometasone 0.1% ointment** applied twice daily can help alleviate the associated erythema and pruritus.

Superficial Bacterial Infections

OVERVIEW

The skin is home to numerous microbes including species of *Corynebacterium, Propionibacterium, Brevibacterium, Streptococcus,* and *Staphylococcus.* These resident microbial organisms have both protective and potentially harmful effects and some have been implicated in infectious and inflammatory skin diseases. For example, the commensal organism *Propionibacterium acnes* and the host reaction to its presence have been shown to contribute to the production of acne. Skin infection usually results from temporary skin invaders either by direct skin invasion or by exotoxins released by the organism itself.

Staphylococcus aureus and *Streptococcus pyogenes* (also known as group A beta-hemolytic streptococcus) account for the vast majority of bacterial skin infections in children. Infections with methicillin-resistant *Staphylococcus aureus* (MRSA) is becoming more common and most often presents as recurrent furunculosis.

In this chapter, the bacterial skin infections most commonly seen in children will be discussed.

IN THIS CHAPTER...

➤ **IMPETIGO**

- Nonbullous impetigo
- Bullous impetigo

➤ **FOLLICULITIS**

➤ **FURUNCOLOSIS**

➤ **PERIANAL STREPTOCOCCAL DERMATITIS**

➤ **PITTED KERATOLYSIS**

BASICS

- Impetigo (see also Chapter 16) is a superficial bacterial skin infection that can occur in all age groups but is most common among infants and children.
- Impetigo is most often caused by *S. aureus,* or, less often by *S. pyogenes* (Group A beta-hemolytic *Streptococcus,* GABHS), although it is often difficult to ascertain the etiologic agent.
- Bullous impetigo occurs when there is infection with the exfoliative toxin producing strain of *S. aureus.*

CLINICAL MANIFESTATIONS

- Impetigo may be transmitted from contact with another child or an infected source.
- It often starts at the site of a minor skin injury such as an abrasion, an arthropod bite reaction, or eczema that has been excoriated and can spread via autoinoculation.

NONBULLOUS IMPETIGO

- Overall, the majority of cases of impetigo in childhood are the **nonbullous** form.
- Nonbullous impetigo begins as a pink macule or papule followed by a transient vesicle or pustule that evolves into a yellow honey-colored crusted plaque (Fig. 5.1).
- In children, nonbullous impetigo tends to occur on the face, especially around the nose and mouth, and also on exposed areas of the body (Fig. 5.2).

BULLOUS IMPETIGO

- The **bullous** form has a predilection for the area of skin under the diaper and body folds and is the more common form of impetigo in infants.
- Bullous impetigo often occurs in the neonatal period but can also occur in children.
- Early in bullous impetigo there are small vesicles that can enlarge into 1- to 2-cm superficial flaccid transparent, bullae. Occasionally bullae may be up to 5 cm in diameter. Bullae rupture easily and leave a collarette of scale but typically there is no thick crust or surrounding erythema (Fig. 5.3).
- Bullous impetigo can also present as a shallow pink, moist, erosion surrounded by remnants of the blister roof.
- Usually there are no associated systemic symptoms but occasionally the bullous form can be associated with weakness, fever, and diarrhea.

DIAGNOSIS

- Diagnosis can be confirmed by culture of the base of the lesion after removal of the crust or from the intact bullae.

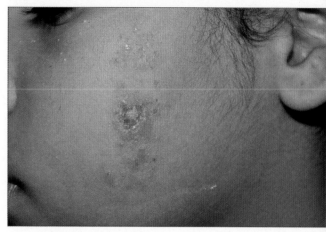

5.1 *Impetigo.* This child has a mixture of superficial moist erosions and a dried yellow crust on her left cheek.

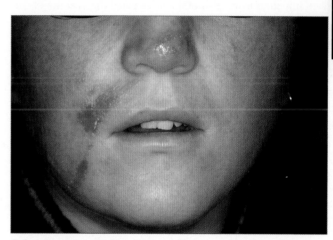

5.2 *Impetigo.* Yellow-orange (honey-colored) oozing lesions are seen here.

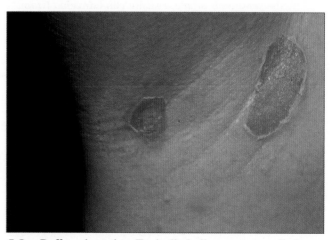

5.3 *Bullous impetigo.* Typically bullae rupture easily leaving a collarette of scale and a pink moist base. Note lack of surrounding erythema.

DIFFERENTIAL DIAGNOSIS

Tinea Corporis
- *The potassium hydroxide examination or fungal culture is positive.*
- *Central clearing of lesions is noted.*
- *Honey-colored crusts are absent.*

Acute Eczematous Dermatitis
- *Dried serous exudate from acute eczema can resemble the yellow crusting of impetigo.*

MANAGEMENT

- Impetigo is a self-limited disease and the vast majority of localized cases in immunocompetent patients clear (even if untreated) in 3 to 6 weeks.
- For localized cases, first-line treatment is a topical antibiotic applied to the affected area twice daily until lesions have completely healed. Effective options include **mupirocin 2% ointment (Bactroban), bacitracin** ointment, **fusidic acid** cream or **retapamulin ointment (Altabax)**.
- In widespread cases, or if there are extensive facial lesions, systemic treatment may be required. Ideally lesions should be cultured to determine the causative agent prior to starting a systemic antibiotic. Empiric treatment should be initiated with a beta-lactamase–resistant penicillin such as **dicloxacillin** or a first- or second-generation cephalosporin such as **cephalexin** (20 to 40 mg/kg/day).
- If cultures show MRSA, treatment will be guided by the sensitivity profile. Usually **clindamycin** (10 to 25 mg/kg/day divided q6–8 hours) or **trimethoprim-sulfamethoxazole** (8 to 10 mg/kg/day divided q12 hours) are effective for cases of community-acquired MRSA.
- In infants with bullous impetigo, oral antibiotics may be required if systemic symptoms are present.
- If lesions are crusted, crusts should be gently removed with a soft washcloth after soaking.
- In cases of recurrent impetigo, patients and close contacts should be tested for the presence of *S. aureus* in the nares, a common place for carriage.
- Carriers can be treated with **mupriocin ointment** to the nares twice daily for 5 days, monthly for 3 months and then the culture should be repeated to check for clearance.

COMPLICATIONS

- **Ecthyma** (see Fig. 16.5), also called ulcerated nonbullous impetigo, is a deep dermal infection that can result from untreated impetigo, usually caused by *S. pyogenes*.
- In immunodeficient patients, the exfoliative toxin in bullous impetigo may disseminate and cause generalized staphylococcal scalded skin syndrome (see Chapter 7).
- Rarely, poststreptococcal glomerulonephritis (but not rheumatic fever) has been reported to follow impetigo caused by certain strains of streptococci.

HELPFUL HINTS

- A young child can usually return to school or a childcare setting as soon as she/he is not contagious—often within 24 hours of starting antibiotic therapy.
- Strains of *S. aureus* are usually resistant to penicillin and amoxicillin and may be resistant to erythromycin.
- Consider MRSA if skin lesions do not improve during treatment intended for methicillin-sensitive *S. aureus*.

POINT TO REMEMBER

- In cases of recurrent impetigo, household members should be questioned about skin infections and bacterial cultures should be taken from the nares of both the patient and all household members to determine carrier status of *S. aureus*.

BASICS

- Folliculitis is a common infection of the hair follicle most often caused by *Staphylococcus*.
- Bacterial folliculitis is also discussed in Chapter 16.

CLINICAL MANIFESTATIONS

- Lesions present as perifollicular pink papules and pustules (Fig. 5.4).
- In children, folliculitis most commonly occurs on the scalp, thighs, back, and buttocks.
- In adolescents, the back and chest are frequently involved (Fig. 5.5).
- In adolescent girls, the legs and axillae are common sites.

CLINICAL VARIANT

- **Irritant folliculitis** commonly occurs on the buttocks or areas of occlusion and friction in children.
- Risk factors for irritant folliculitis are occlusion/maceration, heat/humidity, shaving/plucking/waxing, topical steroids, diabetes, and atopic dermatitis.
- Commonly seen on the buttocks in school-aged children.
- Can be seen on the legs of adolescent girls.

DIAGNOSIS

- Diagnosis is based on clinical recognition.
- Bacterial culture taken from pustule fluid can identify the causative organism.

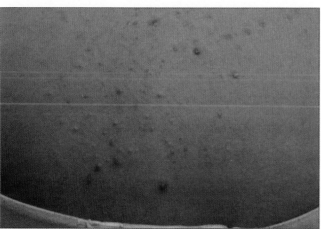

5.4 *Folliculitis.* Erythematous perifollicular papules and pustules on the back.

DIFFERENTIAL DIAGNOSIS

Keratosis Pilaris
- *Grouped keratotic perifollicular papules with rough texture.*
- *Typically located on the arms, lateral cheeks, or extensor thighs in children.*

Acne
- *Open and closed comedones are often admixed with papules and pustules.*
- *Often coexists with folliculitis in adolescents.*

Miliaria Rubra
- *Erythematous papulovesicles seen in occluded areas of the body such as the body folds and the back in infants.*

Pityrosporum Folliculitis
- *Erythematous perifollicular papules on the back and chest of young adults caused by Malassezia furfur.*
- *Resembles acne or folliculitis but is resistant to the typical acne treatments.*

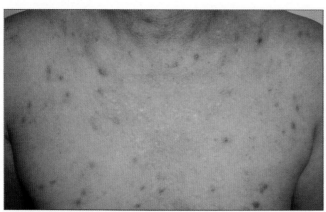

5.5 *Folliculitis.* The chest and back are a common location for folliculitis in adolescents. (Figure courtesy of Miguel R. Sanchez, MD.)

SUPERFICIAL BACTERIAL INFECTIONS

 MANAGEMENT

- Uncomplicated superficial folliculitis can be treated with antibacterial soaps, good hygiene, and topical antibiotics.
- **Mupirocin ointment** applied twice daily to affected areas is useful for localized cases.
- **Clindamycin 1%** solution, gel or lotion twice daily, is commonly used for folliculitis of the chest and back.
- Antibacterial soaps should be used in conjunction with topical antibiotics.
- Benzoyl peroxide 3% to 10% wash (**PanOxyl, Oxy10**) or chlorhexidine wash (**Hibiclens**) are often recommended.
- A novel sodium hypochlorite body wash (**CLn wash**, available at www.clnwash.com) is an effective antibacterial alternative that may be less irritating.
- Refractory, widespread, or deeper infections may require systemic antibiotics.
- First-line treatment is with a beta-lactamase-resistant penicillin, or a cephalosporin such as **cephalexin**.
- Untreated folliculitis can result in a deeper infection including furuncles, carbuncles, or cellulitis.

 POINT TO REMEMBER

- Moisture and occlusion under tight fitting athletic clothes or equipment can be a precipitating factor for folliculitis.

BASICS

- A furuncle, commonly referred to as a boil, is a deep infection of the hair follicle that usually develops from a preceding folliculitis and is most frequently seen in older children and adults (see also Chapter 16).
- Usually caused by *S. aureus* and persons who are chronic carriers of *S. aureus* are particularly predisposed.

CLINICAL MANIFESTATIONS

- Presents as a tender red nodule typically found in hairy areas of the body, especially those that are subject to friction and maceration (Fig. 5.6).
- Gradually the subcutaneous nodule becomes fluctuant and develops central suppuration (Fig. 5.7).
- If untreated, it can drain spontaneously or enlarge and become increasingly tender. When multiple furuncles coalesce the lesion is called a *carbuncle* (Fig. 5.8).

DIAGNOSIS

- Diagnosis is based on clinical recognition.

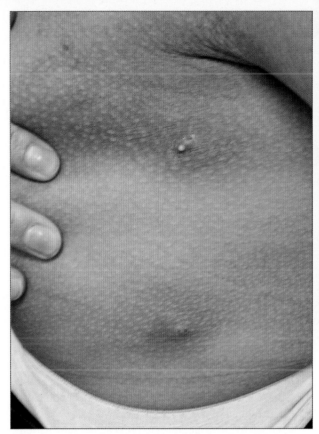

5.7 *Furuncle.* Gradually, lesions become fluctuant and develop central suppuration as noted in the spontaneous drainage of superior lesion in this picture. (Figure courtesy of Miguel R. Sanchez, MD.)

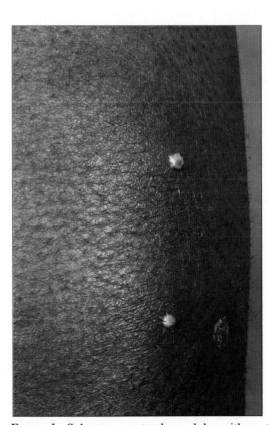

5.6 *Furuncle.* Subcutaneous tender nodules with central puncta. (Figure courtesy of Miguel R. Sanchez, MD.)

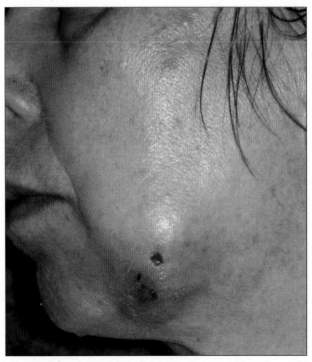

5.8 *Carbuncle.* Multiple furuncles form a carbuncle on this patient's left cheek. (Figure courtesy of Miguel R. Sanchez, MD.)

DIFFERENTIAL DIAGNOSIS

Arthropod Bite Reaction
- *Pink edematous papule or nodule and does not become fluctuant.*

MANAGEMENT

- Incision and drainage is the primary treatment for single, simple boils. Warm compresses or soaks can help to encourage spontaneous drainage.
- Bacterial culture should be sent, especially if the patient will be treated with antibiotic therapy.
- Systemic antibiotics are recommended for extensive disease or for multiple sites of infection, associated systemic symptoms, evolving cellulitis, immunosuppression, very young children or elderly, boils that are located in an area difficult to drain such as the face, hand, or genitalia, and when there is a lack of response to incision and drainage alone.
- In children, first-line antibiotics include **dicloxacillin** (12.5 to 25 mg/kg/day divided q6 hours), or **cephalexin** (25 to 50 mg/kg/day divided q6–12 hours).
- Personal hygiene measures to prevent autoinoculation or transmission include the following:
  - Keep draining wounds covered with clean, dry bandages
  - Regular bathing and cleaning of hands with soap and water or an alcohol-based hand gel, particularly after touching infected skin or an item that has directly contacted a draining wound
  - Similarly, keep high-touch surfaces clean
- Furunculosis may become recurrent in cases where patients are carriers of *S. aureus* or where there is ongoing transmission among close contacts.
- For recurrent furunculosis, treatment includes emphasis on the hygiene measures above and one of the following decolonization strategies:
  - **Mupirocin** ointment intranasally twice daily for 5 to 10 days
  - Skin antiseptic solution (e.g., **chlorhexidine**) for 5 to 14 days or **dilute bleach baths** (see Bleach Baths in The Companion eBook Edition)
  - An oral antibiotic in combination with rifampin (if the strain is susceptible) may be considered for decolonization if infections recur despite above measures
- Close contacts should be evaluated for evidence of infection.

SPECIAL CONSIDERATION: METHICILLIN-RESISTANT *STAPHYLOCOCCUS AUREUS*

- The clinical spectrum of MRSA infection ranges from asymptomatic colonization, to skin and soft tissue infection, to life-threatening invasive infection.
- Skin infections due to MRSA are becoming increasingly prevalent worldwide.
- In children, MRSA commonly presents as recurrent furunculosis or bacterial superinfection of atopic dermatitis.
- Risk factors include skin trauma, frequent skin-to-skin contact, sharing potentially contaminated personal items or equipment, and frequent exposure to antimicrobial agents.
- Consider MRSA in cases of treatment failure.
- Even if caused by MRSA, incision and drainage of a simple abscess is often sufficient as monotherapy.
- Empiric systemic treatment for skin infections secondary to MRSA should be guided by the type and site of infection and the local antibiotic susceptibility patterns.
- Typically, **clindamycin, trimethoprim-sulfamethoxazole, a tetracycline,** and **linezolid** are active against MRSA.

HELPFUL HINT

- Drainage is an essential part of the treatment of a furuncle.

POINTS TO REMEMBER

- Tetracyclines should not be used in children <8 years of age.
- In general, oral antibiotics are used for treatment of bacterial skin infections and not for decolonization.

BASICS

- Perianal streptococcal dermatitis is a superficial infection of the perianal skin, most often caused by group A beta-hemolytic streptococci (GABHS) that typically affects young children.

CLINICAL MANIFESTATIONS

- Clinical findings vary from a very subtle eruption that is overlooked to a well-demarcated area of bright pink to red erythema that extends 2 to 3 cm from anus (Fig. 5.9).
- Typically presents as a sharply demarcated, bright red erythema with a moist, tender surface.
- Occasionally the surface can be moist with an overlying pseudomembrane.
- Can also present with dry pink scaly plaque.
- Infrequently accompanied by itching, fissuring, pain, and mucoid discharge.
- May become more of a cellulitis, with possible pain on defecation.
- Fever is usually absent but sometimes patients also have streptococcal pharyngitis.

DIAGNOSIS

- Bacterial culture of the perianal skin can confirm the diagnosis.

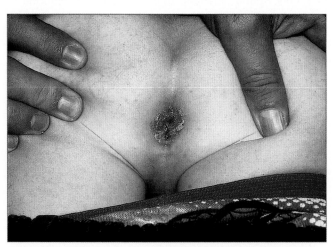

5.9 *Perianal streptococcal dermatitis.* Well-demarcated bright red erythema is characteristic of perianal streptococcal dermatitis.

DIFFERENTIAL DIAGNOSIS

Irritant Dermatitis
- *Pink eczematous plaques or superficial moist erosions caused by excess moisture or contact with urine and stool or heavy wiping and friction.*

Psoriasis
- *Well-demarcated pink scaly plaques.*
- *Typical psoriasis lesions may be present elsewhere.*

Candidiasis
- *Moist, bright pink to red patches often with satellite papules and pustules.*

Pinworm Infestation
- *Significant pruritus.*
- *Pinworms may be detected with the tape test.*

MANAGEMENT

- Topical antibiotics are often used in conjunction with oral antibiotics for symptomatic relief.
- Treatment requires with **penicillin V** (or **erythromycin** for penicillin-allergic patients) is usually effective.
- Oral **cefuroxime** was demonstrated more effective than penicillin in one study, and is another reasonable option.

HELPFUL HINT

- It is important to specify the need to check for GABHS on a rectal swab because labs may use different media for enteric pathogens.

Pitted Keratolysis

BASICS

- Pitted keratolysis is a superficial infection of the plantar feet caused by *Kytococcus sedentarius,* previously called *Micrococcus.*

PATHOGENESIS

- *K. sedentarius* produces proteases that degrade keratin.
- Risk factors for infection include hyperhidrosis, prolonged occlusion, and increased skin pH.

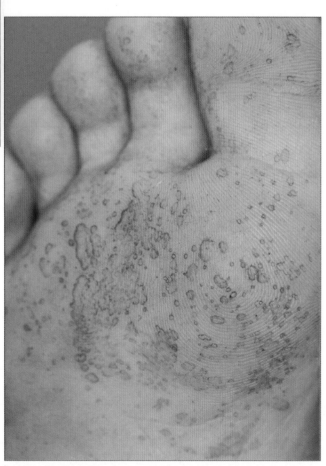

5.10 *Pitted keratolysis.* Shallow, irregular pits and craters forming in a serpiginous distribution on the sole. Malodor and hyperhidrosis are also present in this patient.

CLINICAL MANIFESTATIONS

- Redness and shallow, round and irregular pits or craters; pits coalesce to have serpiginous borders and occur on the weight-bearing parts of the soles (Fig. 5.10).
- Malodor and hyperhidrosis are common.
- Usually asymptomatic but can be associated with painful lesions, especially in children.

DIAGNOSIS

- Based on clinical findings.
- Perform Gram stain of stratum corneum shavings to find gram-positive cocci, if necessary.

 DIFFERENTIAL DIAGNOSIS

Plantar Warts
- *Interrupted dermatoglyphics.*
- *Often hyperkeratotic and firm.*

 MANAGEMENT

- Treatment is aimed at reducing the excess moisture on the skin and treating the underlying infection.
- Prescription strength topical aluminum chloride preparations (>20%) such as **Drysol** can help reduce sweating.
- Topical antibiotics such as **erythromycin, clindamycin, or mupirocin** applied twice daily can clear the infection.

6 Superficial Viral Infections

OVERVIEW

Warts and molluscum contagiosum are among the chief reasons children will visit a dermatologist. Both are the result of a superficial viral infection of the skin. Warts are caused by the human papilloma virus (HPV), and molluscum is due to the molluscum contagiosum virus, a large poxvirus. Both viruses are entirely localized to the skin (dermatotrophic) and do not cause systemic illness. Lesions are spread via skin-to-skin or skin-to-fomite contact and via autoinoculation. Despite frequent parental insistence in finding the source of infection, it is often not possible to discover a definitive source as both of these viruses are ubiquitous in the environment and highly prevalent among school-aged children.

Parents should be reassured that warts and molluscum are benign, albeit annoying, skin conditions that are temporary and usually self-resolve over time. Treatment is often required to prevent further spread or if lesions become symptomatic or are a cosmetic issue.

Superficial cutaneous infection with the herpes simplex virus can present in childhood as herpetic gingivostomatitis, herpes labialis, a focal skin infection or eczema herpeticum. Neonatal herpes simplex is a rare but potentially fatal disease that occurs when a newborn acquires the infection at birth. Oftentimes, the initial infection with herpes simplex in children is asymptomatic but the herpes virus remains latent in the sensory root ganglion and can be reactivated later in life. Superficial skin infections with herpes simplex are characterized by painful vesicles on an erythematous base and may require both antiviral therapy as well as oral analgesics.

IN THIS CHAPTER...

➤ **WARTS**

➤ **MOLLUSCUM CONTAGIOSUM**

➤ **HERPES SIMPLEX VIRUS INFECTIONS**

- Herpes gingivostomatitis
- Herpes labialis
- Cutaneous herpes infections
- Eczema herpeticum
- Neonatal herpes simplex

Warts

BASICS

- Warts are extremely commonplace in children and adolescents. The overall prevalence in school-aged children is 20%. Their prevalence sharply declines with increasing age.
- In children, warts tend to regress spontaneously but this may take several years and in the meantime can be a significant source of emotional distress and a chief reason children seek medical attention.

PATHOGENESIS

- Warts are caused by the human papillomavirus (HPV). The virus infects epidermal keratinocytes, which stimulates cell proliferation.
- Viral transmission occurs primarily through skin-to-skin contact such as handshaking or kissing. The recently shed virus can also be found on moist, warm environments, including doorknobs, hand railings, floors of locker rooms, and around swimming pools.
- Consequently, the virus is virtually impossible to avoid. Often, several family members develop warts. Whether this reflects a genetic susceptibility or is simply a result of the ubiquitous nature of the contagion has not been determined.
- Minor skin abrasions, skin trauma, active dermatitis, or maceration can facilitate viral transmission.
- Autoinoculation from the wart to adjacent skin is often seen especially for flat warts or warts on the fingers.
- It is well documented that HPV can exist in a subclinical or latent state. This latency explains the frequent recurrence of warts at the same site or at an adjacent site, even when the warts had been apparently "cured" many years earlier.

CLINICAL MANIFESTATIONS

- Warts vary widely in shape, size, and appearance and are named according to their clinical appearance and/or location. For example, filiform warts are threadlike; planar warts are flat; and plantar warts are located on the plantar surface of the feet.
- A typical wart is a papillomatous, corrugated, hyperkeratotic growth that is confined to the epidermis. Despite a common misconception, warts have no "roots," and there is no "mother wart."
- Warts may be skin colored to tan and measure 5 to 10 mm in diameter. They may also coalesce into large clusters called *mosaic warts.*
- Warts may develop anywhere on the body, but they are most often found at sites subject to frequent trauma, such as the hands and feet.
- Although HPV can be transmitted during delivery or by autoinoculation, genital warts are uncommon in children and their presence should alert consideration for sexual abuse.

CLINICAL VARIANTS

COMMON WARTS

- Common warts, also called verrucae vulgaris, occur most often on the hands and fingers often around (periungual) and under (subungual) the nails (Figs. 6.1 and 6.2). They are also frequently seen on the knees and elbows, especially in children.
- Common warts are typically verrucose (vegetative) and exophytic and characteristically result in a loss or interruption of dermatoglyphics (fingerprints and handprints).
- "Black dots," representing thrombosed dermal capillaries, are pathognomonic (Fig. 6.3).

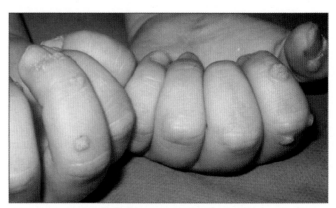

6.1 *Common warts (verruca vulgaris).* Multiple warts on fingers and around the nails (periungual).

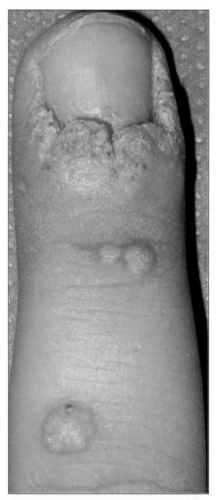

6.2 *Common warts (verruca vulgaris).* Periungual warts.

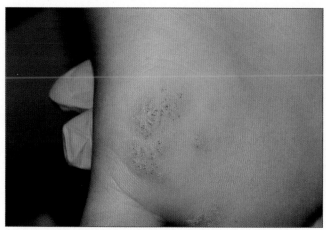

6.3 *Common warts (verruca vulgaris).* Note pathognomonic "black dots," that represent thrombosed dermal capillaries.

- Distribution is generally asymmetric.
- Common warts are usually asymptomatic, but can occasionally be tender and often cause embarrassment.

PLANTAR WARTS

- Plantar warts (verrucae plantaris) occur on and surrounding the plantar surfaces of the feet, most often on the metatarsal area, heels, insteps (Fig. 6.4), and toes in an asymmetric distribution.
- As opposed to common warts, plantar warts are usually endophytic and exhibit inward growth.
- Plantar warts may be solitary or multiple, or they may appear in clusters called *mosaic warts* (Fig. 6.5).
- As with common warts, there is loss of normal skin markings (dermatoglyphics) in the location of the wart, and pathognomonic "black dots" representing thrombosed dermal capillaries, which bleed easily after paring with a no. 15 blade (see Fig. 17.8).
- May be tender and impair ambulation, particularly when present on a weight-bearing surface, such as the sole, heal, or metatarsal areas of the foot.

FLAT WARTS

- Verrucae planae, or flat warts, are commonly found on the face, dorsa of hands, and legs.
- Lesions are small, flat-topped minimally elevated papules that are skin colored or tan (see Fig. 17.10–17.12) to brown in color, and range in size from 1 to 5 mm (Fig. 6.6). Side lighting may be necessary to see them.
- They may appear in a linear configuration due to autoinoculation (see Fig. 17.9).

FILIFORM WARTS

- Lesions present as tan, slender, delicate, finger-like growths that emanate from the skin and most commonly seen on the

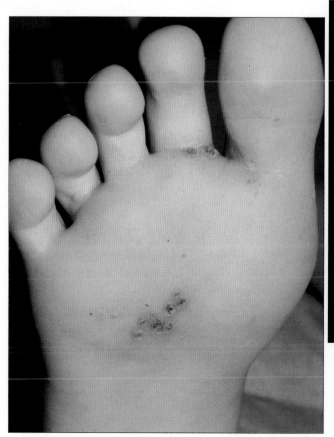

6.4 *Plantar warts (verrucae plantaris).* Note "black dots" and loss of dermatoglyphics.

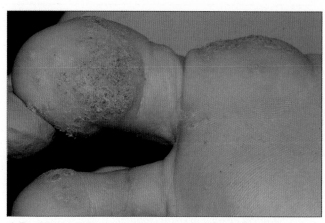

6.5 *Mosaic plantar warts (verrucae plantaris).* Multiple lesions that appear in clusters.

face—usually around the ala nasi (Fig. 6.7), mouth, eyelids, and on the neck.

DIAGNOSIS

- Based on clinical appearance.
- A biopsy to confirm diagnosis is rarely needed.

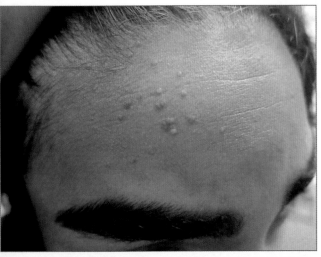

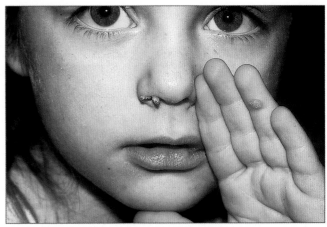

6.7 *Filiform and common warts.* This child has filiform warts on her nose and a common wart on her finger.

6.6 *Verrucae planae (flat warts).* This boy has multiple, tan-colored, flat-topped papules.

DIFFERENTIAL DIAGNOSIS

Common Warts and Flat Warts
Molluscum Contagiosum
- *Dome-shaped shiny papules, central umbilication (see below).*

Plantar Warts
Calluses
- *Broad-based hyperkeratotic plaques commonly found on the soles.*

- *Distinguished from plantar warts because they reveal an accentuation rather than interruption of skin markings.*

MANAGEMENT OF WARTS

General Principles
- The management of warts is often challenging, and there is no ideal, 100% effective treatment (see Table 6.1).
- The method of treatment depends on the following:
  - The age of the patient
  - The patient's pain threshold
  - The type and size of wart
  - The location of the lesion
  - Cosmetic or psychological considerations

Table 6.1 TOPICAL WART MEDICATIONS FORMULARY

AGENT	APPLICATION	FORMS
Topical agents: over-the-counter		
DuoFilm solution	Apply daily under occlusion	17% salicylic acid
DuoFilm patch	Apply daily	40% salicylic acid in rubber-based vehicle
Dr. Scholl's Callus Removers	Apply daily	40% salicylic acid in rubber-based vehicle
Occlusal-HP solution	Apply daily	17% salicylic acid in polyacrylic solution
Compound W gel	Apply daily	17% salicylic acid in flexible collodion
Topical agents: prescription		
Aldara	Nightly as tolerated	5% imiquimod cream
Zyclara	Nightly as tolerated	3.75% imiquimod cream
Tretinoin	Nightly as tolerated	0.025, 0.05, 0.1% cream or gel

continued on page 109

- Treatments listed below are given in a step-wise fashion, beginning with the least painful, least aggressive methods. Oftentimes, multiple treatments with different mechanisms of action are utilized at once which increases efficacy and hasten resolution.

Home Treatment
Benign Neglect
- Because most warts self-resolve, providing no treatment at all ("benign neglect") may be safe and cost effective especially if few lesions are present in cosmetically inconspicuous locations.

Duct Tape ("Ducto-Therapy")
- In some studies, duct tape occlusion for stubborn common warts was as effective as treatment with liquid nitrogen.

Instructions
1. Cut a roll of shiny, electrical (duct) tape into strips slightly larger than the size of the wart.
2. Completely wrap the affected area with two "layers" of the tape (Illus. 6.1), making it airtight, but not wrapped too tightly.
3. If possible, the tape is left on for 6 days (during bathing, working, school, and all activities), and then removed for half a day. In children, the tape will likely need to be changed daily.
4. This procedure is repeated—6 days on, 6 days off; tape is changed daily.
- After several weeks the wart will become smaller, soft, and macerated and hopefully disappears.

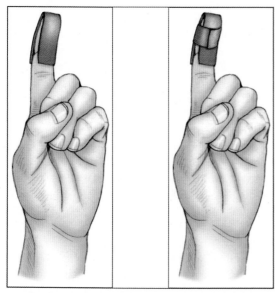

I6.1   Treating warts using "ducto therapy." (Modified courtesy of Jerome Z. Litt, MD.)

Topical Salicylic Acid Preparations
- **Salicylic acid** is a keratolytic (peeling) agent that can be self-administered. It exfoliates the hyperkeratotic "dead skin" of warts and induces inflammation.
- Salicylic acid is available in varying concentrations, in numerous over-the-counter (OTC) trade name preparations such as **Compound** W **gel** and **solution, Duofilm gel, patch**, and **solution** (see Table 6.1 for a detailed list).
- For best results with any keratolytic agent, the affected area should be hydrated first by soaking it in warm water for 5 minutes (or bathing) before application of the agent.
- Topical salicylic acid is often recommended for at home use in between in-office treatments.

Advantages
- Practical for periungual warts
- Nonscarring
- Painless to apply
- Relatively inexpensive
- Do not require office visits

Disadvantages
- Slow response
- Often no response
- Time consuming

Over-the-Counter Cryotherapy
- Salicylic acid preparations and OTC cryotherapy are among the most commonly used OTC treatments patients have tried before seeking medical attention.
- OTC cryotherapy products use the combination of dimethyl ether and propane (**Compound W Freeze Off** or **Dr. Scholl's Freeze Away**) to freeze warts to −57°F.
- Not as effective as cryotherapy with liquid nitrogen.

Immunotherapy: Interferon Induction
- Topical imiquimod, available as a 5% (**Aldara**) or a 3.75% cream (**Zyclara**), induces production of interferons α and γ and other cytokines that results in upregulation of cutaneous cell-mediated immunity.
- **Imiquimod** is approved for the treatment of genital warts (discussed in Chapter 28); however, numerous reports have shown successful off-label use on common and plantar warts, and it is widely used as an adjunctive treatment for them.
- Imiquimod cream is applied directly on the wart under duct tape occlusion after hydrating the area. This is best done at bedtime and washed off after 6 to 10 hours. It can be applied to facial flat warts without occlusion (see later discussion).

continued on page 110

SUPERFICIAL VIRAL INFECTIONS

Topical Retinoids

- Topical retinoids have antiproliferative and anti-inflammatory actions and are best for flat warts or as an adjunctive treatment for common warts as a second- or third-line option.

Topical Chemotherapy

- 5-Fluorouracil (5-FU) is a chemotherapeutic agent that prevents cellular replication and is used as a second- or third-line option for recalcitrant warts.
- 5-FU is applied directly on the wart with or without tape occlusion, which may enhance efficacy.
- It is available in a 0.5% cream (**Carac**), 1% cream (**Fluroplex**), or a 5% cream (**Efudex**) and as a 2% or 5% solution (**Efudex**). 5-FU can also be compounded with salicylic acid at compound pharmacies.

Oral Therapy

- Oral cimetidine (**Tagamet**) has been reported to induce clearance of multiple warts in children and is believed to work by inhibiting suppressor T-cell function and boosting viral specific immunity.
- Some studies have shown up to 80% clearance rates after 2 months of treatment.
- The recommended dose for immunomodulatory effects is 40 mg/kg/day divided into twice-daily doses.
- It is most often used as an adjunctive treatment in children with multiple, widespread warts that have been recalcitrant to other treatments.

In-Office Treatments

Cryotherapy with Liquid Nitrogen (LN₂)

- Liquid nitrogen (LN₂) may be applied with a cotton swab or with a cryotherapy device (**Cryogun**) (discussed in Chapter 35). The goals are a rapid freeze and a slow thaw, which will induce physical destruction of viral infected cells and/or blister formation at the dermal–epidermal junction.
- The treatment should freeze (turning it white) the wart and the surrounding 2- to 3-mm zone of skin. The freeze should last around 5 to 10 seconds. Longer freeze times may be used for thicker lesions.
- Repeated freeze–thaw cycles increase cell damage and efficacy. Three freeze–thaw cycles is ideal.
- The procedure is repeated at 2- to 3-week intervals, based on patient tolerance or on previous treatment results, degree of pain, and posttreatment morbidity.

Advantages

- Treatment is rapid and highly effective.
- Many lesions can be treated during a single office visit.
- It works well for hand warts.

Disadvantages

- Necessitates the availability of an LN₂ unit and a holding tank.
- Treatment is painful and may be unacceptable for some children.
- May result in painful blisters.
- On darkly pigmented skin, cryotherapy can result in hypopigmentation or hyperpigmentation, or even depigmentation, because LN₂ can destroy melanocytes.
- Overaggressive treatment may cause scarring.
- Often requires multiple office visits.

Electrocautery and Blunt Dissection or Curettage

- Electrocautery will burn the wart via the application of direct electrical current that conducts heat through a hot probe.
- The burned wart is then easily removed at its base with a no. 15 blade or a curette and the base is cauterized.
- Best for warts on the knees, elbows, and dorsa of hands; also effective for filiform warts.

Advantages

- Tolerable in most adults.
- Warts are removed on the day of treatment.

Disadvantages

- Local anesthesia is required. Treatment sometimes necessitates a digital block, which can be painful, especially on the fingers and the soles of the feet.
- May result in scarring.

Laser Ablation

- **Carbon dioxide (CO₂) laser** destruction of warts is reserved only for large or refractory lesions.
- **CO₂ laser** is expensive and requires local anesthesia.
- **Pulsed dye laser (PDL)**, targeting the thrombosed capillaries, has also been utilized as an adjunctive treatment of recalcitrant warts.

Sensitizing Agents

- The deliberate induction of allergic reactions by injecting or applying sensitizing agents such as *Candida* skin test antigen (**Candin**), diphencyprone (**DPCP**), and squaric acid dibutylester (**SADBE**), are sometimes used to treat recalcitrant warts.

Vesicants

- Cantharidin (**Cantharone**), or the so-called "blister beetle juice," is a vesicant (blister-producing agent) that was originally derived from the green blister beetle and is most often used for treatment of molluscum contagiosum. It can be used for recalcitrant warts.

continued on page 111

MANAGEMENT OF WARTS *Continued*

- Cantharadin is thinly applied directly on the wart and allowed to dry completely in an office setting. It should be washed off in 4 to 6 hours. In 1 to 2 days a blister or crust will form at the site of application removing the wart.
- **Cantharone Plus** is the combination of cantharidin, salicylic acid, and podophyllin in a flexible collodion and is a very potent alternative to **Cantharone** alone that may cause severe blisters and pain and should be used with caution.

Caustic Agents

- Dichloroacetic acid, trichloroacetic acid, podophyllin, formaldehyde, and glutaraldehyde have all been used, with varying results.

Intralesional Chemotherapeutic Agent

- Intradermal injections of **bleomycin**, a chemotherapy agent that inhibits cell division, is another treatment for highly resistant warts. This agent is expensive and may cause severe pain and tissue necrosis.

Surgical Excision

- Surgical excision of warts is an option
- Used for highly recalcitrant warts or for highly motivated patients

HELPFUL HINTS FOR TREATMENT OF SPECIFIC TYPES OF WARTS

Common Warts

- First line in school-aged children: LN_2.
- In between in-office treatments, use salicylic acid 17% under duct tape occlusion or salicylic acid 40% Band-Aids daily.

Plantar Warts

- Paring with a no. 15 blade parallel to the skin surface often immediately relieves pain on walking.
- The patient should be instructed to apply salicylic acid preparations between visits as follows:
  1. Warts should be "sanded" with an emery board, foot file such as **Dr. Scholl's Callous Removers**, or a pumice stone.
  2. After sanding, an OTC 17% salicylic acid solution (e.g., **Salactic film**) or a 40% salicylic acid plaster (**Mediplast**), cut to the size of the wart, is applied.
  3. This product is left overnight. The plaster may be left on for 5 to 6 days.
- LN_2, blunt dissection, electrodesiccation, and curettage are reserved for more recalcitrant warts or when patients insist on aggressive therapy.

- **Imiquimod cream** under occlusion may also be used (see earlier discussion).

Flat Warts

- First-line in-office treatments: cautious application of LN_2 therapy (e.g., with a cotton-tipped applicator) or low-intensity electrocautery.
- Imiquimod cream (**Aldara**) or tretinoin cream (**Retin-A**), applied daily to lesions, are common first-line agents for flat warts in children; these can also be applied to lesions daily in between the above in-office destructive measures.

Filiform Warts

- A virtually painless method is to dip a mosquito hemostat or a fine-tipped forceps into LN_2 for 10 seconds and then gently grasp the wart for about 4 to 5 seconds. The frozen wart is generally shed in 7 to 10 days (Fig. 6.8A,B). This method may require multiple office visits (see also Chapter 35).

continued on page 112

HELPFUL HINTS FOR TREATMENT OF SPECIFIC TYPES OF WARTS *Continued*

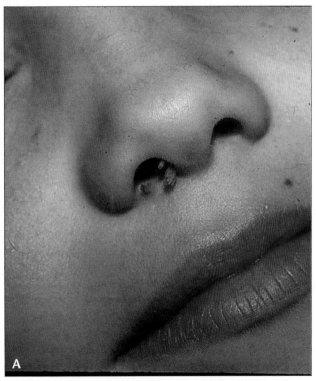

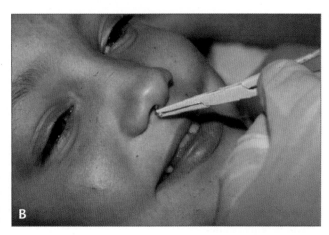

6.8 **A** and **B:** *A gentle method to treat filiform warts.* A relatively painless method is to dip a mosquito hemostat into LN$_2$ for 10 seconds and then gently grab the wart for about 4 seconds. This treatment is repeated four to five times during each visit as tolerated.

HELPFUL HINTS

- In between in-office treatments, use salicylic acid solution or plaster as an adjuvant treatment to help achieve clearance sooner. Occlude the salicylic acid with duct tape.
- Occlusion of topical home treatments such as salicylic acid or imiquimod may aid penetration and contribute to treatment efficacy.
- Warts are highly contagious and are more likely to occur on diseased skin or skin with an impaired barrier. The best way to prevent development of a new wart or spreading of existing warts in patients with atopic dermatitis is to properly treat areas of active dermatitis and maintain a healthy skin barrier with the use of barrier repairing emollients.
- How to avoid getting warts? *Never shake hands. Never kiss anyone. Never walk barefoot. Never share towels. Live in a bubble... and there's still a good chance you'll get one.*

POINTS TO REMEMBER

- Consider psychosocial factors. For example, a 2-year-old child with a filiform wart located emanating from the nostrils, or those with multiple hand warts, should warrant less aggressive treatment than a 6-year-old child with similar lesions who may be subject to teasing by other children in school.
- Freezing and other destructive treatment modalities do not kill the virus but merely destroy the cells that harbor HPV. In other words, when you treat a wart, only the "host" cells are destroyed, not the virus itself.
- Because HPV persists after therapy, some degree of infectivity and the potential for recurrence may remain, even in the absence of clinical lesions.
- Conservative, nonscarring treatments are preferred. A clinical "cure" is achieved when the skin lines are restored to a normal pattern and there is no recurrence.

BASICS

- Molluscum contagiosum (MC) is a common, self-limited superficial viral infection of the epidermis predominantly seen in otherwise healthy toddlers and school-aged children.
- There has been a drastic increase in prevalence of MC among children in the United States over the last several decades.
- MC can also be seen in immunocompromised adults and in sexually active young adults as a sexually transmitted disease. These clinical presentations are discussed in Chapter 17.

PATHOGENESIS

- MC results from a skin infection with the molluscum contagiosum virus (MCV), a member of the poxvirus family, a large DNA virus.
- The virus is spread by skin-to-skin contact or skin to infected fomite contact. Common fomites include wet towels, gym or school equipment, sponges, etc.
- Autoinoculation is a common mode of spread in children.
- Host factors play a role in acquisition of MC because not all children who have prolonged skin contact with an infected person or item develop MC, and immunocompetent adults also rarely get MC.

CLINICAL MANIFESTATIONS

- MC lesions are dome-shaped, "waxy" or "pearly" appearing, 2- to 8-mm papules with a central white core or umbilication (Figs. 6.9 and 6.10).
- Lesions usually appear in clusters or in a linear distribution (autoinoculation) in moist regions of the body such as the axillae, groin, buttocks, posterior thighs, and popliteal fossae.
- However, MC can present anywhere on the body as a single lesion or hundreds of lesions.
- "Giant molluscum," representing several smaller lesions clustered into one larger papule, can also be seen.
- MC can also become red and inflamed or develop a surrounding eczematous dermatitis, termed "molluscum dermatitis," both of which herald their spontaneous resolution (Fig. 6.11).
- In addition, eczematous id reactions or Gianotti–Crosti syndrome-like reactions (GCLRs) may develop at sites distant from the molluscum (usually on the elbows and knees) and also signals impending resolution of the MC.
- The papules of an id or GCLR may resemble molluscum and are often mistaken for a sudden increase in the number of molluscum.
- MC is generally asymptomatic, but on occasion may be slightly itchy.
- Scratching can result in secondary infection as well as spread via autoinnoculation.
- Children with atopic dermatitis are more likely to acquire MC, have a larger number of MC, and more likely to have a prolonged course.

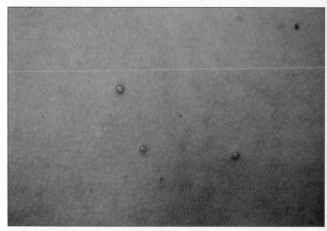

6.9 *Molluscum contagiosum.* Note the characteristic dome-shaped, "waxy" or "pearly" papules with a central white core (umbilication).

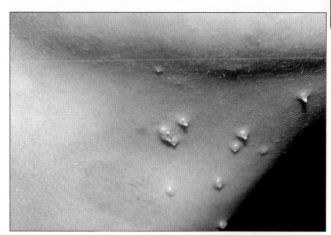

6.10 *Molluscum contagiosum.* The umbilicated centrally located cores are evident in this patient.

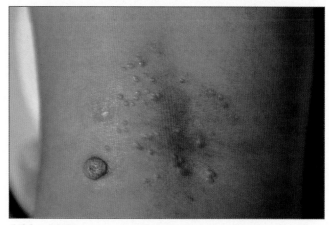

6.11 *Molluscum contagiosum.* Clusters of lesions in a linear distribution (autoinoculation) in the popliteal fossa. The surrounding eczematous dermatitis is termed "molluscum dermatitis." Note the solitary "giant molluscum."

DIAGNOSIS

- Typical molluscum papules are easily recognized and a biopsy is rarely necessary.
- Inspection with a handheld magnifier or dermatoscope often reveals the central core.
- A short application of cryotherapy with LN$_2$ accentuates the central core (Fig. 6.12A,B).

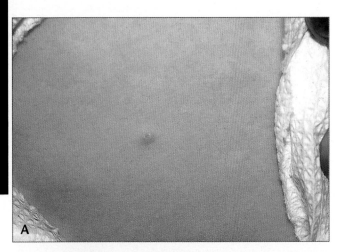

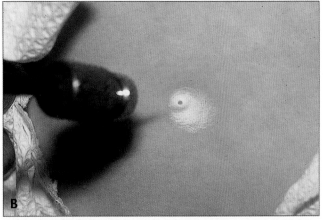

6.12   A and **B:** *Molluscum contagiosum.* A short application of cryotherapy with LN$_2$ accentuates the central core.

 ## DIFFERENTIAL DIAGNOSIS

Flat Warts
- *Skin-colored to tan, flat-topped verrucous papules, lack central umbilication.*

Id (Autoeczematization) Reaction
- *Itchy, skin-colored to slightly pink, monomorphic, eczematous papules usually located on the extensor elbows and knees occurring in response to a strong inflammatory stimulus.*
- *When present in patients with molluscum, it usually represents an immune-mediated response to molluscum and heralds clearance. Can also occur in response to allergic contact dermatitis or dermatophyte infection (e.g., tinea capitis).*

MANAGEMENT

- In the majority of children, the course is self-limiting and lesions of MC resolve within 6 to 24 months.
- Watchful waiting (for lesions to spontaneously resolve) is often appropriate, especially in children with few lesions who do not have atopic dermatitis.
- Patients and parents often seek treatment for several reasons:
  1. To help alleviate pruritus and discomfort
  2. To prevent further spread on their child or to a sibling or friend
  3. Eliminate the associated psychosocial stigma
- There is no gold-standard or FDA-approved treatment for molluscum but there are numerous destructive and immunomodulatory methods that are used to induce clearance of MC. The choice of treatment depends on: (1) the age of the patient, (2) the number of lesions present, and (3) location of the lesions.

MANAGEMENT

In Office Treatment

Cantharadin Therapy

- **Cantharadin**, an extract from the blister beetle *Cantharis vesicatoria,* compounded in a 0.7% or 0.9% solution is a very effective and painless treatment for MC and thus it is often a first-line in-office treatment option for MC in children.
- Cantharadin induces blister formation of the epidermis resulting in extrusion of the molluscum viral bodies.
- Proper application and patient education are essential for the safe use of cantharadin.
- Cantharadin should only be applied in a medical office setting preferably by the physician or other highly trained medical personnel.
- A single drop of cantharadin is applied on each MC taking care not to apply on surrounding skin using the blunt wooden end of a cotton-tipped swab or a toothpick.
- Parents should be instructed to wash off the cantharadin in 4 to 6 hours (less time if prior treatments resulted in large blister reactions) and to expect blistering or crust formation in 24 to 48 hours.
- Cantharadin should be allowed to dry completely before the patient leaves the office. Use of a handheld fan near the area of application is often useful.
- Cantharadin should not be applied on the face (especially perioral or periocular sites), in flexures or occluded areas, on mucosal surfaces or on MC with extensive MC dermatitis.
- Cantharadin is applied every 3 to 4 weeks, or until lesions resolve.
- Parents should be given written instructions that include the time the cantharadin should be washed off, and how to care for blisters and associated pain.
- *Side effects* include large blister formation, pain, pigmentary changes, and scarring.
- Currently in the United States, cantharadin is only available for in-office physician use through specialty compounding pharmacies.

Cryotherapy with Liquid Nitrogen (LN$_2$)

- Typically used to treat MC in older children and adults.
- For MC, **LN$_2$** is applied with a cotton swab or a Cryogun and frozen lightly for 2 to 5 seconds.
- LN$_2$ works by inducing blister formation allowing for extrusion of the molluscum viral bodies.
- *Side effects* include pigmentary changes, pain, and blister formation.
- The associated discomfort is many times not acceptable for young children.

Curettage

- Removal of MC with a curette is a definitive treatment option often used in adolescents and adults, with or without use of local anesthesia.

- For children amenable to this treatment, the application of lidocaine 4% cream (**LMX**) or lidocaine/prilocaine cream (**EMLA**) under occlusion to the areas of molluscum for 30 to 40 minutes prior to curettage can make the procedure painless.

At-Home Treatments

Imiquimod Cream

- Works by inducing cutaneous viral mediated immunity.
- A thin layer of imiquimod should be applied carefully to each lesion three times daily initially and if not irritating should be used daily.
- The main *side effect* is skin redness and irritation, which is more likely to occur in patients with atopic dermatitis.
- Imiquimod is available as a 5% cream (**Aldara**) or 3.75% cream (**Zyclara**).

Tretinoin Cream

- Presumed to work by inducing local skin irritation and is often used for molluscum on the face.
- **Tretinoin cream,** available in varying concentrations as a cream or gel, is applied nightly to each lesion.
- The main *side effect* is redness, irritation, and an eczematous dermatitis at the site of application.

Oral Cimetidine

- Initially found to be effective for the treatment of multiple warts, oral **cimetidine** can also induce clearance of molluscum by presumably increasing viral-mediated immunity.
- For this immunomodulatory effect, a dose of 30 to 40 mg/kg/day in two divided doses is required. The medication is taken until all lesions have resolved.
- Cimetidine is most often utilized as an adjunctive treatment for children with numerous MC.

Potassium Hydroxide

- Application of twice daily **potassium hydroxide** 5% to 10% has been reported to be effective in clearing molluscum after several weeks of use.

Other Treatments

- A plethora of OTC and over-the-internet products are available and marketed as antimolluscum treatments including salicylic acid, α-hydroxy acids, tape stripping, and natural remedies containing plant extracts (**MolluscumRx, ZymaDerm,** or **Emuaid**). Their efficacy is variable.

HELPFUL HINTS

- Parents of infected children rarely get MC.
- Recurrences of MC are rare in immunocompetent persons.
- Inflamed MC may become large, pustular, or fluctuant nodules, but the contents are usually sterile.
- Although MC are contagious, children should not be quarantined or kept home from school because of MC. The virus may be anywhere and chances are they contracted MC at school!

POINTS TO REMEMBER

- In young children with few lesions, aggressive therapy is often not necessary.
- MC in healthy, immunocompetent persons is generally self-limiting and resolves spontaneously within 6 to 24 months.
- A topical anesthetic such as lidocaine cream, applied under occlusion 1 hour before curettage, local anesthetic injection, or cryosurgery can significantly decrease discomfort.
- Redness and inflammation, surrounding eczematous dermatitis, and **Gianotti–Crosti-like reactions** are signs of immune activation and usually signal impending resolution of molluscum.

 SEE PATIENT HANDOUT "Molluscum Contagiosum" IN THE COMPANION eBOOK EDITION.

BASICS

- Infections with the herpes simplex virus can be primary or recurrent and are common in both children and adults.
- Most primary HSV infections occur in childhood and are asymptomatic or subclinical.
- HSV infections can affect mucosal and/or cutaneous surfaces and are characterized by tingling, burning, and painful vesicles on an erythematous base.
- The most common clinical presentations of HSV infection in children are herpetic gingivostomatitis, herpes labialis, or eczema herpeticum, an HSV superinfection of atopic dermatitis.
- The pathogenesis and clinical manifestations of HSV in adults are discussed in Chapter 17.

PATHOGENESIS

- Primary HSV infection results from direct contact with infected secretions or the mucocutaneous lesion itself.
- After an incubation of days to weeks, a mucocutaneous eruption may occur or the infection may be subclinical resulting only in the development of HSV antibodies.
- The virus then remains latent in the sensory root ganglion.

CLINICAL VARIANTS

HERPES GINGIVOSTOMATITIS

- Herpetic gingivostomatitis is most often seen in infants and young children and initially presents with mouth pain, irritability, and not wanting to eat or drink.
- Lesions present as painful, small vesicles on an erythematous base that rapidly evolve into shallow ulcers on the palate, tongue, or gingivae.
- Gums may be red, swollen, and bleed easily and regional lymphadenopathy is often present.
- Is usually self-limited and lesions heal within 1 to 2 weeks.
- Some patients may require IV hydration and systemic pain control in addition to antiviral therapy.

HERPES LABIALIS

- Herpes labialis, also known as a cold sore, is a herpes infection of the lips that usually occurs on the vermilion border. Occasionally, other areas of the face are involved (Fig. 6.13).
- Typically presents with a prodrome of burning, tingling, or itching of the skin that occurs 1 to 2 days before the outbreak.
- An outbreak initially starts with a pink red edematous papule that quickly evolves into a painful vesicle or cluster of vesicles on an erythematous base.
- Self-resolves without sequelae in 1 to 2 weeks; early treatment can hasten resolution.

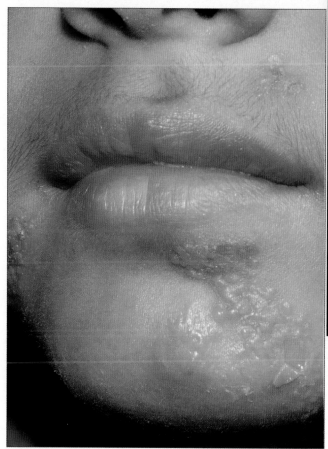

6.13 *Herpes simplex virus.* Lesions on the face consisting of multiple vesicles on an erythematous edematous base.

CUTANEOUS HERPES INFECTIONS

- Grouped small vesicles on an erythematous base can appear anywhere; when deep seated and on the distal finger is termed **herpetic whitlow**.

ECZEMA HERPETICUM

- Also known as **Kaposi varicelliform eruption** (KVE), eczema herpeticum represents a herpetic superinfection of atopic dermatitis or other chronic skin disease.
- Often initially presents with prodrome of fever and malaise.
- Later, the characteristic herpes lesions—painful vesicles and erosions—will appear on the diseased skin (Fig. 6.14).
- Eczema herpeticum can occur in a localized area of diseased skin or be extensive and widespread.
- Complications include bacterial superinfection, dehydration, and herpetic keratoconjunctivitis via direct extension if lesions are present on the face.
- Extensive cases may require hospitalization for IV antiviral therapy and IV hydration.

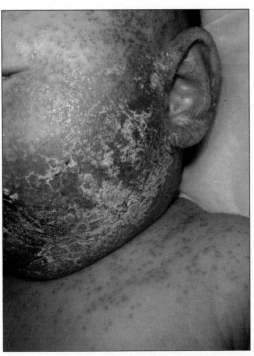

6.14 *Herpes simplex virus. Eczema herpeticum.* This eruption represents a herpetic superinfection of atopic dermatitis.

NEONATAL HERPES SIMPLEX

- Neonatal herpes simplex occurs when newborns are exposed to HSV-2 via the birth canal of an actively infected mother. Less often, infection may occur postnatally or in utero.
- Infection is most likely to occur when the mother has a primary infection during a vaginal delivery.
- Disease usually occurs within the first 4 weeks of life and may present with skin, eye, and/or mucous membrane lesions (*SEM disease*); central nervous system (CNS) involvement; or disseminated disease.
- SEM disease has the best prognosis. Disseminated and CNS disease and can result in serious morbidity and mortality.

DIAGNOSIS

- Diagnosis is based on clinical recognition.
- A Tzanck smear of vesicle contents showing multinucleated giant cells can support the diagnosis.
- The herpes virus can be detected from vesicular fluid or tissue with a viral culture, polymerase chain reaction (PCR), or via direct fluorescent antibody testing.

DIFFERENTIAL DIAGNOSIS

Herpetic Gingivostomatitis
Herpangina
- *Painful oral ulcers usually caused by a strain of the Coxsackie virus; often mistaken for herpetic gingivostomatitis.*
- *Presents with pain, refusal to eat, and high fever.*
- *Lesions present as shallow ulcerations with the rim of erythema clustered on the tonsils and soft palate.*

Hand-Foot-and-Mouth Disease (Discussed in Chapter 7)
- *Characteristic exanthem and enanthem caused by an enterovirus.*
- *Presents with prodrome of fever and malaise followed by characteristic vesicles or shallow erosions often with a rim of erythema on the tongue or buccal mucosa.*
- *On the skin, grayish white tense vesicles on an erythematous base are usually present on the palms, soles, and in the diaper area.*

Aphthous Ulcers (Discussed in Chapter 21)
- *Recurrent round or oval sores or ulcers with erythematous rim on the inside of the lips and cheeks or underneath the tongue.*
- *Lesions are painful.*
- *As with herpes simplex, the lips and gingiva are usually affected, and the back of the throat is spared.*

Stevens–Johnson Syndrome (Discussed in Chapter 27)
- *Severe drug reaction characterized by blisters and erosions in the mouth and lips often accompanied by blisters on the skin and other mucous membranes.*
- *History of medication ingestion.*

Herpes Labialis
Impetigo (Discussed in Chapter 5)
- *Superficial bacterial infection of the skin.*
- *Thin erosions with characteristic honey-colored crusts.*

Recurrent Aphthous Stomatitis (see Chapter 21)

Cutaneous Herpes Infections
Bullous Impetigo (Discussed in Chapter 5)
- *Superficial bacterial infection of the skin.*
- *Causative organism produces an epidermolytic toxin that results in bullae. Bullae easily rupture and a crusted erosion or collarette of scale remains.*

Allergic Contact Dermatitis (Discussed in Chapter 13)
- *Edematous, eczematous pink plaques with overlying vesicles in a geometric distribution corresponding to area of contact with the allergen.*

MANAGEMENT OF PEDIATRIC HSV INFECTIONS

General Principles

- The goals of treatment for any mucocutaneous herpes infection are pain reduction, shortening course of eruption, and preventing dehydration.

Systemic Treatments

- Systemic antiviral therapy with acyclovir or valacyclovir can shorten the duration of the illness especially if initiated within 1 to 2 days of symptoms.
- *Dosage:*

Acyclovir

- 200 mg/5 mL suspension; 200-mg capsules, 400- and 800-mg tablets.
- Initial infection:
  - 2 to 12 years old—1,200 mg/day divided q8h for 7 to 10 days (max 80 mg/kg/day).
  - >12 years old—1,000 to 1,200 mg/day divided q8h for 7 to 10 days (max 1,200 mg/day).
- Recurrence:
  - 2 to 12 years old—1,200 mg/day divided q8h for 5 days (max 80 mg/kg/day);
  - >12 years old—1,000 to 1,200 mg/day divided q8h for 3 to 5 days (max 1,200 mg/day).

Valacyclovir

- 500- and 1,000-mg tablets.
- Initial infection: >12 years old—1 g, twice daily for 7 to 10 days.
- Recurrence: >12 years old—2 g, twice daily × 1 day.

Topical Treatments

- Topical antiviral treatments are overall not as effective as systemic agents and include:
  Acyclovir 5% cream or ointment (**Zovirax**): apply 5×/day × 5 days.
  Penciclovir 1% cream (**Denavir**): apply every 2 hours while awake × 4 days.

  Docosanol 10% cream (**Abreva**): apply 5×/day until healed.
  Xerese (acyclovir 5% and hydrocortisone 1%) cream: apply 5×/day × 5 days.

Pain Control

- Topical anesthetic agents such as lidocaine-containing creams are helpful for pain.
- Compounded mixtures of diphenhydramine elixir, **Kaopectate** or **Maalox**, and viscous lidocaine (often called "magic mouthwash") have been used successfully as a swish and spit or swish and swallow to help lessen oral pain and help facilitate oral intake.
- Oral nonsteroidal anti-inflammatories (NSAIDs) such as ibuprofen taken can also be beneficial for reducing pain and inflammation.

Hydration

- Some children may require hospitalization for IV hydration.

Eczema Herpeticum (Kaposi's Varicelliform Eruption [KVE])

- In addition to systemic antivirals, eczema herpeticum should also be treated with meticulous skin care including using thick bland emollients to all areas with vesicles and erosions.
- Once most healing has occurred, the underlying skin disease should be treated with topical anti-inflammatory agents.

Neonatal Herpes Simplex

- Often requires aggressive inpatient and/or intensive medical care including IV antivirals and supportive care.

 HELPFUL HINT

- Use oral anti-inflammatories such as acetaminophen or ibuprofen to help with HSV associated pain.

 POINT TO REMEMBER

- Initiate antiviral treatment at first sign of prodrome for best chance of shortening course of eruption.

CHAPTER 7
Viral and Bacterial Exanthems

OVERVIEW

In its broadest sense, the term exanthem refers to a widespread cutaneous manifestation of a systemic illness. In children, exanthems are most often the result of a viral infection and less often due to a bacterial infection or a drug reaction. The exanthem can be the initial sign of the illness, can appear as the illness is resolving, or even can appear once it has resolved. The eruption may or may not be pruritic and is usually accompanied by systemic symptoms such as fever, malaise, and headache. Some viruses, such as varicella and measles, trigger specific, well-recognized eruptions, while most viruses result in a nonspecific exanthem, making an exact diagnosis unlikely.

The classic childhood exanthems were numerically designated according to historical appearance in the early 1900s and include measles (first disease), scarlet fever (second disease), rubella (third disease), erythema infectiosum (fifth disease), and roseola infantum (sixth disease).

All have a viral etiology except scarlet fever, which is caused by group A *streptococcus*. Measles and rubella are encountered much less often today because of routine vaccination of young children; however, outbreaks still occur all over the world.

In addition to the classic childhood exanthems, this chapter will discuss the distinct, recognizable presentations of hand-foot-and-mouth disease, the Gianotti–Crosti syndrome, unilateral thoracic exanthem, and the nonspecific viral exanthems, which are clinical characteristics, but can have several viral triggers. The clinical presentation of exanthems associated with toxin-producing *Staphylococcus* and *Streptococcus* will also be presented.

Although exact identification of the infectious agent that has triggered a particular exanthem is not always possible, a definitive diagnosis may be critical, particularly for pregnant and immunocompromised patients in whom certain viral infections can have serious consequences. It is also important to distinguish viral exanthems from rashes caused by treatable bacterial or rickettsial infections and from hypersensitivity reactions to medications. Familiarity with the most common childhood exanthems can aid in prompt recognition, diagnosis, and appropriate management including counseling on avoidance of contact with at-risk persons.

Measles (Rubeola)

BASICS

- Measles is a viral illness characterized by a distinctive exanthem and enanthem.
- The incidence of measles in the United States has decreased dramatically since the introduction of the measles vaccine; however, outbreaks still occur in both industrialized and nonindustrialized nations due to vaccine fears and nonimmunized persons.

PATHOGENESIS

- The measles virus is a single-stranded RNA virus of the Paramyxoviridae family.
- Measles is highly contagious and transmission occurs via respiratory droplets.
- The incubation period lasts from 9 to 11 days.
- The primary site of infection is the respiratory epithelium of the oropharynx.

CLINICAL MANIFESTATIONS

- Measles usually presents with a prodrome of fever, cough, coryza, conjunctivitis, and photophobia.
- Patients appear acutely ill, and often have cervical and preauricular lymphadenopathy.
- Koplik spots, the pathognomonic enanthem composed of small bluish-white macules on the buccal mucosa appear during the prodrome, prior to the exanthem, and provide an opportunity for early diagnosis (Fig. 7.1).
- The exanthem appears 3 to 5 days after the onset of the prodromal illness.
- Lesions begin as discrete erythematous macules and papules which soon coalesce into areas of confluent erythema starting on the forehead and behind the ears and quickly spread to the neck, trunk, and extremities in a cephalocaudal direction over 2 to 3 days (Fig. 7.2).
- The eruption lasts 4 to 7 days and resolves in the same order as it appeared with fine desquamation.

COMPLICATIONS

- Pneumonia is the most common complication. In children, primary measles pneumonitis occurs, whereas in adults, secondary bacterial pneumonias are more common.
- Otitis, encephalitis, and myocarditis can also occur.

DIAGNOSIS

- The diagnosis of measles is usually made on clinical grounds.
- Although usually unnecessary, serologic testing for measles-specific IgM or IgG can help establish the diagnosis.
- The virus can also be detected with PCR techniques from upper respiratory secretions or urine.

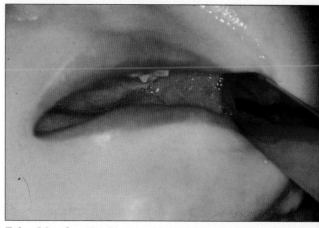

7.1 Measles. Koplik spots have been described as appearing like grains of salt on a red background. These appear 48 hours prior to the classic measles eruption and are pathognomonic for measles. Such lesions are located opposite premolar teeth.

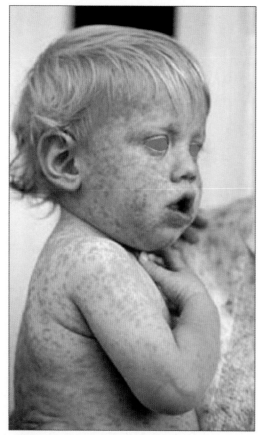

7.2 Measles. The typical measles exanthema begins as discrete erythematous macules and papules that quickly coalesce into areas of confluent erythema, starts on the forehead and behind the ears, and spreads downward to trunk and extremities.

DIFFERENTIAL DIAGNOSIS

Rubella
- *Prodromal symptoms are much more mild.*
- *Koplik spots are absent.*
- *The rash is of shorter duration.*

Scarlet Fever
- *Severe constitutional symptoms and pharyngitis are noted.*
- *Patients have a "strawberry tongue."*
- *A "sandpapery" exanthem occurs.*
- *Marked desquamation is associated with resolution.*

Roseola
- *A high prodromal fever occurs in the absence of other symptoms.*

Drug Hypersensitivity Reaction
- *This is usually associated with marked pruritus.*
- *The exanthem lasts longer than in measles.*

 MANAGEMENT

- In most cases, measles is a benign and self-limited infection. Recovery is usually complete within 14 days of the onset of the prodrome.
- No specific therapy for measles exists. Supportive care should be provided, and patients should be isolated from susceptible persons.
- Routine immunization is recommended for all children with initial dose at 12 to 15 months of age and a second dose at 4 to 6 years of age.
- Measles vaccine or antimeasles immunoglobulin administered within 3 days of exposure can provide some protection to unvaccinated patients.

 HELPFUL HINTS

- A patient with measles becomes contagious 3 days before onset of the rash and remains so until desquamation of the rash.
- All cases should be reported to local public health officials.

Rubella (German Measles)

BASICS

- Rubella is a mild viral illness that, because of its devastating effects on the developing human fetus, is recognized as a major public health issue.
- The incidence of rubella has declined markedly since mass immunization for rubella began in 1969.

PATHOGENESIS

- The rubella virus is an RNA virus of the *Togaviridae* family and is transmitted via respiratory droplets.
- The incubation period is 16 to 18 days.
- Humans are the only known natural hosts where initial infection occurs in the nasopharyngeal mucosa.

CLINICAL MANIFESTATIONS

- Rubella presents with a mild prodromal illness of fever, headache, upper respiratory symptoms, and lymphadenopathy.
- The prodrome is often subclinical in children, but tends to be more severe in older patients.
- One to five days following the prodrome, the exanthem appears as discrete pink to red macules and papules on the face that spreads to the trunk and extremities within 24 hours (cephalocaudal direction; Fig. 7.3).
- Lesions may coalesce to form an erythematous rash reminiscent of scarlet fever.
- The eruption is characteristically short-lived, fading in 1 to 3 days in the same order it appeared sometimes accompanied by fine, branny desquamation.
- Petechiae may also be present on the soft palate and are called Forschheimer spots.
- The exanthem is often accompanied by tender lymphadenopathy especially of the postauricular, suboccipital, and posterior cervical lymph nodes.
- Constitutional symptoms usually resolve within 24 hours of the onset of the rash but in some cases the lymphadenopathy persists for weeks.
- The eruption may be pruritic, particularly in adults.

COMPLICATIONS

- Complications are rare.
- Infection during the first 20 weeks of pregnancy can result in fetal death or the congenital rubella syndrome that is

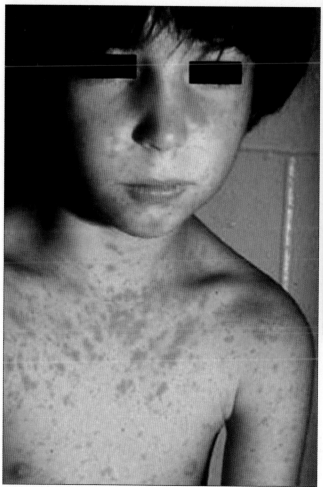

7.3 *Rubella.* The eruption begins on the face and spreads to trunk and extremities within 24 hours and is very short-lived.

characterized by cataracts, deafness, and congenital CNS and heart defects.

DIAGNOSIS

- The clinical features of rubella are not distinctive enough to allow one to make the diagnosis with certainty based on the clinical presentation alone.
- Although unnecessary in most cases, acute and convalescent antibody titers (IgM and IgG) can confirm the diagnosis. These tests are important in pregnant women who may have been exposed to rubella.

DIFFERENTIAL DIAGNOSIS

Measles
- *Prodromal symptoms are of greater severity.*
- *Koplik spots are present.*
- *The rash lasts longer.*

Roseola
- *A high prodromal fever occurs in the absence of other symptoms.*
- *The morphologic appearance and duration of the exanthem are similar to those of rubella.*

Erythema Infectiosum
- *Patients have a distinctive "slapped cheek" erythema.*
- *A lacy, reticular eruption occurs on the extremities.*
- *The exanthem lasts longer than in rubella.*

Scarlet Fever
- *Severe constitutional symptoms and pharyngitis are noted.*
- *Patients have a "strawberry tongue."*
- *A "sandpapery" exanthem occurs.*
- *Marked desquamation is associated with resolution (see Fig. 7.20A,B).*

Drug Reaction
- *May be associated with marked pruritus.*
- *The exanthem lasts longer than rubella.*

 MANAGEMENT

- No specific therapy is available. When necessary, supportive care including antipyretics or anti-inflammatory medications for arthralgias should be provided.
- Rubella immunization is recommended for all children as an initial dose at 12 to 15 months of age and a second dose at 4 to 6 years of age.
- Infected patients should be isolated from susceptible persons.

 HELPFUL HINT

- **Rubella immunization** should be well documented in women of childbearing age; if antirubella antibody titers are negative, rubella immunization should be given.

Erythema Infectiosum (Fifth Disease)

BASICS

- Erythema infectiosum is a common viral illness due to parvovirus B19 that typically occurs in the late winter and spring among school-age children.

PATHOGENESIS

- Parvovirus B19, a single-stranded DNA virus of the Parvoviridae family, is transmitted from person to person through respiratory secretions.
- The incubation period lasts 4 to 14 days, but it may be as long as 3 weeks.

CLINICAL MANIFESTATIONS

- Some patients experience a mild prodrome of low-grade fever, malaise, upper respiratory symptoms, or headache 2 days before the onset of the rash.
- Typically the exanthem of erythema infectiosum progresses through following three phases:
  1. First is the characteristic bright red facial erythema involving the malar surfaces classically sparing the nasal bridge, periorbital, and perioral areas resulting in the so-called "slapped cheeks" appearance (Fig. 7.4).
  2. One to 4 days later, a lacy, reticular erythematous exanthem composed of discrete macules and papules on the extensor surfaces of the extremities appears and later spreads to the trunk and buttocks (Fig. 7.5A,B). The palms and soles are usually spared.
  3. The third phase occurs in only *some* patients and is characterized by periodic recrudescence of the reticular erythema in response to physical stimuli such as heat, friction, sunlight, or warm baths.
- Some children may experience mild joint pain that resolves within several weeks but occasionally can persist for several months.

CLINICAL VARIANTS

- Parvovirus B19 infection can be associated with a **symmetric polyarthropathy**, involving the hands, feet, elbows, and knees usually affecting adult women.
- Infection with parvovirus B19 can also present as **papular-purpuric gloves and socks syndrome (PPGSS)**, which is characterized by painful erythema, petechiae, and purpura involving the palms and soles, occurring most often in older children and young adults.
- PPGSS may be associated with a mild prodrome and an enanthem. Therapy is symptomatic and spontaneous resolution occurs in 1 to 2 weeks.

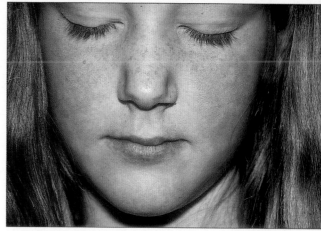

7.4 *Erythema infectiosum.* "Slapped cheeks": The erythema favors the malar surfaces. The slapped cheek appearance on this child is further accentuated by a tendency to spare the nasal bridge and the periorbital and perioral areas.

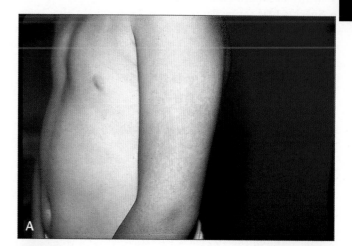

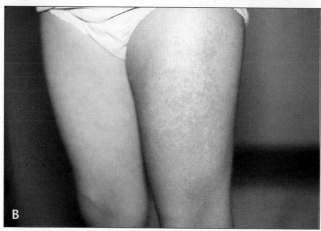

7.5 *Erythema infectiosum.* She also has the characteristic reticular ("lacy") pattern of lesions on her arms (**A**) and similar lesions on her legs (**B**).

COMPLICATIONS

- Due to its affinity for red blood cell precursors, parvovirus B19 infection during pregnancy can lead to varying degrees of fetal anemia and is associated with a 4.2% to 9% risk of hydrops fetalis and fetal death. Risk is greatest with infection during the first 20 weeks of pregnancy.
- In patients with sickle cell disease, hereditary spherocytosis, and thalassemia intermedia, parvovirus B19 infection can lead to aplastic crises.
- Infected immunocompromised patients are at risk of chronic red cell aplasia or generalized bone marrow failure.

DIAGNOSIS

- The diagnosis is based on the characteristic clinical presentation.
- Although usually unnecessary, serologic detection of parvovirus B19 IgM as soon as 3 days after the onset of the exanthem can confirm recent infection.
- Specific IgM antibodies persist for 2 to 3 months after acute infection.

DIFFERENTIAL DIAGNOSIS

Erysipelas on the Face
- *Group A beta-hemolytic streptococcal infection involving the dermis.*
- *Presents as deep erythema with sharply demarcated borders.*

Roseola (Exanthem Subitum)
- *Characteristic clinical course of high fever followed by a morbilliform rash upon defervescence.*
- *Eruption consists of pink macules and papules on the neck and trunk.*

Scarlet Fever
- *Eruption is morbilliform and begins on the neck and trunk and spreads to the extremities.*
- *May have associated pharyngitis.*

Rubella
- *Mild prodrome followed by exanthem.*
- *Exanthem consists of discrete macules and papules that begin on the face and then spread to the trunk and extremities within 24 hours.*

MANAGEMENT

- Erythema infectiosum is benign and self-limited. The exanthem resolves in 1 to 2 weeks.
- Supportive care is all that is required for uncomplicated cases.
- No effective antiviral therapy exists for parvovirus B19.
- Immunocompromised and chronic anemia patients should have blood counts monitored closely.
- Pregnant patients should have appropriate fetal monitoring.

HELPFUL HINT

- By the time the characteristic exanthem of parvovirus B19 appears, the patient is unlikely to be infectious.

POINTS TO REMEMBER

- Facial erythema is often absent in infected adults.
- Because they are at risk for aplastic crisis, all patients with erythema infectiosum who have chronic anemia should have a complete blood cell count.

BASICS

- Roseola infantum, or exanthem subitum, is an acute viral illness marked by a high fever that characteristically resolves with the onset of the rash.
- The majority of cases occur in children 6 months to 3 years and presents more often during the spring.

PATHOGENESIS

- Roseola is caused by herpesvirus type 6 (HHV-6) that is spread via respiratory secretions.
- The incubation period is 7 to 15 days before the onset of symptoms.
- As with other herpesvirus infections, it is likely that HHV-6 establishes a latent infection after the acute illness. The isolation of HHV-6 from the saliva of healthy adults supports this view.

CLINICAL MANIFESTATIONS

- A prodrome of high fever for 3 to 5 days in an otherwise well child typically precedes the exanthem.
- On occasion, the fever is accompanied by coryza, cough, headache, or abdominal pain.
- The exanthem appears 1 day before to 1 day after defervescence and consists of discrete, "rose pink" macules or papules, 1 to 5 mm in diameter, often with a surrounding rim of pallor that frequently coalesce to form areas of confluent erythema (Fig. 7.6).
- A widespread distribution is seen, with lesions appearing on the trunk, buttocks, neck, and, occasionally, the face and limbs.
- The exanthem typically clears within 1 to 2 days, although it may persist for up to 10 days.
- Occipital, cervical, and postauricular lymphadenopathy is commonly present.

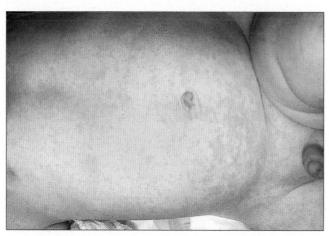

7.6   *Roseola.* The typical exanthem appears 1 day before to 1 day after the fever subsides. (Courtesy of Bernard A. Cohen, MD; http://dermatlas.org.)

- Complications are uncommon and include seizures, encephalitis, and thrombocytopenia.

DIAGNOSIS

- The characteristic clinical presentation is usually sufficient for diagnosis.
- The diagnosis can be confirmed by detection of IgM to HHV-6 or a fourfold rise in IgG titers to the virus over time.

 DIFFERENTIAL DIAGNOSIS

Other Febrile Viral Exanthems
- *Measles, rubella, enteroviral exanthems, and nonspecific viral exanthems can also present with fever and a diffuse rash.*

Scarlet Fever
- *This has severe constitutional symptoms and characteristic oral changes. It resolves with acral desquamation.*

Drug Reaction
- *Typically is not preceded by high fever.*
- *The rash is usually of longer duration (see Chapter 26).*

 MANAGEMENT

- The eruption fades completely without sequelae over a few days.
- During the prodromal phase of illness, antipyretics are often useful, particularly because they may reduce the risk of febrile seizures, which have been reported to occur in up to 10% of patients.

 POINT TO REMEMBER

- Infection with HHV-6 is one of the most common causes of febrile illness in young children.

Hand-Foot-and-Mouth Disease

BASICS

- Hand-foot-and-mouth disease (HFMD) is the most familiar enteroviral exanthem and typically occurs in 1- to 4-year-old children as a vesiculopustular eruption with a characteristic distribution.

PATHOGENESIS

- HFMD is most often caused by coxsackievirus A16 but can also result from other enteroviruses including other coxsackie A and B serotypes, echoviruses, and enteroviruses.
- The virus is spread via the fecal–oral route and the incubation period ranges from 4 to 6 days.
- Outbreaks typically occur in the summer or early fall.

CLINICAL MANIFESTATIONS

- A 1- to 2-day prodrome of fever, malaise, and abdominal pain may be seen.
- The illness most frequently begins as a sore throat or mouth and refusal to eat secondary to the oral lesions (enanthem) of HFMD (Fig. 7.7).
- The enanthem presents as 1- to 5-mm vesicles or shallow erosions often with a rim of erythema.
- The exanthem follows the development of oral lesions and presents as round or angulated, grayish white tense vesicles that are typically 3 to 7 mm in diameter (Fig. 7.8).
- Lesions are usually not pruritic although they may be painful.
- In contrast to most viral illnesses, lymphadenopathy is absent to minimal.
- Although in general complications are rare, the one seen most frequently is aseptic meningitis.

DISTRIBUTION OF LESIONS

- The enanthem appears most commonly on the tongue and buccal mucosa and occasionally on the lips, palate, and gums.
- The exanthem is characteristically present on the palms and soles and less often on the dorsal or lateral aspects of the fingers and toes. All three sites may not be involved at the time of presentation. A typical cutaneous lesion has an elliptical vesicle surrounded by an erythematous halo. The long axis of the lesion is oriented along the skin lines (Fig. 7.9).
- Occasionally the eruption is more widespread on arms and legs.
- The diaper area in infants is also a common area of involvement.
- Occasionally, lesions may extend onto the proximal extremities.

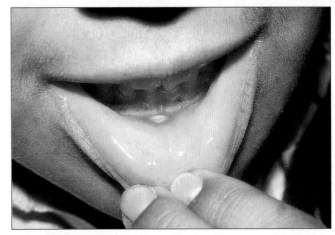

7.7 Hand-foot-and-mouth disease. Oral lesion. Note the oval shape and rim of erythema on this child's oral labial mucosa.

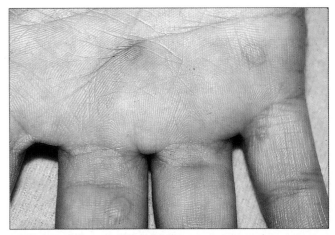

7.8 Hand-foot-and-mouth disease. Oval intact vesicles are noted on the palm.

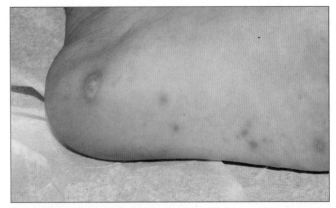

7.9 Hand foot-and mouth disease. Characteristic appearance of HFMD exanthem on the sole of a 5-year-old child.

DIAGNOSIS

- Diagnosis is made on the basis of the characteristic clinical presentation and distribution of lesions.
- Although not routinely indicated, laboratory testing can confirm the diagnosis. The virus can be cultured or detected with PCR from throat washings or stool, with the latter giving a higher yield.
- Acute and convalescent sera show an elevation in antibody titer to the causative virus.

 MANAGEMENT

- Treatment is with supportive care.
- Treat fever and pain with **acetaminophen** and **ibuprofen**.
- It is most important to encourage continued intake of liquids to prevent dehydration.
- Ice pops and cold liquids can help throat pain.

 POINT TO REMEMBER

- The course of HFMD is self-limited, lasting less than a week in most cases.

 DIFFERENTIAL DIAGNOSIS

Primary Oral Herpes Simplex (see Chapters 6 and 17)
- *Typically affects the lips and gingiva, sparing the back of the throat.*
- *Outbreaks tend to be recurrent and occur in the same location.*
- *A Tzanck smear and culture are positive for HSV.*

Aphthous Ulcers
- *Lesions are painful.*
- *As with herpes simplex, the lips and gingiva are usually affected, and the back of the throat is spared.*

Herpangina
- *Small, painful vesicular or ulcerative lesions occur on the roof of the mouth and in the throat.*
- *White to whitish-gray base and a red border.*
- *Usually caused by coxsackie virus, typically coxsackie group A viruses.*
- *Typically occurs during the summer and frequently affects children, but it also may occur in young adults.*
- *Mouth ulcers, high fever, sore throat, and headache are the characteristics.*
- *Systemic symptoms may precede the appearance of lesions.*

BASICS

- Gianotti–Crosti syndrome (GCS) is a clinically distinct viral exanthem, originally thought to occur secondary to hepatitis B, but now known to occur following infection with several viral triggers or after vaccinations.
- The eruption most often occurs in young children in the spring and early summer.

PATHOGENESIS

- GCS is a cutaneous response to various infections and has been linked to numerous viral agents including Epstein–Barr virus (EBV), cytomegalovirus, parvovirus, coxsackie virus, respiratory syncytial virus, rotavirus, and influenza A, among others.

CLINICAL MANIFESTATIONS

- GCS is often preceded by a mild prodrome that can include constitutional symptoms, lymphadenopathy, and/or upper respiratory symptoms.
- The eruption of GCS is characterized by monomorphic skin-colored to pink edematous papules and papulovesicles distributed symmetrically on the extensor surfaces of the upper and lower extremities, buttocks, and face (Figs. 7.10 and 7.11).
- Papules may coalesce to pink edematous plaques.
- The trunk is notably spared.
- It is usually asymptomatic although pruritus may be present.

DIAGNOSIS

- Diagnosis is based on clinical recognition.
- After a thorough history and physical examination, laboratory tests to detect a specific viral etiology should be performed if clinically indicated.

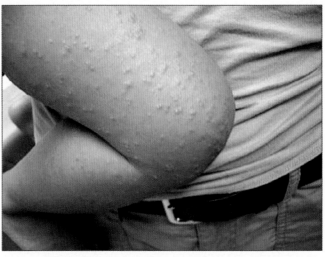

7.10 *Gianotti–Crosti syndrome.* Pink monomorphic edematous papules, characteristic of Gianotti–Crosti on the extensor arm. This eruption resolves without sequelae in 3 to 6 weeks.

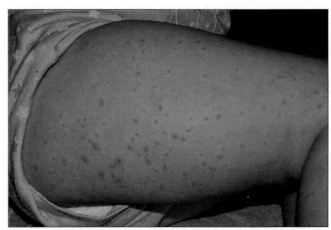

7.11 *Gianotti–Crosti syndrome.* This patient had fever and nonspecific viral symptoms 1 week prior to the appearance of pink edematous papules on her buttocks, posterior thighs, and knees. The lesions were very itchy.

 DIFFERENTIAL DIAGNOSIS

Id Reaction (see Chapter 13)
- *An itchy, eczematous eruption that can present as monomorphic erythematous or skin-colored papules localized to the extensor elbows and knees resembling GCS.*
- *Also called autoeczematization, an Id reaction is usually triggered by a severe inflammatory dermatosis such as allergic contact dermatitis, molluscum contagiosum, or fungal infections.*

Drug Eruption (see Chapter 26)
- *Pink-red blanching macules and papules that begin on the face and neck and spread caudally.*
- *Pruritus is common.*
- *History of inciting drug ingestion in the preceding 7 to 14 days.*

Molluscum Contagiosum (see Chapter 6)
- *Molluscum, particularly when inflamed and located on the extensor knees and elbows, can mimic GCS.*

MANAGEMENT

- Gianotti–Crosti syndrome is self-limited; spontaneous resolution usually occurs within 3 to 4 weeks but may take 8 to 12 weeks.
- Lymphadenopathy may persist for 2 to 3 months.
- Lesions may resolve with postinflammatory hyperpigmentation.
- Treatment is supportive.
- If pruritic, topical corticosteroids and antipruritic creams may provide some benefit.

HELPFUL HINT

- A Gianotti–Crosti syndrome-like eruption can also occur as a response to molluscum contagiosum and often heralds resolution of molluscum. This eruption is often pruritic.

POINT TO REMEMBER

- The extent and intensity of the eruption can be impressive and recognition of the characteristic distribution and morphology of GCS can help to quickly reassure parents.

Unilateral Laterothoracic Exanthem

BASICS

- Unilateral laterothoracic exanthem (ULE), also called unilateral periflexural exanthem of childhood, is a peculiar unilateral eruption that typically occurs on the trunk in young children.
- It is most often seen in the winter or spring.

PATHOGENESIS

- The exact etiology of ULE is unknown, but it is thought to be a distinct reaction pattern to a variety of potential infectious triggers, most likely viral.

CLINICAL MANIFESTATIONS

- A prodrome of low-grade fevers with respiratory or gastrointestinal symptoms may occur.
- The eruption begins on one side of the trunk, usually near the axilla, but occasionally on the inguinal creases. Initially lesions are pink morbilliform or eczematous macules and papules that sometimes have a surrounding pale halo. The lesions may coalesce (Fig. 7.12).

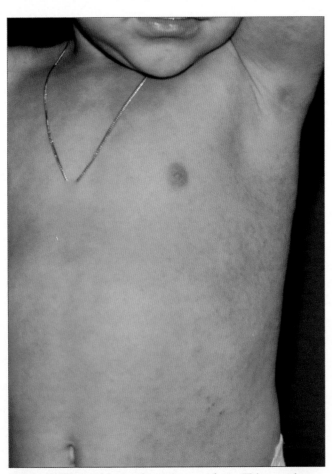

7.12 *Unilateral laterothoracic exanthem.* This eruption of pink eczematous papules began near the axilla and spread downward on the trunk. ULE usually remains localized to one side of the body and resolves in 3 to 6 weeks.

- The eruption spreads centrifugally and may become bilateral but always maintains predominance on the originating side.
- Over time, lesions become scaly and may develop a central dusky or gray color.
- Pruritus may occur and is usually mild.
- Resolves with desquamation.

DIAGNOSIS

- Diagnosis is based on clinical recognition.

 DIFFERENTIAL DIAGNOSIS

Contact Dermatitis (see Chapter 13)
- *Eczematous, edematous papules, and plaques often in a geometric distribution coinciding with areas of contact to the allergen.*
- *Often very pruritic.*

Nonspecific Viral Exanthem
- *Constitutional symptoms may be present.*
- *Resolves quickly within 1 to 2 weeks and is usually asymptomatic.*

Drug Eruption
- *Pink-red blanching macules and papules that begin on the face and neck and spread caudally.*
- *Pruritus is common.*
- *History of inciting drug ingestion in the preceding 7 to 14 days.*

 MANAGEMENT

- ULE resolves spontaneously without sequelae in 3 to 6 weeks.
- Sometimes complete resolution is delayed up until 8 weeks.
- Treatment is symptomatic with topical corticosteroids and antipruritics as necessary.

 POINT TO REMEMBER

- ULE can be bilateral and more widespread but usually maintains unilateral predominance.

BASICS

- The vast majority of viral exanthems in children are nonspecific and lack a distinctive prodrome, lesion morphology, enanthem, or distribution.
- The exanthem often presents abruptly as a widespread, generalized, asymptomatic eruption.

PATHOGENESIS

- Numerous viruses have been associated with nonspecific viral exanthems, most commonly enteroviruses, adenovirus, parainfluenza virus, respiratory syncytial virus, and influenza virus.

CLINICAL MANIFESTATIONS

- A prodrome or concurrently associated features may include low-grade fever, myalgias, headache, rhinorrhea, or gastrointestinal symptoms.
- In children the prodrome may be mild or subclinical and the exanthem is the most prominent feature, which brings the child to medical attention.
- The eruption usually begins abruptly with blanchable erythematous macules and papules on the trunk and extremities, usually sparing the face (Fig. 7.13).
- The exanthem is typically asymptomatic.

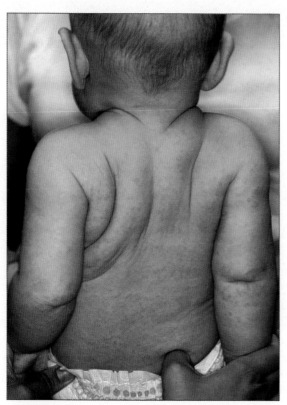

7.13 *Nonspecific viral exanthem.* The eruption shown here was preceded by 3 days of upper respiratory viral symptoms.

DIAGNOSIS

- Diagnosis is based on clinical recognition and ruling out other eruptions that may require treatment or further investigation.
- Identification of the exact etiologic agent is oftentimes not necessary or clinically feasible.

 DIFFERENTIAL DIAGNOSIS

Drug Eruption
- *Pink-red blanching macules and papules that begin on the face and neck and spread caudally.*
- *Pruritus is common.*
- *History of inciting drug ingestion in the preceding 7 to 14 days.*

Id Reaction or Id Dermatitis
- *An acute eczematous eruption characterized by itchy skin-colored to pink papules symmetrically distributed on the extensor extremities and trunk.*
- *Also called autoeczematization, it is usually triggered by a severe inflammatory dermatosis such as allergic contact dermatitis, molluscum contagiosum, or fungal infections.*

Kawasaki Disease
- *A small vessel vasculitis characterized by fever (lasting at least 5 days), conjunctivitis, oral mucosal erythema, cervical lymphadenopathy, and erythema of the palms and soles in addition to a widespread, nonspecific eruption.*

 MANAGEMENT

- Nonspecific viral exanthems are usually self-limited and the eruption resolves over 1 to 2 weeks.
- Supportive treatment with antipyretics, hydration, and use of bland emollients is generally sufficient.
- If pruritus is present, topical corticosteroids are occasionally helpful.

 POINT TO REMEMBER

- Nonspecific viral exanthems are the most common viral exanthems seen in children and are one of the chief reasons for pediatric urgent care visits.

Varicella (Chickenpox)

BASICS

- Varicella, or chickenpox, is an infection caused by the varicella-zoster virus (VZV).
- The incidence of chickenpox has drastically decreased with the introduction of routine vaccination in 1996.
- Nonetheless, chickenpox is still seen in areas of the world where vaccination is not routine mostly in young children.
- In countries with routine vaccination, chickenpox is still seen in immunocompromised patients and the elderly due to waning immunity.

PATHOGENESIS

- Varicella zoster virus, also called human herpesvirus-3 (HHV-3), is transmitted via aerosolized droplet and initially presents as an upper respiratory infection.
- Primary viremia occurs 3 to 4 days after infection followed by a secondary viremia that occurs cyclically over a period of approximately 3 days and results in successive crops of lesions.
- The incubation period is 2 weeks (range 10 to 21 days) after contact with an infected person.

CLINICAL MANIFESTATIONS

- Chickenpox often begins with a prodrome of fever, chills, malaise, headache, arthralgia, and myalgia. This prodrome may be very mild or undetectable in young children.
- One to two days later, the characteristic lesions begin as red macules, which progress rapidly to form papules that evolve into vesicles and/or pustules that eventually rupture and crust (Fig. 7.14). This entire cycle may occur within 8 to 12 hours.
- The eruption typically begins on the face, scalp, and trunk and then spreads to involve the extremities (cephalocaudal spread).
- The typical vesicles are superficial and thin-walled, and they are surrounded by an irregular area of erythema, giving them the appearance of "a dewdrop on a rose petal" (Fig. 7.15).
- The lesions are usually pruritic.
- An enanthem may occur, most commonly on the palate as a vesicle or as shallow erosion.
- Lesions characteristically appear in successive crops over 3 to 5 days. Thus, lesions in varying stages of development will be present simultaneously (Fig. 7.16).
- Most lesions crust within 1 week and crusts usually fall off within 1 to 3 weeks, depending on the depth of involvement.
- Large blisters or hemorrhagic lesions can also be seen.
- Scarring is not unusual in uncomplicated varicella and appears as "punched-out" skin lesions on the face (Fig. 7.17) or hypertrophic scars on the trunk (Fig. 7.18).

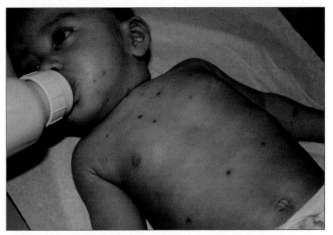

7.14 *Varicella.* Discrete crusts scattered on the trunk. Crusts usually fall off within 1 to 3 weeks depending on the depth of involvement.

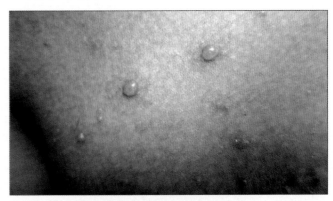

7.15 *Varicella.* Thin-walled vesicles on a base of erythema often referred to as "dewdrops on rose petals."

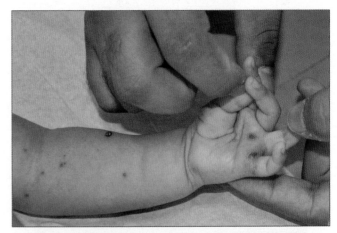

7.16 *Varicella.* Lesions in various stages of healing is characteristic of varicella. Note pink papules on the forearm, an intact vesicle on the palm, a weeping vesicle as well as dried crusts on the forearms.

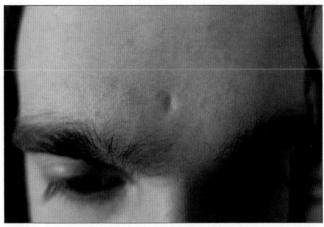

7.17 *Varicella atrophic scar.* The scars on this boy's face resulted from a healed chickenpox lesion.

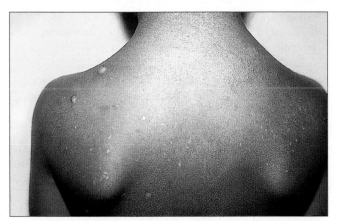

7.18 *Varicella hypertrophic scars.* The scars on this boy's shoulders resulted from healed chickenpox lesions.

COMPLICATIONS

- The most common complication in children is bacterial superinfection with *Staphylococcus aureus* and Group A beta-hemolytic *Streptococcus* which will present with fever and localized skin symptoms.
- Neurologic complications such as encephalitis, meningoencephalitis, cerebellar ataxia, transverse myelitis, or Guillain–Barré syndrome can rarely occur.
- Varicella pneumonia is typically seen as a complication of adult onset varicella and is rare in children.

- Pregnant patients who develop varicella in the first trimester have a 2.3% to 4.9% risk of delivering a child with the **fetal varicella syndrome,** a congenital malformation complex with features such as intrauterine growth retardation, prematurity, cicatricial lesions in a dermatomal distribution, limb paresis and hypoplasia, chorioretinitis, and cataracts.

DIAGNOSIS

- The diagnosis of varicella is usually straightforward, based on the characteristic presentation and clinical findings.
- A Tzanck smear showing characteristic herpesvirus-induced multinucleated giant cells can be helpful in establishing the diagnosis.
- Direct immunofluorescence, which uses fluorescent-labeled antibodies to detect VZV in skin cells obtained from the base of active lesions can provide rapid and accurate results.
- The scrapings from the base of an active lesion and the vesicle contents can be sent for culture of the VZV virus.
- PCR and in situ hybridization on tissue samples of active lesions
- Serologic tests include varicella IgM and IgG can also be helpful in confirming the diagnosis.

 DIFFERENTIAL DIAGNOSIS

Other Viral Exanthems
- *Vesicular exanthems of coxsackievirus and echovirus infections may be mistaken for varicella.*
- *These exanthems may show a characteristic distribution, as in hand-foot-and-mouth disease.*

Eczema Herpeticum (Kaposi Varicelliform Eruption, see Fig. 4.13)
- *Atopic dermatitis that becomes secondarily infected with HSV.*
- *Direct immunofluorescence or culture results indicative of HSV infection.*

Impetigo
- *The patient generally feels well.*
- *Typical moist, honey-colored crusts are present, often in a periorificial distribution (see Chapter 5).*

MANAGEMENT

Acute Varicella

- Uncomplicated varicella in otherwise healthy children is usually a mild self-limited disease and is generally treated with supportive care such as antipruritics and antipyretics. Aspirin should be avoided because of the risk of Reye syndrome.
- **Oral acyclovir** is warranted in patients who are at an increased risk of complications, and, in general, it should be started within 24 hours of the onset of the rash.

These patients include the following:
- Otherwise healthy, nonpregnant patients 13 years of age or older.
- Children older than 12 months of age with chronic skin or pulmonary conditions.
- Children receiving chronic corticosteroids or salicylates.
- **Intravenous acyclovir** is indicated in immunocompromised patients or in patients with virally mediated complications of varicella.
- Varicella-zoster immune globulin (**VariZIG**) or the varicella vaccine can be given prophylactically to immunocompromised individuals with known exposure to VZV.

Varicella Vaccine

- The **VZV vaccine** is recommended for universal immunization in all children.

- Given the occurrence of breakthrough varicella with the one dose regimen, the current recommendation is for a two-dose VZV vaccine schedule. Initial dose is optimally given between 12 and 18 months of age; and a booster immunization should be given between 4 and 6 years of age.
- However, the vaccine may be administered at any time before 13 years of age as two doses given at least 3 months apart.
- Unimmunized older adolescents or adults should receive two doses of the vaccine administered at least 28 days apart.

Varicella and Pregnancy

- Peripartal maternal varicella poses a particular risk to the newborn. Neonates born 2 days before or 5 days after the onset of maternal varicella should be given **varicella immunoglobulin (VZIG)**. Newborns who develop varicella should be treated with intravenous acyclovir.
- **Oral acyclovir** is not recommended in pregnant women with uncomplicated varicella because the risks and benefits to the fetus are unknown.

 HELPFUL HINTS

- In the United States, two varicella-containing vaccines are licensed for use—**Varivax**, a monovalent vaccine and **ProQuad**, which combines varicella and measles–mumps–rubella virus (MMRV). When possible the combination should be used to decrease the number of injections.
- Children can still get herpes zoster after VZV immunization, although the risk seems to be lower than after wild-type varicella infection.

 POINT TO REMEMBER

- Patients with chickenpox remain contagious until all cutaneous lesions are crusted.

BASICS

- Scarlet fever (SF) is a mucocutaneous eruption most commonly triggered by an erythrogenic exotoxin-producing strain of group A beta-hemolytic *streptococci*.
- The incidence and disease associated mortality has markedly declined due to the development of antibiotics and a reduction in the virulence of disease-associated streptococci.
- SF is typically seen in children in the late fall, winter, or spring.

PATHOGENESIS

- SF usually follows a streptococcal pharyngitis or tonsillitis but occasionally follows a wound infection, burn, or upper respiratory tract infection.
- SF is most often caused by the erythrogenic toxins A, B, and C produced by group A beta-hemolytic streptococci.
- Less often, an exotoxin-producing *S. aureus* can trigger scarlet fever.
- The exotoxins lead to immune activation and the characteristic exanthem.

CLINICAL MANIFESTATIONS

- SF typically begins with the abrupt onset of fever, sore throat, headache, and chills.
- The rash begins 12 to 48 hours later as generalized blanchable erythema on the neck and chest that quickly becomes generalized. Shortly thereafter the eruption becomes finely papular, covered with tiny papules, developing a distinctive "sandpapery" or "scarlatiniform" texture (Fig. 7.19).
- The skin around the mouth may show a characteristic pallor (circumoral pallor).
- Linear streaks of petechiae called Pastia lines may develop in the flexures.
- Mucosal findings include erythema and edema of the pharyngotonsillar area, punctate erythematous macules and petechiae on the palate, and a "strawberry tongue."
- The characteristic strawberry tongue is initially white with bright red papillae and then becomes beefy red with prominent papillae.
- During the convalescent phase of the illness, the skin of the palms and soles frequently desquamates. Desquamation may be sheetlike (Fig. 7.20A,B).

COMPLICATIONS

- Complications are uncommon but may include pneumonia, pericarditis, arthritis, meningitis, hepatitis, glomerulonephritis, and rheumatic fever.
- Erythema nodosum and acute guttate psoriasis may also follow or accompany an infection with group A beta-hemolytic streptococci (see Chapter 34).
- SF can recur, with reported recurrence rates as high as 18%.

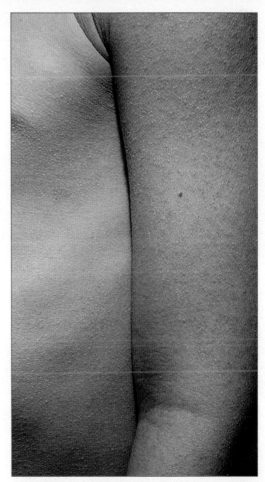

7.19   *Scarlet fever.* The exanthem appears as diffuse redness with numerous overlying tiny (1 to 2 mm) rough, blanchable papules resulting in a "sandpaper" like feel to the skin. Lesions resemble a "sunburn with goose bumps."

DIAGNOSIS

- The diagnosis of SF is often made on clinical grounds.
- The isolation of group A streptococci from the pharynx, or the presence of elevated antistreptolysin-O titers and anti-DNase B antibodies, can help confirm the diagnosis.

 MANAGEMENT

- First-line treatment is with **penicillin** or **amoxicillin** for 10 to 14 days. Alternatives include **erythromycin, cephalosporins, ofloxacin, rifampin**, and newer **macrolide antibiotics**.
- Improvement should be seen within 1 to 2 days of starting antibiotics.
- Prompt and complete treatment is essential to prevent the development of rheumatic fever.
- Emollients can be used to soothe the scarlatiniform eruption.

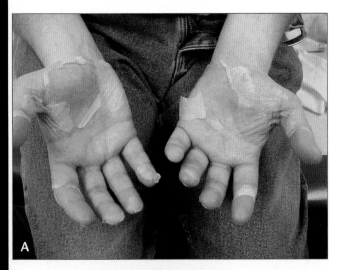

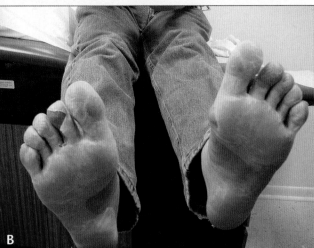

7.20 *Scarlet fever.* Skin peeling from this boy's palms (**A**) and soles (**B**) during the convalescent phase of his illness. This exuberant desquamation occurred 2 weeks after he had fever and a truncal exanthem that began as a streptococcal throat infection.

DIFFERENTIAL DIAGNOSIS

Streptococcal or Staphylococcal Toxic Shock Syndromes
• *Distinguished by hypotension and multiorgan system involvement.*

Kawasaki Syndrome
• *A small vessel vasculitis characterized by fever (lasting at least 5 days), conjunctivitis, oral mucosal erythema, cervical lymphadenopathy, and erythema of the palms and soles in addition to a widespread, nonspecific eruption; lymphadenopathy.*

Febrile Drug Reactions
• *Pink-red blanching macules and papules that begin on the face and neck and spread caudally. Eruption is itchy.*
• *Pastia lines and strawberry tongue are not present.*

Viral Exanthem
• *Eruption is not as erythematous, but rather pink to skin colored.*
• *Pastia lines and strawberry tongue are not present.*

HELPFUL HINT

• Sometimes the original streptococcal infection and eruption may have passed unnoticed and patients may seek medical attention solely for the desquamation of the palms and soles.

Toxin-Mediated Streptococcal and Staphylococcal Disease

BASICS

- Some streptococcal and staphylococcal species are capable of producing circulating toxins. Patients infected with these toxin-producing bacteria exhibit clinical manifestations distant from the site of local infection. Several distinct syndromes related to these toxins have been recognized, including toxic shock syndrome (TSS) and staphylococcal scalded skin syndrome (SSSS).
- The responsible toxins act as superantigens, bypassing the normal sequence of immune system activation to stimulate an immune response in a general, nonspecific manner. This nonspecific immunologic activation leads to damage in various organ systems.
- Both toxic shock syndrome and staphylococcal scalded skin syndrome have characteristic cutaneous features that will be discussed next.

TOXIC SHOCK SYNDROME

BASICS

- TSS is a systemic illness caused by infection with toxin-producing strains of *S. aureus* or less often streptococci.
- Originally described in association with tampon use, TSS now occurs more commonly secondary to a local wound infection.

CLINICAL MANIFESTATIONS

- TSS is the constellation of fever, rash, hypotension, and multisystem organ involvement (at least three organ systems) and its presentation ranges from mild to fatal disease.
- TSS typically presents with the sudden onset of high fever, muscle aches, vomiting, diarrhea, and headache.
- A diffuse macular erythema or a "scarlatiniform" (i.e., sandpaper-like feel) exanthem with accentuation in flexures develops first on the trunk and quickly spreads to the extremities.
- Other skin features that may be present include erythema and edema of the palms and soles, hyperemia of the conjunctiva and mucous membranes, and "strawberry tongue."
- Desquamation of the palms and soles may occur 1 to 3 weeks after the onset of illness (Fig. 7.21).

COMPLICATIONS

- Hypotensive shock may occur.
- Decreased renal function, prolonged muscle aches, paresthesias, arthralgias, and amenorrhea can occur as a result of TSS.
- Months after recovery some patients may develop Beau lines, nail shedding, or telogen effluvium.

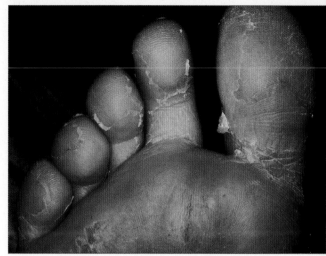

7.21 Toxic shock syndrome. Desquamation of the foot after toxic shock. (From Lugo-Somolinos A, McKinley-Grant L, Goldsmith L, et al. *Visual Dx: Essential Dermatology in Pigmented Skin*. Philadelphia, PA: Lippincott Williams & Wilkins, 2011.)

DIAGNOSIS

- Diagnosis is made when the characteristic clinical findings of fever, rash, and hypotension are present in patients who have an infection with *S. aureus* or *Strepococcus*.
- Blood urea nitrogen, creatinine, liver enzymes, and the white blood cell count may be elevated and thrombocytopenia may be present.
- Gram stain and cultures of vaginal exudate or wounds positive for *S. aureus* or, rarely, group A streptococci can support the diagnosis.

🔵 DIFFERENTIAL DIAGNOSIS

Scarlet Fever
- *The skin eruption may appear similar to TSS but hypotension does not occur.*

Kawasaki Syndrome (see Chapter 10)
- *Usually occurs in children and causes prominent cervical lymphadenopathy and prolonged fever of at least 5 days.*

Staphylococcal Scalded Skin Syndrome
- *Occurs in newborns and in infants younger than 2 years.*
- *Nikolsky sign is positive; exfoliation is prominent in the flexures.*

MANAGEMENT

- Treatment of TSS includes removal foreign bodies (i.e., surgical mesh, gauze, or tampons) that may be sources of infection and drainage of any abscesses.
- Patients should be treated with **penicillinase-resistant antibiotics.**
- Supportive care may include **hydration** and **vasopressors** for hypotension and **antipyretics**.
- Intravenous gamma globulin has been reported to be effective in treating STSS, but it is not yet in widespread use.

 HELPFUL HINTS

- Look for a cutaneous site of infection or for a forgotten or retained vaginal tampon.
- TSS due to *Streptococcus* (STSS) may be clinically identical to TSS, but it is usually distinguished by a more marked soft tissue infection at the site of origin, with localized pain in an extremity the most frequent initial complaint.
- Blood cultures are positive in more than 50% of patients with STSS.
- Antibiotic coverage for both staphylococci and penicillin-resistant streptococci should be given.
- MRSA is responsible for only a small portion of TSS cases.

STAPHYLOCOCCAL SCALDED SKIN SYNDROME (SSSS)

BASICS

- Staphylococcal scalded skin syndrome (SSSS) is a generalized red, blistering eruption caused by infection with an exfoliative toxin-producing strain of *S. aureus* and primarily occurs in infants and young children.

PATHOGENESIS

- The exfoliative toxin derived from *S. aureus* spreads from the initial site of infection, usually the nasopharyx or conjunctiva, via the bloodstream.
- The toxin is epidermolytic and cleaves desmoglien 1, an important protein necessary for cell-to-cell adhesion in the granular layer of the epidermis, resulting in blister formation.

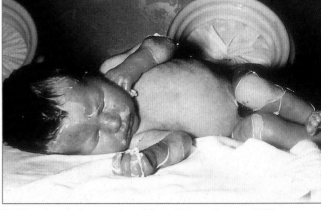

7.22 *Staphylococcal scalded skin syndrome.* Diffuse erythema and sloughing of the skin.

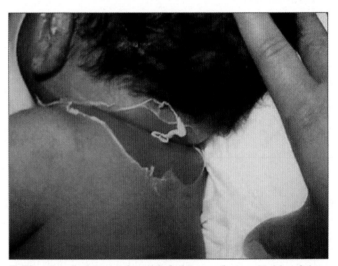

7.23 *Staphylococcal scalded skin syndrome.* Folds of the body are usually the first to exfoliate.

CLINICAL FEATURES

- The prodrome consists of fever, irritability, and skin pain.
- Sometimes evidence of the staphylococcal infection in the conjunctiva or nose may be present as conjunctivitis or rhinorrhea.
- The skin eruption begins as diffuse redness of the skin starting on the head and neck (with or without facial swelling) and flexures and becomes generalized over 1 to 2 days (Fig. 7.22).
- Soon thereafter, flaccid bullae develop that easily rupture with minimal pressure leaving behind moist superficial erosions (Fig. 7.23).
- Nikolsky sign, the easy separation of epidermis with minimal lateral pressure, is positive.

- Periorificial crusting and radial fissuring with sparing of the oral mucosa is a characteristic clinical feature.
- Desquamation can last 3 to 5 days, followed by complete healing without scarring.

DIAGNOSIS

- The diagnosis of SSSS is generally made clinically.
- Cultures taken from the bullae and erosions on the skin are negative but *S. aureus* may be cultured from the conjunctiva, nasopharynx, or perianal skin.

 DIFFERENTIAL DIAGNOSIS

Sunburn
- *No Nikolsky sign.*
- *Patients are usually well appearing.*

Toxic Shock Syndrome
- *No Nikolsky sign.*
- *Hypotension and multiorgan involvement.*

 MANAGEMENT

- In mild cases, treatment with an oral beta-lactamase–resistant antibiotic such as **dicloxacillin** or **cephalexin** for at least 1 week together with supportive care is all that is necessary.
- In severe and generalized cases, patients may require hospitalization for **IV antibiotics** and **hydration**.
- Supportive care should include **hydration, antipyretics**, and meticulous **wound** and **skin care**.
- With proper and prompt treatment SSSS resolves completely without sequelae in 1 to 2 weeks.

HELPFUL HINT

- Nikolsky sign occurs when apparently normal epidermis is easily separated at the basal layer and rubbed off with the application of minimal lateral pressure. It is used as an indication of pemphigus vulgaris, toxic epidermal necrolysis, and SSSS.

Lumps, Bumps, and Linear Eruptions

OVERVIEW

Children are often brought medical attention for evaluation of various "lumps" or "bumps" on the skin. Infectious and neoplastic conditions that present with bumps such as molluscum contagiosum, folliculitis, and pyogenic granuloma, are discussed elsewhere. The lumps and bumps discussed in this chapter result from cyst formation (epidermal cysts and pilomatricomas) and benign tumors (Spitz nevus, mastocytomas, and juvenile xanthogranulomas). Linear and inflammatory conditions (lichen striatus, lichen nitidus, and frictional lichenoid dermatitis) are also discussed.

Many of these lesions are self-limited and only require symptomatic treatment. For example, typical juvenile xanthogranuloma are expected to involute over several years. Likewise, lichen striatus will also spontaneously resolve. However, pilomatricomas usually do not involute and may require surgical excision. Similarly, Spitz nevi that are clinically or histologically atypical require removal.

Distinguishing these lesions is necessary for prediction of the course of the eruption and for optimal management. This chapter will point out the key clinical features that can help establish the precise diagnosis and avoid unnecessary procedures or anxiety.

IN THIS CHAPTER...

- ➤ **EPIDERMAL CYSTS**
- ➤ **PILOMATRICOMA**
- ➤ **JUVENILE XANTHOGRANULOMA**
- ➤ **SPITZ NEVUS**
- ➤ **MASTOCYTOMA**
- ➤ **INSECT BITE REACTIONS**
- ➤ **SPIDER ANGIOMA**
- ➤ **LICHEN NITIDUS**
- ➤ **LICHEN SPINULOSUS**
- ➤ **FRICTIONAL LICHENOID DERMATITIS**
- ➤ **LICHEN STRIATUS**

BASICS

- An epidermal cyst (aka epidermal inclusion cyst or epidermoid cyst) is a well-demarcated subcutaneous nodule that typically occurs after puberty.

CLINICAL MANIFESTATIONS

- Presents as a round, mobile, slow-growing subcutaneous nodule seen most commonly on the face, scalp, back, or scrotum.
- Often a visible overlying pore or punctum through which white keratinaceous debris is extruded is typical.
- Vary in size from a few millimeters to several centimeters.
- Occasionally develop surrounding redness secondary to an inflammatory response to cyst wall rupture (Fig. 8.1).

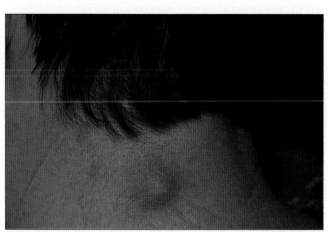

8.1   *Epidermal cyst, inflamed.* Note surrounding erythema.

DIAGNOSIS

- Diagnosis is based on clinical recognition.
- A biopsy would show an epithelial lining with keratinaceous debris.

 MANAGEMENT

- If the cyst is small and asymptomatic, no treatment is necessary.
- Large cysts or those that become recurrently inflamed or are in a cosmetically sensitive area may warrant excision.

HELPFUL HINTS

- Multiple epidermal cysts in childhood can be the presenting sign of Gardner syndrome, a form of familial adenomatous polyposis (FAP).
- The term "sebaceous cyst" is often inaccurately used to describe epidermal cysts.
- Epidermal cysts on the scalp are called pilar cysts and those on the eyelids are referred to as chalazions.

Pilomatricoma

BASICS

- Pilomatricomas are a common benign tumor in children.

PATHOGENESIS

- Pilomatricomas (aka calcifying epithelioma of Malherbe) arise from the outer root sheath of the hair follicle and are thought to be caused by mutations in the b-catenin gene.

CLINICAL MANIFESTATIONS

- Presents as a skin-colored or bluish subcutaneous nodule that may be rock hard to the touch (Fig. 8.2).
- Characteristic secondary calcification is often present and contributes to its firmness.
- Lesions are mobile and often have irregular contours.
- Most are asymptomatic but some are associated with mild tenderness or pain.
- Typically found on the head and neck and less often are seen on the upper extremity or trunk in children (Fig. 8.3).
- On the face pilomatricomas are most often found in the periorbital, lateral cheek and preauricular areas.
- Most pilomatricomas are solitary, although multiple pilomatricomas do occur.

DIAGNOSIS

- Diagnosis is based on clinical recognition.
- The "tent sign" is a useful clinical test that will show the irregular contours of the nodule when the skin is stretched taut.

DIFFERENTIAL DIAGNOSIS

Epidermal Cyst
- *Soft to the touch if not fibrosed or calcified; often has central punctum.*

MANAGEMENT

- Surgical excision is the treatment of choice as these lesions usually do not resolve spontaneously.
- Small, asymptomatic lesions in cosmetically insignificant locations can be clinically observed.

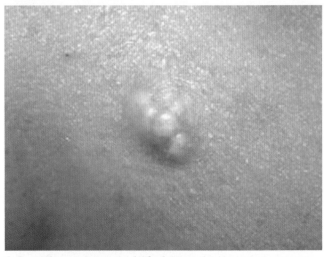

8.2 *Pilomatricoma/calcified.* Note the irregular contours. These lesions are often rock hard on palpation.

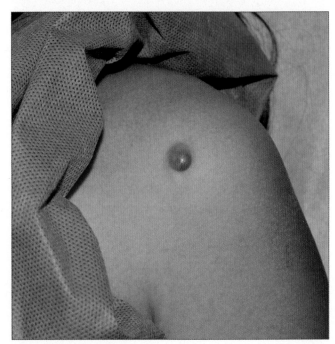

8.3 *Pilomatricoma.* Rock hard nodule on the shoulder with some surrounding erythema.

BASICS

- A juvenile xanthogranuloma (JXG) is the most common type of non-Langerhan cell histiocytosis and typically presents as a well-demarcated, dome-shaped, yellow-brown or reddish-orange papule or nodule on the head and neck of an infant or child.

CLINICAL MANIFESTATIONS

- Most JXGs occur early in life on the head, neck, or trunk.
- Sometimes JXG can present at birth or develop rapidly in the first few years of life.
- JXGs present as a small firm, round, papule or nodule, ranging from 0.5 cm to 2 cm but larger ("giant") lesions have been described.
- Early on, lesions are erythematous or skin colored (Fig. 8.4), but with time they become yellow (Fig. 8.5).
- Usually presents as a single lesion but occasionally multiple JXGs occur.
- Lesions are typically asymptomatic but sometimes ulceration or crusting may be seen.
- Occasionally extracutaneous lesions may be present (0.3% to 0.5% of cases) and the eye is the most frequent site affected.
- Risk factors for ocular involvement include onset of lesions within the first 2 years of life and when multiple cutaneous JXGs appear.
- Other affected extracutaneous sites include the liver and lungs. Most visceral lesions spontaneously regress with time.

DIAGNOSIS

- Diagnosis is based on clinical features.
- If in doubt, the diagnosis can be confirmed with a skin biopsy that shows a dense infiltrate of foamy histiocytes within the dermis and the classic Touton giant cells (a wreath of nuclei surrounded by eosinophilic cytoplasm).

 DIFFERENTIAL DIAGNOSIS

Spitz Nevus
- *Pink papule commonly found on the head and neck of children (see below).*

 MANAGEMENT

- JXGs are benign growths that spontaneously regress over 3 to 6 years and have an excellent prognosis.
- Parents can be reassured; however, residual atrophy or pigmentary changes are possible.
- Ophthalmologic evaluation is needed if multiple cutaneous lesions are present, especially in patients under the age of 2 years.

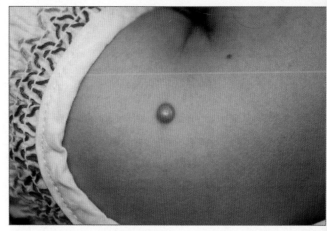

8.4 *Juvenile xanthogranuloma.* A small firm, round, reddish papule on this child's arm.

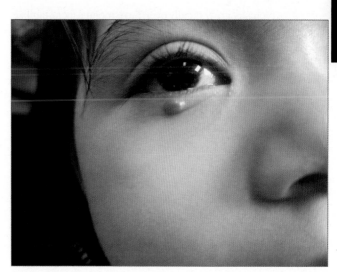

8.5 *Juvenile xanthogranuloma.* Firm, yellow-orange papule of the lower eyelid.

 POINTS TO REMEMBER

- Multiple JXGs on physical examination, even in the absence of ocular symptoms, should prompt an ophthalmologic evaluation.
- Children with neurofibromatosis and multiple JXGs have a higher risk for juvenile chronic myelogenous leukemia (JCML).

Spitz Nevus (also Called Spindle and Epithelioid Cell Nevus)

BASICS

- A spitz nevus is a distinct type of melanocytic neoplasm that most often develops in children. Spitz nevi are benign neoplasms, but their management has historically been controversial because of their histologic resemblance to melanoma.
- Formerly referred to as "benign juvenile melanoma," and "Spitz juvenile melanoma," these terms are no longer used as they are misleading.

CLINICAL MANIFESTATIONS

- Classic Spitz nevi present as a pink- or flesh-colored, dome-shaped papule or nodule that appears most frequently on the head/neck region or lower extremities, and is most often noted in childhood or adolescence (Fig. 8.6).
- A pigmented Spitz nevus appears as a smooth dark brown to black papule (Fig. 8.7).
- Lesions typically grow rapidly over 3 to 6 months then stabilize.
- They are usually less than 6 mm but can vary in size from 2 mm to >2 cm.
- Most often are well circumscribed with a smooth surface; telangiectasias may be present.
- Multiple Spitz nevi arising within a nevus spilus has been described.

DIAGNOSIS

- Clinical features and the use of dermoscopy can help identify Spitz nevi on physical examination.
- Histopathologic features of classic Spitz nevi include large spindle and/or epithelioid cells, usually in the paucity or absence of melanin, the so-called Kamino bodies, and uniform architecture and absence of mitoses.

DIFFERENTIAL DIAGNOSIS

Juvenile Xanthogranuloma (see above)
- *Firm yellowish papule or nodule.*

Pyogenic Granuloma (Discussed in Chapter 30)
- *Rapid growth, epidermal collarette.*
- *Friable and bleeds easily.*

Dermal Nevus (Discussed in Chapter 30)
- *Skin-colored or light brown papule can look pink in fair-skinned persons.*

POINTS TO REMEMBER

- Initial growth of a Spitz nevus is usually rapid, which can be alarming to parents and physicians.
- In children, Spitz nevi may involute over time.

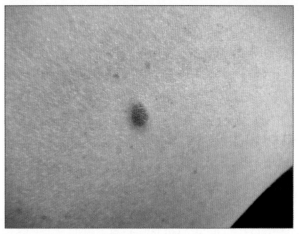

8.6 *Spitz nevus.* A pink dome-shaped papule is the typical presentation of a Spitz nevus in childhood.

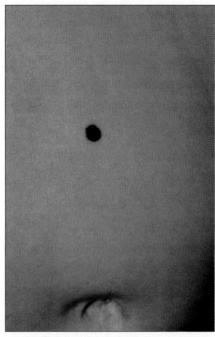

8.7 *Pigmented Spitz nevus.* Darkly pigmented Spitz nevi such as this are often mistaken for melanoma clinically.

MANAGEMENT

- Management of Spitz nevi in children is different than in adults (see Chapter 30).
- In children, complete excision is only recommended for Spitz nevi with any atypical features (clinically or histologically).
- A large survey–based study of pediatric dermatologists published in 2012 supports this conservative management.
- When lesions are excised, complete excision is warranted and specimens should be examined by a dermatopathologist or pathologist experienced in the diagnosis of melanocytic lesions and Spitz nevi.

BASICS

- Solitary mastocytoma represents a collection of mast cells in the skin and is at one end of a clinical spectrum that includes urticaria pigmentosa (UP) and diffuse cutaneous mastocytosis.
- Activating mutations in *KIT*, a key regulator of mast cells, have been implicated in the pathogenesis of all forms of mastocytosis.

CLINICAL MANIFESTATIONS

SOLITARY MASTOCYTOMA

- Presents at birth or within the first year of life as a skin-colored to yellow-orange-red papule or plaque (Fig. 8.8).
- Lesions develop an itchy erythematous urticarial wheal when rubbed or stroked; this change is referred to as Darier sign, and represents mast cell degranulation induced by physical stimulation (Fig. 8.9A,B). This reaction can be elicited after gentle mechanical irritation such as with rubbing of a tongue blade or the blunt end of a cotton tip swab.
- A similar reaction may be provoked by other everyday triggers (see Table 8.1).
- Occasionally, stroking or rubbing can result in blistering or systemic symptoms including flushing or gastrointestinal disturbance.
- Lesions tend to spontaneously involute over several years.
- Sometimes multiple mastocytomas may be present.

URTICARIA PIGMENTOSA (ALSO CALLED MACULOPAPULAR CUTANEOUS MASTOCYTOSIS)

- This is the most common presentation of childhood mastocytosis.
- Presents with multiple tan to red-brown macules and papules usually on the thighs, arms, trunk, and genitalia, but may occur anywhere, including the mucous membranes.

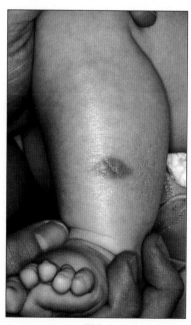

8.8 *Solitary mastocytoma.* This lesion presented as a pruritic erythematous plaque.

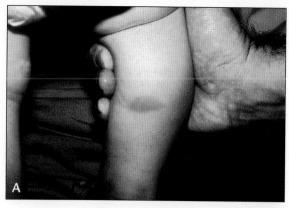

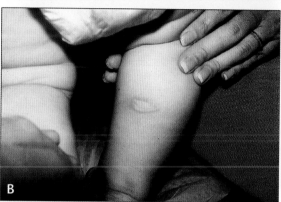

8.9 *Solitary mastocytoma.* A: Tan-colored lesion. **B: Darier sign.** An erythematous edematous, urticarial wheal is noted after the lesion was gently stroked with the blunt end of a cotton-tipped swab.

Table 8.1 TRIGGERS OF MAST CELL DEGRANULATION

Exercise
Changes in temperature—cold exposure or hot baths
Emotional stress
Medications: aspirin, opiates (morphine, codeine), dextromethorphan, NSAIDs, topical polymyxin B
General anesthesia agents: d-tubocurarine, scopolamine, pancuronium
Iodine-containing contrast media
Foods: egg white, seafood, chocolate, strawberries, tomatoes, citrus, and ethanol

- Lesions can also present as flat macules resembling café au lait spots (Fig. 8.10).
- The palms and soles are usually spared.
- In children the face and scalp may be involved.
- Affected persons may have tens to hundreds of lesions that range in size from a few millimeters to several centimeters.
- Darier sign is positive and dermatographism (see Chapter 27) may be present.
- Pruritus is the most common symptom resulting from mast cell degranulation and occurs in response to triggers such as changes in temperature, hot showers, friction or emotional stress (see Table 8.1).

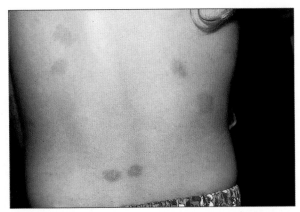

8.10 *Urticaria Pigmentosa.* Numerous tan macules on the trunk is typical of UP.

- Occasionally associated with systemic mastocytosis. The most commonly involved extracutaneous site is the gastrointestinal tract followed by the skeletal system.
- In most cases, lesions improve or resolve completely by adolescence.

DIFFUSE CUTANEOUS MASTOCYTOSIS

- Least common, this is a systemic variant of childhood mastocytosis characterized by diffuse infiltration of the skin by mast cells manifested as thickened doughy, yellowish skin.
- Usually accompanied by intense pruritus and flushing and is often associated with systemic symptoms including elevated temperature, vomiting, diarrhea, abdominal pain, or occasionally shock.

DIAGNOSIS

- Eliciting the Darier sign can aid in the diagnosis of all forms of cutaneous mastocytosis.
- If the diagnosis is in doubt, a skin biopsy will show an accumulation of mast cells in the dermis, which can be highlighted by Giemsa, toluidine blue, or tryptase antibodies.
- A serum tryptase level and/or urinary n-methylimidazoleacetic acid, a histamine metabolite, are useful chemical markers for the disease and will be elevated in systemic involvement or be suggestive of a high disease burden.

POINTS TO REMEMBER

- Risk factors for systemic disease include: children with the onset of skin lesions beyond 2 years of age and those who have persistence of skin lesions beyond adolescence.
- Avoid physical irritation of a solitary mastocytoma to prevent symptoms.
- Information for patients and families about mastocytosis and mast cell degranulators can be found at www.mastokids.com.

DIFFERENTIAL DIAGNOSIS

Solitary Mastocytoma
Insect Bite Reaction
- *Pink edematous itchy papule or plaque at the site of a bite.*
- *Occurs on exposed areas of skin and usually resolves in days to weeks.*

Herpes Simplex
- *Recurrent bullous reactions can mimic a recurrent herpes infection.*
- *HSV culture and/or Tzanck preparation may be positive and lesions are generally painful.*

Urticaria Pigmentosa
- *Café au lait macules.*
- *Asymptomatic macules.*
- *Negative Darier sign.*

MANAGEMENT

- Solitary mastocytomas usually involute after several years and the lesions of urticaria pigmentosa resolve completely or improve during adolescence in the vast majority of patients. The tendency for a blistering reaction disappears in 1 to 3 years.
- Families should be educated on the natural history of the condition and its tendency to spontaneously resolve by adolescence, often much sooner.
- Families should be counseled on the triggers of mast cell degranulation and on avoiding these triggers if possible.
- Patients with extensive cutaneous disease or elevated baseline tryptase levels may be at increased risk of anaphylaxis from a variety of triggers. These patients should have a yearly serum tryptase level, complete blood count (CBC) with differential, and a chemistry panel including alkaline phosphatase.
- Treatment is primarily symptomatic. Patients with higher tryptase levels (>6 ng/mL) are more likely to be symptomatic and require daily treatment.
- Potent topical steroids under occlusion such as **clobetasol 0.05% cream** have been noted to improve solitary mastocytomas.
- Nonsedating antihistamines such as **cetirizine, loratidine, or fexofenadine** are a good initial treatment of choice.
- In patients with extensive involvement or symptoms the addition of the classic H1 antagonists, **diphenhydramine** or **hydroxyzine**, or H2 antagonists such as **cimetidine** or **ranitidine** may be considered.
- Oral **cromolyn sodium** has been beneficial in patients with gastrointestinal involvement.

Insect Bite Reactions (see Discussion in Chapter 29)

BASICS

- Insects are a specific class of arthropods that are distinguished by having three body parts—a head, thorax, and an abdomen. Insects include flies, fleas, mosquitoes, bees, wasps, ants, lice, and beg bugs.
- Insects are important because they are disease vectors and can induce significant skin reactions, particularly in children.

CLINICAL MANIFESTATIONS

- Initially, an insect bite can cause a local area of erythema, edema, and pruritus at the site of the bite. The reaction is triggered by irritant substances in insect saliva and often occurs within minutes of the offending bite.
- This initial localized inflammatory reaction is short-lived and may go unnoticed.
- In sensitized individuals, a local reaction may be followed by a delayed skin reaction consisting of urticarial wheals, itching, swelling, redness, firm red papules or nodules that may last for hours to several days.
- The area of redness and swelling can extend several centimeters from the bite.
- An overlying central punctum may be present.
- Occasionally, especially in young children, a vesicular, bullous, indurated, or hemorrhagic lesion can occur (Fig. 8.11).
- Lesions are characteristically grouped and when in a linear distribution are referred to as the insect's "breakfast, lunch, and dinner" (Fig. 8.12 [see also Fig. 29.2]) on exposed areas of skin, typically the extremities.
- It is often not possible to determine the exact type of offending insect from the skin reaction.

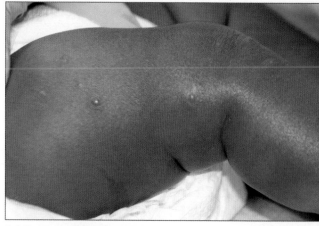

8.12 *Insect Bite Reaction.* Note the linear distribution of lesions referred to as the insects' "breakfast, lunch, and dinner," on the extremities.

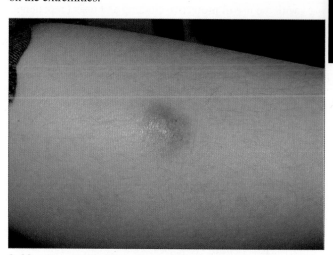

8.13 *Insect bites/Papular(nodular) urticaria.* This nodule presumably arose secondary to an insect bite.

PAPULAR URTICARIA

- Papular urticaria occurs when there are recurrent and chronic itchy papules on exposed areas of skin that are triggered by a hypersensitivity reaction to a variety of insect bites. Papular urticaria typically occurs in young children in the late spring and summer.
- Lesions present as grouped, 3 to 10 mm urticarial or firm pink papules some with central punctum or with an overlying excoriation or crusting.
- Typically found on face, and exposed areas of the extremities (Fig. 8.13). Covered areas and body folds are typically spared.
- Individual lesions usually heal over 1 to 2 weeks but scratching may lead to reactivation and persistent itching of older lesions, which leads to a chronic itch–scratch cycle that can last from months to years.

DIAGNOSIS

- Diagnosis is based on history and clinical examination and ruling out other etiologies.

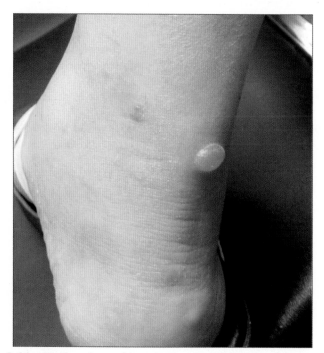

8.11 ***Bullous insect bite reaction.*** Vesicobullous plaque that is the result of an insect bite.

DIFFERENTIAL DIAGNOSIS

Infantile Acropustulosis (see Chapter 2)
* *Recurrent crops of itchy papulovesicles usually on palms and soles.*

Eosinophilic Pustular Folliculitis (see Chapter 2)
* *Recurrent crops of itchy papules usually on the scalp in infants.*

Cellulitis
* *Bacterial infection of the skin and subcutaneous tissues characterized by expanding erythema, warmth and tenderness.*
* *Often accompanied by fever.*
* *As opposed to bite reactions erythema expands and deepens in color if the cellulitis is untreated.*

MANAGEMENT

Prevention
* Management should primarily emphasize prevention with the use of protective clothing and insect repellents.
* Scented hair products, perfumes, and colognes should be avoided as they may attract insects. Mosquitoes are attracted to bright clothing as well as human odors.
* **DEET (N,N-diethyl-3-methylbenzamide)** is the most effective and most widely used insect repellent and is recommended by the American Academy of Pediatrics at concentrations <30%.
* The duration of protection is directly related to DEET concentration. Concentrations between 10% and 30% will provide adequate protection in most circumstances.
* Multiple DEET–containing insect repellants are available in varying concentrations and vehicles including: **Off! Deep Woods® Insect Repellent** (25% DEET), **Off! FamilyCare Smooth** (15% DEET), and **3M Ultrathon Insect Repellant** (25% DEET).
* **Picaridin** is a newer insect repellent that is odorless and has comparable efficacy to DEET. It is used in concentrations up to 20%. Examples include **Natrapel 8-Hour** (20% picaridin), **Sawyer Premium Insect Repellent** (20% picaridin), **Repel Sportsmen Gear Smart Pump Spray** (15% picaridin).
* Extensive studies of DEET and picaradin found no significant toxicologic risks from the typical use of these repellents.

Treatment
* For insect bite reactions, cooling (with an ice or cold pack) can reduce local edema.
* Potent topical corticosteroids such as **mometasone 0.1% ointment** or **fluocinoinde 0.05% gel** can be helpful for decreasing inflammation and relieving pruritus.
* Topical antipruritic creams, gels, and lotions, such as those containing calamine or pramoxine (**Sarna sensitive lotion** or **Caladryl**) may be beneficial.
* Topical anesthetic and antihistamine preparations can induce allergic contact sensitivity and routine use should be avoided.
* Nonsedating oral antihistamines such as **cetirizine** or **loratadine** may be helpful for itching but ideally should be taken prophylactically to help prevent pruritus and whealing.

Papular Urticaria
* Management of **papular urticaria** is particularly challenging because parents need to be persuaded that the condition is the result of insect bites. Many times the bites occurred days to weeks before, and in addition constant scratching and picking at the lesions contributes to their persistence.
* Treatment for papular urticaria includes education of parents and prevention of bites as well as mid to potent topical corticosteroids such as **mometasone 0.1% ointment** or **triamcinolone 0.1% ointment** applied to individual lesions and antihistamines.
* **Cordran tape** provides the added benefit of occlusion and a physical impediment to scratching.
* If itching and scratching is interfering with sleep, a sedating antihistamine such as **hydroxyzine** (0.5 mg/kg/dose every 6 hours and prior to sleep) may be helpful.
* Papular urticaria can be frustrating for both affected families and physicians because of its significant associated itch and chronic nature; however parents should be reassured of its benign nature and eventual resolution.

BASICS

- Appear as a bright red papule with branching telangiectasias on the face or upper trunk of children.
- In adults, spider angiomas can be associated with liver disease and high estrogen states such as pregnancy, but in children they are idiopathic and common occurring in up to 15% of normal children and young adults.

CLINICAL MANIFESTATIONS

- A spider angioma typically appears suddenly and is characterized by a central bright red vascular papule with symmetrically radiating thin telangiectasias (resembling the legs of a spider) (Fig. 8.14).
- Most commonly on the face but can also appear on the exposed areas of the upper trunk, arms, or hands.

DIAGNOSIS

- Diagnosis is based on clinical recognition.
- Lesions will usually blanch completely with firm pressure or diascopy.

MANAGEMENT

- In children, spider angiomas may regress spontaneously usually by puberty.
- For angiomas that persist or when treatment is desired, **pulsed-dye laser** or **electrocoagulation** are the treatment of choice.

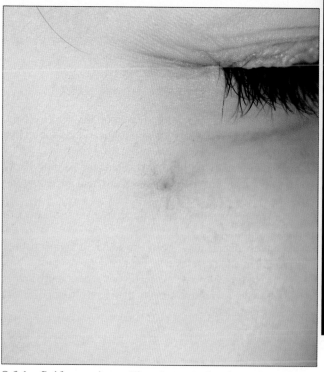

8.14 *Spider angioma.* Note the central red papule with feeding capillary legs.

Lichen Nitidus

BASICS

- Lichen nitidus (LN) is an idiopathic, inflammatory skin disease primarily seen in school-aged children.

CLINICAL MANIFESTATIONS

- Presents as tiny (1 to 2 mm), monomorphic, skin-colored, shiny, flat-topped papules often in a linear distribution that are the result of *Köebnerization* (Fig. 8.15).
- The lesions usually occur in groups, and are seen primarily on the abdomen, chest, back, glans penis, and upper extremities.
- The *Köebner* phenomenon is invariably present and is a clinical hallmark of LN (Fig. 8.16).
- Nail involvement may occur in patients with palmar involvement and presents with linear ridges and pits.
- Lesions are typically asymptomatic but occasionally itch.
- LN is slowly progressive initially then tends to stabilize and regress spontaneously.

DIAGNOSIS

- Diagnosis is easily made by clinical recognition.
- Biopsy will show the very characteristic "ball in claw" pattern where elongated rete ridges at the margins appear to be grasping a focal circumscribed infiltrate of lymphocytes and histiocytes in the papillary dermis.

DIFFERENTIAL DIAGNOSIS

Molluscum Contagiosum (see Chapter 6)
- *Skin-colored, pearly papules with central umbilication; may be spread by autoinoculation of viral particles (pseudo-Köebnerization).*
- *Molluscum lesions are larger than those of LN and often are of various sizes.*

Flat warts (see Chapter 6)
- *Light brown flat-topped papules, may also be spread by autoinoculation (pseudo-Köebnerization).*
- *Often variably sized lesions present.*

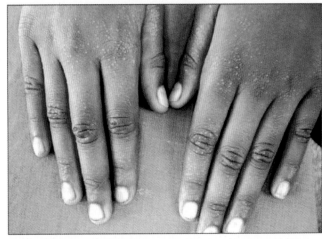

8.15 *Lichen nitidus.* Tiny (1 to 2 mm), monomorphic, skin-colored, shiny, flat-topped papules.

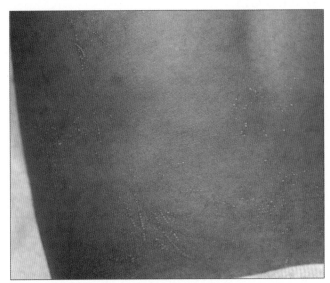

8.16 *Lichen nitidus.* The **Köebner** reaction is evident here. Note linear distribution of many lesions.

MANAGEMENT

- Localized asymptomatic cases may go unnoticed or be an incidental finding.
- If asymptomatic no treatment is necessary.
- Mid- to high-potency topical corticosteroids such as **triamcinolone 0.1% ointment** can alleviate pruritus symptoms, if present, and may hasten resolution.
- Parents should be reassured of its benign nature and the tendency for spontaneous regression.

BASICS

- Lichen spinulosus is a skin disorder characterized by round or oval collections of tiny, dry, monomorphic papules that is commonly seen in children and adolescents with dry skin.
- Most commonly occurs in dark-skinned individuals.

CLINICAL MANIFESTATIONS

- Lichen spinulosus presents as discrete round plaques that are made up of numerous tiny, monomorphic keratotic skin-colored to slightly hypopigmented papules (Fig. 8.17).
- Individual lesions have a keratotic spine protruding from their surface, which results in a rough texture on palpation.
- Most often located on the neck, buttocks, abdomen, or the extremities of a child with dry skin or atopic dermatitis.
- Plaques may be distributed symmetrically.
- May be asymptomatic or mildly itchy.

DIAGNOSIS

- Diagnosis hinges on clinical recognition.

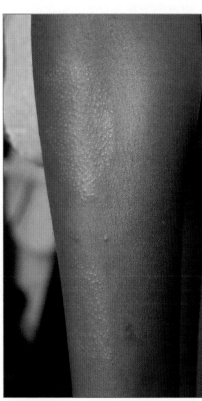

8.17 *Lichen spinulosus.* Note pretibial oval plaques comprised of numerous tiny, monomorphic keratotic skin-colored papules. (Figure courtesy of Lawrence Schachner, M.D.)

 DIFFERENTIAL DIAGNOSIS

Keratosis Pilaris (see Chapter 4)

- *Common condition seen in children with an atopic predisposition.*
- *Keratotic perifollicular papules typically distributed on the cheeks, lateral arms, and thighs of children and adolescents.*

Frictional Lichenoid Dermatitis (see below)

- *Grouped, monomorphic skin-colored papules usually symmetrically distributed on the extensor elbows and dorsal hands.*

 MANAGEMENT

- Lichen spinulosus may persist unchanged for years or come and go; however there is a tendency for lesions to spontaneously disappear at puberty.
- The treatment is similar to what is used for keratosis pilaris and involves keratolytics and emollients.
- Lotions or creams containing salicylic acid, glycolic acid, or ammonium lactate such as **AM Lactin** (12% ammonium lactate) or **Cerave SA** (6% salicylic acid) may help improve appearance and alleviate symptoms.
- **Topical vitamin A** has been used in resistant and extensive cases.
- Most patients are asymptomatic and require no therapy.
- Lichen spinulosus runs a variable course. There is a tendency for lesions to spontaneously disappear at puberty.

 POINTS TO REMEMBER

- Lichen spinulosus is a condition of follicular hyperkeratosis and is regarded as a variant of keratosis pilaris by some.
- Lichen spinulosus often goes unnoticed by the patient or family.

Frictional Lichenoid Dermatitis

BASICS

- Frictional lichenoid dermatitis is an itchy eruption of grouped flat-topped papules on the hands, elbows, and knees that most commonly occurs in children during the spring and summer.
- The condition is more likely to occur in children with an atopic predisposition and is thought to be caused by friction on the affected area.
- Frictional lichenoid dermatitis has also been called *frictional lichenoid eruption, recurrent papular reaction of childhood,* and *summertime pityriasis of the elbows and knees.*

CLINICAL MANIFESTATIONS

- Eruption consists of grouped, 1- to 2-mm, skin-colored, flat-topped papules some coalescing into larger papules or plaques.
- The distribution is very characteristic and typically occurs on the back of the hands, fingers, extensor elbows and knees, although it may occur elsewhere on the body (Fig. 8.18).

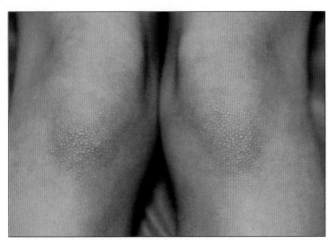

8.18 *Frictional lichenoid dermatitis.* Grouped, 1- to 2-mm, skin-colored, flat-topped papules in a typical location on the knees.

- Often accompanied by mild pruritus.
- Typically, there is a history of contact with an abrasive material such as sand, grasses or wool carpet, or a history of friction on the affected area.

DIAGNOSIS

- Diagnosis is based on clinical recognition of the characteristic lesions in the typical distribution.

 DIFFERENTIAL DIAGNOSIS

Lichen Nitidus (see above)
- *Tiny monomorphic flat-topped papules often in a linear configuration due to Köebnerization.*
- *Common on trunk.*

Molluscum Contagiosum
- *Skin-colored umbilicated papules with central umbilication.*
- *Are usually scattered.*

Id Dermatitis
- *Itchy eruption of eczematous papules that occurs in response to a strong antigenic trigger such as a fungal skin infection or molluscum contagiosum.*

 MANAGEMENT

- Investigating and avoiding the inciting frictional trauma can lead to resolution of the condition.
- Emollients and topical corticosteroids can help alleviate the associated pruritus.

BASICS

- Lichen striatus (LS) is an idiopathic, acquired, linear inflammatory eruption of childhood.
- Although the etiology is unknown, both genetic and environmental factors play a role as LS has been reported to occur in outbreaks and more often in the spring and summer. Also, there is a strong association between LS and atopy.

CLINICAL MANIFESTATIONS

- Most often seen in children 5 to 15 years of age with a median age of 2 to 3 years.
- Individual lesions are tiny, 1- to 2-mm, flat-topped, scaly erythematous papules that coalesce to linear plaques (Fig. 8.19).
- LS most commonly occurs on the extremities but can also be seen on the face (Fig. 8.20), trunk, and buttocks.
- The most characteristic feature is the linear configuration of the lesions along Blaschko lines, the lines of embryonic skin migration. The linear band may be continuous or interrupted (Fig. 8.21).
- Length can vary from several centimeters to involvement of an entire extremity.
- Presents abruptly and reaches its maximum length within several weeks and then regresses spontaneously within 4 to 12 months or occasionally longer.
- In dark-skinned children the eruption may present as linear hypopigmentation.

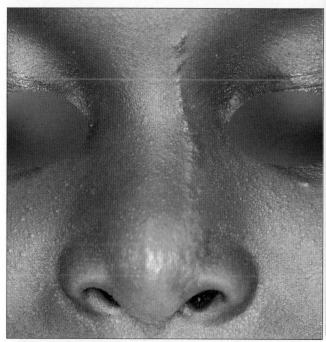

8.20 *Lichen striatus.* Flat-topped, scaly erythematous papules that coalesce into a linear plaque on this boy's nose.

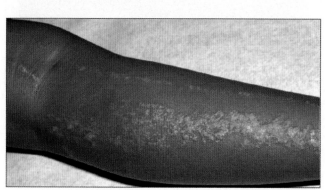

8.21 *Lichen striatus.* Plaques are evident as multiple linear bands in this young girl.

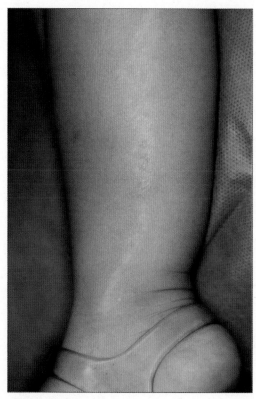

8.19 *Lichen striatus.* Note the linear hypopigmented configuration in this patient.

- Nail involvement may occur as an extension of the skin lesion.
- Usually the eruption is asymptomatic.
- Post-inflammatory hypopigmentation may last months to years.

DIAGNOSIS

- History of abrupt onset and clinical examination will determine the diagnosis.
- If diagnosis is in doubt, a skin biopsy will show the characteristic features including a bandlike lymphohistiocytic infiltrate in the dermis and surrounding the eccrine sweat glands and ducts, epidermal hyperkeratosis and focal parakeratosis.

DIFFERENTIAL DIAGNOSIS

Epidermal Nevus
- *Usually presents at birth or shortly thereafter.*
- *Epidermal nevi can be flat and hypopigmented, verrucous, or pink and scaly (such as in an inflammatory linear verrucous epidermal nevus [ILVEN]) and are linear along Blaschko lines.*

Segmental Vitiligo
- *Type of vitiligo frequently seen in children that presents as a linear depigmented patch along Blaschko lines often on an extremity (Fig. 8.22).*
- *Not palpable, that is, entirely macular.*

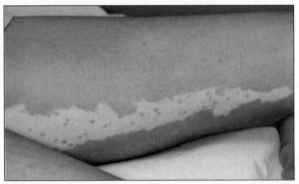

8.22 *Segmental vitiligo.* This linear lesion is not palpable.

 MANAGEMENT

- Usually resolves spontaneously without sequelae in 1 to 3 years thus no therapy is required.
- **Topical corticosteroids** can alleviate pruritic symptoms, if present, and may hasten resolution.
- Parents should be reassured of its benign nature and the expected complete resolution without sequelae.

9 Hair and Nail Disorders

OVERVIEW

Disorders of the hair and nails can cause a considerable amount of emotional distress and anxiety for both the child and family. Hair has significant psychosocial implications and children with hair disorders, particularly hair loss, are often subject to teasing at school. Accurate diagnosis and treatment are essential.

Telogen effluvium is the most common cause of hair loss in children and is often triggered by illness or other stressors. Similarly, onychomadesis or nail shedding most commonly occurs after severe illness. Both conditions are self-limited and discussion with parents about the favorable prognosis and eventual resolution suffices.

Alopecia areata may show spontaneous regrowth but many times parents and/or patients opt for treatment. Tinea capitis should be recognized early and treated with appropriate weight-based systemic antifungals. Intervention for head lice should be prompt so as to avoid epidemics in the classroom. Trichotillomania, categorized as an impulse control disorder, may also require treatment. This chapter will review common pediatric hair and nail conditions and discuss their management.

Alopecia Areata (Also Discussed in Chapter 19)

BASICS

- Alopecia areata (AA) has an estimated lifetime risk of 1.7%, with a peak occurrence in childhood and adolescence. AA is a common autoimmune form of hair loss characterized by one or more focal patches of complete nonscarring alopecia that most often presents in childhood or adolescence.
- AA is discussed in detail in Chapter 19, but the clinical features and its management in childhood will be discussed here.

CLINICAL MANIFESTATIONS

- The most common presentation in children is the sudden onset of a single well-circumscribed, localized patch of smooth alopecia (Fig. 9.1).
- The preceding associated hair shedding may go unnoticed by the patient and/or parent.
- Multiple alopecic patches, sometimes coalescing into larger geometric areas, may be present (Fig. 9.2) or; alopecic patches may be present elsewhere on the body such as the eyebrows (Fig. 9.3), eyelashes, beard, arms, or legs.
- There is usually no associated redness or scaling.
- In the initial active stage of the condition, peripheral hairs are short and thin, appear as "exclamation point hairs" (hairs with tapered ends) under dermoscopy, and are easily plucked from the scalp.
- Initial hair regrowth often appears as white depigmented hairs.
- Nails will show pitting in a grid-like pattern or trachyonychia in 10% to 20% of patients.

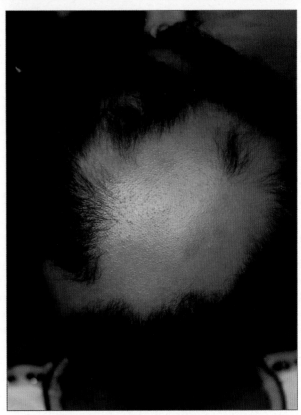

9.2 *Alopecia areata.* Large area of smooth alopecia on the vertex scalp with regrowing hair on posterior scalp.

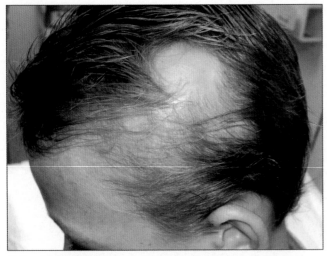

9.1 *Alopecia areata.* A single localized patch of nonscarring, smooth alopecia on the scalp is the most common presentation in children.

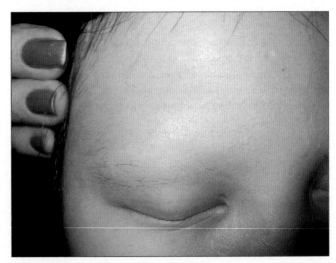

9.3 *Alopecia areata.* Alopecia areata can involve eyebrows and eyelashes.

CLINICAL VARIANTS

- Progression to *alopecia totalis* (complete loss of scalp hair) occurs more commonly in children than adults and is estimated to occur in 5% of children with AA (Fig. 9.4).
- *Alopecia universalis* occurs when there is complete loss of scalp and body hair and is the most severe form of alopecia areata.

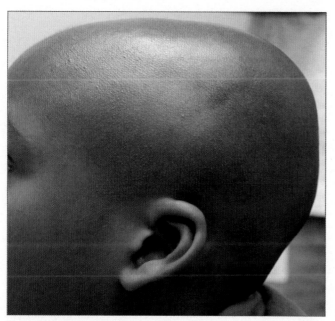

9.4 *Alopecia totalis.* Complete absence of scalp hair but, eyebrows and eyelashes are not affected in this child. (Figure courtesy of Lawrence Schachner, M.D.)

- The *ophiasis* pattern of alopecia areata describes a band-like distribution of hair loss along the hairline of the posterior occipital scalp and the inferior parietal scalp. This pattern occurring in <5% of children has a worse prognosis (see Fig. 19.9).

POOR PROGNOSTIC FACTORS IN AA

- Early age at onset (<2 years)
- Coexisting atopy
- Family history of autoimmune conditions
- Presence of nail abnormalities

DIAGNOSIS

- Diagnosis is made by recognizing the characteristic features on physical examination.
- If in doubt, a skin biopsy showing peribulbar inflammation would be helpful at establishing the diagnosis.

 DIFFERENTIAL DIAGNOSIS

Tinea Capitis
- *Presents as a scaly alopecic patch oftentimes black dots are visible.*
- *KOH or fungal culture will be positive.*

Trichotillomania (Compulsive Hair Pulling)
- *Seen most often in young girls.*
- *Hairs tend to be broken at different lengths.*
- *Occasionally, the alopecia has a telltale geometric shape (see discussion below and in Chapter 19).*

Congenital Triangular Alopecia (Triangular Temporal Alopecia [TTA])
- *Triangular-, oval-, or lancet-shaped alopecic patches typically located on the frontotemporal scalp (Fig. 9.5).*
- *Nonprogressive, nonscarring alopecia in which mature hair follicles have been replaced with vellus-like hair follicles.*
- *Despite the name, the alopecia more typically becomes apparent at 2 to 6 years of age when the surrounding hair becomes thicker.*
- *TTA is typically sporadic but few familial occurrences have been reported.*

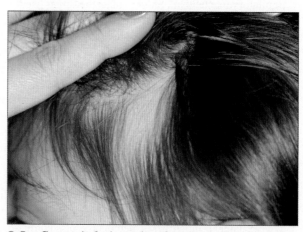

9.5 *Congenital triangular alopecia.* This congenital alopecic patch is typically lancet shaped and unilateral and can mimic alopecia areata. Usually becomes apparent at 2 to 6 years of age.

MANAGEMENT

- In the vast majority of children with AA, complete spontaneous regrowth is expected. Thus, therapy is often unnecessary.
- Alopecia areata can become recurrent in up to 30% of patients.
- Associated autoimmune disorders in affected children are quite rare, if a family history of other autoimmune disorders is elicited then an evaluation of autoimmune conditions, especially thyroiditis, may be indicated.
- Treatment can help hasten regrowth but does not cure the condition and does not prevent new patches from developing.

Topical Treatments

- First-line treatment in children is potent or superpotent topical corticosteroids such as **clobetasol 0.05% cream** or **ointment** with or without occlusion. Foams or solutions may be more practical.
- Occlusion can be achieved with a shower cap.
- If using superpotent topical steroids for a prolonged period on a large area of the scalp, it is important to watch closely for signs of cutaneous atrophy and systemic absorption.
- **Anthralin 1% cream** works by a nonspecific immunostimulatory mechanism. Short contact therapy is used, initially applied to the affected area on the scalp and left on for 30 minutes then washed. The duration of contact is increased gradually to a maximum of 2 hours. The presence of a mild dermatitis is required for regrowth and can be treated with topical corticosteroids.
- Anthralin can be irritating to the skin and can stain skin and clothes.
- Immunotherapy with **squaric acid** induces an allergic contact dermatitis and works by driving away the perifollicular T cells allowing hairs to grow.
- Squaric acid is useful in cases with large alopecic areas. Patients are sensitized to squaric acid (2%) with the application of the chemical on the inner right arm. Then 1 week later, a much lower percentage of squaric acid, usually 0.001%, is applied to the alopecic areas on the scalp and increasing concentrations are applied weekly until a mild low-grade dermatitis occurs. Therapy is continued until cosmetically acceptable regrowth occurs.

- **Excimer laser** therapy (308 nm) targeted twice to three times per week to the alopecic area has been effective in some patients.
- **Topical minoxidil** in a 2% or 5% concentration, scalp massage, heat, aloe vera, vitamins, hypnotherapy, oral psoralens combined with exposure to ultraviolet light in the A range (PUVA), narrow band UVB are other treatments that have varying success rates.

Intralesional Treatment

- Older children and adolescents may tolerate intralesional injections with triamcinolone acetonide (5 mg/cc for scalp, 2.5 mg/cc for eyebrows).
- Injections should be distributed evenly throughout the alopecic patch with a 30-gauge needle in aliquots of 0.1 mL, 1 cm apart; and administered every 4 to 6 weeks for best results.
- The following *pain-reducing techniques* can help children tolerate the discomfort associated with the injections:
  - Topical anesthetics such as **EMLA cream** (lidocaine 2.5% and prilocaine 2.5%) cream or **LMX** (lidocaine 4% cream) applied to area to be injected 30 minutes prior to treatment.
  - **Gebauer's Ethyl Chloride** spray, a skin coolant, sprayed directly on the area to be injected immediately prior to the injection provides instant temporary anesthesia.
  - **Buzzy** is a palm-sized high-frequency vibration device that is placed on the skin next to the injection site and decreases the perception of pain.

Systemic Treatments

- High-dose pulse therapy with PO **prednisone** or IV **methylprednisolone** is reserved for patients with severe (>50% scalp hair) and recurrent disease.
- Corticosteroid pulses are more likely to be effective in patients with a short disease duration (≤6 months), younger age at disease onset (<10 years), and multifocal disease (as opposed to severe, diffuse variants).
- Relapse rate is high.
- **Cyclosporine** and **methotrexate** have been tried with variable success. Treatment with the biologics such as adalimumab, alefacept, etanercept, and infliximab, has been uniformly disappointing.

HELPFUL HINTS

- The vast majority of children have mild or moderate alopecia areata involving <50% of scalp hair.
- Children using superpotent topical steroids under occlusion may absorb sufficient corticosteroids to have systemic effects; absorption can be evaluated with an 8 AM cortisol level.

- Locks of Love is a nonprofit organization that provides hair prostheses to children under the age of 18 years (www.locksoflove.org).
- The National Alopecia Areata Foundation (www.alopeciaareata.com) is a national support group that can be a valuable resource for families.

BASICS

- Telogen effluvium (TE) is the most common type of alopecia in children and is characterized by diffuse hair thinning.
- TE occurs when a triggering event results in the simultaneous shifting of a large number of hairs into the telogen (shedding) phase.
- In children, TE is seen in certain clinical scenarios: during the newborn period, after a severe acute illness, a major trauma, surgery, malnutrition or restricted diets, or rarely, in association with medications such as oral contraceptives and isotretinoin.

CLINICAL MANIFESTATIONS

- Hair shedding and generalized thinning throughout the scalp occurs 3 to 4 months after the triggering event.
- Young children rarely notice a change in hair density.
- Affected adolescents and parents of young children may report an increased shedding as noted by an increased number of hairs on a brush or comb, on pillows or clothing, or a smaller ponytail size.
- Clinical spectrum is variable and may go unnoticed; in general medical attention is sought when >25% of hair is lost.

CLINICAL VARIANTS

OCCIPITAL ALOPECIA OF THE NEWBORN (TELOGEN EFFLUVIUM OF THE NEWBORN)

- Occipital alopecia of the newborn occurring at 3 to 4 months of age is an asymptomatic, ill-defined patch of alopecia localized to the posterior occipital scalp (Fig. 9.6).

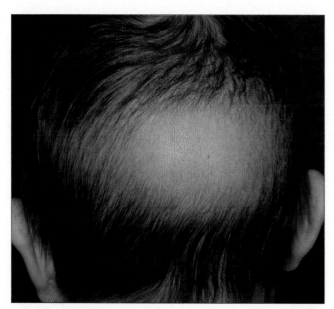

9.6 Occipital alopecia of the newborn. Physiologic telogen effluvium can present as alopecia localized to the posterior occipital scalp in young infants.

- After the first few days of life, anagen hairs convert into telogen hairs and as a result a higher proportion of occipital scalp hairs are shed during the first 4 months of life, creating a noticeable patch of alopecia on the posterior scalp.
- Friction created by rubbing the posterior scalp on the pillow or mattress is also a factor.
- Clinically, the presentation varies from a small patch of relative alopecia to a larger area of complete alopecia.
- Spontaneous complete recovery occurs within months, no treatment is required.

DIAGNOSIS

- Clinical examination of the hair and scalp should include a gentle hair pull of 30 to 60 hairs, if telogen effluvium is present >6 hairs will come out easily.
- A trichogram showing >20% to 25% of hairs in telogen phase can help establish the diagnosis.

 MANAGEMENT

- If the trigger has been removed, complete regrowth is expected within months.
- If the underlying trigger is sustained, telogen effluvium can become chronic.
- Careful discussion with parents about the cause of the condition and its favorable natural history is usually all that is needed.
- Shedding typically stops in 3 to 6 months and complete regrowth may take another 6 months.
- No treatment is necessary and no treatment is uniformly effective.
- However, topical **minoxidil** 2%, 1 mL applied to the scalp twice daily can promote transition back to anagen.

 HELPFUL HINTS

- Occasionally TE can unmask androgenetic alopecia in predisposed individuals and a new baseline hair density is set when the TE episode resolves.
- Blood tests for a possible underlying cause should be guided by history and physical examination if there are no obvious triggers.
- Rate of scalp hair growth is 0.3 mm/day or 1 cm/month.

Trichotillomania

BASICS

- Trichotillomania (TTM) is considered an impulse disorder in which there is self-induced plucking or breakage of hair resulting in noticeable hair loss.
- There is a wide clinical spectrum and not all patients with TTM meet the DSM-IV diagnostic criteria.
- The highest incidence of TTM is in childhood and adolescence and is most commonly seen in girls of age 5 to 12 years.

CLINICAL MANIFESTATIONS

- TTM can present as an irregularly shaped patch of alopecia.
- Bizarre shapes with irregular or telltale geometric shapes (Fig. 9.7) or borders can be seen; some start at a single point and go out centrifugally in a wave-like manner.

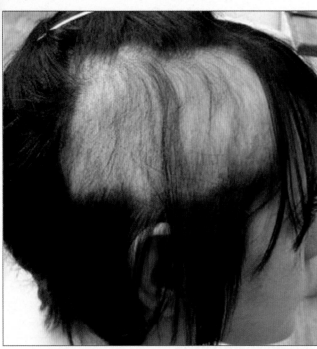

9.7 *Trichotillomania.* Can present as an irregularly shaped patch of alopecia and can take on bizarre or geometric shapes as noted in this patient.

- Typically, hairs in occiput are spared; occasionally the whole scalp is involved.
- Patients with TTM pluck scalp hair most frequently but they may also pluck hair from other hair-bearing areas of the body such as eyebrows.
- Oftentimes, the patient is unaware of the behavior.

DIAGNOSIS

- The clinical diagnosis can be supported by making a "hair growth window" by shaving a small area of involved scalp (at least weekly) to demonstrate normal dense hair regrowth.

 MANAGEMENT

- First-line treatment is behavior modification which can be achieved through cognitive behavioral therapy, specifically habit reversal training.
- Among pharmacologic therapy, **clomipramine** has been most effective in clinical trials.
- **Selective serotonin reuptake inhibitors** (SSRIs) are most commonly prescribed and are beneficial for some patients.
- Hypnosis has also been reported to be helpful in some cases.

BASICS

- Tinea capitis most commonly occurs in prepubertal children.
- In the United States, African-American children are disproportionately affected by this superficial fungal infection of the hair shaft. Tinea capitis appears most often in overcrowded, impoverished inner-city communities.
- *Trichophyton tonsurans* is, by far, the most common etiologic agent; more than 90% of cases are caused by it. Other species, such as *Microsporum audouinii,* which is spread from human to human, and *Microsporum canis,* which is spread from animals (cats and dogs), are more often seen in white children. Patients frequently have a family member, pet, or playmate with tinea.
- Tinea capitis is quite contagious and is generally spread by person-to-person contact. Studies have demonstrated a 30% carrier state of adults exposed to a child with *T. tonsurans.* The organism has also been isolated from such inanimate objects as hairbrushes and pillows.

CLINICAL MANIFESTATIONS

There are essentially five clinical expressions of tinea capitis, with some overlapping physical presentations:

- **Inflamed, scaly**, often alopecic patches, mimicking seborrheic dermatitis, are especially common in infancy until the age of 6 to 8 months (Fig. 9.8).
- A diffuse scaling is seen with multiple round areas, characterized by alopecia that occurs secondary to broken hair shafts, leaving residual black stumps (**"black dot"** ringworm) (Fig. 9.9A,B). It is seen uncommonly and is often mistaken for alopecia areata.

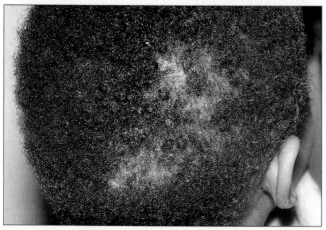

9.8 *Tinea capitis.* Scaly, alopecic patches mimic seborrheic dermatitis; however, there is alopecia and lesions tend to be more localized in tinea capitis.

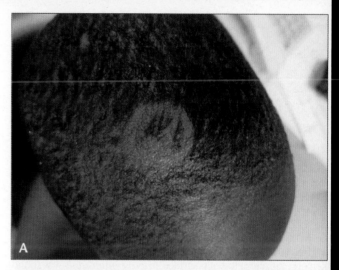

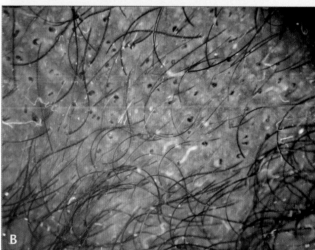

9.9 **A** and **B:** *Tinea capitis.* **A:** "Black dot" ringworm. **B:** A close-up dermoscopic view* of black dot tinea capitis demonstrates the short broken hairs within the alopecic patch. (*A dermoscope is an optical instrument that magnifies and allows inspection of skin lesions unobstructed by skin surface reflections.)

- The **"gray patch"** type (Fig. 9.10) consists of round, scaly plaques of alopecia in which hairs are broken off close to the surface of the scalp.
- A **kerion** is a boggy, pustular, indurated, tumor-like mass, which represents an inflammatory hypersensitivity reaction to the fungus. It typically appears on the scalp. Such inflammation can result in localized scarring (Fig. 9.11).
- Secondary bacterial invaders such as *Staphylococcus aureus* and some gram-negative organisms may sometimes be recovered from a kerion. Often, there is accompanying nontender regional adenopathy.
- Occasionally, a **pustular variety**, with or without alopecia, can mimic a bacterial infection.

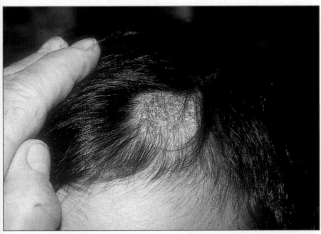

9.10 *Tinea capitis.* "Gray patch type." Note alopecia with broken off hairs close to scalp surface. *Microsporum canis* was found on culture, and the area fluoresced green with a Wood lamp.

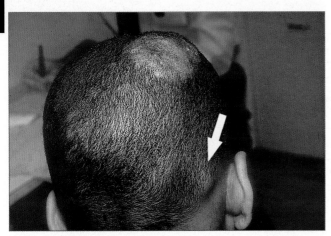

9.11 *Tinea capitis with kerion.* There is also a palpable, asymptomatic, nontender right occipital lymph node (*arrow*).

DIAGNOSIS

- A KOH preparation or fungal culture confirms the diagnosis.
- When in doubt, or when a KOH preparation is negative, a fungal culture placed on Sabouraud's agar should be done. This can be performed by obtaining broken hairs and scale by stroking the affected area with a sterile toothbrush, a familiar object to a child and one that is less frightening than a surgical blade or forceps (see Chapter 35). The collected material is then tapped onto the surface of Sabouraud's agar.
- An alternative method of harvesting broken hairs is by rubbing a moistened gauze pad on the involved area of scalp and then using forceps to place the hairs on the culture medium or slide. Pustules generally are sterile or grow bacterial contaminants.
- A biopsy is rarely necessary.
- In the past, Wood's light examination was a valuable screening tool to diagnose tinea capitis easily (because *Microsporum* species are usually fluorescent), but it has largely lost its usefulness because most cases are caused by the nonfluorescing *T. tonsurans*.

DIFFERENTIAL DIAGNOSIS

Alopecia Areata
- *Has a well-demarcated, symmetric patch of alopecia.*
- *Smooth and free of scale.*
- *KOH is negative.*

Atopic Dermatitis
- *A common cause for an itchy, scaly scalp in children.*
- *No hair loss.*

Seborrheic Dermatitis
- *Infants have "cradle cap" with thick scale.*
- *Alopecia is absent in adults who have scalp involvement.*

Tinea amiantacea
- *KOH-negative local patch or plaque of thick adherent scale ("tinea" is a misnomer for this condition)* (Fig. 9.12).

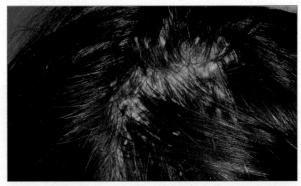

9.12 *Tinea amiantacea.* An inflammatory condition of the scalp in which heavy white or yellow (from sebum) scales extend onto the hairs and bind the proximal portions together; it is not caused by a fungus despite its name. "Pityriasis amiantacea" is probably a better name for this condition.

MANAGEMENT

- Topical therapy is of little or no value in treating tinea capitis; although an adjunctive antifungal shampoo such as ketoconazole 1% to 2% (**Nizoral**) or selenium sulfide 1% to 2.5% (**Selsun**) may be used by the infected person and contacts to prevent reinfection and spread.

Griseofulvin

- In children, systemic therapy with a **liquid suspension of griseofulvin** has been the mainstay of therapy.
- *Dosing:* The effective dose of **microsized griseofulvin** = 20 to 25 mg/kg/day; sometimes as high as 25 mg/kg/day in divided doses. **Ultramicrosized griseofulvin** = 15 to 20 mg/kg/day.
- Should be given with milk or food to increase its absorption and continued until the patient is clinically cured, generally 6 to 8 weeks. Some patients may require longer therapy.
- Treatment failure may indicate inadequate doses or duration of therapy, drug resistance, reinfection from another family member, poor compliance, or immune incompetence.
- **Terbinafine, itraconazole**, and **fluconazole** are more efficacious agents. They have been used in some cases of griseofulvin treatment failure.

Terbinafine (Lamisil)

- Available as a 250 mg tablet or a 125 or 187.5 mg granule packet.
- *Dosing:* weight-based, <20 kg take 62.5 mg/day; 20 to 40 kg take 125 mg/day; >40 kg take 250 mg/day.
- Granules are child friendly and parents can be instructed to sprinkle it on the food.

Itraconazole (Sporanox)

- Available as 100 mg capsules or as an oral suspension of 10 mg/mL.
- *Dosing:* 5 mg/kg/day (maximum 500 mg) for 4 to 8 weeks.

Fluconazole (Diflucan)

- Available in 100, 150, and 200 mg tablets and as an oral solution of 10 and 40 mg/mL.
- *Dosing:* 6 mg/kg/day for 3 to 6 weeks
- Occasionally, concomitant systemic steroid therapy is warranted in addition to griseofulvin or other systemic antifungal when the patient is experiencing a severe, tender, or painful kerion. A short course (usually 5 to 7 days) of **oral prednisone**, 1 mg/kg/day, is sufficient.

HELPFUL HINTS

- A pustular presentation of tinea capitis can mimic a bacterial infection.
- When a child has scaling alopecia and enlarged lymph nodes in the posterior auricular or occipital area, obtain a fungal culture and consider starting empiric antifungal treatment.
- In many instances, therapy may have to be initiated in a patient with negative KOH examination and fungal cultures, based solely on clinical appearance.
- Siblings of tinea capitis patients should be evaluated, or else the infection might be "ping-ponged" back and forth within the family.
- Occasionally, an "id-like" reaction occurs shortly after the initiation of griseofulvin therapy. This consists of multiple small sterile papules on the face or body, and it probably represents a hypersensitivity response.

POINTS TO REMEMBER

- The standard of diagnosis is a positive KOH examination or culture.
- Topical therapy is ineffective for tinea capitis.
- Systemic therapy must be in an adequate dosage and duration.

BASICS

- Pediculosis capitis (head lice) is a common parasitic infestation in school-aged children, occasionally occurring in epidemics.
- Lice spend their entire life cycle on the human and feed exclusively on human blood.
- Transmission occurs by head-to-head contact or via shared combs, brushes, hats, or other personal items.
- Head lice occur more often in girls and women; they are unusual in African-Americans, but not in African blacks.

CLINICAL MANIFESTATIONS

- Patients usually complain of intense scalp itch but occasionally children with head lice may be asymptomatic.
- There are no primary lesions; however, secondary crusts and eczematous dermatitis resulting from scratching may be present.
- Itching may be delayed 4 to 6 weeks.
- Female louse lays 10 eggs per day → the egg (nit) tightly adheres to the hair shaft at the scalp → eggs hatch in 7 to 12 days → becomes an adult (after three nymph stages) in 9 to 12 days. Female lice live for 3 to 4 weeks.
- Nits (louse eggs) are firmly stuck on to scalp hairs and can be easily visualized with side lighting. Nits can be seen at varying distances from the scalp.
- Occasionally live living lice can also be seen on the scalp (Fig. 9.13).

DIAGNOSIS

- Knowledge of an epidemic at school generally alerts parents or school nurses to look for evidence of lice.
- White nits may be very obvious on a background of darker hair.
- A hair may be plucked and examined for nits using the low power of a microscope (Fig. 9.14).
- A nit is attached to the base of a hair shaft when the egg is first laid and remains cemented to the growing hair so in general the distance from the scalp can give an idea of how long the infestation has been present.

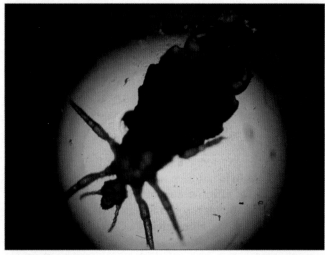

9.13 **_Head lice._** Occasionally the adult female louse can be found on the scalp. The female louse can lay up to 10 eggs per day and lives 3 to 4 weeks on the human scalp.

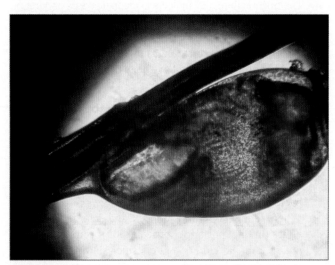

9.14 **_Head lice._** Nits adhere firmly to the hair shaft.

 DIFFERENTIAL DIAGNOSIS

Atopic Dermatitis of the Scalp
- _Should be considered if there is a positive atopic history._

Seborrheic Dermatitis or Dandruff
- _White flakes on hair will easily fall away when patted._
- _Redness and typical greasy yellow scaling throughout scalp._

 HELPFUL HINTS

- Patients being treated for lice should be instructed to wear hair pulled back.
- In a patient who has been treated for lice, nits attached more than 1 cm from the scalp are typically nonviable.
- Items that cannot be washed or dry cleaned should be placed in a sealed bag for 2 weeks.

MANAGEMENT

General Principles

- First-line treatment for head lice is a topical pediculicide.
- **All treatments should be repeated after 1 week** (regardless of what package instructions suggest), in order to assure killing any nits that may have survived and prevent reinfestation from fomites.
- Pediculicides have two modes of action: neurotoxic or physical.
- Despite recommendations against it by the American Academy of Pediatrics, many schools still have a "no nit" policy whereby a child will not be allowed back to school unless the scalp is completely nit free; thus, manual removal of nits is important part of the treatment.
- Nits are best removed manually with a fine-tooth metal comb.
- All recently used clothing, hats, bedding, and towels as well as combs, brushes, and hair clips should be washed in hot water.
- Other household members should be evaluated for lice and treated simultaneously.

Topical Treatments: Neurotoxic Mode of Action

Permethrin 1% cream or rinse (Nix Creme Rinse, Acticin) is available over the counter.
- *How to use:* Wash hair, towel dry, apply cream rinse leave on for 10 minutes then rinse, repeat in 7 days.

Permethrin 5% Cream (Elimite Cream) is available as a prescription.
- *How to use:* Apply to dry hair, leave on overnight (12 hours) under an occlusive shower cap, repeat in 7 days.
- High rates of resistance (even to the higher concentrations) have limited its usefulness.

Pyrethrins with piperonyl butoxide (RID, Pronto, Licide) available over the counter.
- *How to use:* Apply to dry hair, leave on for 10 minutes then rinse off, repeat in 7 days.
- Treatment failures are now commonplace due to resistance.
- Allergic reactions can develop in patients sensitive to chrysanthemums, ragweed, and related plants.

Malathion 0.5% Lotion (Ovide) available as a prescription.
- This agent is considered the most effective treatment for head lice.
- *How to use:* Apply to dry hair, massage into the scalp and leave on for 8 to 12 hours, repeat in 7 days.
- Caution: Ovide Lotion is flammable. Treated areas that are wet with this product should be kept away from open flames and electric heat sources such as hair dryers.

- Some resistance has been reported in the United Kingdom, but not in the United States.

Lindane 1% shampoo (Kwell, Scabene), available as a 1% prescription shampoo.
- *How to use:* Apply for 4 minutes to clean, dry hair then add water to lather and rinse, repeat in 7 days.
- Reserved for patients who fail to respond to other approved lice therapies due to risk of CNS side effects and associated FDA black box warning.
- Resistance is commonly observed.

Ivermectin 0.5% lotion (Sklice) available as a prescription.
- *How to use:* Apply to dry hair, leave on for 10 minutes, repeat in 7 days.
- Approved for use in people 6 months of age and older.

Spinosad 0.9% cream rinse (Natroba) available as a prescription.
- A newer pediculicide, Spinosad is a fermentation product of the bacterium *Saccharopolyspora spinosa* that induces muscle spasms and paralysis in lice.
- *How to use:* apply to dry hair, leave on for 10 minutes then rinse, repeat in 7 days.

Topical treatments: Physical mode of action

Benzyl alcohol 5% lotion (Ulesfia) available as a prescription.
- Benzyl alcohol is thought to act via asphyxiation by preventing lice from closing their respiratory spiracles, which become blocked by the lotion; it is not ovicidal.
- FDA approved for the treatment of head lice in children ≥6 months of age.
- *How to use:* Two 10-minute applications administered 1 week apart.

Other occlusive agents: **Vaseline Petroleum Jelly, mayonnaise, or Cetaphil cleanser**
- Quite messy and difficult to remove, but it is an inexpensive and sometimes effective method that asphyxiates the lice and nits.
- *How to use:* Apply to entire scalp and is left on under a shower cap overnight, repeat in 7 days.

Oral Pediculicide

Ivermectin via prescription as 3 mg tabs.
- *How to use:* Take 200 to 400 mcg/kg of ivermectin on days 1 and 8.
- Ivermectin is an option for patients whose disease is resistant to topical treatments.
- Children who weigh less than 33 pounds (15 kg) and pregnant or breastfeeding women should not receive oral ivermectin since safety data on these populations are not available.

Trachyonychia

BASICS

- Trachyonychia (derived from the Greek *trakos* for rough) is an acquired condition of rough nails and is characterized by ridging, longitudinal grooves, opaque discoloration and roughness, and an increased tendency for nail breakage (see also Chapter 22).
- Trachyonychia can occur in one or multiple nails. When all 20 nails are involved the condition is called *20-nail dystrophy,* although this term is often used when the typical changes are present even in only a few nails.
- In children, trachyonychia most commonly occurs as an isolated condition, but it may be seen in association with skin diseases such as atopic dermatitis, alopecia areata, or psoriasis.

CLINICAL MANIFESTATIONS

- Clinical presentation varies from mild disease presenting as thin brittle nails with excessive longitudinal ridging and pits to severe disease manifesting as thick, opaque, sandpaper-like nails (Figs. 9.15 and 9.16).
- The cuticle is usually hyperkeratotic and ragged.
- Koilonychia (spoon-shaped nails) may be present.
- It may involve one, several, or all digits.

DIAGNOSIS

- Made on clinical grounds and ruling out of causative conditions.

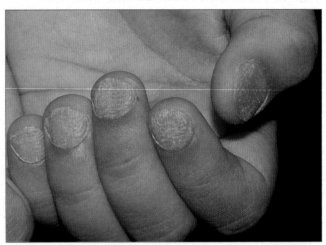

9.15   *Trachyonychia.* Longitudinal ridging and a rough sandpaper-like texture are characteristic of this condition.

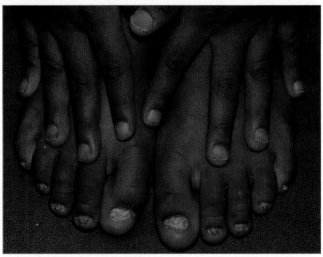

9.16   *Trachyonychia.* When all 20 nails are involved, the condition is termed 20-nail dystrophy. Spontaneous resolution over time typically occurs.

 DIFFERENTIAL DIAGNOSIS

Onychomycosis (see discussion Chapter 22)
- *Positive KOH examination or fungal culture* (Fig. 9.17).

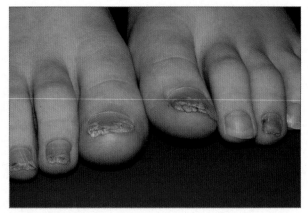

9.17   *Onychomycosis.* The nails are dystrophic and discolored, and there is a buildup of keratin underneath them (subungual hyperkeratosis).

 MANAGEMENT

- The majority of cases of pediatric trachyonychia are isolated and improve with time.
- Spontaneous improvement may take months to years.
- Potent topical steroids with or without occlusion such as **clobetasol 0.05% ointment** or **flurandrenolide tape (Cordran tape)** may improve the appearance of the nails.
- Topical tazarotene cream or gel has been used with some success.

- Regular nail care such as filing and using a clear nail polish can help smoothen the texture of the nail plate surface.
- Biotin supplementation is often recommended and has been reported to be useful in some cases.
- In severe cases, systemic retinoids and intralesional steroids have been tried.

BASICS

- Onychomadesis is a spontaneous nail shedding that most often results as a reaction to a viral exanthem, most commonly the enteroviral exanthems.
- A Beau line is a transverse depression in the nail plate that grows distally with the growth of the nail.
- Both onychomadesis and beau's lines result from a temporary interruption of nail formation.
- Most common associations in children include: coxsackie infection, febrile illnesses, Kawasaki disease, periungual inflammation, or trauma.

CLINICAL MANIFESTATIONS

- When there is only partial interruption of the nail matrix activity a single transverse groove appears at the proximal nail fold that moves outward with nail growth. This is referred to as a Beau line (Fig. 9.18).
- When the trigger interrupts nail matrix function completely then there is onychomadesis where there is complete separation of the nail plate (Fig. 9.19).
- Normal fingernail growth is 1 mm per week. The Beau line or the completely separated nail will move outward as normal new nail grows. New nail growth is usually complete by 4 to 6 months.

 MANAGEMENT

- Reassurance of complete normal nail growth is expected.

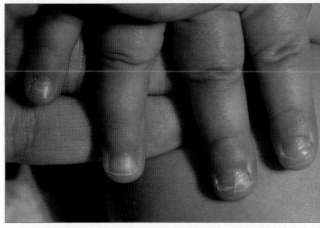

9.18 *Beau line.* Transverse groove in the nail plate that represents partial interruption of the nail matrix.

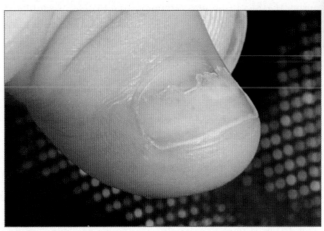

9.19 *Onychomadesis.* When there is temporary complete arrest of nail matrix activity there is shedding of the distal nail.

Cutaneous Manifestations of Systemic Disease

OVERVIEW

Characteristic skin features can be clues to more serious underlying systemic illnesses in children. Henoch–Schönlein purpura (HSP) is the most common small vessel vasculitis in children and can be associated with considerable morbidity. Recognition of the associated palpable purpura on the skin can help make the diagnosis quickly. Similarly, identifying the skin features of Kawasaki disease (KD) in a patient with a conjunctivitis and fever can alert the clinician to the diagnosis. The diagnosis of juvenile dermatomyositis (JDM) is often delayed because the skin findings may be brushed off as an eczematous dermatitis. In the correct clinical context, redness of the face and scaly plaques on the hands and wrists should prompt consideration of dermatomyositis.

Early recognition of the skin findings is key to aid in prompt diagnosis and treatment. In this chapter HSP, KD, and JDM will be discussed with particular attention to the associated skin features. Correctly recognizing the skin findings and associating them with the other clinical features may help prevent unnecessary tests and delay in diagnosis.

IN THIS CHAPTER...

➤ **HENOCH–SCHÖNLEIN PURPURA**

➤ **KAWASAKI DISEASE**

➤ **JUVENILE DERMATOMYOSITIS**

Henoch–Schönlein Purpura

BASICS

- Henoch–Schönlein purpura (HSP) is the most common systemic vasculitis in children and is thought to occur in 10 to 20 per 100,000 children.
- Incidence is highest among children of Asian descent.
- Mean age at onset is 4 to 6 years and it is more common in males, primarily in the fall and winter.

PATHOGENESIS

- HSP is a systemic immune-mediated small vessel vasculitis characterized by IgA deposition within affected organs.
- The underlying cause remains unknown but suspected etiologic agents include infections (viral or Group A *streptococcus*), vaccinations, or insect bites.

CLINICAL MANIFESTATIONS

- Signs and symptoms develop over the course of days to weeks and vary in order of presentation.
- Typically, the skin eruption is the first sign followed by arthralgia/arthritis, abdominal pain or GI bleeding, and renal involvement.
- Early skin lesions may be pink urticarial papules that evolve into deep red to purple nonblanching macules or petechiae.
- The characteristic finding is palpable purpura, which is the result of swelling and extravasation of red blood cells.
- Lesions are nonblanching meaning that they do not disappear when pressure is exerted on them.
- Skin lesions are more common on dependent areas of the body including the legs and buttocks. The lateral malleolus is almost invariably involved (Fig. 10.1).
- Lesions can vary in size and coalesce. Occasionally, vesicles, bullous lesions, and/or ulcers occur (Fig. 10.2).
- If the scrotal vessels are affected, there may be acute scrotal swelling with or without erythema or purpura and is associated with severe pain.
- Systemic involvement is common and occurs in 80% of affected children, most often in the GI tract and presents with colicky abdominal pain with or without vomiting.
- The joints are the second most common site of systemic involvement.
- Rarely, seizures, headaches, or intracerebral bleeding occurs.

DIAGNOSIS

- The diagnosis of HSP is made clinically by and requires the presence of palpable purpura on the skin in addition to at least one of the following findings:
  - Diffuse abdominal pain
  - ANY biopsy showing predominant IgA deposition

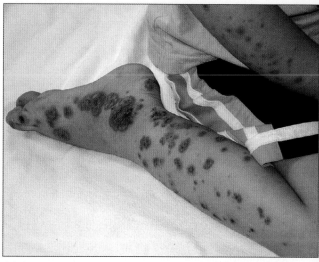

10.1 *Henoch–Schönlein purpura.* Palpable purpura on the lower extremities, some lesions have developed overlying bullae. Note involvement of the lateral malleolus.

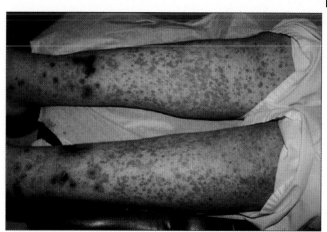

10.2 *Henoch–Schönlein purpura.* Severe eruption of palpable purpura on the lower extremities with ulcerations.

  - Arthritis or arthralgia
  - Renal involvement
- For atypical presentations, a skin biopsy with direct immunofluorescence showing leukocytoclastic vasculitis and IgA deposition can help solidify the diagnosis.

 DIFFERENTIAL DIAGNOSIS

Hypersensitivity Vasculitis (i.e., Secondary to a Drug, etc.)
- *Systemic symptoms usually absent.*
- *History of a trigger.*

MANAGEMENT

- Most patients with HSP recover fully without sequelae in 4 to 6 weeks.
- Supportive care with oral hydration, bed rest, elevation of swollen areas is often sufficient.
- Pain can be managed with acetaminophen or NSAIDs.
- Skin lesions fade over 5 to 7 days with postinflammatory hyperpigmentation.
- Hospitalization is warranted if patient is unable to maintain adequate hydration or if there is severe abdominal or joint pain, significant GI bleeding, or renal insufficiency.
- Patients with kidney involvement require long-term follow-up.
- Occasionally, patients may have recurrent flares of HSP.

 HELPFUL HINTS

- Systemic steroids are reserved for cases of HSP with severe abdominal or joint pain.
- In pediatric patients, biopsy is only necessary for patients with an unusual presentation of HSP (i.e., no rash, or an atypical rash) or those with significant renal disease.

 POINT TO REMEMBER

- In mild cases of HSP, the lateral malleolus may be one of the few areas where the skin eruption is present.

Kawasaki Disease

BASICS

- Kawasaki Disease (KD), also known as mucocutaneous lymph node syndrome, is an acute, febrile, multisystem illness that primarily affects young children.
- Its most serious complications are the result of systemic vasculitis.
- The peak incidence of KD is between 1 and 2 years of age and mostly occurs before 5 years of age. It is more common in boys.
- In the United States, children of Asian ancestry are affected six times more often than are white children.
- KD occurs sporadically and in epidemics. A seasonal predilection has been observed, with cases occurring more often in the winter and spring.

PATHOGENESIS

- KD is a generalized vasculitis that involves small- to medium-sized arteries.
- Although the exact cause of KD is unknown, it is most likely the result of a superantigen produced by an infectious agent such as *Staphylococcus aureus,* resulting in massive cytokine release.

CLINICAL MANIFESTATIONS

- *Fever.* Usually marks the onset of KD and is present for at least 5 days straight. Elevated temperature shows a remittent pattern, with spikes to 103°F and even up to 105°F. The average duration of the fever is 11 days.
- *Cervical lymphadenopathy.* A single, enlarged, nonsuppurative lymph node on the side of the neck (cervical chain) is the least common diagnostic feature of KD, seen in 75% of patients.
- *Bilateral conjunctival injection.* Characterized by bilateral, nonpurulent, limbic sparing conjunctival injection. Patients may exhibit signs of photophobia (Fig. 10.3).
- *Oral mucous membrane changes.* The earliest manifestations are seen on the lips, with bright red erythema accompanied by fissuring and swelling. Prominent papillae create the appearance of a "strawberry tongue" (Fig. 10.4). Examination of the oropharynx reveals a diffuse erythema without vesicles, erosions, or ulcers.
- *Changes in the extremities.* An intense erythema appears on the palms and soles on days 3 to 5 of the illness, followed by an indurated edema. A sharp demarcation may be seen at the wrists and the sides of the hands and feet.
- *Polymorphous rash.* The truncal rash of KD is polymorphous and can be macular, papular, urticarial, erythrodermatous, targetoid, or composed of fine micropustules, but it is never vesicular or bullous. The eruption is usually pruritic and favors the trunk and proximal extremities, but it may be generalized (Fig. 10.5).
- The presence of scarlatiniform erythema in the perianal or inguinal area may be a useful diagnostic sign. The rash in

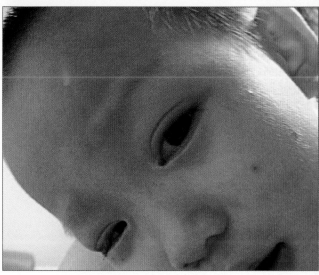

10.3 *Kawasaki disease.* Nonpurulent, limbic sparing conjunctival injection typical of KD.

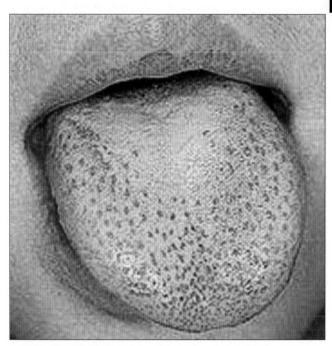

10.4 *Kawasaki disease.* "Strawberry tongue."

this area progresses to desquamation before the palms and soles begin to peel (Fig. 10.6).

CLINICAL SEQUELAE

- Cardiac involvement is the most worrisome complication of KD.
- During the acute phase of the illness, tachycardia may develop, with gallop rhythm, subtle electrocardiographic changes, pericardial effusion, tricuspid insufficiency, or mitral regurgitation.
- Coronary artery aneurysms have been reported to occur in approximately 25% of untreated patients and may result in thrombosis with subsequent infarction.

DIAGNOSIS

- The diagnosis of KD is based on recognition of its clinical features and is supported by compatible laboratory findings.
- Diagnosis requires fever persisting 5 days or more plus 4 out of 5 of the following features:
  - Polymorphous rash
  - Bilateral conjunctival injection
  - Oral mucous membrane changes
  - Cervical lymphadenopathy
  - Changes of peripheral extremities: Erythema of palms and soles, indurative edema of the hands and feet, desquamation of the fingertips.

LABORATORY FINDINGS

- During the acute phase of the illness, leukocytosis with a predominance of immature and mature granulocytes is common, with 50% of patients having a white blood cell count >15,000/mL.
- Nonspecific abnormalities of acute phase reactants, such as the erythrocyte sedimentation rate and C-reactive protein levels are usually present.

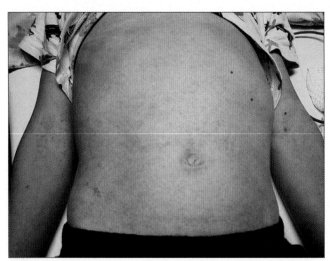

10.5 *Kawasaki disease.* Polymorphous rash on the trunk in a patient with KD.

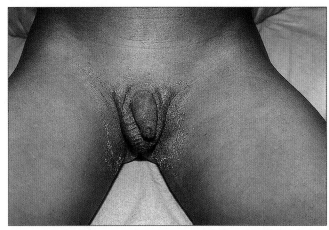

10.6 *Kawasaki disease.* Desquamation in the genital area. This sheet-like desquamation occurred 2 weeks after the original infection.

 DIFFERENTIAL DIAGNOSIS

- **Staphylococcal** or **Streptococcal Toxic Shock Syndrome (TSS)** (see Chapter 7)
- **Scarlet fever** (see Chapter 7)
- **Rubella and rubeola** (see Chapter 7)
- **Febrile viral exanthems**
- **Mononucleosis**
- **Hypersensitivity reactions** (including Stevens–Johnson syndrome)
- **Drug eruptions** with accompanying fever (see Chapter 26)
- Infantile **polyarteritis nodosa**

MANAGEMENT

- Most children with KD must be hospitalized for a complete workup and supportive care. Because high temperatures and irritability make feeding difficult, intravenous fluids are often needed for hydration.
- The initial goals of therapy are to reduce the fever and the inflammation of the myocardium and to prevent subsequent cardiac sequelae.
- Children with evidence of cardiac disease may require intensive support.
- Once the diagnosis of KD has been established, therapy with **intravenous immune globulin (IVIG)**, or **gamma globulin**, and **aspirin** should be started.
- **High-dose aspirin** at a dose of 80 to 100 mg/kg/day PO in four equally divided doses is continued during the acute phase for its anti-inflammatory effects. It is continued at this dose until day 14 of the illness or until the patient has been afebrile for 48 to 72 hours.
- **IVIG** has a synergistic effect with aspirin and reduces acute inflammation, with the maximal benefits seen when it is given within the first 10 days of the illness. IVIG has been shown to reduce the rate of coronary aneurysms from greater than 25% in untreated patients to 1% to 5% in treated patients. IVIG may decrease autoantibody production and increase solubilization and removal of immune complexes.

HELPFUL HINTS

- KD should be considered in children with an unexplained fever lasting more than 5 days who have a polymorphous rash that may look like scarlet fever or measles, and conjunctivitis without pus.
- Some children may present with an incomplete clinical picture and may not exhibit sufficient clinical signs to fulfill the diagnostic criteria; therefore, a high level of suspicion is required to recognize these patients.
- The extent of the coronary vascular involvement is so significant that KD has now surpassed rheumatic fever as the leading cause of acquired heart disease in children from developed nations.
- All patients with KD should have an echocardiogram during the acute illness and 3 to 6 weeks after the onset of fever.

POINTS TO REMEMBER

- Prompt treatment with aspirin and IVIG significantly decreases the risk of cardiac complications.
- Although most patients recover with little to no limitations on physical activity, a delay in diagnosis results in a greater likelihood of coronary lesions and related complications.

Juvenile Dermatomyositis

BASICS

- Dermatomyositis in adults is discussed in detail in Chapter 34. The juvenile form for dermatomyositis and its characteristic distinguishing features will be discussed in this section.
- Juvenile dermatomyositis (JDM), the most common inflammatory myopathy in children, occurs in 3 per million children, and more often in girls.
- Incidence of JDM peaks between 2 and 5 years of age and at 12 to 13 years of age.

KEY DIFFERENCES BETWEEN ADULT-ONSET DERMATOMYOSITIS AND JDM

- JDM is rarely paraneoplastic.
- Children tend to have more severe muscle inflammation.
- Calcinosis cutis occurs more frequently in JDM.
- JDM is associated with lower mortality.
- Adults have higher frequency of myositis-specific antibodies

PATHOGENESIS

- Not exactly known, but thought to be an autoimmune systemic small vessel vasculopathy, where the primary lesion occurs in the endothelial cell.
- Infectious agents and genetic factors likely play a role.

CLINICAL MANIFESTATIONS

- Onset is usually gradual with subtle symptoms including low-grade fever, malaise, weight loss, poor appetite, pruritus, and photosensitivity of affected skin areas. Occasionally, the onset is rapid with fevers and severe muscle weakness.
- The cutaneous features are seen at presentation in the vast majority of patients with JDM and range from very subtle to striking.
- Violaceous telangiectatic erythema with or without scaling on the sun-exposed areas of the body is characteristic (Fig. 10.7). When present around the eyes and eyelids it is called the heliotrope rash (see Fig. 34.25). When present on the dorsal knuckles it is called Gottron sign and on shoulders and chest it is referred to as the Shawl sign (see Figs. 34.27 and 34.28).
- Gottron papules are a pathognomonic sign of JDM and appear as grouped erythematous or violaceous, flat-topped papules on the dorsal metacarpal phalangeal and proximal phalangeal joints (Fig. 10.8 [see Fig. 34.26]).
- Periungual telangiectasias and erythema with thickened, unkempt appearing cuticles are also characteristic of JDM (Fig. 10.9 [see Figs. 34.17 and 34.30]).

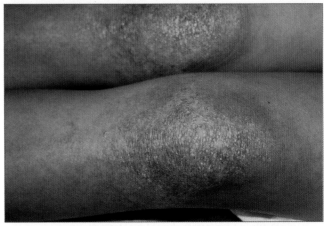

10.7   *Juvenile dermatomyositis.* The scaly violaceous plaques on the knees of a patient with JDM can resemble subacute eczema. (Figure courtesy of Lawrence A. Schachner, MD.)

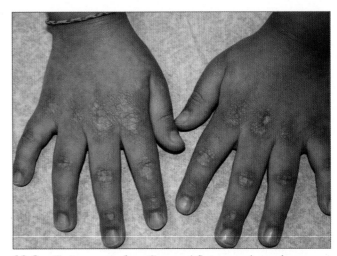

10.8   *Gottron papules.* Grouped flat-topped papules on the dorsal hand in a child with JDM. (Figure courtesy of Lawrence A. Schachner, MD.)

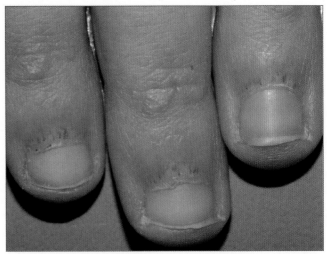

10.9   *Periungual telangiectasias.* Characteristic of JDM, course parallels improvement of systemic disease. Note gottron papules over distal interphalangeal joints.

- Calcinosis cutis occurs in up to 40% of patients with JDM and presents as firm, yellow- or flesh-colored nodules, often over bony prominences.
- Other skin features that occur less often include palmar erythema and thickening, panniculitis presenting as tender, indurated plaques and nodules on the arms, thighs, and buttocks, and nonscarring alopecia.
- With long-standing disease some affected children develop very itchy dry skin with poikiloderma (telangiectasia, atrophy, hyperpigmentation, and hypopigmentation), and lipodystrophy may occur especially if condition is not well controlled.
- Pitted ulcerations of distal aspects of the limbs are a sign of severe disease.
- Muscle weakness affects the large proximal muscles and is bilateral and progressive.
- Patients may report an inability to comb hair or difficulty climbing stairs and young children may show more demanding behavior or complaints of fatigue and not wanting to walk or reach for things.
- Arthritis usually is asymptomatic and of the large joints occurs in half of the affected children.

DIAGNOSIS

- Diagnosis is usually made on clinical grounds by identifying the characteristic clinical features and the muscle weakness.
- One or more muscle enzymes including serum aldolase, aspartate aminotransferase, lactic dehydrogenase, and serum creatine phosphokinase will be elevated.
- A muscle MRI will show muscle inflammation.
- A skin biopsy is not necessary.

 MANAGEMENT

- The course of JDM is variable and can be chronic in up to 60% of cases.
- Limited skin disease and short duration of disease before treatment is initiated portends a better prognosis.
- First-line treatment is **high-dose systemic corticosteroids** preferably given IV, as pulses, every 1 to 2 days until muscle enzymes normalize.
- **Methotrexate** in addition to systemic steroids is more effective than either treatment alone.
- Methotrexate alone is second-line treatment when corticosteroids cannot be given.
- Other systemic agents that have shown efficacy for JDM include the following:
  - **IVIG**
  - **Azathioprine**
  - **Cyclosporine**
  - **Rituximab**
- Skin disease may persist despite improvement in muscle disease.
- In general, patients should avoid excessive sun exposure and use broad-spectrum sunscreens.
- The antimalarial, hydroxychloroquine **(Plaquenil)**, 5 mg/kg/day can help the cutaneous manifestations.
- Topical corticosteroids may help with itching but do little to improve the skin changes associated with JDM.
- Calcinosis cutis is difficult to treat and can lead to significant morbidity.
- The bisphosphonates and surgical excision have both been helpful for problematic calcinosis.

 HELPFUL HINT

- Patients on hydroxychloroquine long term should have regular ophthalmologic examinations every 6 months.

 POINTS TO REMEMBER

- Sun exposure is known to trigger both cutaneous and muscle signs.
- Presence of periungual telangiectasias and erythema on the skin correlates with disease activity.

11 Neurocutaneous Syndromes

OVERVIEW

Skin lesions are often the initial clue seen in neurocutaneous syndromes. As discussed in this chapter, identifying multiple café au lait spots or hypopigmented macules on a skin examination should prompt a more thorough history taking and a directed physical examination.

A definitive diagnosis of neurofibromatosis type 1 (NF1) can be made with a clinical examination that identifies six or more characteristic café au lait macules (CALMs) and axillary freckling. Identifying one of these two findings on a skin examination should raise suspicion for the NF1 and lead to further workup. Similarly the typical hypopigmented macule (*ash-leaf spot*) and the *shagreen patch* on the lower back, representing a connective tissue nevus are among the earliest signs of tuberous sclerosis. Neurofibromatosis and tuberous sclerosis are autosomal dominantly inherited neurocutaneous syndromes with variable clinical features a wide spectrum of clinical presentations. Early recognition is essential for proper surveillance and early interventions as necessary.

IN THIS CHAPTER...
➤ **NEUROFIBROMATOSIS**
➤ **TUBEROUS SCLEROSIS**

Neurofibromatosis

BASICS

- Neurofibromatosis type 1 (NF1), also called von Recklinghausen disease, and neurofibromatosis type 2 (NF2), also called bilateral acoustic or central neurofibromatosis, are autosomal dominantly inherited diseases characterized by the propensity to develop tumors, especially of the nerve sheath.
- NF1 occurs in 1 out of 3,500 births and demonstrates variable expressivity and significant clinical heterogeneity ranging from a severe course with malignant brain tumors and profound mental retardation to mild disease with few skin tumors.
- The incidence of NF2 is 1 per 40,000 births.

PATHOGENESIS

- There are two types of NF:
  - NF1 is caused by a mutation in the gene for neurofibromin, a tumor suppressor gene, located on chromosome 17q11.2. Fifty percent of cases are the result of spontaneous new mutations.
  - NF2 is caused by a mutation in the gene that codes for merlin, a protein important for cell division, localized to chromosome 22q11.

CLINICAL MANIFESTATIONS

NEUROFIBROMATOSIS TYPE 1

- **Café au lait macules** (CALMs), often called café au lait spots, are the earliest clinical manifestation of NF.
- A CALM is a light brown to tan macule or patch. The CALMs that are associated with NF1 typically have smooth borders (Fig. 11.1).
- Axillary or inguinal freckling (**Crowe sign**) consists of small, pigmented tan macules and when present is considered to be pathognomonic for NF1 (Fig. 11.2).
- **Cutaneous neurofibromas** are soft, rubbery, skin-colored or tan-pink papules and nodules (Figs. 11.3 and 11.4) and usually present after puberty.

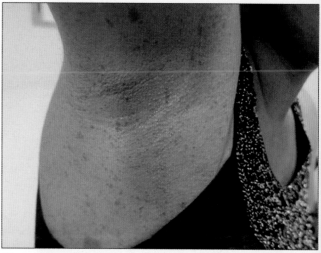

11.2 *Neurofibromatosis.* Axillary freckling is a major criterion for NF1.

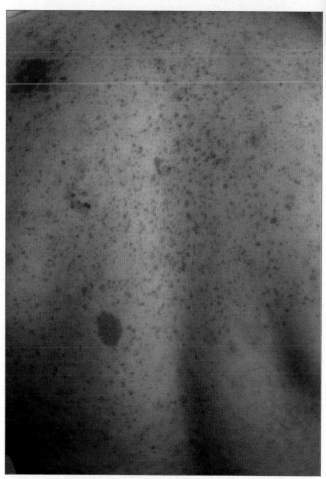

11.3 *Neurofibromatosis.* Multiple variably sized café au lait macules and several neurofibromas on the back. (Figure courtesy of Miguel R. Sanchez, M.D.)

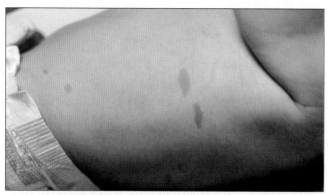

11.1 *Neurofibromatosis.* Café au lait spots with smooth borders, typical of NF1, on the abdomen of this 4-month-old boy.

- **Plexiform neuromas** manifest as large drooping tumors, which on palpation feel like a "bag of worms" and occur in 30% to 50% of patients with NF1 (Fig. 11.5).
- Ocular lesions (**Lisch nodules**) are asymptomatic, pigmented iris hamartomas seen in 80% of patients with NF.

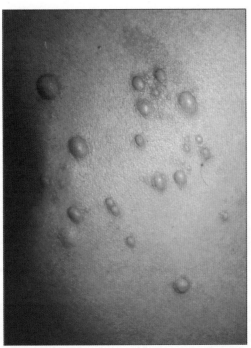

11.4 *Neurofibromatosis.* Multiple variably sized neurofibromas and a large café au lait on the back. (Figure courtesy of Miguel R. Sanchez, M.D.)

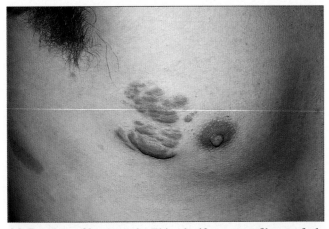

11.5 *Neurofibromatosis.* This plexiform neurofibroma feels like a "bag of worms."

- Macrocephaly is also an early sign of NF1 and may be present in up to 16% of patients.
- Benign and malignant tumors of the CNS and peripheral nervous system may occur in up to 10% to 20% of patients with NF1.
- An optic glioma is the most common benign tumor associated with NF1. Other tumors include malignant peripheral nerve sheath tumors, meningiomas, and glioblastomas.
- Many patients with NF1 have seizure disorders and mental retardation.
- Musculoskeletal findings can occur including osteopenia, scoliosis, sphenoid wing dysplasia, congenital tibial dysplasia, and pseudarthrosis.
- Endocrine disorders occur; 3% to 5% of affected children have sexual precocity associated with short stature.

- Gastrointestinal symptoms may result from stromal tumors in the GI tract.
- Patients with NF1 have an increased risk of malignancies including breast cancer, leukemia and lymphoma, and pheochromocytoma (<1% of patients with NF1).

NEUROFIBROMATOSIS TYPE 2

- CALMs occur less frequently in NF2, but are found in 33% of patients. Usually affected patients have <5 lesions.
- Skin tumors including schwannomas or neurofibromas are often the presenting sign of NF2 and can occur in 30% to 50% of patients.
- Tumors including vestibular and cranial schwannomas, cranial meningiomas, and spinal cord tumors.
- Hearing loss and visual impairment may occur as a result of tumor burden. Hearing impairment occurs in 75% of affected children.
- Presentation in childhood is associated with a worse prognosis.

DIAGNOSIS

NEUROFIBROMATOSIS TYPE 1

- The diagnosis of NF1 can be made based on clinical findings and requires two or more of the following:
  - ≥6 café au lait macules (must be >5 mm if prepubertal and >15 mm if postpubertal)
  - Axillary or inguinal freckling
  - ≥2 neurofibromas or ≥1 plexiform neurofibroma
  - Optic glioma
  - ≥2 Lisch nodules
  - Bony lesions (sphenoid dysplasia, pseudarthrosis)
  - First-degree relative with NF1

NEUROFIBROMATOSIS TYPE 2

- Diagnostic criteria for NF2 include the following:
  - Bilateral vestibular schwannomas seen by magnetic resonance imaging (MRI) scan *OR* a first-degree relative with NF2
    AND
  - Unilateral vestibular schwannoma *OR* two of the following:
    - Meningioma
    - Glioma
    - Schwannoma
    - Juvenile posterior subcapsular cataract

LABORATORY EVALUATION

- Genetic testing is now more readily available through commercial laboratories and is often covered by insurance. Laboratories that perform genetic testing for NF1 and NF2 can be found on www.genetests.org
- MRI studies of the brain and cervical spine may be helpful in NF1 patients with symptoms of CNS disease and in patients with suspected NF2 disease.

DIFFERENTIAL DIAGNOSIS

Café au lait macules

- *CALMs are a common birthmark seen in 10% to 20% of the general population (see Chapter 1), most persons have one to three lesions.*
- *Isolated CALMs usually have irregular or smudgy borders.*

Segmental Neurofibromatosis

- *CALMs and neurofibromas localized to one segment of the body.*
- *Absence of CNS tumors.*
- *Lack of inheritance (somatic mutation).*

McCune–Albright Syndrome (also called Polyostotic Fibrous Dysplasia)

- *A genetic condition caused by mutations in GNAS that results in skin, bone, and endocrine problems.*
- *Associated with a large pigmented macular lesion (resembling a CALM) that is usually located on the trunk or abdomen and has a typical geographic ("coast of Maine") border.*
- *Precocious puberty and bone lesions usually occur.*

NF1-like Syndrome (or Legius Syndrome)

- *Most patients with Legius syndrome have six or more CALMs and intertriginous freckling, thus meeting the criteria for NF1. However, patients never develop neurofibromas, Lisch nodules, optic gliomas, or bony lesions.*
- *Macrocephaly and learning disabilities are common.*
- *Caused by mutations in SPRED1 gene.*

MANAGEMENT

- Education on neurofibromatosis, its natural history and clinical heterogeneity is key.
- It is often helpful to inform parents of the estimated relative risk of the different associations. For example, not all patients with NF1 will develop a glioblastoma or severe mental retardation.
- Children with NF1 should have complete physical examinations including head circumference, height, weight, and blood pressure twice yearly.
- Surveillance for learning disabilities, tumors, and ophthalmologic examinations should occur yearly.
- Symptomatic or disfiguring neurofibromas can be removed surgically.
- Treatment of NF2 is primarily surgical.
- Genetic counseling for patients and their families is an important aspect of treatment.

HELPFUL HINTS

- At present, genetic testing is used for unusual presentations and for reproductive counseling.
- Numerous support networks exist for NF patients and their families including the National Neurofibromatosis Foundation, Inc. and the Children's Tumor Foundation (http://www.ctf.org).

Tuberous Sclerosis

BASICS

- Tuberous sclerosis (TS; **Bourneville disease**) is an autosomal dominant disorder characterized by typical skin lesions and the growth of hamartomatous tumors of the CNS and other organs.
- The classic triad of TS includes the following:
  - **Adenoma sebaceum**
  - **Epilepsy**
  - **Mental retardation**, although at least 50% of affected persons show no evidence of mental retardation
- TS has an incidence of 1 per 6,000 births.

PATHOGENESIS

- TS results from mutations in *TSC1* or *TSC2*, which encode for hamartin and tuberin, respectively.
- Hamartin and tuberin act together to regulate cell differentiation and proliferation. Defects in these gene products may result in the growth of multiple hamartomas in TS.
- An estimated 70% of patients with TS have a new mutation.

CLINICAL MANIFESTATIONS

- Ash-leaf macules are hypopigmented, characteristically oval, and sometimes linear or "confetti-shaped" macular lesions that are the earliest clinical feature of TS (Fig. 11.6).
- The so-called adenoma sebaceum (actually angiofibromas) are pink to reddish-brown, dome-shaped papules most commonly located on the nose, nasolabial folds, and cheeks (Fig. 11.7).
- Periungual fibromas (Koenen tumors) are smooth, firm, skin-colored papules (Fig. 11.8).
- The characteristic "shagreen patch" is a pebbly, skin-colored *"peau d'orange"* or "pigskin-like" dermal plaque (collagenoma) that has fine hypopigmentation resembling confetti and most often appears in the lumbosacral region.
- A fibrous forehead plaque may occur on the forehead, face or scalp and is usually present from birth (Fig. 11.9).

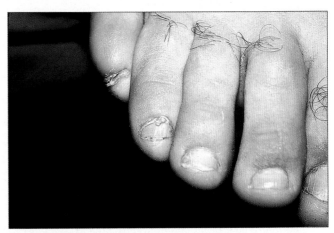

11.8   *Tuberous sclerosis.* Periungual fibromas (Koenen tumors) characteristic of tuberous sclerosis.

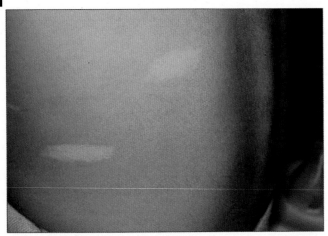

11.6   *Tuberous sclerosis.* Multiple ash-leaf macules on the back.

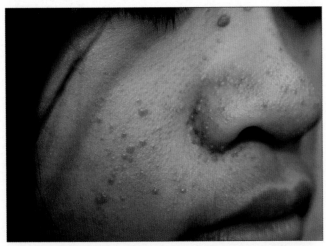

11.7   *Tuberous sclerosis.* Facial angiofibromas (often, but incorrectly referred to as adenoma sebaceum) typical of TS. (Figure courtesy of Lawrence A. Schachner, MD.)

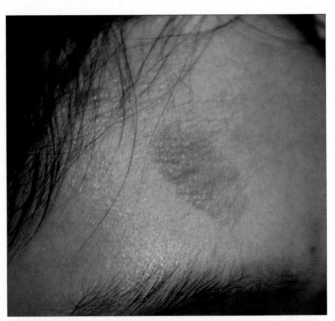

11.9   *Tuberous sclerosis.* The characteristic fibrous forehead plaque seen in up to 25% of TS patients. (Figure courtesy of Lawrence A. Schachner, MD.)

- Ash-leaf macules and the fibrous forehead plaque are usually present at birth.
- Adenoma sebaceum may begin to develop in late childhood and adolescence.

CENTRAL NERVOUS SYSTEM LESIONS

- Gliomatous brain tumors (tubers), which may calcify in 50% of patients
- Seizure disorders in 70% to 80% of patients, with fewer than 50% showing evidence of mental retardation
- Retinal and optic nerve gliomas

OTHER FINDINGS

- Renal involvement is common and is usually apparent in the first decade. Typically presents as renal hamartomas (angiomyolipomas) or less often as renal cysts.
- Bone changes, mostly bone cyst formation and sclerosis, are also common in TS.
- Cardiac rhabdomyomas of the atrium occur in 50% to 60% of patients but rarely cause cardiac obstructive disease and tend to regress spontaneously.
- Less common clinical findings include retinal hamartomas (called phakomas), gastrointestinal tumors, and pulmonary lymphangioleiomyomatosis.
- Pits in the tooth enamel are another marker of TS.

DIAGNOSIS

- Diagnosis of TS requires the presence of two major or one major and two minor criteria:

MAJOR DIAGNOSTIC CRITERIA

- Adenoma sebaceum
- Hypopigmented ash-leaf macules (three or more)
- Shagreen patch
- Periungual fibroma
- Cortical tuber
- Cardiac rhabdomyosarcoma
- Subependymal nodule
- Subependymal giant cell astrocytoma
- Lymphangiomatosis
- Renal angiolipoma

MINOR DIAGNOSTIC CRITERIA

- Multiple dental enamel pits
- Hamartomatous rectal polyp
- Bone cyst
- Gingival fibroma
- Nonrenal hamartoma
- Retinal achromic patch
- Confetti skin lesions: fine, hypopigmented macules (2 to 4 mm) that look as though they are "sprinkled" on the lower legs
- Multiple renal cysts

LABORATORY EVALUATION

- Cranial MRI to identify cortical tubers
- Posteroanterior and lateral skull films (for adults) to demonstrate calcifications of gliomas of the brain
- Echocardiography to detect rhabdomyomas
- Renal ultrasonograms to search for tumors
- Skin biopsy of cutaneous lesions

DIFFERENTIAL DIAGNOSIS OF ADENOMA SEBACEUM

Acneiform papules
- *They often resemble adenoma sebaceum.*
- *Acne has a waxing and waning course.*
- *A skin biopsy is necessary only if the diagnosis is in doubt.*

DIFFERENTIAL DIAGNOSIS OF ASH-LEAF MACULES

Nevus depigmentosus (see Chapter 1)
- *An ND is often difficult to distinguish from an ash-leaf macule.*
- *NDs are well-demarcated hypopigmented patches often seen at birth or within the first years of life.*
- *ND is usually a solitary lesion but occasionally multiple lesions or a segmental lesion is present.*

Vitiligo
- *Depigmented patches variably sized, that will appear "chalk white" with Wood lamp examination.*

MANAGEMENT

- Prognosis of TS depends on the severity of the condition and the presence of neurologic involvement.
- Parents should be educated about association and genetic basis of condition.
- Patients should have close surveillance for development of seizures and mental retardation.
- Patients with TS should also be monitored for the development of brain, cardiac, renal, bony, lung, or eye tumors.
- Removal of cosmetically objectionable or disfiguring adenoma sebaceum by **excision, electrocautery, dermabrasion,** or laser resurfacing.
- **Rapamycin** has shown promising results for the treatment of tumors associated with TS. The topical form is effective for facial angiofibromas (adenoma sebaceum).
- Painful periungual fibromas can be removed surgically.
- **Genetic counseling** of patients with TS and their families after computed tomographic scanning is performed on the parents and siblings of the affected patient (these studies have demonstrated CNS lesions in asymptomatic parents of TS patients).

 HELPFUL HINTS

- In general, patients with mutations in *TSC1* have a milder course.
- Ash-leaf macules are hypopigmented not depigmented.
- Families dealing with TS should be made aware of support networks including the Tuberous Sclerosis Alliance (www.tsalliance.org).

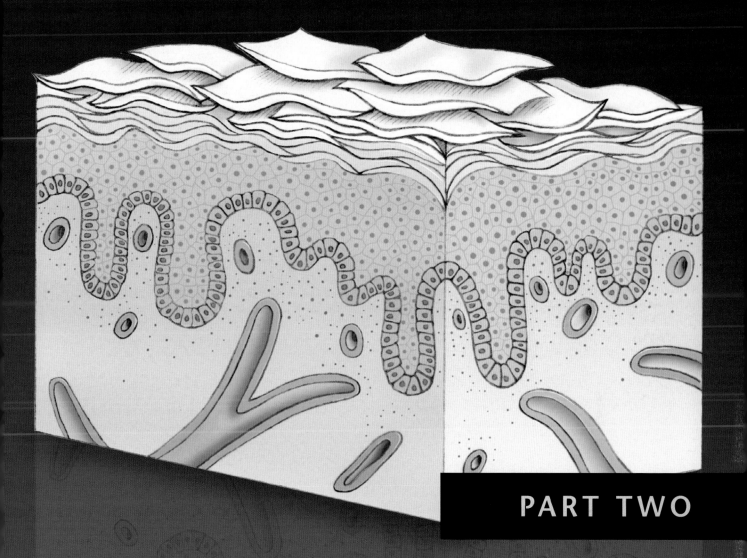

PART TWO

Common Adult/Elderly Skin Conditions: Diagnosis and Management

OVERVIEW

Acne, the most common skin disorder in the United States, is an embarrassing problem for many teenagers, but it is not limited to that age group. It may develop before puberty in either sex, or it may first present in adulthood, particularly in women.

Acne is a disease of the pilosebaceous apparatus of the skin. Acne vulgaris, or common acne, begins in the teen or preteen years. In general, it becomes less active as adolescence ends but may continue into adulthood.

Acne that initially occurs in adulthood is designated postadolescent acne or adult-onset acne. Despite the clinical similarities and occasional overlapping of adolescent and postadolescent acne, the pathogenesis and treatment of each are somewhat different.

The pathogenesis and treatment of acne vulgaris, postadolescent acne, rosacea, drug-induced acne, and other acneiform conditions will be discussed in this chapter. Neonatal and infantile acne are discussed in Chapter 3.

IN THIS CHAPTER...

➤ **ACNE VULGARIS (ADOLESCENT ACNE)**

➤ **POSTADOLESCENT ACNE**

➤ **ROSACEA**

➤ **ROSACEA VARIANTS**

- Perioral dermatitis
- Steroid-induced rosacea
- Rhinophyma

➤ **ACNE: OTHER TYPES**

- Systemic drug-induced (or drug-exacerbated) acne
- Acne Excoriée des Jeunes Filles
- Endocrinopathic acne

ACNE MYTHS VERSUS FACTS

Myth: Blackheads are caused by dirt.
Fact: They are black because of oxidized melanin. Blackheads, or open comedones, are collections of sebum and keratin that form within follicular openings, and when exposed to air, become oxidized and turn black.

Myth: Acne should disappear by the end of adolescence.
Fact: Some women have acne that persists well past adolescence. Others have an initial episode in their 20s or 30s.

Myth: Acne is caused, or worsened by certain foods, such as chocolate, sweets, and greasy junk food.
Fact: Despite occasional personal anecdotes and persistent cultural myths, acne is probably not significantly influenced by diet.

Myth: A dirty face exacerbates acne; therefore, scrubbing the face daily helps clear it up.
Fact: Scrubbing and rubbing a face that has acne, particularly inflammatory acne, will only serve to irritate and redden an already inflamed complexion. Instead, the face should be washed daily with a gentle cleanser and patted (not rubbed) dry.

Myth: Frequent facials are beneficial.
Fact: Frequent professional facials and at-home scrubs, astringents, and masks are generally not recommended because they tend to aggravate acne.

Acne Vulgaris (Adolescent Acne)

BASICS

- Teenage acne (acne vulgaris) has a strong tendency to be hereditary and is less likely to be seen in Asians and dark-skinned people.
- Acne is common; more than 90% of teenagers will have some degree of acne.
- Acne is classified according to the predominant type of lesion present and the degree of involvement.

PATHOGENESIS

- Lesions begin during puberty when androgenic hormones cause increased sebum production and abnormal follicular keratinization that blocks the follicular orifice, forming a microcomedo, the primary acne lesion.
- The microcomedo enlarges to become the visible comedo: the "blackhead" or "whitehead."
- Enlargement and/or rupture of the comedone triggers inflammation and results in an acne papule or pustule.
- The anaerobe *Propionibacterium acnes* plays a significant role in the pathogenesis of acne. The gram-positive rod is found in the sebaceous gland and hair follicle and releases enzymes that contribute to comedo rupture and inflammation (Illus. 12.1–12.4).

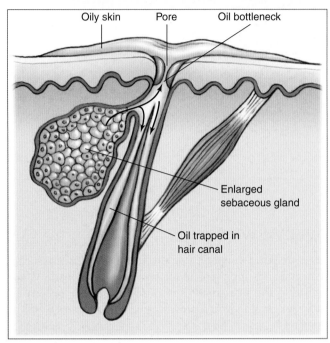

I12.2 *Follicular occlusion.* Pores become clogged and the follicular canal narrows.

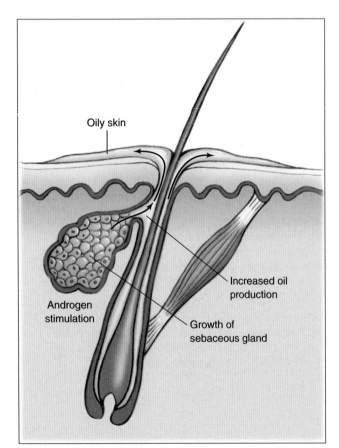

I12.1 *Androgenic stimulation.* The sebaceous gland over-reacts to androgen stimulation.

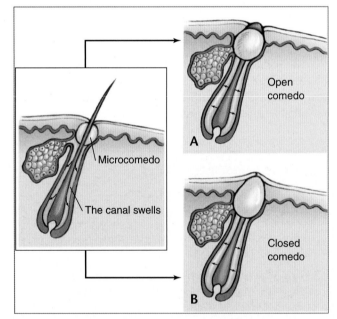

I12.3 *Comedogenesis.* The microcomedo forms and becomes either an open (**A**) or closed comedo (**B**).

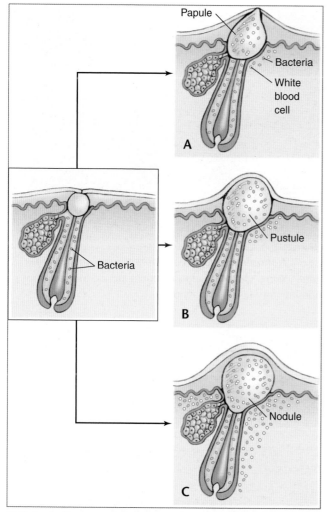

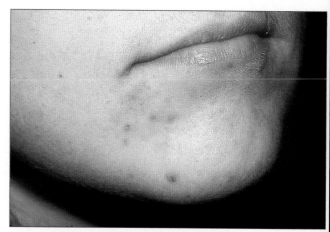

12.1 *Inflammatory acne (mild).* Papules.

I12.4 *Inflammatory acne.* The microcomedo becomes an inflammatory papule (**A**), pustule (**B**), or nodule (**C**).

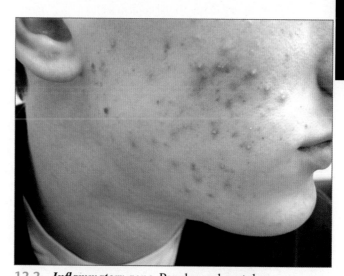

12.2 *Inflammatory acne.* Papules and pustules.

CLINICAL MANIFESTATIONS

- Acne most commonly erupts in areas of maximal sebaceous gland activity: the face, neck, chest, shoulders, back, and upper arms.
- Individual acne lesions are designated as inflammatory (papules and pustules) or as comedones. A patient's acne can be primarily comedonal, primarily inflammatory, or a combination of the two.

INFLAMMATORY LESIONS

- **Papules:** Superficial red "pimples" that may have become crusted (scabbed surfaces caused by dried pustules or by picking or squeezing) (Figs. 12.1–12.3).
- **Pustules:** Superficial raised lesions containing purulent material, generally found in the company of papules (Figs. 12.1–12.3).
- **Macules:** The remains of formerly palpable inflammatory lesions that are in the process of healing from therapy or spontaneous resolution. They are flat, red or sometimes

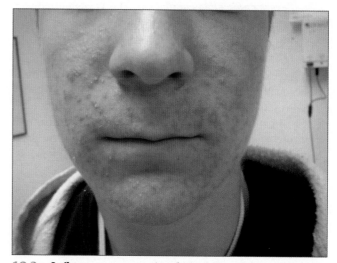

12.3 *Inflammatory acne (moderate).* Papules and pustules.

Chapter 12 • Acne and Related Disorders **189**

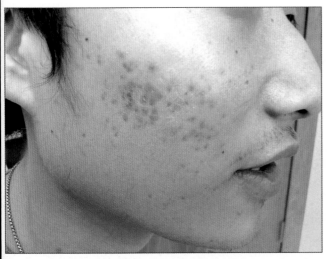

12.4 *Inflammatory acne.* Violaceous macules.

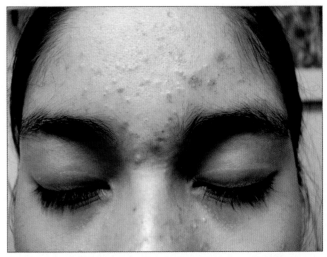

12.6 *Noninflammatory (comedonal) acne and inflammatory acne.* Open and closed comedones, as well as a few inflammatory lesions are evident.

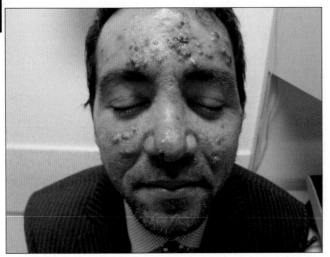

12.5 *Severe cystic acne conglobata.* This is an unusually severe form of acne characterized by multiple abscesses and scars (both keloidal and atrophic).

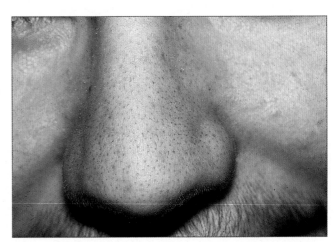

12.7 *Follicular prominence.* These are blackhead-like, dilated ostia (pores) that are frequently seen on the nose.

purple (violaceous) blemishes that slowly heal and may occasionally form depressed, atrophic scars (Fig. 12.4).

- **"Acne cysts" (nodules):** Persistent deep papules or pustules (0.5 to 1 cm in size). Acne "cysts" are not really cysts (true cysts are neoplasms that have an epithelial lining). Instead, acne cysts are composed of poorly organized conglomerations of inflammatory material (Fig. 12.5).

COMEDONAL LESIONS

- A comedo is a collection of sebum and keratin that forms within follicular ostia (pores) (Figs. 12.6).
- **Open comedones (blackheads)** have large ostia that are black as a result of oxidized melanin.
- **Closed comedones (whiteheads)** are small (usually 1 to 2 mm) skin-colored papules that have small or no ostia and little to no associated erythema.

- **Follicular prominence.** These blackhead-like, dilated pores are frequently seen on the nose and cheeks in acne patients (Fig. 12.7).

SEVERITY

- Acne may be further classified as mild, moderate, or severe.
- **Mild acne** consists of comedones and/or occasional papules and pustules.
- **Moderate acne** is more inflammatory, with relatively superficial papules and/or pustules (papulopustular acne); comedones may also be present. Lesions may heal with scars.
- **Severe acne** ("cystic" or nodular acne, acne conglobata) has a greater degree, depth, and number of inflammatory lesions: papules, pustules, nodules, "cysts," and possibly abscesses. Sinus tracts, significant scarring, and keloid formation may also be evident.

CLINICAL SEQUELAE

- The more severe inflammatory lesions of acne are prone to heal with atrophic or pitted ("ice-pick") scars on the face, and hypertrophic scars or keloids on the trunk (Figs. 12.8–12.11).
- Postinflammatory hyperpigmentation may occur, particularly in patients with darker skin.
- Having acne can lead to feelings of diminished self-esteem and be a source of anxiety particularly in teenagers who are just beginning to confront the outside world.
- The negative psychological effects of acne and its impact on limiting employment opportunities and social functioning are among the overriding concerns of individuals who have moderate to severe acne.

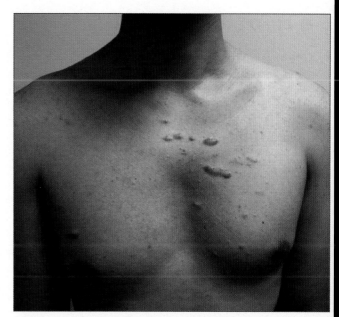

12.10   *Acne scars.* These presternal keloids arose secondary to acne.

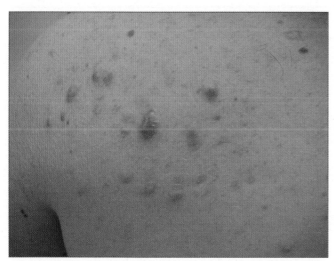

12.8   *Acne scars.* Hypertrophic scars are seen on the shoulder of this patient.

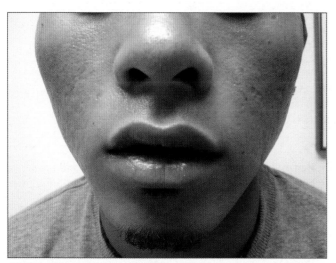

12.9   *"Ice-pick scars."* Inflammation of acne have healed with depressed atrophic pitted scars.

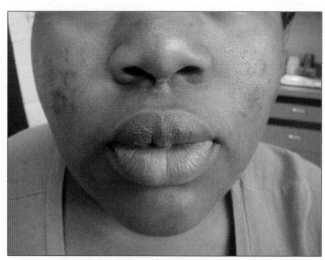

12.11   *Postinflammatory hyperpigmentation secondary to acne.* Resolving acne lesions often leave dark macules such as those seen in this African-American patient. (From Goodheart HP. *Goodheart's Same-Site Differential Diagnosis.* Philadelphia, PA: Lippincott Williams & Wilkins; 2011.)

DIAGNOSIS

- Adolescent acne is typically easy for both the patient and practitioner to recognize.
- Specific underlying causes of acne (e.g., hyperandrogenism) should be considered in certain female patients (see polycystic ovary syndrome later in this chapter).

DIFFERENTIAL DIAGNOSIS

Keratosis Pilaris (see Chapter 13)

- *Appears on upper and outer arms, consists of small, follicular, horny spines. The tiny papules may resemble acne when they are inflamed.*
- *In children, the lateral sides of the cheeks are frequently involved and are commonly mistaken for acne.*

Folliculitis (see Chapter 16)

- *Refers to inflammation of the hair follicle, particularly the upper portion of its structure.*
- *Characterized by papules and/or pustules with or without obvious emerging hairs.*

- *Follicular papules and pustules may be indistinguishable from acne.*

Rosacea (see below)

- *Noted primarily in adults.*
- *Typically involves central face and is characterized by redness.*
- *No change with menses.*

Perioral/Periorificial Dermatitis (see below)

- *Seen in young children or adults.*
- *Distribution is perinasal, periorbital, or perioral.*

 MANAGEMENT

Goals

- To prevent scarring.
- To help improve the patient's appearance.
- Hasten resolution of lesions and prevent new lesions.

General Principles

- Treatment of acne should be individualized and frequently involves a trial-and-error approach that begins with those agents that are known to be most effective, least expensive, and have the fewest side effects.
- Acne is a multifactorial disease; therefore, appropriate therapy often involves the use of more than one agent, each of which targets a different pathogenic factor.
- Mild acne can often be managed successfully by topical treatments, including over-the-counter (OTC) remedies. More severe, widespread acne often requires systemic treatment in combination with topical therapy.
- Oral medications should be tapered or discontinued as soon as control is achieved.
- A patient should be advised not to squeeze or pick lesions.

Topical Therapies

Despite the testimonials seen on infomercials, no "one-size-fits-all" treatment for acne exists. In fact, the active ingredients in most advertised preparations can be obtained less expensively in many OTC products.

Benzoyl Peroxide

- Benzoyl peroxide is a potent antibacterial agent that has comedolytic properties and is effective against both inflammatory (papules/pustules) and noninflammatory lesions (comedones) (see Table 12.1).

Table 12.1 BENZOYL PEROXIDE–CONTAINING PREPARATIONS	
OVER-THE-COUNTER PREPARATIONS	
5%, 10% benzoyl peroxide	**Oxy-5, Oxy**-10
2.5% benzoyl peroxide gel	**Clear by Design**
10% benzoyl peroxide lotion	**Clearasil** 10%
3.5% benzoyl peroxide wash	**Neutrogena Clear Pore Cleanser/Mask**
5%, 10% benzoyl peroxide wash, 10% gel	**Clean & Clear**
PRESCRIPTION FORMULATIONS	
5%, 10% benzoyl peroxide gel (water based)	**Desquam-X**
2.5%, 5%, 10% benzoyl peroxide gel (water based)	**Desquam-E**
4%, 8% benzoyl peroxide gel (water based)	**Brevoxyl**
3%, 6%, 10% benzoyl peroxide gel (water based)	**Triaz pads**

- Benzoyl peroxide may be used alone to treat mild acne, but it is most effective when used in conjunction with other topical and systemic therapies.
- Benzoyl peroxide is available OTC in many different strengths and formulations including bar soaps, washes, gels, lotions, creams, foams, and pads. **Clearasil, Oxy, Pan-Oxyl,** and **Clean & Clear** are several brands that make benzoyl peroxide–containing products.
- Benzoyl peroxide is also available by prescription in combination with clindamycin, erythromycin, and adapalene.

continued on page 193

MANAGEMENT *Continued*

Table 12.2A TOPICAL RETINOIDS FOR ACNE

GENERIC NAME	BRAND NAME	STRENGTHS	SIZES
Tretinoin	**Retin-A cream, gel**	Creams: 0.025%, 0.05%, 0.1% Gels: 0.01%, 0.025%	20 g, 45 g
Tretinoin	**Retin-A Micro topical gel**	0.04%, 0.1%	20-, 45-, 50-g pump dispenser
Tretinoin	**Avita cream, gel**	0.025%	20 g, 45 g
Adapalene	**Differin cream, gel**	0.1%, 0.3%	15 g, 45 g 30 mL, #60
Tazarotene	**Tazorac cream, gel**	0.05%, 0.1%	30 g, 100 g

Table 12.2B TOPICAL COMBINATIONS CONTAINING RETINOIDS

GENERIC NAME	BRAND NAME	SIZES (g)
Clindamycin 1.2%/tretinoin 0.25% gel	**Ziana**	30, 60
Clindamycin 1.2%/tretinoin 0.25% gel	**Veltin**	30
Adapalene 0.1%/benzoyl peroxide 2.5%	**Epiduo gel**	45

- Lower-strength (e.g., 2.5%) preparations are less irritating and probably as effective as the higher 5% and 10% concentrations.

How to Use Benzoyl Peroxide
- Beginning with a lower-strength preparation, benzoyl peroxide is applied sparingly once or twice daily, in a thin layer on acne-prone areas.
- *Side effects:* Irritation and burning are not uncommon but usually resolve in 2 to 3 weeks; bleaching of colored clothing and bedding.

Topical Retinoids
- Topical retinoids are primarily comedolytic (i.e., they treat comedones) but they also have potent anti-inflammatory effects (see Tables 12.2A and 12.2B).
- In addition, retinoids facilitate the penetration of other topical antiacne agents such as benzoyl peroxide.
- These agents help "plump up" the skin and make enlarged pores (follicular prominence) less obvious.
- They should not be used during pregnancy or breastfeeding (although no studies have shown them to be harmful to the fetus).
- Topical retinoids used for acne include (listed in increasing potency) the following:
  - Adapalene (**Differin**), available as 0.1% cream or gel, or 0.3% gel
  - Tretinoin (**Retin-A Micro**), available as 0.025%, 0.04%, 0.05%, or 0.1% in cream or gel
  - Tazarotene (**Tazorac**), available as 0.05% or 0.1% cream or gel, or 0.1% foam

- Newer products that combine topical retinoids with topical antibiotics, can help simplify treatment regimens. Examples include **Ziana** (tretinoin 0.025% and clindamycin 1.2% gel), **Veltin** (tretinoin 0.025% and clindamycin 1.2% gel), and **Epiduo** (benzoyl peroxide 2.5% and adapalene 0.1% gel).

How to Use Topical Retinoids
- Topical retinoids are applied once daily, as a thin layer to acne-prone areas at bedtime.
- Patients who exhibit sensitivity may use it every other day, or less frequently, until they develop a tolerance to it.
- The area of application should first be washed and thoroughly dried.
- *Side effects:* May include erythema, dryness, and peeling—these usually resolve after 3 weeks; photosensitivity (or "sun sensitivity") in some patients, thus concurrent daily use of sunscreen should be advised.

Topical Antibiotics
- Preparations that contain the topical antibiotics, clindamycin and erythromycin, are active against *P. acnes* and have anti-inflammatory action against papules and pustules (see Table 12.3).
- Topical clindamycin and erythromycin are considered equally effective.
- Drug resistance has been reported with these antibiotics so monotherapy with these agents should be avoided.

continued on page 194

MANAGEMENT *Continued*

Table 12.3 TOPICAL ANTIBIOTICS*a*

GENERIC NAME	BRAND NAME	STRENGTHS (%)	SIZES
Erythromycin	**A/T/S solution, gel**	2	60 mL, 30 g
Erythromycin	**Akne-Mycin ointment**	2	25 g
Clindamycin	**Cleocin T solution, gel, lotion**	1	30, 60 mL
Clindamycin	**Evoclin foam**	1	50, 100 g
Dapsone	**Aczone gel**	5	30 g

*a*Bacterial resistance is possible with all of these agents.

How to Use Topical Antibiotics
- These agents are applied once or twice daily, in a thin layer across the acne-prone areas.
- *Side effects:* Irritation and burning are uncommon and may be avoided by using an ointment-based erythromycin such as **Akne-Mycin** or clindamycin (**Cleocin**) in a lotion preparation.
- Topical antibiotics are available in a variety of vehicles, including creams, lotions, ointments, gels, and solutions.

Combination of Topical Antibiotic and Benzoyl Peroxide
- The combination of erythromycin or clindamycin with benzoyl peroxide helps prevent bacterial resistance and has a synergistic effect (the combination appears to be more effective than either drug used alone) (see Table 12.4).
- **Benzamycin** (Benzoyl peroxide 5% and erythromycin 3%), **BenzaClin** (benzoyl peroxide 5% and clindamycin 1%), **Duac** (benzoyl peroxide 5% and clindamycin 1.2%), and **Acanya** (benzoyl peroxide 2.5% and clindamycin 1.2%) are the most commonly prescribed formulations.

How to Use Combination of Topical Antibiotics and Benzoyl Peroxide
- These agents are applied sparingly once daily to acne-prone areas.
- *Side effects:* The same cautions apply as for benzoyl peroxide. Dryness, erythema, and pruritus are the most common side effects.

Alternative Topical Prescription Drugs
- Azelaic acid: antibacterial and anticomedone, available as a 20% cream (**Azelex**) or 15% gel (**Finacea**).
- Sulfur and sodium sulfacetamide preparations: antibacterial and keratolytic properties, available as 10% sodium sulfacetamide in lotion, cream, or wash (**Ovace, Klaron**) and together with 5% sulfur as a cleanser, cream, or lotion (**Avar Cleanser, Clenia, Plexion, Sulfacet-R, Novacet**).
- Dapsone: antibacterial and antineutrophil, available as 5% gel (**Aczone**).

Topical Nonprescription Agents
Alpha- and Beta-Hydroxy Acids
- Many OTC products contain ingredients that have been used for acne for many generations without great success.
- For children just beginning to develop acne or for patients with very mild acne, gentle OTC washes or creams containing the topical peeling agents **salicylic acid** or **glycolic acid;** or the anti-inflammatory agents **resorcinol** or **sulfur,** may be helpful.

Systemic Therapies
- Systemic therapy is added to topical treatment, in patients with moderate to severe acne, moderate acne unresponsive to topical treatment, acne that tends to scar, or those with significant acne on the chest and back.

Table 12.4 COMBINATION TOPICAL ANTIBIOTIC AND BENZOYL PEROXIDE AGENTS*a*

GENERIC NAME	BRAND NAME	SIZES (g)
Erythromycin 3%/benzoyl peroxide 5%	**Benzamycin gel**	23.3, 46.6
Clindamycin 1%/benzoyl peroxide 5%	**BenzaClin gel**	25, 50
Clindamycin 1%/benzoyl peroxide 5%	**Duac gel**	45
Clindamycin 1.2%/benzoyl peroxide 2.5%	**Acanya gel**	50
Clindamycin 1.2%/benzoyl peroxide 3.75%	**Onexton gel**	50

*a*No bacterial resistance is reported with these agents.

continued on page 195

⚙ **MANAGEMENT** *Continued*

Table 12.5 SYSTEMIC ANTIBIOTICS FOR ACNE AND ROSACEA

GENERIC NAME	BRAND NAME	DELIVERY	COMMON STARTING DOSE
Tetracycline		Capsules	250 or 500 mg bid
Doxycycline		Capsules, tablets, liquid	50, 75, or 100 mg bid
Doxycycline hyclate	**Adoxa**	Tablets	75 or 100 mg bid
Doxycycline hyclate	**Doryx**	Extended-release tablets	75, 100, or 150 mg daily
Doxycycline monohydrate	**Oracea**	Capsules	40 mg QD
Doxycycline monohydrate	**Monodox**	Capsules	50, 75, or 100 mg bid
Minocycline			50, 75, or 100 mg bid
Minocycline	**Solodyn**	Tablets	1 mg/kg/day
		Extended-release tablets	45, 65, 90, 115, 135 mg once daily (1 mg/kg/day)
Minocycline	**Minocin**	Capsules, oral suspension	50 or 100 mg bid
Minocycline	**Dynacin**	Capsules, tablets	50 or 100 mg bid

- Systemic therapy results in a more rapid improvement, which may serve to enhance patient compliance. However, side effects, drug allergy/intolerance, drug interactions, and fetal exposure in women who are, or may become pregnant, must be carefully considered before initiating systemic treatment.
- **Systemic agents** for acne include oral antibiotics, hormonal agents, such as oral contraceptives and antiandrogenic drugs and oral retinoids (isotretinoin or **"Accutane"**) which is usually reserved for more severe, recalcitrant disease (see discussion below).

Oral Antibiotics
Tetracyclines
- The tetracycline derivatives—minocycline and doxycycline—are the mainstay and the first-line antibiotic drugs of choice for moderate to severe acne (see Table 12.5).
- Tetracycline derivatives inhibit the growth of *P. acnes,* which decreases free fatty acid production and pustule formation and have a significant anti-inflammatory action via inhibition of the neutrophil chemotactic response.
- The use of any of the tetracyclines during a child's tooth development (before 8 years of age) may cause a permanent discoloration of the teeth. Unborn fetuses and nursing children are also at risk.

Tetracycline
- Tetracycline is not readily available in the United States and is less commonly used today.

- The following dosing is advised where it is available: 250 to 500 mg twice a day and taken on an empty stomach (1 hour before or 2 hours after a meal). Dairy products such as milk or divalent cations that contain iron, magnesium, zinc, or calcium may interfere with tetracycline's absorption from the stomach.

Minocycline
- *Dosing:* 50 mg twice a day, 75 mg once or twice a day, or 100 mg once or twice a day.
- An extended-release formulation of minocycline tablets, **Solodyn,** is available in doses ranging from 45 to 135 mg, given in a weight-based dosage of 1 mg/kg daily (see Table 12.5). It has been shown to have anti-inflammatory effects without acting on *P acnes,* the bacteria involved in causing acne. This approach is intended to prevent bacterial resistance.
- The drug's excellent absorption allows it to be taken with food.
- It causes few, if any, phototoxic problems and appears to be less likely to induce candidal vulvovaginitis than tetracycline.
- *Side effects:* Nausea, vomiting, and, in high doses (those that approach 200 mg/day), dizziness owing to vestibular dysfunction (dizziness usually diminishes after a few days or when the dosage is lowered). Reversible discoloration of the skin—muddy brown in sun-exposed areas, bluish color in scars or normal skin (usually the shins), and a grayish-blue discoloration of the oral or ocular mucosa can occur. It can also lead to blue gray staining of adult teeth. Risk of discoloration increases with prolonged treatment.

continued on page 196

MANAGEMENT *Continued*

• In rare cases, minocycline is associated with benign intracranial hypertension, hepatitis, and a lupus-like syndrome that is antinuclear antibody positive. This syndrome, which occurs most often in young women, usually develops late in the course of therapy.

Doxycycline
• *Dosing:* ranges from 50 mg twice a day, 75 mg once or twice a day, or 100 mg once or twice a day.
• Doxycycline is absorbed well and may be taken with food.
• Its main disadvantage is its phototoxic potential—the highest of the tetracyclines. Patients should be advised regarding careful sun protection.
• *Side effects:* Higher incidence of gastrointestinal upset—patients should be advised not to swallow without liquid and not to take right before lying down.
• Vestibular dysfunction, hyperpigmentation, and the lupus-like syndrome associated with minocycline have not been reported.

Alternative Antibiotics
• **Azithromycin, clarithromycin, trimethoprim-sulfamethoxazole**, or **amoxicillin** are used as second-line alternatives when a tetracycline derivative fails or is not tolerated.

Hormonal Treatment
• Oral contraceptives or systemic antiandrogens (such as **spironolactone**) are used in women with hormonally triggered acne as an alternative or adjuvant to antibiotics and oral retinoids (see discussion later in this chapter).

Oral Retinoids (Isotretinoin)
• Isotretinoin (13-*cis*-retinoic acid) is an oral synthetic derivative of vitamin A that promotes long-term remissions in severe acne and is used for patients with severe, recalcitrant nodulocystic acne.
• Isotretinoin is also highly effective in patients with moderate to severe acne that was previously unresponsive to topical and systemic acne therapies.
• While isotretinoin is still commonly referenced by its original trade name in the United States, **Accutane**, it is currently only sold under several generic brand names **Amnesteem, Claravis, Absorica**, and **Sotret**. It is available as **Roaccutane** outside of the United States.

Mechanism of Action
• Dramatically reduces the size and output of sebaceous glands.
• Normalizes the shedding dead skin cells (stabilizes keratinization), the process through which keratinocytes (epidermal cells) produce the protein keratin. Consequently, the keratinocytes are less likely to clog pores (comedogenesis).

Dosage
• Oral isotretinoin is available as capsules in strengths of 10, 20, 30, and 40 mg.
• **Absorica (isotretinoin-Lidose)** is a formulation which enhances absorption of isotretinoin in the absence of dietary fat. It is available in strengths of 10, 20, 25, 30, 35, and 40 mg.
• Patients are dosed based on weight and usually given 0.5 to 1 mg/kg/day until a total dosage of 120 to 150 mg/kg is reached (which equates to 4 to 6 months of treatment). There is some evidence that longer courses with lower doses (0.25 to 0.4 mg/kg/day) can also be effective while minimizing the dose-related side effects.

Side Effects
General
• Isotretinoin **can cause severe birth defects in pregnant women** or a woman who becomes pregnant while taking the drug, even if for a short time. Teratogenic birth defects include skull abnormalities, heart defects, deafness, cleft palate, and central nervous system defects. Because the drug remains in the body for a long time, it can cause birth defects for 1 month *after* a woman has stopped taking it. It also carries an increased risk of miscarriage when used during pregnancy or up to 1 month prior to pregnancy. Many prescribers require that women use oral contraceptives before starting treatment, during treatment, and for 1 month after isotretinoin treatment is completed.
• Isotretinoin's ability to shut down the oil production in the body accounts for some of its less serious side effects, such as cheilitis (dryness and inflammation of the lips), conjunctivitis, dry skin, nose bleeds, dry eyes, increased sun sensitivity, and itching. In general, these reactions are well tolerated because the drug is so effective that patients want to continue taking it despite these mild side effects.
• Approximately 25% of patients experience serum triglyceride elevations, and 15% experience decreases in high-density lipoprotein levels.
• Less commonly, a patient may experience musculoskeletal and joint pains, or hair thinning (usually reversible upon drug discontinuation).
• Allergic reactions, decreased night vision, persistent headaches, benign intracranial hypertension, and hearing impairments, are rare findings. Skeletal hyperostosis is limited to those who take a high dosage (much higher than is used to treat acne), and those undergoing long-term isotretinoin therapy.

continued on page 197

MANAGEMENT *Continued*

- Studies performed in men taking isotretinoin showed no significant effects on their sperm and no long-term damage to a man's ability to have healthy children.
- Isotretinoin has also been under scrutiny for a possible link to inflammatory bowel disease (IBD). A case-control study showed that this drug may be associated with a very small risk of developing ulcerative colitis, but no connection to Crohn disease was found.

Depression and Suicide
- In the United States, the Food and Drug Administration (FDA) has received reports of depression and suicide in patients who take isotretinoin, and there is concern about a possible link between the drug, psychiatric disorders, and suicide.
- Depression is unfortunately a common problem and the onset tends to occur between 12 and 24 years of age when acne is most prevalent.
- Increased incidence of emotional problems in adolescence coupled with the stress of having severe acne makes it difficult to determine whether isotretinoin can trigger depression and suicide or whether successful treatment may thwart such problems. Because suicide is a major cause of death in teenagers, particularly in boys, it has been difficult to determine a causal relationship between isotretinoin and these events, there is a great need for further study.

ALERT

If a patient taking isotretinoin is showing signs of moodiness, depression, or psychosis, the drug should be discontinued and the patient should be evaluated!

THE iPLEDGE PROGRAM
- **Due to isotretinoin's potential for serious toxicity during pregnancy, the Federal Drug Administration established an isotretinoin federal registry program called iPLEDGE. The registry keeps tabs on all isotretinoin prescriptions in the United States. Manufacturers, wholesalers, pharmacists, prescribers, and patients are linked through a centralized computer registry. The registry also connects to the laboratories that perform the required pregnancy testing in this system.**

PROCEDURES ALL iPLEDGE PATIENTS MUST FOLLOW
- *Everyone* in the United States who is prescribed isotretinoin must register with iPLEDGE. After registration, a female patient of childbearing potential must receive ongoing counseling and pregnancy testing each month

---

while taking the drug. All patients, male or female, are allowed only a 30-day supply of isotretinoin at each office visit. These prescriptions are only valid for 7 days after they are prescribed (unless the patient is unable to become pregnant).

Adjuvant Therapeutic Modalities

Comedo Extraction (Acne Surgery) (see Chapter 35)
- Manual extraction of comedones with a comedone extractor can quickly improve the appearance of acne.
- Comedones may be removed more easily if the patient is pretreated with a topical retinoid for 3 to 4 weeks before comedo removal.

Intralesional Corticosteroid Injection
- Intralesional injections of glucocorticosteroids, introduced with a 30-gauge needle, can reduce the inflammatory response and decrease the size of nodular inflammatory lesions.
- The recommended dose of intralesional triamcinolone acetate suspension is a concentration of 2.5 mg/mL to avoid local steroid atrophy. For patients with severe disease and considerable hypertrophic scarring, the concentration can be increased to 5 or 10 mg/mL.

Office-Based Chemical Peels
- Chemical peels have become popular as antiaging facial rejuvenation procedures; however, they are sometimes used to treat acne as well.
- In this procedure, a chemical acid solution is applied to the skin, causing the skin to peel off so that new skin can regenerate.
- Chemical peels are probably not effective for the treatment of inflammatory lesions of acne. They seem to work best in the elimination of comedonal acne and post-inflammatory hyperpigmentation.
- Deeper peels, with stronger concentrations of acids, are sometimes used to treat acne scars.
- The two most commonly used chemicals for peels are the alpha-hydroxy acids (glycolic, lactic, and mandelic acids) and the beta-hydroxy acids (salicylic acid).

Lasers, Lights, and Other New Technologies
- Laser and light therapies offer a promising, noninvasive treatment alternative and are most effective when used in combination with traditional acne medication treatments.
- They improve inflammatory acne and acne scarring.

Photodynamic Therapy
- **Photodynamic therapy (PDT)** involves applying a photosensitizing agent (aminolevulinic acid—ALA) to the

continued on page 198

MANAGEMENT *Continued*

skin, which accumulates in the sebaceous glands, followed by exposure to a high-intensity light source.

- Light sources used in PDT include visible (nonlaser, e.g., blue, red, intense pulsed) or laser light (e.g., 585 to 595 nm pulsed dye, 635 nm red diode). The *P. acnes* that reside in sebaceous glands produce porphyrins as a by-product of their metabolism. The light activates these porphyrins and kills the bacterial cells.

Lasers

- Lasers that are used in dermatology are devices that produce light at a specific wavelength to target and destroy specific chromophores in the skin (hemoglobin, water, melanin, etc.).
- Lasers and light devices used for acne target blood vessels, and sebaceous glands; and fractionated laser devices are beneficial for treatment of acne scarring. Below is a list of some laser and light devices that have been used for acne:

- **Intense pulsed light (IPL):** These devices emit a wider range of wavelengths (500 to 1,200 nm). Selective UV filters allow for versatility and customization to reach the specific targets such as blood vessels and sebaceous glands.
- **Pulsed dye laser (PDL):** This laser is "tuned" to a specific wavelength of light (585 to 95 nm) and is effective at removing redness and telangiectasias in acne, acne scars, and rosacea.
- **Pulsed light and heat energy (LHE) therapy:** This treatment combines pulses of light and heat, which may target both *P. acnes* and sebaceous glands.
- **Diode laser:** This laser uses longer infrared wavelengths (1,450 nm) and targets water and the sebaceous glands. It appears to be effective for acne and acne scars.

HELPFUL HINTS

- Compliance is often a problem for teenagers, so it is important to clearly explain the treatment regimen, make it simple, and give written instructions. The teenager should be advised to call the health care provider with any questions or concerns.
- Because topical retinoids may *appear* to make acne worse initially, the concurrent use of BenzaClin, Duac, or Benzamycin gel may help treat inflammatory lesions and make acne look better more rapidly.
- For patients who experience irritation and excessive dryness, topical retinoids may be applied for 2 to 3 minutes (increasing duration as tolerated) and then washed off. This "short-contact" treatment works quite well and minimizes irritation. Alternatively, retinoids can be applied every other night to lessen irritation.
- Titrating or fine tuning the dosage of oral antibiotics may help minimize potential side effects. For example, a dosage schedule can begin as 50-mg minocycline capsules—two in the morning and one in the afternoon. This

method lessens the total dosage, and lowers the total cost. In addition, the dose can be increased by 50 mg (maximum dose = 200 mg/day) if not improved, or decreased by 50 mg if there is marked improvement.
- For patients who experience premenstrual flares of acne, increasing the dosage of the antibiotic 5 to 7 days before a period (then lowering the dose afterward) reduces the total amount of drug used.
- Because patients frequently take tetracyclines on a long-term basis (in some instances for years), there is understandably a concern about their consequences. Studies have indicated that routine laboratory supervision of healthy young people receiving long-term tetracycline therapy is not necessary. However, when treatment extends for more than 1 to 2 years, some dermatologists recommend periodical monitoring via appropriate blood tests. This is particularly important if the patient has a history of liver, kidney, or autoimmune disease.

POINTS TO REMEMBER

- The patient should be informed that a significant therapeutic response requires 6 to 8 weeks.
- Every effort should be made to try tapering oral medications as soon as acne is controlled.
- If there is evidence of scarring, acne should be treated more aggressively (even mild acne can heal with significant scarring).
- The two Hs—hormones and heredity—underlie teenage acne (one or both parents probably had acne), and not the proverbial poor diet and dirty face (the two Ds)—although, there may be a connection between certain dairy products, glycemic load, and acne.
- In the treatment of females of childbearing potential, isotretinoin should be used concurrently with two methods of birth control to prevent pregnancy while on isotretinoin.

 SEE PATIENT HANDOUTS, "Acne: How to Apply Topical Retinoids" AND "Acne: How to Apply Duac, BenzaClin, and Benzamycin Gel" IN THE COMPANION eBOOK EDITION.

ACNE FACTS

- In most people, acne tends to improve temporarily during the summer months. Exposure to the sun in small doses diminishes acne, and tanning promotes a blending of skin tones.
- Fall and winter acne flare-ups are quite common and are often influenced by mood swings.
- Some women may note improvement of acne during pregnancy or while taking birth control pills. Others may note a worsening of acne or no change at all.
- Moderate to severe involvement of the chest and back is more difficult to treat. Severe, unremitting, scarring acne is more prevalent among men.
- Because acne is a visible disease, acne patients may suffer from impaired self-image, depression, anxiety, employment insecurities, social withdrawal, self-destructive behaviors, and even suicidal ideation.
- Acne, hirsutism, and irregular periods may be associated with hyperandrogenism and/or polycystic ovaries.
- Some drugs, including systemic steroids, lithium, epilepsy agents, and antituberculosis medicines, can cause or exacerbate acne.
- Stress seems to worsen acne. College students at examination time, teenagers about to go to the prom, or someone going for a first job interview often provide testimony to this phenomenon.
- Patients with darker skin tones are sometimes more, or just as, concerned about acne-related pigmentary changes as they are about the acne itself.

Postadolescent Acne (Adult-Onset Acne)

BASICS

- Dermatologists regularly hear the lament "acne, at my age!" expressed by women in whom acne suddenly appears or in whom acne has not resolved by 20 years of age.
- Adult-onset acne is overwhelmingly a condition of women and occurs when acne develops for the first time in the 20s or early 30s. In some cases, teenage acne persists into adulthood or disappears but then recurs later.
- The prevalence of female adult acne has increased significantly in the past several generations.
- Adult-onset acne in men has traditionally been unusual but it is now increasingly seen in men who participate in athletic activities particularly those who use hormonal supplementation.
- There is little question that acne is influenced by hormones. Many women report premenstrual or (less commonly) midcycle flares of inflammatory acne. Pregnancy, oral contraceptives, and hormonal supplementation also appear to affect a woman's complexion and cause fluctuations in acne.

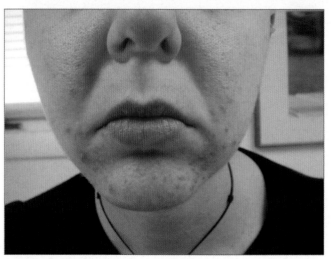

12.12 *Postadolescent acne.* Characteristic location of inflammatory acne papules on the chin and along the jawline in a female adult.

CLINICAL MANIFESTATIONS

- Acneiform lesions tend to appear and reappear like clockwork, typically recurring premenstrually or at ovulation.
- Lesions may last several days or sometimes persist for a month or longer.
- In some women, lesions occur without any pattern.

DESCRIPTION OF LESIONS

- Postadolescent acne is relatively free of comedones and consists of evanescent, inflammatory red papules and/or pustules.
- In general, there are fewer lesions than in typical teenage acne.

DISTRIBUTION OF LESIONS

- In women, lesions occur on the face, most often in the perioral area, along the jawline, or on the chin, that is, the lower part of the face (Fig. 12.12). Also, the hairline, neck, and upper trunk may be affected.
- In men, lesions tend to be limited to the trunk.

DIAGNOSIS

- The diagnosis is made clinically.
- In female patients whose acne is not responding to treatment, or for those who have other signs of hormonal excess such as male characteristics (e.g., facial hair) or irregular menstrual periods, hormonal tests are indicated. More often than not, these levels are normal, and it appears that these women may have an end-organ hypersensitivity to their endogenous androgens.

 DIFFERENTIAL DIAGNOSIS

Rosacea/Perioral/Periorificial Dermatitis (see below)
- *Background redness and telangiectasias also present.*

Folliculitis
- *Monomorphic perifollicular pustules usually on back, arms, or legs.*

Acne Cosmetica
- *Traditional name for acne that is supposedly caused by cosmetics.*
- *May look like inflammatory acne; however, it is often the result of skin irritation.*

MANAGEMENT

Topical Treatment

- Skin care should be kept simple and gentle with the use of mild soaps (**Cetaphil gentle cleanser** or **Purpose facial wash**).
- Postadolescent acne in female patients is treated with many of the same agents used for adolescent acne; however, care should be taken in choosing a topical because aging skin is often more sensitive than teenage skin and may become dry or irritated more easily.

Systemic Treatment

Oral Antibiotics

- Oral antibiotics are effective and commonly used for postadolescent acne (see the earlier discussion in this chapter and in Table 12.5).
- Need to be used with caution in women of childbearing potential. Patients should be advised to stop the treatment if they become pregnant.

Hormonal Treatment

Indications include the following:

- Normal serum androgens and intractable acne that flares with menses or midcycle
- Ovarian or adrenal excess
- When indicated, during a course of oral isotretinoin
- Relapse after taking a course of oral isotretinoin

Oral Contraceptive Pills

- By suppressing gonadotropins, reducing ovarian androgen secretion, and increasing sex hormone–binding globulin levels, oral contraceptives decrease serum testosterone concentrations. They also block the androgenic stimulation of sebaceous glands.
- **Ortho-Tri-Cyclen** (ethinyl estradiol/norgestimate), **Estrostep** (ethinyl estradiol/norethindrone), and **Yaz** (ethinyl estradiol/drospirenone) are FDA approved to treat acne vulgaris. **Alesse** and **Yasmin** are other oral contraceptive pills (OCPs) that are effective for acne.

- *Antibiotics and the "Pill"*—studies have shown that the antibiotics used to treat acne do not interfere with the efficacy of oral contraceptives.

Oral Antiandrogens

- Before oral antiandrogens (androgen receptor blockers) are prescribed, a hormonal and gynecologic evaluation is appropriate for certain patients, particularly women who have treatment-resistant acne, women with the sudden onset of severe acne, virilizing signs or symptoms, irregular menstrual periods, or hirsutism.
- Oral antiandrogens may also be considered for those women who are reluctant to take oral contraceptives for moral or religious reasons.

Spironolactone (Aldactone)

- Spironolactone is the antiandrogen used most frequently to treat acne. It has potent antiandrogenic effects and works by decreasing sebum production.
- *Dosing:* Usually started at 25 to 50 mg/day and then titrated upward according to response (dose range 50 to 200 mg/day).
- It may take 3 months for any positive effects to become visible, but results may appear sooner. The dosage may need to be adjusted during the first 6 months of treatment.
- *Side effects:* Most are dose dependent and include breast tenderness, irregular menstrual periods, headaches, and potential hyperkalemia (rare in young healthy patients).

Other Androgen Receptor Blockers

- **Cyproterone** is an acetate steroidal androgen receptor blocker and competitively inhibits testosterone and dehydroepiandrosterone. It is not available in the United States but is sold outside the United States in combination with ethinyl estradiol as **Diane-35**.
- **Flutamide**, a nonsteroidal androgen receptor blocker approved for prostate cancer, has been used for acne at doses of 62.5 to 500 mg/day.

HELPFUL HINTS

- A minimum of 3 to 6 months of therapy is required to evaluate the efficacy of oral contraceptives and antiandrogen agents in treating adult-onset acne.
- The birth control patch and ring have an unpredictable effect on acne and can actually provoke acne. **Depo-Provera**, an injectable form of birth control–containing synthetic progesterone, can also worsen or trigger acne.
- In women with predicable premenstrual flares of acne, a short course of an oral antibiotic can be given 5 to 7 days before her next menstrual period ("pulse therapy").

POINT TO REMEMBER

- Every female patient with acne should be questioned about her menstrual history and possible virilizing symptoms.

Rosacea

BASICS

- Rosacea is a common disorder that is frequently mistaken for acne. In fact, as recently as 20 years ago, rosacea was referred to as "acne rosacea." Both conditions look alike, they often respond to the same treatments, and often coexist.
- Rosacea arises later in life than does acne, usually between 30 and 50 years of age and women are three times more likely to be affected than men.
- Rosacea has been traditionally described as occurring predominantly in fair-skinned people from Great Britain (Scotland and Wales), Ireland, Germany, Scandinavia, and certain areas of Eastern Europe; however, a greatly underreported incidence of rosacea is also seen in Hispanic populations.

PATHOGENESIS

- The precise cause of rosacea remains unknown, it is believed that multiple factors contribute to its development and progression, including:
  - Genetic predisposition
  - Defects in the skin's innate immunity (decreased cathelicidins)
  - Overstimulation of cutaneous nerves and blood vessels
  - Damage from ultraviolet light
  - Demodex, a species of mite that is often found in the hair follicle
- Rosacea is not caused by drinking excessive amounts of alcohol and does not appear to have any relationship to androgenic hormones.
- Recognized environmental factors may trigger flushing and exacerbate rosacea.

COMMON TRIGGERS OF ROSACEA FLARES

- Sun exposure
- Excess alcohol ingestion. *Drinking alcohol does not cause rosacea nor does it worsen the condition; however, it may trigger flushing (particularly with red wine).*
- Spicy foods, smoking, and caffeine
- Cooking over a hot stove or oven
- Emotional stress
- Physical exertion

CLINICAL MANIFESTATIONS

- Burning and flushing, in some patients, can become quite uncomfortable.
- Patients may also have ocular involvement, typically blepharoconjunctivitis. They may complain of eye stinging, burning, dryness, photophobia, excessive tears, or a foreign

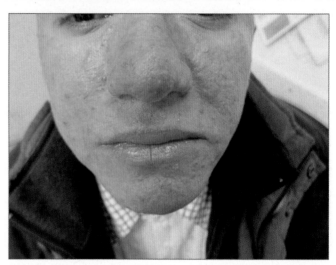

12.13 *Rosacea.* Severe inflammation in a Hispanic patient.

body sensation. Episcleritis and keratoconjunctivitis sicca are rare complications.
- Ocular rosacea may precede the skin manifestations in up to 20% of people.

DESCRIPTION OF LESIONS

- Rosacea is a facial eruption that consists of acne-like erythematous papules, pustules, and telangiectasias.
- At first, rosacea begins with erythema on the cheeks and forehead that later spreads to the nose and chin. This is referred to as *erythematotelangiectatic rosacea.*
- As rosacea progresses, telangiectasias, papules, and sometimes, pustules begin to arise against a background of erythema and can be severe (Fig. 12.13). The papules and pustules (*papulopustular rosacea*) may tend to come and go, but the erythema and telangiectasias are likely to remain.
- Lacks the comedones ("blackheads" or "whiteheads") that are seen in acne and in general, no scarring or nodules/cysts are present (unless the patient has concomitant acne).
- Ocular lesions include erythema of the lid margins and conjunctival injection (Fig. 12.14).

DISTRIBUTION OF LESIONS

- Lesions are typically seen on the central third of the face—forehead, nose, cheeks, and chin (the so-called "flush/blush" areas) (Fig. 12.15).
- Lesions tend to be bilaterally symmetric, but they may occur on only one side of the patient's face.

DIAGNOSIS

- Rosacea is diagnosed clinically.
- A biopsy may be necessary in atypical cases.

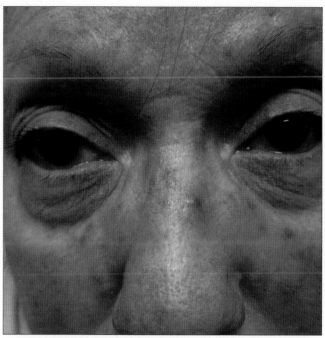

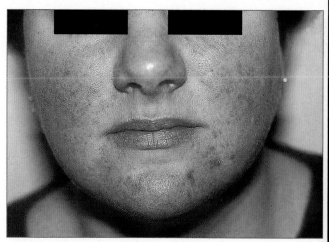

12.15   *Rosacea.* As seen here, rosacea involves inflammatory papules and pustules and telangiectasias that are located on the central third of the face.

12.14   *Ocular rosacea.* Note the conjunctivitis as well as the typical facial papules of rosacea.

DIFFERENTIAL DIAGNOSIS

Adult-onset Acne
- *Tends to occur on the lower part of the face (in females) and often has a much wider distribution than rosacea, such as on the chest and back.*

Seborrheic Dermatitis (see also Chapter 13)
- *The presence of scale and erythema, without acne-like lesions (papules and pustules).*
- *Appears on the nasolabial area, eyebrows, and scalp.*

Systemic Lupus Erythematosus (see Chapter 34)
- *"Butterfly" distribution of rash.*
- *Absence of papules and pustules.*
- *Presence of antinuclear antibodies in addition to other manifestations of lupus.*

"Flusher/Blushers"
- *Physiologic "flusher/blusher" redness occurs on the sides of the cheeks, the front and side of the neck, and the ears, rather than the central area of the face (Fig. 12.16).*

Sun-Damaged Skin (Dermatoheliosis) and "Rosy Cheeks"
- *In many instances, rosacea can be difficult to distinguish from weathered, sun-damaged skin that is seen in many fair-skinned farmers, gardeners, sailors, or in people who have worked or spent long periods of their lives outdoors.*

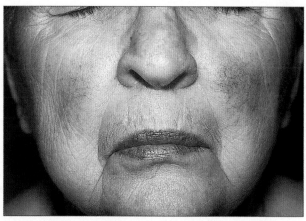

12.16   *Facial erythema.* Frequently misdiagnosed as rosacea, this woman has "rosy cheeks" and telangiectasias.

MANAGEMENT

General Principles

- Topical therapy and lasers are helpful for erythrotelangiectatic rosacea, and systemic treatments in addition to topicals are often required for papulopustular rosacea.
- Patients should be advised to avoid environmental triggers and to apply a sunscreen prior to sun exposure.

Topical Therapy

- Some of the topical medications used to treat acne are also very effective for rosacea; however, precautions must be taken because many with rosacea have very sensitive skin. Consequently, standard acne medications such as topical retinoids and benzoyl peroxide can be drying and/or irritating, and sensitize the skin to the sun and exacerbate rosacea (Table 12.6).
- If possible, long-term control of rosacea should be attempted with topical therapy alone, and oral antibiotics should be reserved for initial control and for breakthrough flares.
- The preparations described in this section can be used in combination with oral antibiotics and other topical medications. It may take 6 to 8 weeks before significant improvement is noted.

Metronidazoles

- The "metros" are the most frequently prescribed first-line topical therapy for rosacea.
- Metronidazole, available as 0.75% to 1% cream or gel (**Noritate** 1% cream, **MetroGel** 1% gel), is applied once daily on rosacea-prone areas.

Azelaic Acid

- Available as a 15% gel (**Finacea**) or 20% cream (**Azelex**)
- **Skinoren** is available in Europe and elsewhere
- Application is twice a day

Sodium Sulfacetamide and Sulfur

- Available as 5% to 10% cream, lotion, suspension cleanser, foam, and cloths (**Klaron, Ovace, Clenia, Avar, Sulfacet-R**)
- Application is twice a day

Brimonidine Tartrate Gel 0.33% (Mirvaso)

- New topical vasoconstrictor indicated for the treatment for moderate to severe facial erythema of rosacea and significantly improves redness and flushing associated with rosacea. It is an alpha$_2$-adrenergic receptor agonist with vasoconstrictive activity.
- Application is once daily.

Ivermectin (Soolantra)

- Topical ivermectin 1% cream has both anti-inflammatory and anti-parasitic activity and is indicated for the inflammatory lesions of rosacea. Application is once daily.

Systemic Therapy
Oral Antibiotics

- The same systemic oral antibiotics used to treat acne are also used to treat the papules and pustules of rosacea. Most cases can be treated and controlled with topical agents alone; however, if topical treatment is ineffective, an oral antibiotic is generally prescribed (see Table 12.5).

Tetracycline Derivatives

- **Minocycline** and **doxycycline** are the first-line oral drugs of choice in the management of moderate to severe rosacea. The mechanism of action of these drugs is more likely anti-inflammatory than antibiotic, because no microorganisms have been definitively identified as a cause of rosacea or its variants.
- Improvement of rosacea is usually noticeable in a week or two. The papules and pustules begin to flatten and disappear, and new ones stop appearing. The antibiotic is tapered when this improvement persists (usually after 3 to 4 weeks).
- *Dosing:* Minocycline—50 to 100 mg bid, doxycycline—50 to 100 mg twice a day. Taper when the inflammation has improved (usually after 3 to 4 weeks).
- **Oracea,** an anti-inflammatory low-dose (subantimicrobial) doxycycline, is available as a 40-mg capsule that contains 30-mg immediate-release and 10-mg delayed-release beads. It is taken once daily.

Table 12.6 TOPICAL AGENTS FOR ROSACEA		
GENERIC NAME	**BRAND NAME**	**SIZES (g)**
Metronidazole 1%	**Noritate cream**	30
Metronidazole 1%	**MetroGel, MetroCream**	60
Metronidazole 0.75%		45
Azelaic acid 15%, 20%	**Azelex, Finevin, Skinoren creams**	30, 50
Azelaic acid 15%	**Finacea gel**	30
Sodium sulfacetamide 10%/sulfur 5%	**Rosac cream**	45
Sodium sulfacetamide 10%	**Sulfacet-R lotion**	25
Ivermectin 1%	**Soolantra**	30, 45, 60
Brimonidine Tartrate gel 0.33%	**Mirvaso**	30, 45

continued on page 205

MANAGEMENT *Continued*

Alternative Antibiotics

- **Azithromycin, clarithromycin, erythromycin** (250 mg twice to four times daily), or **amoxicillin** are used as second-line alternatives when a tetracycline fails or is not tolerated.

Other Treatment Options

Electrocautery

- Electrocautery with a small needle is used to destroy small telangiectasias.

Pulse Dye Lasers and Intense Pulsed Light

- These light-based treatments are highly effective for redness, flushing, and the larger telangiectasias associated with rosacea.

Camouflaging Cosmetics

- Green-tinted creams available OTC (**Eucerin Redness Relief** and **Clinique Redness Solutions**) can help reduce the appearance of redness.

 HELPFUL HINTS

- Initial treatment with oral antibiotics typically delivers a rapid therapeutic response and helps confirm the diagnosis of rosacea.
- Telangiectasias, flushing, and erythema tend to persist and respond minimally, if at all, to antibiotic therapy.
- Patients with rosacea should avoid irritating cosmetics, astringents, and exfoliating agents. Instead, water-based moisturizers and cosmetics are recommended.
- Sunscreens that contain zinc oxide or titanium dioxide—the barrier sunscreens—should be used, especially if other sunscreens irritate or worsen rosacea.
- Rosacea is a condition that is regularly overdiagnosed by health care providers; sometimes these patients may simply have "rosy cheeks" (see Fig. 12.16) or a persistent red face that is the result of long-term sun exposure.

 POINTS TO REMEMBER

- Rosacea is a chronic condition with no known cure.
- Acne and rosacea share similar clinical manifestations and overlapping management strategies, yet each has a distinctive course and prognosis; consequently, an attempt at making a specific diagnosis should be made.
- If possible, long-term control of rosacea should be attempted with topical therapy alone, with oral antibiotics used only for breakthrough flares.

PERIORAL DERMATITIS

- This condition, also known as *periorificial dermatitis,* is a rosacea-like eruption seen primarily in young women and children (see Chapter 3).
- It is usually found circling the mouth (Fig. 12.17), but it may be noted around the eyes and nose (which explains the more inclusive term, "periorificial") (Fig. 12.18).
- As with rosacea, the etiology is unknown but the application of potent topical steroids and the use of fluoridated toothpaste have been implicated.

Clinical features that may help distinguish perioral dermatitis from rosacea include the following:

- Perioral dermatitis appears in children, and in women between 15 and 40 years of age.
- It manifests as small, erythematous papules or pustules without telangiectasias.
- It characteristically circles the mouth and spares the vermilion border of the lips.
- Occasionally, there is superimposed scaling.
- Usually it does not recur after successful treatment.

TOPICAL STEROID-INDUCED ROSACEA

- Rosacea induced by topical steroids is often clinically indistinguishable from ordinary rosacea, but a history of long-term, indiscriminate misuse of a potent topical steroid on the face helps confirm the diagnosis. It is sometimes referred to as "steroid use/abuse/misuse/dermatitis" (Fig. 12.19).
- The topical steroid may have been prescribed for another family member or for another skin condition and then overused by the unsuspecting person, who continues to apply it.
- The condition typically worsens when the topical steroids are discontinued (an occurrence known as "rebound rosacea").
- In an unfortunate cycle, the steroid is sometimes reapplied to diminish the erythema, which only worsens the condition.
- This condition is treated by stopping the offending topical steroid and by taking a tetracycline derivative for a few weeks or more to get over the "hump" of the rebound.

> **HELPFUL HINT**
>
> - Topical steroid-induced rosacea may worsen with the discontinuation of topical steroids ("one step forward, two steps backward").

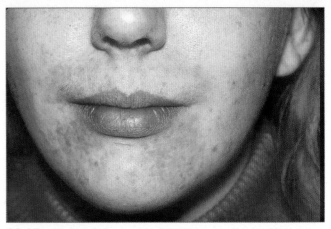

12.17 *Perioral dermatitis.* Multiple, small, acneiform papules can be seen on this young woman. Note the characteristic sparing around the lips. (From Goodheart HP. *Goodheart's Same-Site Differential Diagnosis*. Philadelphia, PA: Lippincott Williams & Wilkins; 2011.)

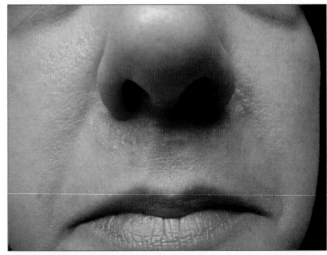

12.18 *Periorificial dermatitis.* Note multiple papules surrounding the nares in this patient.

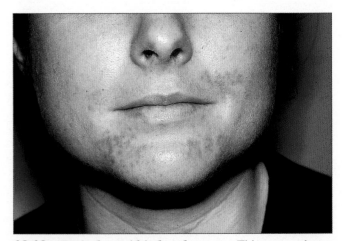

12.19 *Topical steroid-induced rosacea.* This woman has been applying a potent topical steroid every day to her face for 8 months.

RHINOPHYMA

- Rhinophyma is an uncommon yet unsightly manifestation of rosacea and usually occurs in men over 40. It is rarely seen in women.
- It consists of knobby nasal papules that tend to become larger and swollen over time (Fig. 12.20).
- The usual treatments for rosacea are not effective for rhinophyma.
- Recontouring procedures with a scalpel or a carbon dioxide laser have been used successfully to remove ("sculpt") the excess nose tissue, resulting in a more normal shape and appearance. This may also be accomplished by electrocautery and dermabrasion.

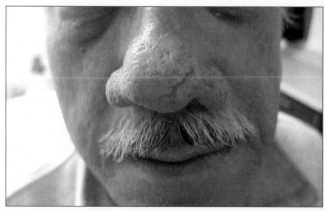

12.20 *Rhinophyma.* This man's enlarged nose is caused by marked sebaceous hyperplasia.

Acne: Other Types

SYSTEMIC DRUG-INDUCED (OR DRUG-EXACERBATED) ACNE

Several drugs are known to provoke acneiform reactions.

- **Oral corticosteroids** and **adrenocorticotropic hormone** produce acne-like lesions that are usually more monomorphic and symmetric in distribution than those seen in adolescent and postadolescent acne. Lesions are located primarily on the trunk. The precise mechanism is uncertain.
- **Lithium** may exacerbate acne.
- Androgens, including **anabolic steroids** and **gonadotrophins**, may precipitate acne, especially in athletes who take such drugs.
- Antiepileptic drugs, especially **phenytoin**, have been held responsible for causing or exacerbating acne; however, modern anticonvulsants do not appear to have acne as a potential side effect.
- Patients taking **isoniazid**, especially those who slowly inactivate the drug, appear to be prone to develop acne.
- The management of drug-induced or drug-exacerbated acne includes discontinuation of the causative drug, decreasing the dosage, or substituting the drug with another agent. Then, proceed with the treatment of acne as described earlier in this chapter.

ACNE EXCORIÉE DES JEUNES FILLES

- This refers to acne that is routinely picked at by the patient, who is almost invariably is female (Fig. 12.21).
- Many of these patients deny that they manipulate their skin, but it is rather obvious because there are usually no primary lesions present and all, or most, have crusts.
- Some of these patients may benefit from selective serotonin receptor inhibitors and/or psychotherapy.

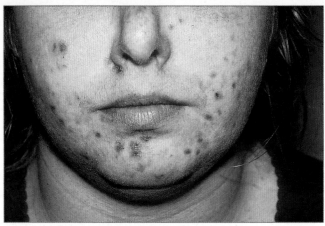

12.21 *Acne excoriée des jeunes filles.* This type of acne has obviously been picked at by the patient.

ENDOCRINOPATHIC ACNE

- The presence of acne, coupled with other signs or symptoms, may indicate an endocrinopathy.
- Hormonal disorders that can produce excessive androgens (e.g., polycystic ovary syndrome), as well as those that can manifest with elevated cortisol levels (e.g., congenital adrenal hyperplasia) can be responsible for producing or aggravating pre-existing acne (see Chapter 20).

OVERVIEW

The term "eczema," often referred to redundantly as "eczematous dermatitis," casts a wide net and tends to be confusing to most nondermatologists. Despite being the most common inflammatory skin condition, eczema is the most confusing skin ailment for both patients and their nondermatologic health care providers. Eczema is very difficult to define. United States Supreme Court Justice Potter Stewart once said that he could not define pornography, but he knew it when he saw it. Such is the case with eczema, a condition that is best understood through repeated viewing (see Chapter 4 for a more precise definition).

At one end of its clinical spectrum there is acute eczema (e.g., poison ivy), manifested by itchy red patches, edema, plaques, or papules that may become intensely inflamed and often develop into vesicles and bullae (Fig. 13.1). *Subacute eczema* is an intermediate stage between acute and chronic eczema. The term has little clinical value but is sometimes used to describe the stage when the acute oozing lesions become dry crusts (Fig. 13.2). On the other end is chronic eczema (e.g., lichen simplex chronicus) whose hallmark is "lichenification," a thickened plaque with an accentuation of the normal skin lines. It is the result of repeated rubbing of the skin. Lichenification was so named because it resembles the lichens found on tree trunks (actually, it more closely resembles the bark of a tree) (Figs. 13.3 and 13.4).

IN THIS CHAPTER...

- ➤ **CONTACT DERMATITIS**
- ➤ **ATOPIC DERMATITIS**
- ➤ **HAND-AND-FOOT ECZEMA**
- ➤ **LICHEN SIMPLEX CHRONICUS**
- ➤ **PRURIGO NODULARIS**
- ➤ **NUMMULAR ECZEMA**
- ➤ **ASTEATOTIC ECZEMA AND NONSPECIFIC ECZEMATOUS DERMATITIS IN THE ELDERLY**
- ➤ **SEBORRHEIC DERMATITIS**
- ➤ **STASIS DERMATITIS**

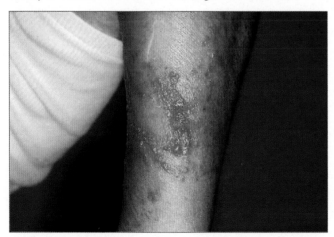

13.1 *Acute allergic eczematous eruption of poison ivy.* The red color and linear blistered appearance suggest an acute "boiling," bubbling, second-degree burn.

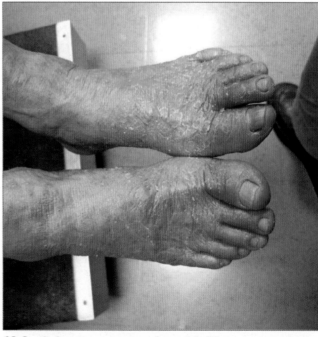

13.2 *Subacute eczematous dermatitis.* There are acute (scale, erythema, and crusts) and chronic (lichenification) findings here.

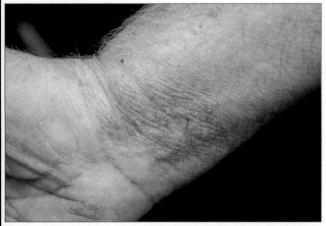

13.3 *Chronic eczematous dermatitis.* This is an example of lichenification, an exaggeration of the skin markings caused by repeated rubbing and scratching.

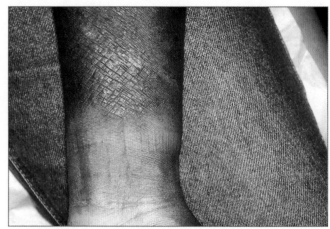

13.4 *Chronic eczematous dermatitis.* This lesion shows no evidence of active inflammation. Lichenification and post-inflammatory hyperpigmentation are apparent.

BASICS

- Contact dermatitis is a type of eczema that is caused by an external agent that produces an inflammatory reaction of the skin. The appearance of the eruption and a careful history often provide clues as to the offending agent.
- Contact dermatitis is divided into two major types based on etiology: *irritant* and *allergic contact dermatitis.*

IRRITANT CONTACT DERMATITIS

- Also known as nonallergic contact dermatitis, irritant contact dermatitis (ICD) is an inflammatory cutaneous eruption that is *not* caused by an allergen, but rather results from a direct toxic effect of a single or repeated application of a chemical or physical insult to the skin. Irritants are often found in the home and workplace and include water, soaps, detergents, solvents, acids, alkalis, and friction. For example, underarm shaving, deodorants, and antiperspirants can produce an irritant contact dermatitis after repeated contact.
- ICD may affect anyone, providing they have had enough exposure to the irritant. Patients who have atopic dermatitis are more likely to develop ICD as a result of their inherent skin sensitivity and defective barrier function.
- The eruption of ICD is confined to the area(s) of exposure or insult, as exemplified by diaper rash (see Chapter 4, Fig. 4.28), scaly dry hands from overwashing, habitual lip licking, or areas where a topical medication or an adhesive was applied (Figs. 13.5–13.8).
- The **diagnosis** and cause of ICD is based on a careful history and ruling out of allergic contact dermatitis (ACD).
- **Management** consists of avoidance or minimizing contact with the offending agent and treatment, if necessary.

ALLERGIC CONTACT DERMATITIS

- Allergic contact dermatitis (ACD) is a true allergic or hypersensitivity reaction that precipitates an eczematous dermatitis. ACD is a delayed-type (type IV) hypersensitivity

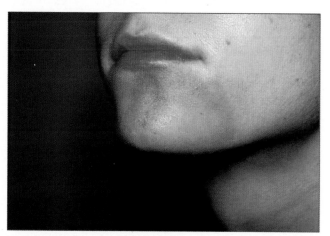

13.5 *Irritant contact dermatitis.* The erythema on this boy's chin face was caused by irritation from benzoyl peroxide in an acne preparation.

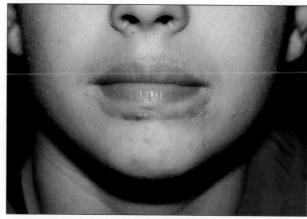

13.6 *Irritant contact dermatitis.* The perioral erythema is obviously due to this child's habit of licking her lips.

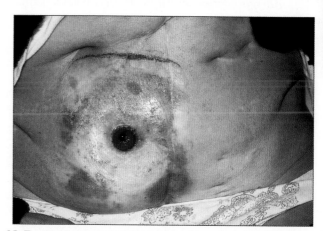

13.7 *Irritant contact dermatitis.* Chronic irritation from a stoma was the cause of this reaction.

reaction that occurs when the skin comes in contact with an allergen (antigen) to which an individual has previously been sensitized.
- Poison ivy and oak (discussed below) and nickel are the most common contact allergens. Other common allergens found in home and work environments include components of jewelry, metals, cosmetics, topical medications, and rubber compounds; namely, thimerosal (a mercurial preservative), neomycin (a topical antibiotic), formaldehyde (found in shampoo and cosmetics), paraphenylenediamine (found in certain hair dyes) (Fig. 13.8), and quaternium-15 (a preservative often found in cosmetics) are also potential allergens.
- ACD occurs only in sensitized persons. ACD is not dose dependent, and it may spread extensively beyond the site of original contact. ACD is seen less commonly in infants, the elderly, and African-Americans.

POISON IVY/POISON OAK DERMATITIS

- In the United States, poison ivy and poison oak are the principal causes of ACD. Poison ivy is found throughout the country, whereas poison oak is found more commonly in the western United States and poison sumac (a small related

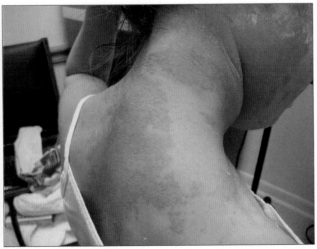

13.8 *Allergic contact dermatitis.* This is a contact dermatitis due to paraphenylenediamine in this patient's hair dye.

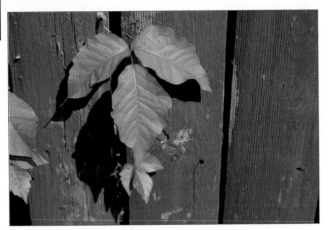

13.9 *Poison Ivy.* This plant has the following four characteristics: (a) clusters of three leaflets, (b) alternate leaf arrangement, (c) lack of thorns, and (d) each group of three leaflets grows on its own stem, which connects to the main vine.

tree), is found only in woody, swampy areas. Poison ivy, oak, and sumac were formerly members of the genus *Rhus* (hence the term *Rhus* dermatitis) but now are classified into the genus *Toxicodendron,* a member of the Anacardiaceae family (Figs. 13.9 and 13.10).

- Pentadecylcatechol and heptadecylcatechol are the sensitizing allergens in the plants' resinous oils (urushiol). These invisible oils may reach the skin not only from direct contact, but also through garden tools, pet fur, golf clubs, or the smoke of a burning plant. Identical or related antigens are found in the resin of the Japanese lacquer tree, ginkgo trees, cashew nut shells, the dye of the India marking nut (used as a clothing dye in India), and the skin of mangoes. All cause similar skin rashes in sensitized people.
- In the eastern United States, poison ivy dermatitis occurs mainly in the spring and summer. In the western and southeastern United States, where outdoor activity is common all year, it may occur in any season.

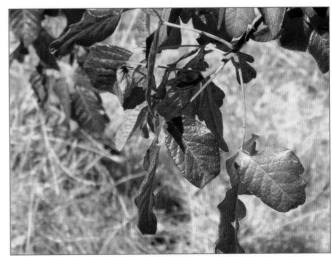

13.10 *Poison oak.* Widespread throughout the mountains and valleys of California. It commonly grows as a climbing vine with leaves that look like oak leaves.

CLINICAL MANIFESTATIONS

- The characteristic eruption consists of intensely pruritic *linear* streaks of erythematous papules, "juicy" vesicles, and bullae (blisters), which give the appearance of having been caused by an outside agent (Fig. 13.11). The rash typically occurs 2 days after contact with the plant, but initial reactions have been noted within 12 hours of contact and as long as 1 week later.
- The distribution of lesions is characteristic. Generally, exposed areas of the body are affected first. The rash may later involve covered areas that have come into contact with the plant oil. The external vulva or perianal areas may be affected in women (Fig. 13.12). In men, involvement of the penis is sometimes a diagnostic sign.
- Further dissemination, or **autoeczematization** (see later in this chapter), is believed to occur through hematogenous spread and subsequent immune-complex deposition in the skin. This spread may occur within 5 to 7 days after the initial exposure, and the resulting rash may last for 3 weeks or more.

🧑 DIFFERENTIAL DIAGNOSIS

Plant Dermatitis other than *Toxicodendron* (e.g., Reactions to Meadow Grass and other Plants) Scabies (see Chapter 29)
- *Has characteristic distribution (finger webs, flexor wrists); generally spares the head and neck in those who are immunocompetent.*
- *May have other family members or intimate persons with similar symptoms.*

Herpes Zoster (see Chapter 17)
- *Dermatomal distribution.*
- *Often painful.*

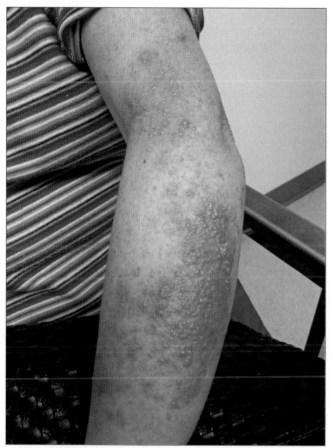

13.11 *Allergic contact dermatitis. Poison ivy.* Contact with poison ivy caused this fiery red eruption. Note the "outside job" appearance of the linear streaks of vesicles and bullae.

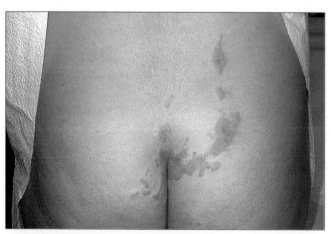

13.12 *Allergic contact dermatitis. Poison ivy.* Note the buttocks which became involved 24 hours after this patient used toilet paper that had been contaminated by the resin of poison ivy.

 MANAGEMENT

A **limited eruption** and mild itching may be relieved by the following:

- The application of frozen vegetable packages (e.g., frozen peas) and **Calamine lotion**
- Cool baths with colloidal oatmeal agents such as **Aveeno Oatmeal Bath**
- Cool compresses with Burow solution help dry vesicles and bullae
- Oral antihistamines are helpful, particularly at bedtime

In **severe cases** with widespread eruption and marked pruritus, topical therapy may require supplementation with systemic agents, as follows:

- **Prednisone** in a tapering dosage schedule that often starts at 1 mg/kg and decreases by 5 mg every 2 days for at least 2 weeks and for as long as 3 weeks. Prednisone tablets should be taken with meals, and the entire daily dose may be taken all at once, rather than in divided doses throughout the day. (Possible side effects of short-term systemic corticosteroids include gastrointestinal upset, sleep disturbances, and mood changes. Hyperactivity, anxiety, depression, and even paranoid reactions have been reported.) **Medrol Dosepaks** (methylprednisolone) usually *do not* provide enough days of treatment for most patients with severe reactions.
- **Intramuscular triamcinolone diacetate** or **hexacetonide** may be used if the patient has gastrointestinal intolerance to oral corticosteroids.
- For corticosteroid intolerant patients, **cyclosporine**, 4 to 5 mg/kg/day in two divided daily doses for 2 to 3 weeks, is rapidly effective.

 SEE PATIENT HANDOUT "Burow Solution" IN THE COMPANION eBOOK EDITION.

 HELPFUL HINTS

- Learn to recognize "leaves of three, let it be."
- If work or hobbies involve frequent exposure to poisonous plants, a barrier cream may be applied before exposure. Use of gloves may also be helpful.
- After contact with the plant or its oil, one should wash with soap and cold water as soon as possible. All exposed clothing should be laundered.
- Contrary to common belief, the fluid in blisters does not contain the resinous oil, and it cannot transfer the rash to others or cause the rash to spread on the affected person. During the tapering course of the prednisone regimen for treatment of severe poison ivy dermatitis, patients may experience a rebound of the eruption and itching. When this rebound occurs, patients may be advised to increase the dosage back to the dosage that worked effectively the day before and then be slowly weaned thereafter.

OTHER COMMON EXAMPLES OF ALLERGIC CONTACT DERMATITIS

- **Eyelid contact dermatitis:** The thin skin of the eyelids contributes to its sensitivity and susceptibility to allergic and irritant reactions (e.g., poison ivy, cosmetics, nickel). Not uncommonly, ACD of the eyelids, as well as on the face and fingers, may occur from the application of artificial acrylic nails. Patients generally touch their face and eyelids often without being aware of it (Fig. 13.13).
- Airborne contact dermatitis: Chemicals in the air may produce airborne CD which usually manifests on the eyelids, but may affect other exposed areas, particularly the head and the neck.

DIAGNOSIS OF ACD

- Patients should be questioned regarding their daily habits and occupational exposures.

- The distribution and shape of the eruption may point to a specific allergen. For example, dermatitis from rubber in underpants (Fig. 13.14), neomycin in eardrops (Fig. 13.15), hair dyes, nickel in earrings (Fig. 13.16), or to an adhesive (Fig. 13.17).
- Patch testing is used to identify specific allergens in patients with histories suggestive of ACD (Fig. 13.18A,B). The standardized, commercially available allergens are fixed in dehydrated gel layers, taped against the skin of the patient's back for 48 hours and are then removed. A final reading is performed after 96 hours. The presence of erythema, papules, or vesicles (i.e., an acute eczematous reaction) at the

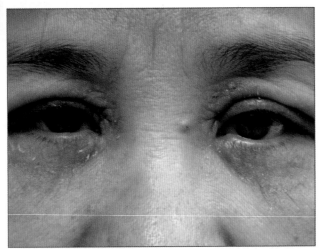

13.13 *Allergic contact dermatitis.* Eyelid dermatitis from artificial acrylic fingernails. (Figure courtesy of Miguel R. Sanchez, M.D.)

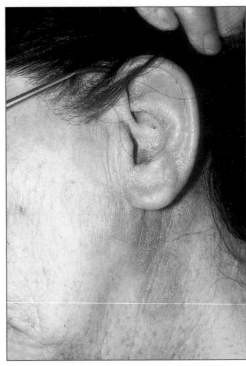

13.15 *Allergic contact dermatitis.* This contact dermatitis was caused by neomycin in this patient's ear drops.

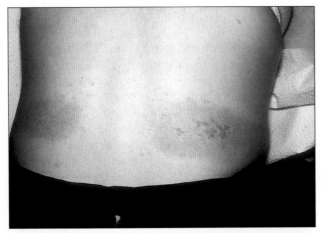

13.14 *Allergic contact dermatitis.* This patient reacted to the rubber in the elastic waistband of her underpants. Note sparing at the sites where the garment did not come into constant contact with her skin.

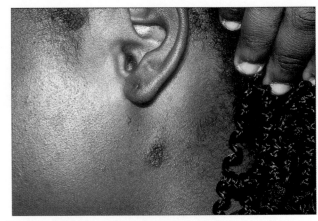

13.16 *Allergic contact dermatitis.* Nickel caused the dermatitis on the earlobe and neck of this woman who wore long earrings.

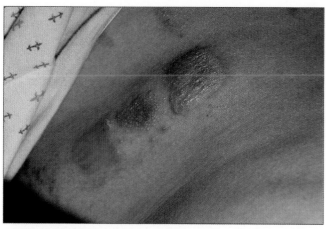

13.17 *Allergic contact dermatitis.* This a reaction to an adhesive dressing (Band Aid).

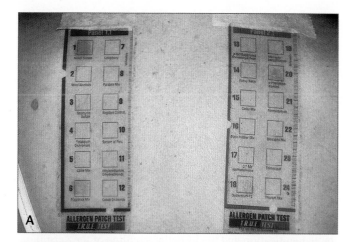

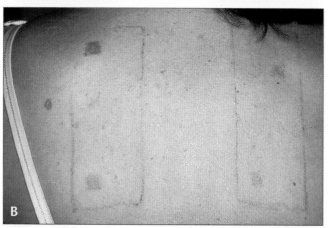

13.18 *Allergic contact dermatitis.* Test patches. **A:** These test patches will be removed after 48 hours. **B:** The final reading at 96 hours shows positive reactions to various allergens.

site where the chemical is applied is a strongly positive reaction. A bullous reaction is extremely positive.
- Interpretation of patch test results and correlation with clinical findings require experience and are generally performed by dermatologists.

 DIFFERENTIAL DIAGNOSIS

Irritant Contact Dermatitis
- *Eruption may be identical to ICD; however, the history and a negative patch testing result may distinguish ICD from ACD.*

Other Types of Acute and Chronic Eczematous Dermatitis (e.g., Atopic Dermatitis)
- *No history of exposure to a contactant and often the patient will have a positive atopic history.*

Systemic Drug Reactions (see Chapter 26)
- *More likely to present as a morbilliform eruption or with erythema and/or urticaria.*

 MANAGEMENT

- Identification and removal of the inciting agent.
- Advice on how to avoid the inciting agent that is, providing a list of alternative products that do not contain the allergen, reading labels, etc.
- Treatment with topical or systemic corticosteroids, if necessary.

 HELPFUL HINT

- Patients are often asked whether they are using any "new soaps or detergents." These agents can certainly trigger or exacerbate ICD, but are unlikely to be the cause of ACD.

BASICS

- Although most cases of atopic dermatitis (AD) begin in childhood (often in infancy), AD may start at any age. The disease frequently remits spontaneously—reportedly in 40% to 50% of children—but it may persist, or return in adolescence or adulthood and possibly endure for a lifetime. Traditionally, patients and their families were advised that children "will outgrow eczema"; however, this optimistic prognosis is not always realized.
- AD is a type of eczema that occurs in association with a personal or family history of atopy (asthma or allergic rhinitis). In adults, AD often displays a variety of clinical manifestations that are often quite different in appearance and location than seen in the pediatric age group.

PATHOGENESIS
(Discussed in Chapter 4)

CLINICAL MANIFESTATIONS

- The distribution of lesions may be similar to that seen in early childhood (i.e., in flexural folds); however, adult and adolescent AD tends to also arise on extensor locations: the posterior neck (Fig. 13.19), dorsa of the hands (Fig. 13.20), wrists, shins, ankles, and feet. AD may be limited to the lips (Fig. 13.21), areolae (Fig. 13.22), eyelids, as well as vulvar or scrotal areas (Figs. 13.23 and 13.24).

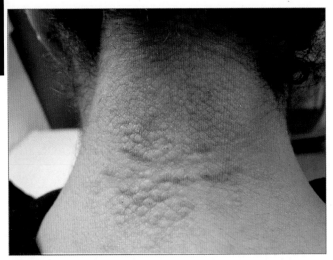

13.19 *Atopic dermatitis (lichen simplex chronicus).* The nape of the neck is a common site of involvement. Note lichenification.

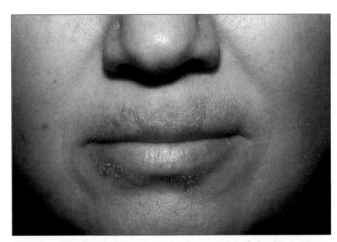

13.21 *Atopic cheilitis (atopic dermatitis of the lips).* Note the lichenification and the ill-defined outline of the vermilion border of the upper lip.

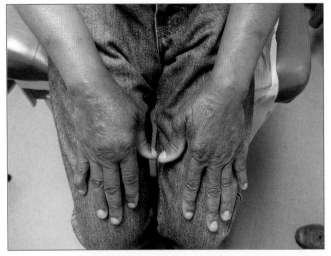

13.20 *Atopic dermatitis (lichen simplex chronicus).* Dorsal hands in a senior. Note postinflammatory hyperpigmentation.

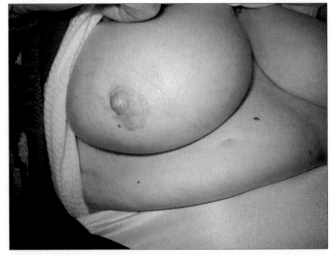

13.22 *Atopic dermatitis of breast and areola.* This woman has periareolar atopic dermatitis. When localized to one breast, Paget disease (see Fig. 31.47) should be considered if the lesion does not improve with topical steroid therapy.

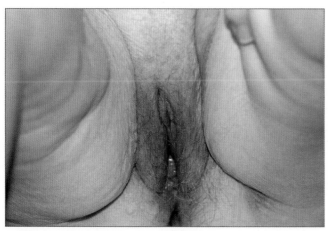

13.23 *Atopic dermatitis of vulvar, perineum, and inguinal areas.* This eruption was initially diagnosed and treated as a fungal infection by the patient's health care provider.

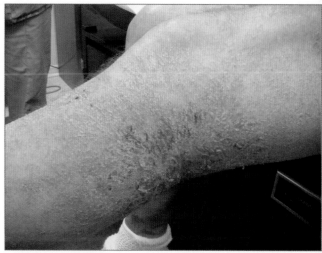

13.25 *Eczematous dermatitis (impetiginized).* Note scale, erythema, and "honey-colored" crusts. Staphylococcal infection from fissured areas of the skin.

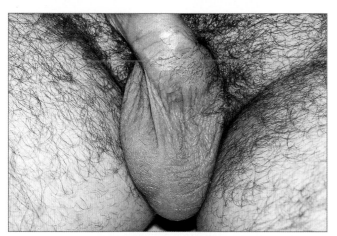

13.24 *Atopic dermatitis (lichen simplex chronicus) limited to the scrotum.* As above, this eruption is often diagnosed as a fungal infection. Note the lichenification.

CLINICAL SEQUELAE AND POSSIBLE COMPLICATIONS

- Pruritus leading to rubbing and scratching may result in lichenification, oozing, and secondary bacterial infection (impetiginization), typically caused by *Staphylococcus aureus*. One should suspect staphylococcal infection if honey-colored crusting or weeping from cracked areas of the skin occurs (Fig. 13.25).
- Postinflammatory hyperpigmentation and postinflammatory hypopigmentation are frequent sequelae after lesions resolve.
- Eczema herpeticum (Kaposi varicelliform eruption) (Fig. 13.26), a secondary infection with herpes simplex virus, is more commonly seen in childhood (See Chapter 4).

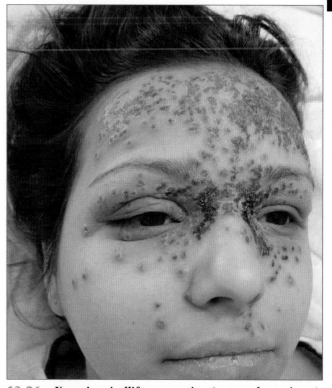

13.26 *Kaposi varicelliform eruption (eczema herpeticum).* Most cases are due to *Herpes simplex virus* type 1 or 2. The virus infects the skin because those with AD appear to have reduced immunity to herpes infection as well as breakdown of the skin barrier in eczematous skin. (Image courtesy of Joseph Eastern, MD.)

DIAGNOSIS

- The diagnosis of atopic dermatitis is generally made clinically, especially in those patients with an atopic history.
- A skin biopsy is performed if the diagnosis is in doubt.

DIFFERENTIAL DIAGNOSIS

Contact Dermatitis (see above)

• *Location and shape of lesion(s) may be suggestive and the history may reveal an irritant or allergic contactant.*

Scabies (see Chapter 29)

• *History may reveal exposure. Tends to involve wrists and web spaces of fingers and is less likely to occur above the neck in adults.*

Psoriasis (see Chapter 14)

• *At times, psoriasis can be clinically and histopathologically indistinguishable from eczema. Psoriasis is less likely to itch and tends to occur more often on extensor areas.*

Tinea Pedis, Corporis, Manuum, and Capitis (see Chapter 18)

• *KOH or fungal culture is positive.*

 MANAGEMENT

Topical Therapy (see Chapter 4, and "Introduction: Topical Therapy")

General Principles

• The application of an appropriately chosen topical steroid—potent or super potent may be necessary for exuberant flares or for chronic lichenified areas—evenly and sparingly one or two times daily to the affected area(s) until the skin is clear of dermatitis.

• As the dermatitis improves, the frequency of application may be decreased, or a less potent topical corticosteroid may be prescribed.

• "Stronger" is often preferable to "longer."

Face and Body Folds (Intertriginous Regions)

• Use a low-potency corticosteroid cream or ointment or a topical calcineurin inhibitor such as **Protopic ointment** (tacrolimus) **0.1%** or **Elidel cream 1%** (pimecrolimus).

• In more severe cases of atopic dermatitis, initial therapy may be with a higher-potency steroid, followed by a less potent preparation or a topical calcineurin inhibitor for maintenance.

Body (Trunk, Arms, Legs, Scalp)

• Treatment can be initiated with a midstrength (class 4) cream, ointment, foam, or a midstrength (class 3) agent. Even a superpotent (class 1) agent, such as **clobetasol 0.05%**, may be used for limited periods until control is achieved.

• A 1-lb jar of **triamcinolone acetonide cream** or **ointment 0.1%** is economical.

Topical Immunomodulators

• **Protopic ointment** (tacrolimus), a nonsteroidal immunomodulator, is as effective as a class 4 or 5 topical steroid in the treatment of atopic dermatitis and is often used as an alternative to topical steroids, particularly for AD on the face or intertriginous areas (axillae and groin), where the long-term use of high-potency steroids is limited.

• When applied twice daily, **Protopic** may cause transient side effects, such as burning and itching.

• The 0.1% concentration has been approved for the treatment of atopic dermatitis in those >16 years of age.

• Elidel cream (pimecrolimus), a nonsteroidal immunomodulator, is considered equipotent to a class 5 or 6 topical steroid.

Infection

• Open, weeping, crusted, impetiginized lesions may be treated with a drying agent, such as **Burow solution**, before topical steroids are applied.

• **Clorox bleach**—1/2 to 1 cup per tubful of water for 2 to 3 days, then 2 to 3 times per week.

• Topical antibiotics—2% mupirocin cream or ointment (**Bactroban**) and 1% retapamulin ointment (**Altabax**).

• For patients with secondary herpes simplex infection (Kaposi varicelliform eruption), oral antiviral therapy and possibly hospitalization may be required.

Phototherapy

• Natural sunlight or phototherapy with ultraviolet B rays is often very effective for widespread skin involvement.

Systemic Treatments

• Before resorting to systemic treatments, a "soak-and-smear" regimen may be used. (See "Introduction: Topical Therapy.")

• Systemic steroids should be used in only exceptional circumstances as they can lead to severe rebound flares upon discontinuation.

• Immunosuppressive therapy with systemic agents such as **cyclosporine**, or short-term hospitalization is sometimes necessary in patients with severe unresponsive generalized atopic dermatitis.

• **Mycophenolate mofetil, azathioprine, and methotrexate** are sometimes utilized for chronic, severe refractory atopic dermatitis.

continued on page 219

MANAGEMENT *Continued*

General Management (see also Chapter 4)
Bathing
Frequency of bathing in atopic dermatitis has been the subject of controversy and misunderstanding. There are many reasons not to restrict frequent bathing:
- Bathing removes crusts, irritants, potential allergens, and infectious agents.
- Bathing provides pleasure and reduces stress.
- Bathing hydrates the skin and allows better delivery of corticosteroids and moisturizers.
- The addition of Clorox bleach to bath water ("bleach baths") can be effective (see earlier discussion) for oozing or infected atopic dermatitis.

Bathing Tips
- Mild, moisturizing soaps such as **Dove** or nonsoap cleansers such as **Cetaphil Gentle Skin Cleanser** should be used.
- The patient should be cautioned not to scrub or use harsh soaps on lesional skin (many people are erroneously led to believe that scrubbing with "good soaps" may actually help inflamed skin).
- Excessive bathing that is not followed immediately by application of a moisturizer tends to dry the skin.
- Excessive toweling and scrubbing should be avoided.

Prevention of Atopic Dermatitis
The following measures may help the patient to avoid or reduce exposure to triggers such as dry skin, irritants, overheating and sweating, and allergens.
- **Moisturize dry skin:** A cream or ointment should be applied immediately after bathing to "trap" water in the skin. However, in warm climates or in the summer, moisturizers may actually be irritating or may interfere with healing.
- Suggested ointments: **Vaseline Petroleum Jelly, Aquaphor**
- Suggested creams and lotions: **Eucerin, Cetaphil, Lubriderm, Curel, Moisturel**
- **Barrier repair: Atopiclair, MimyX**, and **Epiceram** are multiple-ingredient prescription, nonsteroidal barrier creams that are applied two or three times per day. The barrier cream and lotion **CeraVe** can be purchased OTC.
- **Avoid irritants:** Use nonirritating fabrics, such as cotton. Avoid wool clothing, overheating and sweating, and excess dryness or humidity.
- **Avoid known contact and airborne allergens:** Common allergens include nickel, pollen, and fragrances.

 SEE PATIENT HANDOUTS, "Burow Solution" and "Soak and Smear Instruction Sheet" IN THE COMPANION eBOOK EDITION.

 POINTS TO REMEMBER

- Topical steroids should be applied only to active disease (inflamed skin) and used until the skin is completely smooth.
- When topical steroids are applied immediately after bathing, their penetration and potency are increased.
- Low-potency topical steroids or topical immunomodulators are recommended for use on the face and in skin folds, such as the perineal area and underarms.
- "Soak and smear" therapy can often be substituted for, or limit the use of, systemic steroids.

 HELPFUL HINTS

- It should be kept in mind that both irritant and allergic contact dermatitis can coexist when atopic dermatitis is present.
- Contact dermatitis is eczema that comes from the outside is and eczema that comes from the *inside* is atopic dermatitis.
- The "gooiest" and cheapest moisturizer is petrolatum.
- "Bleach showers" for patients who are unable to take baths an empty spray bottle (like one that used to contain "Windex" spray) can be used as follows:
  1. Nearly fill the bottle with warm water
  2. Add a capful of Clorox bleach
  3. Shake well
  4. Spray affected, crusted sites during the shower
  5. Rinse well

Hand-and-Foot Eczema

BASICS

- Hand-and-foot eczema, a common problem in adults, has various clinical manifestations.
- Both, **dyshidrotic eczema**, or the *"wet" type;* and the scaly, patch/plaque hand-and-foot eczema, or the *"dry" type*, are thought to be triggered by various endogenous or exogenous factors.
- Frequently, both exogenous (i.e., irritants, allergens, or microbes) and endogenous (i.e., a personal or family history of atopy) factors are at work in the same patient.

CLINICAL MANIFESTATIONS

- For descriptive purposes, atopic hand-and-foot eczema may be divided into two clinical types that may overlap in the same patient: a "wet" type and a "dry," scaly type. The clinical course of both types may be acute, recurrent, or chronic.

"WET" TYPE

Dyshidrotic eczema, the wet type (Figs. 13.27 and 13.28), was formerly referred to as *pompholyx* (the Greek word for bubble), and describes the following:

- An itchy, clear, vesicular eruption on the hands and/or feet.
- The vesicles are typically located on the sides of the fingers, but they can also occur on the palms and, less commonly, on the soles of the feet and the lateral aspects of the toes.
- Initially, lesions are small, deep seated, clear vesicles that resemble little bubbles.
- Later, as they dry and resolve without rupturing, they generally turn into a golden-brown appearance ("sago grain vesicles") without surrounding erythema.
- Secondary *impetiginization* may occur.

"DRY," SCALY TYPE

In nondyshidrotic hand eczema—the dry, scaly type—the following are noted:

- Lesions are scaly and often erythematous.
- Hyperkeratotic, lichenified plaques may be apparent.
- The central palm or palmar aspect of the hands and fingers are also commonly affected.
- Fingertips may become dry, wrinkled, and red, with resultant painful fissures and erosions (Fig. 13.29).
- As with the dyshidrotic type of hand eczema, secondary bacterial infection ("honey-crusted" skin) may occur.
- With long-standing disease, patients' fingernails may reveal dystrophic changes (e.g., irregular transverse ridging, pitting, thickening, discoloration) when the nail matrix (root) becomes involved (Fig. 13.30).

DIAGNOSIS

- The diagnosis of atopic hand eczema is usually made on clinical grounds when other causes are excluded. A diligent history must be taken to rule in or rule out contact dermatitis.

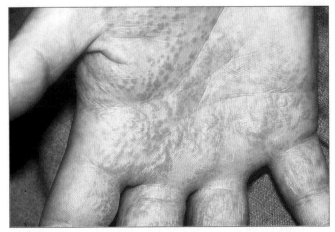

13.27 *Atopic hand eczema, dyshidrotic or "wet" type.* The characteristic vesicles (pompholyx) are apparent in this patient's palm.

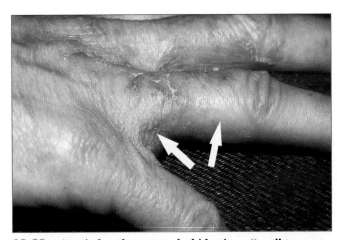

13.28 *Atopic hand eczema, dyshidrotic or "wet" type.* The vesicles on the sides of the fingers are shown here.

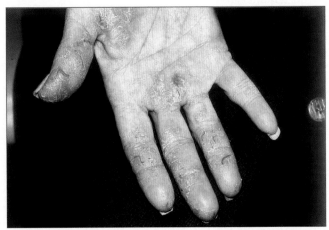

13.29 *Atopic hand eczema ("dry," scaly type).* The fingers have become dry and fragile, with resultant painful fissures.

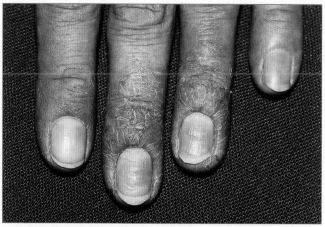

13.30 *Atopic dermatitis (nail dystrophy).* This patient's middle fingernails show dystrophic changes, transverse ridging, and cuticle loss solely on those fingers where eczema is present in the proximal nail folds.

DIFFERENTIAL DIAGNOSIS

Contact Dermatitis

- *This is suspected, particularly if the eruption is on the dorsum of the hands or feet.*
- *Patch testing with putative allergens (see earlier in this chapter) may be performed if an exogenous cause is suspected.*

Inflammatory Tinea Manuum or Pedis

- *Suggested by well-demarcated plaques on the palms (often on one palm only) and soles with an advancing edge of scale; or a positive KOH examination or fungal culture.*

Palmoplantar Psoriasis

- *Often indistinguishable from hand-and-foot eczema.*
- *The patient may have evidence of psoriasis elsewhere on the body or a personal or family history of psoriasis.*

Scabies (see Chapter 29)

- *Considered if there is an acute pruritic vesicular eruption in the web spaces of the fingers.*

MANAGEMENT

Mild Cases

- Nonirritating cleansers or soap substitutes.
- Protective cotton-lined gloves should be used for washing dishes or similar tasks.
- Fastidious hand protection, emollient barrier creams, protective gloves, and the avoidance of irritants and allergens.
- For oozing and infected lesions, compresses with **Burow solution** (aluminum acetate) are applied. This treatment promotes drying and has an antibacterial effect. The solution is applied in a 1:40 dilution two or three times daily until bullae resolve.
- **Topical corticosteroids:** Ointments penetrate skin better than creams do, but patients may prefer to use creams during the day. Most patients require at least medium-potency (class 3) corticosteroids (e.g., **triamcinolone 0.1%**), with or without occlusion. However, higher-potency (class 2) corticosteroids (e.g., **fluocinonide 0.05%**) can be used on an as-needed basis. Lower-strength (class 5) corticosteroids (e.g., **hydrocortisone valerate 0.2%**) may sometimes be applied for long-term maintenance.
- **Protopic ointment** (tacrolimus) 0.1% or **Elidel cream** (pimecrolimus) 1% may also be effective as maintenance but may be less effective for treating an acute flare.

Severe Cases

- Application of potent corticosteroids applied under plastic or vinyl occlusion, as well as superpotent topical corticosteroids can be used intermittently and for short periods, because they increase the risk of skin atrophy.
- Systemic antibiotics should be administered for obvious or suspected secondary infection.
- Short-term use of systemic corticosteroids may be required for very severe flares.
- Treatment of hyperkeratotic palmar eczema is notoriously difficult. Acitretin (**Soriatane**), an aromatic retinoid, may help control hyperkeratosis.
- Other measures, such as **oral psoralen plus topical ultraviolet A (PUVA), oral cyclosporine, azathioprine**, and low-dose **methotrexate** are used for severe, refractory cases.
- Botulinum toxin A injection may be effective, particularly in those patients in whom hyperhidrosis is considered to be an aggravating factor.

 SEE PATIENT HANDOUTS "Burow Solution" and "Hand Eczema" IN THE COMPANION eBOOK EDITION.

Lichen Simplex Chronicus

BASICS

- Lichen simplex chronicus (LSC) is a common, chronic, often solitary, pruritic eczematous eruption caused by repetitive rubbing and scratching. LSC can appear *de novo* on areas of previously normal skin or it can arise as a variant of atopic dermatitis.

CLINICAL MANIFESTATIONS

- Patients with LSC have single or multiple, well-demarcated lichenified plaque(s) that are slightly erythematous (early lesions) or hyperpigmented, and thickened (older lesions) with accentuation of the skin lines. LSC is typically seen on areas of skin that are easily reached to scratch such as the nape of the neck, scalp, external ear canals, upper back wrists, extensor forearms, ankles (Figs. 13.31 and 13.32),

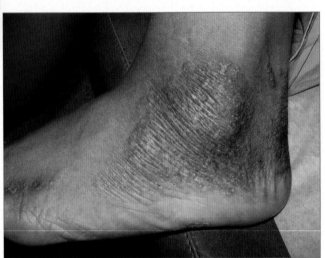

13.31 *Lichen simplex chronicus.* A large lichenified plaque is seen on the lateral malleolar area.

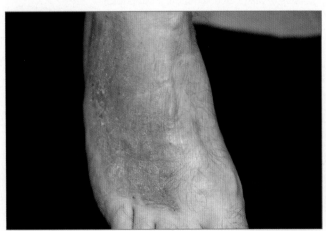

13.32 *Lichen simplex chronicus.* This focal lichenified plaque involves the distal lower leg and ankle. This patient not only scratched the lesion, but he also persistently rubbed it with his contralateral heel.

pretibial areas, or inner thighs. LSC may also involve the vulvae, scrotum (see Fig. 13.24), intragluteal area, and perianal area (pruritus ani).
- Chronic or paroxysmal pruritus with scratching and rubbing is the primary symptom.

DIAGNOSIS

- The diagnosis is readily apparent and is made on clinical grounds.

DIFFERENTIAL DIAGNOSIS IN GENITAL AREA

Tinea Cruris and Candidiasis (see Chapter 18)
- *A chronic itchy vulvar or scrotal rash may also suggest a fungal infection such as tinea cruris or candidiasis.*
- *KOH examination or fungal culture is positive.*

Inverse Psoriasis and Intertrigo (see Chapter 14)
- *Should be considered when lesions involve the inguinal creases and perianal area.*

MANAGEMENT

- The most important aspect of therapy is the elimination of scratching and rubbing.
- LSC may be treated with an intermediate-strength (class 3 or 4) topical corticosteroid, or if necessary, a high-potency (class 1) topical corticosteroid.
- Occlusion, when required, has the added advantage of preventing patients from scratching or rubbing—or, at least, reminding them not to do so.
- Oral antihistamines may be helpful at bedtime because of their sedative effect.
- **Protopic ointment** (tacrolimus) **0.1%** or **Elidel cream 1%** (pimecrolimus) may prove beneficial in patients with vulvar or perianal LSC.

HELPFUL HINT

- There is a potential for stinging and burning when **Protopic** ointment is applied to sensitive, intertriginous (e.g., genital) areas. This can be lessened by refrigeration prior to its application.

BASICS

- **Prurigo nodularis (also called picker's nodule)** is another chronic variant of atopic dermatitis that is often seen in the same clinical context as lichen simplex chronicus (see above).
- It is characterized by intensely pruritic nodules that are difficult to treat, occurring mainly on the extensor aspect of the lower extremities. It is more common in adults but may affect both children and adolescents.

CLINICAL MANIFESTATIONS

- Lesions are reddish, brown, or hyperpigmented dome-shaped firm, papules or nodules that typically resolve with prominent postinflammatory hyperpigmentation (Figs. 13.33 and 13.34).
- Lesions are most commonly noted on the pretibial shafts and sometimes on the extensor areas of the arms as well as the upper and lower back and are often crusted or excoriated—pruritus may be intense.

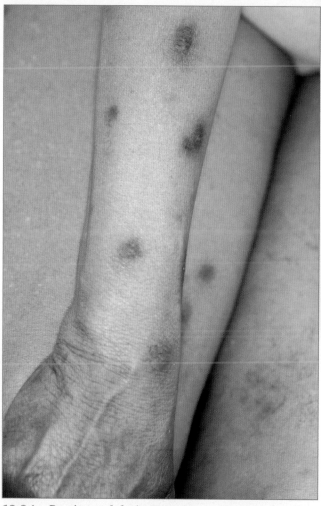

13.34 *Prurigo nodularis.* These intensely pruritic excoriated papules and nodules on the thighs and arms show marked postinflammatory hyperpigmentation.

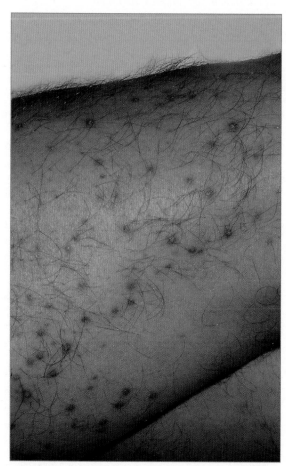

13.33 *Prurigo nodularis.* Pruritic papules on the thighs.

⚒ MANAGEMENT

- Prurigo nodularis tends to be very resistant to topical corticosteroids.
- Occlusion topical steroid therapy with **Cordran tape** or a class 1 topical steroid is sometimes effective.
- In recalcitrant cases, intralesional corticosteroid injections may be helpful.

Nummular Eczema

BASICS

- Nummular eczema is a recurrent and chronic eruption that may appear at any age, although it is most common in people in their 60s. It does not appear to be hereditary. The coin-shaped patches or plaques can affect any part of the body, but the legs and buttocks are the most common areas. Flare-ups are typically associated with the winter season.

CLINICAL MANIFESTATIONS

- The word "nummular" comes from the same root as "numismatic," meaning "coin-shaped," and indeed, the round lesions of nummular eczema often have the shape of coins.
- Lesions are usually itchy eczematous patches and plaques that often occur in clusters (Fig. 13.35).
- Lesions are seen mainly on the legs; less commonly, they may also arise on the arms, trunk, and buttocks. The patches or plaques sometimes clear centrally and resemble tinea corporis ("ringworm").

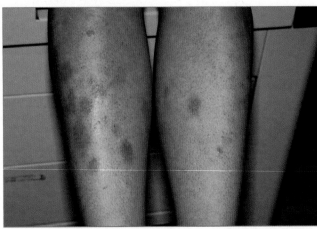

13.35 *Nummular eczema.* These are characteristic erythematous coin-shaped lesions.

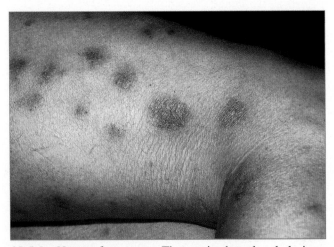

13.36 *Nummular eczema.* These coin-shaped scaly lesions demonstrate postinflammatory hyperpigmentation.

- Healing or resolving lesions often display postinflammatory hyperpigmentation, particularly in dark-skinned patients (Fig. 13.36).

DIAGNOSIS

- The diagnosis of nummular eczema is based on the clinical appearance and, if necessary, negative results of a KOH examination.

 DIFFERENTIAL DIAGNOSIS

Tinea Corporis
- *KOH examination or fungal culture is positive.*

Psoriasis
- *Psoriatic lesions frequently occur on elbows and knees and may have a whitish or micaceous scale.*

Lichen Simplex Chronicus (see above)
- *Focal lichenified plaques are noted.*
- *Often, a there is a history of atopy.*

 MANAGEMENT

- Nummular eczema can often be controlled by an intermediate-strength (class 3 or 4) topical corticosteroid, such as **triamcinolone acetonide cream 0.1%**, applied sparingly two to three times daily.
- If necessary, for thicker lesions, a high-potency (class 1) topical corticosteroid, such as **clobetasol cream 0.05%** once or twice daily, may be used.
- Recalcitrant cases may require occlusion—provided by a polyethylene wrap (Saran wrap) or **Cordran tape** (flurandrenolide)—or intralesional corticosteroid injections.

 HELPFUL HINT

- Nummular eczema is frequently misdiagnosed as tinea corporis ("ringworm") and is often inappropriately treated with topical antifungals.

BASICS

- *Asteatotic eczema* and *nonspecific eczematous dermatitis* are common forms of dermatitis in the elderly that tend to occur in the dry, cold winter months. These eruptions tend to worsen with aging as the skin loses some of its barrier function and lubrication. Both of these conditions are sometimes referred to as "winter itch" and "senile pruritus." (See also Chapter 25.)

CLINICAL MANIFESTATIONS

ASTEATOTIC ECZEMA

- Scaly patches with superficial fissures that resemble a cracked antique China vase (also called *erythema craquelé*) (Figs. 13.37 and 13.38).
- Often manifest in geometric shapes such as squares, rectangles, and rings (Fig. 13.39).
- May be somewhat pruritic.
- Lesions are located most commonly on the shins, arms, hands, and trunk.

NONSPECIFIC ECZEMATOUS DERMATITIS IN THE ELDERLY

- Ill-defined, dry (xerotic), itchy, scaly, erythematous lesions.
- Itching with or without specific lesions tends to occur on the arms, legs, and upper back.

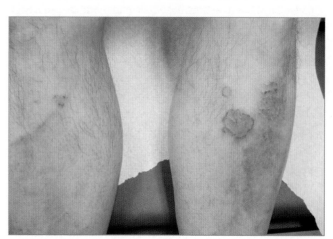

13.38   *Asteatotic eczema.* Typical pretibial lesions.

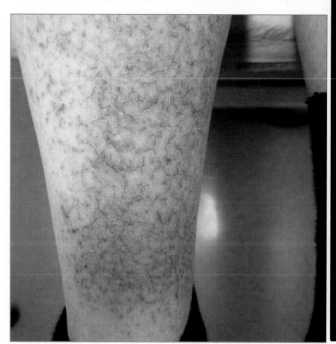

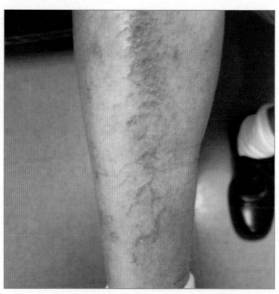

13.37   *Asteatotic eczema (erythema craquelé).* The scaly patches on this patient's shin demonstrate superficial fissures that resemble a cracked antique China vase or a dry riverbed.

13.39   *Asteatotic eczema.* Note the scaly patches that have square and ring-like geometric shapes.

 HELPFUL HINT

- Dry skin and persistent pruritus—especially in elderly patients—may be evidence of a systemic condition (e.g., hypothyroidism or hypoparathyroidism), renal disease, or an underlying malignancy.

MANAGEMENT

- Asteatotic eczema is managed readily by the use of shorter and/or less frequent showers or baths, using only tepid (not hot) water and the application of moisturizers regularly. Preparations such as **Sarna** (an anti-itch lotion) or **Eucerin Calming Creme**, moisturize the skin while soothing the itch.
- For both of these conditions, low- to medium-potency (class 4 to 6) **topical corticosteroids** are valuable. In severe cases, more potent topical corticosteroids (class 1 to 3) may be applied for brief periods when necessary.

Seborrheic Dermatitis ("Seborrheic Eczema")

BASICS

- Seborrheic dermatitis (SD) is a very common, chronic inflammatory dermatitis. Its characteristic distribution involves areas that have the greatest concentration of sebaceous glands: the scalp, face, presternal region, interscapular area, umbilicus, and body folds (intertriginous areas).
- Many people experience some degree of dandruff—a whitish scaling of the scalp that is sometimes itchy and is fairly easily controlled with antidandruff shampoos. When dandruff is accompanied by erythema, a sign of inflammation, it is referred to as seborrheic dermatitis.
- SD is seen more commonly in males and often begins after puberty. There appears to be a hereditary predisposition to its development. When it appears in patients who are infected with the human immunodeficiency virus, SD may serve as an early marker of the acquired immunodeficiency syndrome. SD is also seen commonly in patients with Parkinson disease and in patients taking phenothiazines.
- SD has many features in common with chronic eczema and psoriasis. Typical lesions of SD often appear in patients with psoriasis, and its histologic features resemble those of both eczema and psoriasis. In fact, some dermatologists do not consider SD as a distinct nosologic entity but instead assign it to various forms of eczema or psoriasis. In the latter case, the term "seborrhiasis" has been used. In the United Kingdom, seborrheic dermatitis is referred to as "seborrhoeic eczema."

PATHOGENESIS

- Described as idiopathic, some evidence indicates that an abnormal response to *Malassezia*, a small yeast, may play a part in its pathogenesis because SD occasionally responds to antifungal medications. *Malassezia* organisms are probably not the cause but are a cofactor in SD. Because SD occurs only where the sebaceous glands are found, sebum has also been thought to play a role, although no link has yet been shown.

CLINICAL MANIFESTATIONS

- The eruption of SD tends to be bilaterally symmetric in its distribution and the appearance of the lesions varies depending on their location.
- On the **face**, lesions are red, with or without an overlying whitish scale, or they may appear as orange-yellow greasy patches and are typically found on the forehead, eyebrows, eyelashes, cheeks, beard, and nasolabial folds (Figs. 13.40 to 13.42). Lesions can also occur behind the ears and in the external ear canal.
- On the **scalp**, SD may range from a mild erythema and scaling to thick, armor-like plaques that are indistinguishable from psoriasis ("sebopsoriasis"). There may be itching and scale with resultant dandruff that, embarrassingly, often falls on clothing.

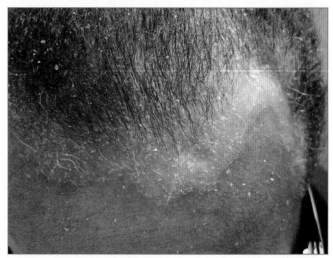

13.40 *Seborrheic dermatitis.* Scale and erythema are evident along the frontal hairline.

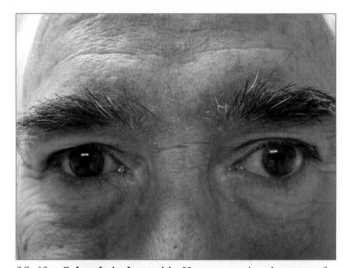

13.41 *Seborrheic dermatitis.* Here we see involvement of the eyebrows, and eyelashes (*seborrheic blepharitis*).

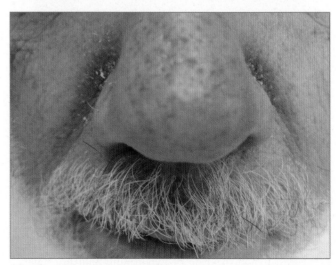

13.42 *Seborrheic dermatitis.* This patient has involvement nasolabial creases.

- When lesions occur in **body folds**, they often consist of sharply defined, bright red plaques that may develop fissures. Typically involved areas include inframammary, axillae, inguinal creases, intragluteal crease, perianal area, and umbilicus. In these areas, SD is often clinically indistinguishable from tinea, intertrigo, and inverse psoriasis.
- **Presternal lesions** are scaly or papular (Fig. 13.43).
- Facial SD usually flares in the winter and improves in the summer. However, some patients report provocation of the condition *after* sun exposure.
- When fissures develop in the body folds and umbilicus, symptoms may consist of burning, itching, oozing, and pain.

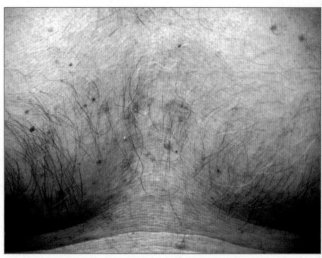

13.43 *Seborrheic dermatitis.* This patient has scaly presternal lesions.

 ## DIFFERENTIAL DIAGNOSIS

The differential diagnosis of SD varies depending on the age, sex, and ethnic background of the patient and, particularly, on the location of lesions.

Scalp and External Ears
Psoriasis
- *Psoriatic lesions will be present elsewhere on the body and there may be a family history of psoriasis.*

Eczematous Dermatitis
- *Eczematous lesions present elsewhere on body. There may be an atopic history and onset is often before adolescence.*

Tinea Capitis
- *Usually seen in the preteen age group. Prevalent in African-American toddlers. Positive KOH and/or fungal culture.*

Face
Erythrotelangiectatic Rosacea, Rosacea
- *Prominent telangiectasias and acne-like papules and pustules will be present.*

"Butterfly" Rash of Systemic Lupus Erythematosus
- *Positive antinuclear antibody test and other features of lupus erythematosus.*

Tinea Faciale (see Chapter 18)
- *Lesions are generally annular (ring-shaped) with an asymmetric distribution.*
- *KOH examination or positive fungal culture.*

Body Folds and Genitalia
Inverse Psoriasis (see Chapter 14)
- *Often indistinguishable from SD. Negative KOH examination or no growth on fungal culture.*

Tinea Cruris (see Chapter 18)
- *Arcuate shape with advancing "active border" with central clearing. Positive KOH examination or fungal culture.*

Cutaneous Candidiasis (see Chapter 18)
- *"Beefy" red plaques and "satellite pustules."*
- *Positive KOH examination and fungal culture will be positive for Candida species. Most common in patients with diabetes mellitus.*

Eczematous Dermatitis (such as Atopic Dermatitis)
- *Eczematous lesions will be present elsewhere on the body. Sometimes there will be an atopic history and marked pruritus.*

MANAGEMENT

- Treatment options for SD vary according to the location of lesions (Table 13.1). In general, antiseborrheic shampoos and topical antifungals alone, or in combination with topical corticosteroids, are the treatments of choice.

Scalp

- **Mild scalp** SD generally responds to the numerous commercially available antidandruff, or antiseborrheic shampoos that contain one or more of the following ingredients: **zinc pyrithione, coal tar, salicylic acid, selenium sulfide**, and/or **sulfur**, as well as the antifungals **ciclopirox** and **ketoconazole**.
- The shampoos should be left on for at least 5 minutes after lathering.
- For itching and inflammation, a medium-strength (class 3 or 4) topical steroid in a gel or solution, such as

betamethasone dipropionate lotion 0.05% (**Diprosone**) or betamethasone valerate foam 0.1% (**Luxiq foam**), may be used, but only if necessary.

- **Severe scalp** SD ("sebopsoriasis") is often managed in the same manner as psoriasis of the scalp (see also Chapter 14).
- Potent (class 2) agents such as fluocinonide gel 0.05% (**Lidex**) and superpotent (class 1) clobetasol propionate gel/lotion/foam 0.05% (**Temovate, Olux foam, Clobex lotion**) may be used. These topical steroids should be preceded by keratolytic agents to remove thick scale, allowing the medications to penetrate the scalp.
- Scale may be removed with a keratolytic preparation (e.g., **Salex, Keralyt**) as often as necessary, usually two to three times per week initially and then whenever scale builds up again.

Table 13.1 SEBORRHEIC DERMATITIS FORMULARY

SCALP

Shampoos/gels/lotions

Antiseborrheics and antifungals	Pyrithione zinc (**Head & Shoulders**[a]) shampoo
	Coal tar (**Neutrogena T-Gel**[a]) shampoo
	Coal tar (**Zetar**[a]) shampoo and emulsion
	1% Selenium sulfide (**Selsun Blue**[a]) shampoo
	13.5% Selenium sulfide shampoo
	1% Ketoconazole shampoo (**Nizoral**[a])
	2% Ketoconazole shampoo (**Nizoral**), ciclopirox 0.77% (**Loprox** shampoo and gel)
Keratolytics *(agents that remove excessive scale)*	Sulfur 2%, salicylic acid 2% (**Sebulex**[a]) shampoo, or **Salex** cream or lotion, or **Keralyt** gel
	Salicylic acid (**Neutrogena T-Sal**[a]) shampoo

Topical corticosteroids

Medium potency (class 4)	Betamethasone valerate 0.1% (**Valisone**)
	Desoximetasone (**Topicort**) gel 0.05%, betamethasone valerate 0.12% (Luxiq foam)
	Fluocinolone acetonide (**Capex**[b]) shampoo 0.01%
High potency (class 2)	Fluocinonide (**Lidex**) gel or solution 0.05%
Superpotency (class 1)	Clobetasol gel, foam, or solution 0.05%

FACE AND INTERTRIGINOUS AREAS

Topical steroids

Very low potency (class 7)	Hydrocortisone cream or ointment 0.5% to 1%[a]
Low potency (class 6)	Desonide (**DesOwen**) cream, lotion 0.05%, desonide 0.05% foam (**Verdeso**)
Medium potency (classes 4 and 5)	Hydrocortisone valerate (**Westcort**) cream, or ointment 0.2%

Topical creams/ointments

Antifungals	Ketoconazole (**Nizoral**[a]) 1% cream, ciclopirox 0.77% (**Loprox** gel), and econazole cream 1% (**Spectazole**)[a]
	Ketoconazole (**Nizoral**) 2% cream, gel (**Xolegel**), foam (**Extina**)
Immunomodulators	Tacrolimus 0.03% and 0.1% (**Protopic**) ointment
	Pimecrolimus 1% (**Elidel**) cream

[a]Available over the counter.
[b]This shampoo contains a midpotent topical steroid. It is used two or three times weekly, as needed.

continued on page 229

MANAGEMENT *Continued*

Intertriginous/Body Fold Areas
- Body folds and genital areas are similarly treated with low-potency (class 4 to 7) topical steroids.

Face
- SD of the face responds quickly to topical steroids, but this treatment requires long-term maintenance and vigilance to avoid atrophy, telangiectasias, and rosacea-like side effects.

- To minimize these unwanted reactions, low-potency topical steroids may be alternated with antifungals such as ketoconazole cream 2% (**Nizoral**), ketoconazole gel 2% (**Xolegel**), or ciclopirox 0.77% gel (**Loprox**). Topical immunomodulators (**Protopic or Elidel**) can be used for long-term maintenance.

 SEE PATIENT HANDOUT IN THE COMPANION eBOOK EDITION.

 HELPFUL HINT

- SD of the scalp is not seen in preadolescent children; therefore, excessive use of antidandruff shampoos should *not* be encouraged in this age group. The child may actually have atopic dermatitis, which is only aggravated by frequent shampooing.

Stasis Dermatitis

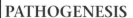

ECZEMA AND RELATED DISORDERS

BASICS

- Stasis dermatitis (also called gravitational dermatitis) is an eczematous eruption that is most commonly located on the lower legs. It often appears on the medial ankles of middle-aged and elderly patients and rarely occurs before the fifth decade of life.
- The dermatitis is a consequence of chronic venous insufficiency ("leaky valves") and is seen more often in women, particularly those with a genetic predisposition to develop varicosities. It may also occur in patients with acquired venous insufficiency resulting from surgery (e.g., vein stripping or harvesting of saphenous veins for coronary bypass), deep venous thrombosis, or other types of traumatic injury to the lower venous system.
- Contributing factors include: congestive heart failure (CHF), dependent leg edema, long-standing hypertension.

PATHOGENESIS

- Traditionally, the following sequence of events has been proposed to explain the pathogenesis of stasis dermatitis:

> Varicose veins ➤ Reversed flow through incompetent valves ➤ Diminished venous return ➤ Increased hydrostatic capillary pressure ➤ Pooling of blood ➤ Peripheral edema and relative tissue hypoxia

- **Fibrin Cuff Theory:** The preceding schema may account for the pruritic, eczematous eruption seen in the early stages of stasis dermatitis; however, the *fibrin cuff theory* offers an explanation at the tissue level.
  - Instead of pooled, stagnant blood with low oxygen tension, leg veins in patients with venous insufficiency have *increased* flow rates and *high* oxygen tension.
  - An increase in permeability of dermal capillaries enables macromolecules, such as fibrinogen, to leak out into the pericapillary tissue, polymerization of fibrinogen to fibrin results in the formation of a fibrin cuff around the capillaries serving as a barrier to oxygen diffusion, with resulting tissue hypoxia and cell damage.

CLINICAL MANIFESTATIONS

- Lesions begin with erythema and scale (eczematous dermatitis) (Fig. 13.44). Later, the rash may become subacute, with more intense erythema, edema, erosions, crusts, and secondary bacterial infection (Fig. 13.45). The eruption may progressively lead to the chronic stages of stasis dermatitis, in which pigmentary changes occur. After an initial redness (from extravasated red blood cells), affected areas turn reddish brown (from iron that is left from the breakdown of red blood cells).

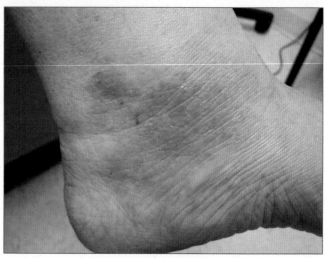

13.44 *Acute stasis dermatitis.* This patient has the earliest signs of stasis dermatitis—pruritus, erythema, scale (eczematous dermatitis), and slight distal hyperpigmentation.

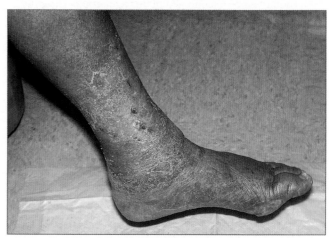

13.45 *Subacute stasis dermatitis.* This patient shows symptoms of more advanced stasis dermatitis—increased scale, peripheral edema, erosions, crusts, and secondary bacterial infection ("impetiginization").

- Postinflammatory hyperpigmentation (from melanin) also occurs. These colors may overlie a cyanotic background.
- Ultimately, the skin may thicken and become less supple and nonpitting, and feel permanently bound down and fibrotic ("woody") on palpation.
- Most cases of stasis dermatitis and associated ulcers are located on the medial malleolus. When symptoms progress, lesions may spread to the foot or calf.

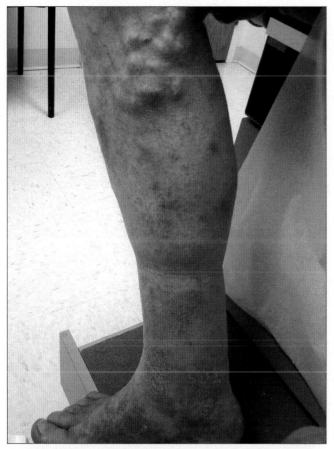

13.46 Chronic stasis dermatitis. Large venous varicosities are evident proximal to the eruption, and superficial varicosities surround the affected area.

- Large venous varicosities may be evident proximal to the eruption, and superficial varicosities may surround the affected area (Fig. 13.46).
- Pruritus may occur.
- Ankle edema that is initially pitting later may become fibrotic and nonpitting.

CLINICAL SEQUELAE AND POSSIBLE COMPLICATIONS

- **Venous stasis ulcers** may develop and be exacerbated by trauma (e.g., scratching), bacterial infection, or improper care of the eczematous rash (Fig.13.47). Ulcers are often asymptomatic but can sometimes produce a dull pain.
- Induration may progress to **lipodermatosclerosis**, which has a classic "inverted water bottle" appearance (Fig. 13.48).

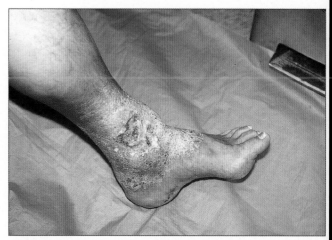

13.47 Stasis dermatitis with venous stasis ulcer. Note the eczematous eruption, the nonpitting edema ("woody" fibrosis) surrounding the ulcer (lipodermatosclerosis).

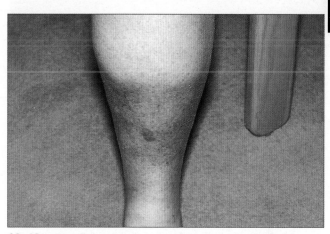

13.48 Lipodermatosclerosis. Chronic stasis dermatitis has produced a circumferential fibrosis that gives the leg an "inverted water bottle" appearance.

- **Autoeczematization** is a widespread, often explosive, acute eczematous eruption that is presumably triggered by secondary bacterial infection (impetiginization) of eczema, with resultant circulating immune complexes released from the site of the stasis dermatitis lesions (Figs. 13.49A,B). It is hypothesized that patients become sensitized to their own tissue breakdown products.

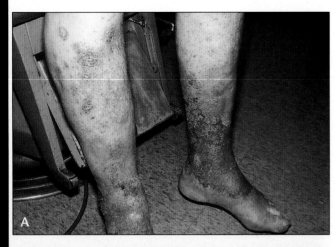

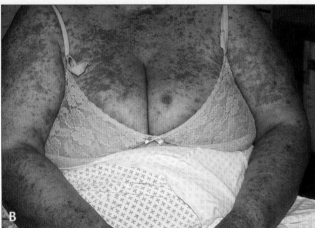

13.49 **A and B:** *Stasis dermatitis with secondary impetiginization. Autoeczematization.* The same patient as in the previous figure. This patient's ankle eruption has become widespread as a result of impetiginization of the eczema on her legs.

DIAGNOSIS

- The diagnosis is made clinically. Skin biopsy of stasis dermatitis is rarely indicated.
- Blood tests may be helpful only rule out underlying hypercoagulable states.
- Radiologic/Doppler studies can rule out deep venous thrombosis or severe valve damage due to past thrombosis.

DIFFERENTIAL DIAGNOSIS

Cellulitis

- *Stasis dermatitis is often confused with cellulitis (Fig. 13.50), an acute infection of skin and soft tissues characterized by localized pain, swelling, tenderness, erythema, and warmth. It is usually caused by gram-positive aerobic cocci (e.g., S. aureus, S. pyogenes).*

Other Diagnoses

- *When ulcerations are present, the differential diagnosis includes vasculitis, arterial disease, cryoglobulinemia, the antiphospholipid syndrome, protein C deficiency, skin cancer, or pyoderma gangrenosum.*

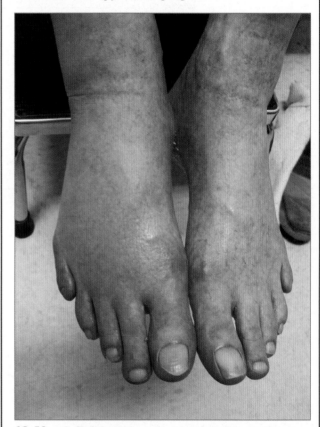

13.50 *Cellulitis.* This patient has painful, swollen tender, edematous involvement of his dorsal foot.

MANAGEMENT

Stasis Dermatitis (Eczematous Eruption): Topical Therapy

- Weeping, oozing, or infected areas may be soaked with Burow Solution followed by a midpotency topical corticosteroid such as triamcinolone 0.1% ointment for reducing inflammation and itching during acute flares.
- Higher-potency topical corticosteroids should be avoided.
- Patients should be advised not to apply topical corticosteroid preparations directly to stasis ulcers because the preparations may interfere with healing.
- Plain white petrolatum (**Vaseline Petroleum Jelly**) is a cheap occlusive moisturizer/dressing with no potential to develop ACD.
- Possible OTC sensitizers such as lanolin, neomycin, and bacitracin should be avoided since patients with stasis dermatitis tend to develop ACD quite readily.

Edema

- Significant edema may be managed with **compressive therapy**, the mainstay of therapy for venous insufficiency.
- **Support hose**, elastic bandages, and specialized compression stockings (**Jobst, Sigvaris**) that deliver a controlled gradient of pressure should be strongly recommended.
  The patient's peripheral arterial circulation should be assessed clinically or with a Doppler or Duplex study before compression is recommended. Adding compression to a leg with compromised arterial circulation could increase claudication and put the patient at risk for ischemic damage.

Infection

- Obvious superficial infections (impetiginization) should be treated with systemic antibiotics that have activity against *S. aureus* and *Streptococcus* species (e.g., **dicloxacillin, cephalexin**, or a **fluoroquinolone**).
- A widespread autoeczematized eruption may require treatment with both systemic corticosteroids and oral antibiotics.

Stasis Ulcers

- Stasis ulcers are managed by treating the underlying eczematous dermatitis, controlling weight, preventing infection, and using compression. Venous ulcers at times produce a dull pain that is relieved by elevation.

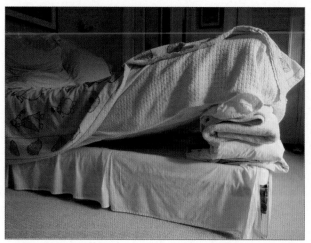

13.51 *Leg elevation.* Here the foot of the bed is propped up by sheets and towels.

- An **Unna boot** is best applied in the morning, before edema progresses. After application, the bandage hardens into a cast. The boot decreases edema, promotes healing, and serves as a barrier from trauma (e.g., scratching). It should be changed weekly until the ulcer heals.
- If feasible, corrective surgery, such as skin grafts or vascular procedures, may be another option.

Prevention of Diminished Venous Return

- Venous return can be increased by engaging in regular exercise, such as brisk walking and bicycling. Such activities augment the "calf pump."
- Furthermore, the affected leg(s) should be elevated above the level of the heart or at least to hip level if the patient has congestive heart failure (sitting with the leg elevated by a stool is inadequate).
- At night, leg elevation can be accomplished by propping up the foot end of the bed with 2 to 3 in of plywood or a bedding fabric such as sheets (Fig. 13.51).
- Compression of lower extremities with support hose or elastic bandages can help venous return and should be strongly encouraged as an essential component of prevention.

 SEE PATIENT HANDOUT "Burow Solution" IN THE COMPANION eBOOK EDITION.

HELPFUL HINTS

- Stasis dermatitis is often misdiagnosed as cellulitis.
- Infected stasis dermatitis should be considered in patients who develop a sudden onset of extensive generalized eczematous dermatitis (autoeczematization).
- Compression is the mainstay of therapy for venous insufficiency and venous leg ulceration.

HELPFUL HINTS

- Sitting in a reclining chair while reading or watching television can help promote venous return.
- Compression stockings should be applied early in the morning, before the patient rises from bed, to facilitate application when leg edema is at its lowest point.
- Walking regularly at a brisk pace should be encouraged.
- Physical therapy should be considered.
- Smoking and long periods of standing or sitting should be discouraged.

14 Psoriasis

OVERVIEW

Psoriasis (psoriasis vulgaris) is a chronic, immune-mediated skin condition characterized by red, scaly plaques that are most often found on the scalp, elbows, and knees. Psoriasis is common and is estimated to affect 1% to 2% of the world's population. The condition is more common in whites and occurs less often in West Africans, African-Americans, Native Americans, and Asiatic people. Psoriasis is found equally in men and women and most frequently begins in the second or third decade of life, but can first present in infants or in the elderly.

Psoriasis is considered a systemic disease. Psoriatic arthritis will develop in 5% to 30% of patients and it may precede or follow the onset of skin lesions. Patients with moderate to severe psoriasis are at increased risk for developing diabetes, obesity, hyperlipidemia, and hypertension (components of the *metabolic syndrome*). There also appears to be an increased risk of myocardial infarction, particularly in those who have severe psoriasis at an early age.

The primary concern to most patients is the unsightly appearance of lesions whose visibility and persistence often lead to feelings of self-consciousness and uncleanliness. The emotional toll and the personal struggle to come to terms with psoriasis are expressed in an autobiographic short story, "At War with my Skin," by John Updike, who had severe psoriasis. After undergoing an operation for a broken leg, Updike reflected, "I chiefly remember amid my pain and helplessness being pleased that my shins, at that time, were clear and I would not offend the surgeon."

The clinical features, differential diagnoses, and management of the most common clinical forms of psoriasis will be discussed in this chapter:

IN THIS CHAPTER...

➤ **PSORIASIS**

➤ **LOCALIZED PLAQUE PSORIASIS**

➤ **GENERALIZED PLAQUE PSORIASIS**

➤ **ACUTE GUTTATE PSORIASIS**

➤ **SCALP PSORIASIS**

➤ **INVERSE PSORIASIS**

➤ **PSORIASIS OF THE PALMS AND SOLES**

➤ **PSORIATIC NAILS**

➤ **PSORIATIC ARTHRITIS**

➤ **EXFOLIATIVE DERMATITIS SECONDARY TO PSORIASIS**

Psoriasis

BASICS

- Psoriasis is a common, chronic skin condition that has a characteristic clinical and histologic appearance but has various clinical presentations.
- The severity of psoriasis ranges from asymptomatic thin localized plaques that are an incidental finding, to widespread generalized plaques, or rarely, complete erythroderma.
- Severity is often assessed as total-body surface area (BSA) affected, where the patient's palm = 1% BSA. Greater than 10% BSA is considered to be severe. However, less BSA involvement can still be severe if it significantly interferes with an individual's quality of life.

PATHOPHYSIOLOGY

- Psoriasis is an immunologically based inflammatory skin condition that results in abnormal epidermal differentiation and hyperproliferation.
- Psoriasis is more likely to occur in persons with a genetic predisposition. Genome-wide association studies have revealed that psoriasis susceptibility genes have immune-related functions.
- The inflammatory process is triggered and maintained by Th1, Th17, and Th22 cells and their corresponding proinflammatory cytokines, tumor necrosis factor alpha (TNF-α) and IFN-γ, IL-17, and IL-22.

- The lesions of psoriasis result from a dramatic activation of keratinocyte proliferation.
- Such a "turned-on" epidermis, with a rapid accumulation of cells and no time for shedding, accounts for the characteristic lesion of psoriasis: a red papule or plaque (Fig. 14.1) with a buildup white or silvery (micaceous) scale (Figs. 14.2 and 14.3). Uncommonly, lesions may be very thick and verrucous (Fig. 14.4).
- Ongoing vigorous investigation into the pathogenesis of psoriasis has resulted in a multitude of new, effective, targeted therapies.

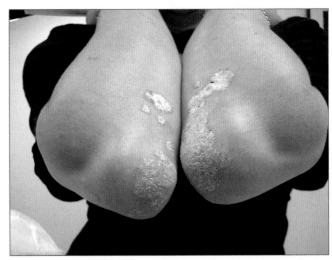

14.2 *Psoriasis.* Here the scale is thicker (hyperkeratotic) and white in color.

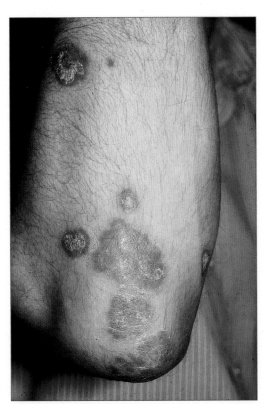

14.1 *Psoriasis.* This is a typical location for the characteristic lesions of psoriasis. Note the well-circumscribed erythematous plaques surmounted by a fine scale.

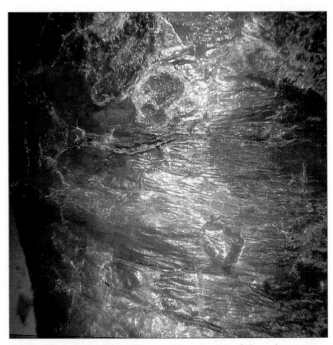

14.3 *Psoriasis.* The silvery, shiny luster of the micaceous scale is obvious.

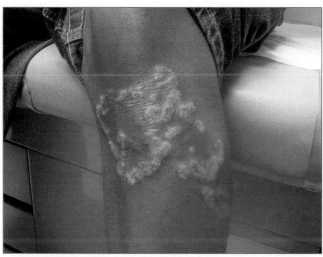

14.4 *Psoriasis.* Thick, wart-like (verrucous) lesions are present in this patient.

HISTOPATHOLOGY

The histopathologic findings demonstrate the altered cell kinetics of psoriasis (Illus. 14.1):

- Marked thickening (acanthosis) as well as thinning of the epidermis with resultant elongation of the rete ridges
- Parakeratosis (nuclei retained in the stratum corneum)
- Dermal inflammation (lymphocytes and monocytes) and dilation of dermal blood vessels
- Epidermal inflammation (polymorphonuclear cells) in the stratum corneum that may form the so-called *microabscesses of Munro*

CLINICAL MANIFESTATIONS

- Lesions of psoriasis are characterized by well-demarcated pink papules or plaques with silvery-white scale.
- Lesions tend to be remarkably symmetric in their distribution.

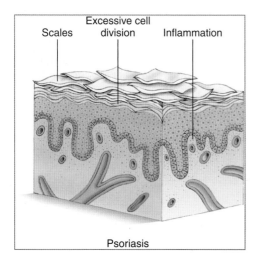

I14.1 *Psoriasis.* Scales, excessive cell division, and inflammation.

- Psoriasis can present in various clinical forms (listed below) and a single patient may have multiple forms throughout his or her lifetime.
  - Localized plaque psoriasis
  - Generalized plaque psoriasis
  - Guttate psoriasis
  - Inverse psoriasis
  - Palmoplantar psoriasis
  - Scalp psoriasis
  - Nail psoriasis

CLINICAL SEQUELAE

PRURITUS

- Psoriasis is generally asymptomatic, but can occasionally become quite pruritic and uncomfortable, particularly during acute flare-ups or when lesions involve the scalp or intertriginous areas.

THE KÖBNER REACTION (ISOMORPHIC RESPONSE)

- Those who have psoriasis commonly recognize the "Köbner" phenomenon in which new lesions appear at sites of injury or trauma to the skin.
- Noxious stimuli, such as scratching and rubbing, or sunburn can elicit a Köbner reaction (Figs. 14.5 and 14.6).

FISSURING OF PLAQUES

- Painful fissures may occur when lesions are present over joints, in the axillae or intragluteal fold, or on the palms and soles.

PSYCHOSOCIAL PROBLEMS

- Psoriasis can be a major blow to one's ego. It may stifle social activities and sexual spontaneity, interfere with job

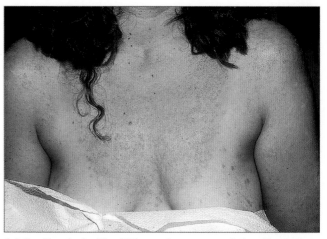

14.5 *Psoriasis.* The Köbner phenomenon is localized to the area of sunburn. The region that had been covered by the patient's bathing suit is almost free of lesions.

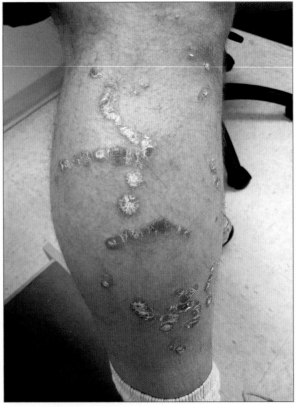

14.6 *Psoriasis.* The Köbner phenomenon is evident in this patient, who developed psoriatic plaques at the sites where he repeatedly scratched and picked the lesions.

opportunities and inhibit participation in sports, and the use of beaches and public swimming pools.

- The psychological ramifications of psoriasis—anxiety, social isolation, alcoholism, depression, suicidal ideation— are possible associations and outcomes of this essentially benign skin disease.

TRIGGERS

Factors that may adversely influence psoriasis include the following:

- **Stress.** Stress has been implicated as a trigger in acute exacerbations and in progression of psoriasis.
- **Alcohol.** Alcohol overindulgence has been reputed to exacerbate psoriasis.

- **Drugs.** Antimalarials, beta-blockers, angiotensin-converting enzyme inhibitors, certain nonsteroidal anti-inflammatory drugs (e.g., indomethacin), systemic interferon, and lithium carbonate have been reported to worsen psoriasis; however, pre-existing psoriasis is not necessarily a contraindication to their use. Both systemic, and less likely, potent topical steroids have been known, albeit rarely, to trigger a severe, acute, potentially fatal pustular psoriasis (*pustular psoriasis of von Zumbusch*) that tends to occur after withdrawal of the medication.
- **Physical trauma.** Surgery, thermal and chemical burns, and infections potentially exacerbate psoriasis. For example, an increase in psoriasis activity has been observed in patients who are, or become, infected with the human immunodeficiency virus (HIV).
- **Sunlight.** A small minority of patients find that their psoriasis is worsened by strong sunlight, probably via the Köbner reaction (see Figs. 14.5 and 14.6), whereas the vast majority of patients generally discover that sunlight is beneficial.

COURSE

- Psoriasis is an erratic condition with an unpredictable, waxing-and-waning course. It has no known cure; however, there are numerous methods to keep it under control.
- Many patients tend to improve during the summer and worsen during the colder periods of the year. This fluctuation is presumably the result of the positive influence of sunlight.

DIAGNOSIS

- The diagnosis of psoriasis is usually made on clinical grounds.
- A skin biopsy or fungal studies may be performed to rule in or rule out other possible diagnoses.

 DIFFERENTIAL DIAGNOSIS

The differential diagnosis of psoriasis is extensive and varies, depending on the type and location of lesions. The differential diagnoses to consider for each clinical type of psoriasis will be discussed separately in this chapter.

 SEE PATIENT HANDOUT, "Psoriasis" IN THE COMPANION eBOOK EDITION.

BASICS

- In its mildest manifestation, psoriasis is an incidental finding and consists of mildly erythematous, scaly patches on the elbows or knees.
- Localized plaque psoriasis, the most common presentation of psoriasis, may remain limited and localized (Figs. 14.7 and 14.8), or it may become unstable and widespread (Figs. 14.9 and 14.10).

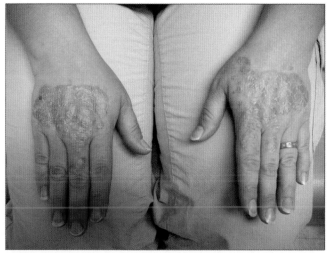

14.7 *Psoriasis.* Note the symmetrical distribution of the plaques.

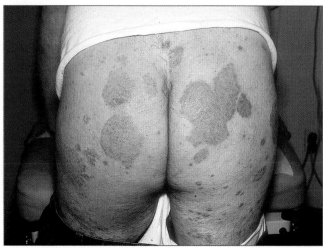

14.8 *Psoriasis.* Larger plaques.

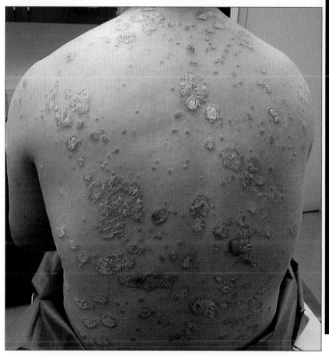

14.9 *Psoriasis.* Widespread plaques are evident on this patient.

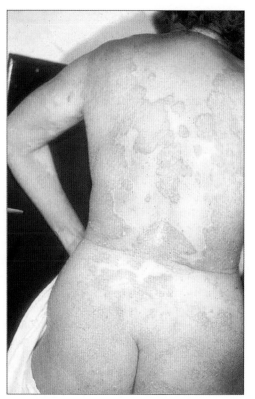

14.10 *Psoriasis.* Extensive, large plaques covering 70% of body surface area.

CLINICAL MANIFESTATIONS

- Lesions can be present anywhere but are most commonly located on:
  - Large extensor joints (elbows, knees, and knuckles).
  - Scalp.
  - Anogenital region (perineal and perianal areas, glans penis).
  - Palms and soles.

DIAGNOSIS

- When the typical well-demarcated whitish or silvery plaques are present in the usual locations, the diagnosis of psoriasis is quite evident.
- Other helpful diagnostic features include a family history of psoriasis and nail findings (see later in this chapter and also Chapter 22).
- If necessary, other tests, such as a skin biopsy and fungal examinations, can be performed to rule out other conditions (e.g., Bowen disease, tinea corporis, parapsoriasis, and mycosis fungoides).

DIFFERENTIAL DIAGNOSIS

Eczematous Dermatitis (Lichen Simplex Chronicus and Atopic Dermatitis)
- *Poorly defined plaques; they blend gradually into normal surrounding skin.*
- *Lichenification is often present.*
- *Usually pruritic.*
- *Possible atopic diathesis.*

Nummular Eczema
- *Coin-shaped eczematous lesions.*
- *Scale is not micaceous or silvery white.*

Tinea Corporis
- *Lesions typically are annular ("ringlike")—round and clear in the center.*
- *The potassium hydroxide (KOH) examination or fungal culture is positive.*

Bowen Disease (Squamous Cell Carcinoma in situ)
- *A solitary lesion may resemble a typical psoriatic plaque.*
- *Unresponsive to topical steroids.*

MANAGEMENT

General Principles
- Therapy is aimed at decreasing size and thickness of plaques, reducing pruritus, alleviating arthritic symptoms, if present, and improving emotional well-being.
- Treatment regimens must be individualized according to age, sex, occupation, personal motivation, and other health-related conditions.
- Treatment selection is determined by some of the following factors:
  - **Age of patient.** Oral agents that are used to treat severe psoriasis are less likely to be used in children. Very young children, particularly infants, are not able to cooperate with phototherapy treatment (described later in this chapter).
  - **Type of psoriasis.**
  - Site and **extent of involvement.**
  - Health care provider's **experience in managing psoriasis.** Mild to moderate psoriasis can be managed by primary care clinicians and moderate to severe psoriasis is best treated by dermatologists.
  - **Availability** of facilities, such as a phototherapy unit.
  - **Concurrent psychosocial problems**, such as anxiety, depression, alcoholism, and substance abuse.

Available Treatment Modalities
- Three basic treatment modalities are available for the overall management of psoriasis: (a) topical agents, (b) phototherapy, and (c) systemic agents, including biologic therapies. Treatments may be used alone or in combination.
- **Topical therapy** is the first-line approach in the treatment of plaque psoriasis (Tables 14.1 and 14.2) and options include topical corticosteroids, coal tar, anthralin, calcipotriene, calcitriol, and tazarotene. No single agent is ideal, and many are often used concurrently in a combined approach. Auxiliary agents such as scale-removing keratolytics can also be used.
- **Phototherapy** and **systemic therapy** are sometimes initiated after topical treatments have been tried unsuccessfully (see also the later section titled "Generalized Plaque Psoriasis").

Specific Treatment of Localized Plaque Psoriasis
Topical Corticosteroids
- A potent topical steroid for a limited period, followed by a less potent topical steroid for maintenance, is the most common method for treating localized plaque psoriasis.

continued on page 241

MANAGEMENT *Continued*

Table 14.1 SHORT LIST OF TOPICAL STEROIDS USED TO TREAT PSORIASIS

POTENCY	GENERIC NAME	BRAND NAME
Class I	Clobetasol propionate 0.05% cream/gel/ointment/foam, lotion	**Temovate, Olux foam, Clobex lotion, Cormax scalp solution**
	Flurandrenolide	**Cordran tape** small or large roll
Class II	Desoximetasone 0.05% gel	**Topicort**
	Fluocinonide 0.05% cream/ointment/solution/gel	**Lidex**
Class III	Fluticasone 0.005% ointment	**Cutivate**
Class IV	Triamcinolone acetonide 0.1% ointment	**Kenalog**
	Betamethasone valerate 0.12%	**Luxiq foam**
	Hydrocortisone valerate 0.2% cream	**Westcort**
Class V	Triamcinolone acetonide 0.1% cream	**Kenalog**
	Desonide 0.05% ointment	**DesOwen**
Class VI	Desonide 0.05% cream, foam	**DesOwen, Verdeso foam**
Class VII	Hydrocortisone cream/ointment/lotion 0.5%, 1.0%[a]	**Hytone, Cortizone-10**, and many other brands

Most preparations are available in tubes of 15, 30, or 60 g. Lotions and solutions are available in bottles of 20 to 60 mL.
[a]Available over-the-counter.

Table 14.2 OTHER TOPICAL AGENTS USED TO TREAT PSORIASIS

GENERIC NAME	BRAND NAME
Keratolytic agents	
Salicylic acid 6%	**Keralyt gel (1 oz)**
Salicylic acid 6%	**Salex cream (400 g) and lotion (441 mL)**
Topical vitamin D_3 analogs	
Calcipotriene 0.005%	**Dovonex cream, scalp solution**
	Sorilux foam
Calcitriol 0.003%	**Vectical ointment**
Tacalcitol	**Curatoderm, Bonalfa**
Topical vitamin D_3–topical steroid combination	**Taclonex ointment or scalp solution**
Topical retinoids	
Tazarotene 0.05%, 0.1%	**Tazorac cream, gel**
Anthralin preparations	
Anthralin 0.1%, 0.25%, 0.5%	**Drithocreme, Dritho-Scalp**
Anthralin 1% cream	**Psoriatec**
Tar preparations	**Estar[a], PsoriGel[a], Balnetar[a], Doak tar oil[a]**

Note: All tar preparations (except liquor carbonis detergents) must be used in grease- or oil-based vehicles. Tar is commonly available in shampoos and is often combined with salicylic acid. Liquor carbonis detergens is an alcohol-extracted tar.
[a]Available over-the-counter.

Advantage
- Rapid onset in decreasing erythema, inflammation, and itching.

Disadvantages
- Drug tolerance (tachyphylaxis) is not uncommon.
- Potential side effects of topical steroids (see "Introduction: Topical Therapy").
- Expensive and time consuming, especially when extensive areas are involved.

Occlusion of Topical Corticosteroids
- Occlusion can improve penetration and lead to a quicker therapeutic effect.
    - **At-home occlusion.** Generally, a medium- or high-potency agent is applied and then covered with polyethylene wrap (e.g., **Saran Wrap**) for several hours or overnight, if tolerated. For scalp psoriasis, a plastic shower cap can be used during treatment with topical steroids.
    - **Prescription occlusion. Cordran tape** (see "Introduction: Topical Therapy") is similarly effective.

Advantage
- Increases the absorption, and thus potency, of topical steroids.

Disadvantage
- Increases risk of topical steroid side effects.

continued on page 242

⚙ **MANAGEMENT** *Continued*

Intralesional Steroids

- Intralesional **triamcinolone acetonide** (**Kenalog,** 2.5 to 5 mg/mL) is delivered intradermally with a 30-gauge needle. May be repeated at 4- to 6-week intervals.

Advantages
- Useful with limited number of lesions.
- Acts rapidly.
- Provides longer periods of remission.

Disadvantages
- Painful.
- Possible local skin atrophy and telangiectasias.
- Requires office visits to administer injections.

Topical Vitamin D₃ Derivatives

- Calcipotriene (**Dovonex***) and calcitriol (**Vectical**) are synthetic forms of vitamin D_3, which slow down the rate of skin cell growth.
- **Calcipotriene** is available as a cream, ointment, and scalp solution in 0.005% strength.
- Calcitriol, available as **Vectical ointment**, is similar to calcipotriene, but is less irritating.

*Dovonex in the United States, "Daivonex" outside of North America, and "Psorcutan" in Germany

- **Taclonex** is a combination product containing calcipotriene and betamethasone ointment 0.064% and is available as **Taclonex ointment** and **Taclonex scalp solution**.

Advantages
- Calcipotriene and calcitriol do not have side effect of thinning of the skin.
- May enhance the effectiveness of ultraviolet (UV) treatments.
- A combined maintenance treatment of daily Dovonex or Vectical plus weekend use of a superpotent topical steroid (called *pulse therapy*) may prolong remissions and reduce tachyphylaxis (drug tolerance).
- Taclonex combines a vitamin D_3 analog, which reduces scale and slows skin cell growth with the anti-inflammatory effects of a steroid and is applied once daily.

Disadvantages
- Not as effective at decreasing inflammation and works more slowly than topical steroids.

- Most common minor side effects are skin irritation, stinging, or burning.
- Taclonex is expensive and because it contains a potent topical steroid, it should not be applied to the face, axillae, groin, or other skin folds.

Topical Tar Preparations

- Before the advent of topical steroids, tar preparations such as crude tar oil were the mainstay of therapy for psoriasis and most inflammatory dermatoses. Currently, they are used much less often.
- Coal tar can be compounded in concentrations of 0.5% to 10% into a variety of vehicles including an ointment or a shampoo. Agents such as liquor carbonis detergens, **Balnetar, Doak Tar oil, Estar gel, PsoriGel,** and **T/Derm tar oil** are the traditional tar preparations. **Neutrogena T-Gel therapeutic shampoo** contains 0.5% coal tar.

Topical Anthralin

- Anthralin is a coal tar derivative without the side effects of crude coal tar.
- Anthralin is used for shorter periods than coal tar, sometimes several minutes at a time; this is referred to as short-contact anthralin therapy (SCAT).
- Major drawbacks are the possible occurrence of skin irritation and a reversible brownish-purple staining of the skin.

Innovative Management Strategies

Rotational Therapy

- An innovative approach consists of cycling or rotating different treatment modalities. This strategy presumably decreases cumulative side effects and drug tolerance; and it often allows for lower dosages and shorter durations of therapy for each agent.
- For example, a superpotent (class 1) topical steroid, such as **clobetasol**, may be applied for 2 weeks, discontinued for 1 or 2 weeks, and then restarted. Alternatively, clobetasol may be used on weekends only, and **Dovonex cream** or **Vectical ointment** may be used during the week.

BASICS

- Generalized psoriasis occurs when psoriatic plaques are present in a more widespread fashion.
- Psoriasis can flare very quickly and unexpectedly to cover 20% to 80% of the body.

CLINICAL MANIFESTATIONS

- Well-demarcated, variably sized thick pink to red plaques with silvery-white micaceous scale in a generalized distribution.
- Extent can range from only a few lesions on elbows, knees, and trunk to numerous large plaques that cover extensive areas of the body.

 DIFFERENTIAL DIAGNOSIS

Eczematous Dermatitis (Lichen Simplex Chronicus and Atopic Dermatitis)
- *Poorly defined plaques; they blend gradually into normal surrounding skin.*
- *Lichenification is often present.*
- *Usually pruritic.*
- *Often have atopic diathesis.*

Nummular Eczema
- *Coin-shaped eczematous lesions.*
- *Scale is not micaceous or silvery white.*

Tinea Corporis
- *Lesions typically are annular ("ringlike")—round and clear in the center.*
- *The KOH examination or fungal culture is positive.*

Mycosis Fungoides (Cutaneous T-cell Lymphoma)
- *"Smudgy" patches and plaques or tumors usually seen on buttocks and trunk.*
- *Often pruritic.*

Pityriasis Rubra Pilaris
- *Reddish-orange lesions.*
- *"Islands of sparing".*

 MANAGEMENT—GENERALIZED PLAQUE PSORIASIS

General Principles
- When quantifying disease severity, it is important to consider both the extent of body surface involvement as well as impact on a patient's quality of life. Even mild disease can warrant systemic therapy if it is causing significant disruption in daily life and/or employment.
- Treatment should aim to clear psoriatic plaques and improve quality of life.
- Choice of systemic treatment should be individualized and take into account the patient's medical history, current medications, as well as extent of psoriasis and comorbidities such as psoriatic arthritis.

Topical Therapy
- For extensive psoriasis, topical therapy alone becomes less effective, more expensive, time consuming, and labor intensive, but is often continued alongside phototherapy or systemic therapy.

Phototherapy
- The observation that most cases of psoriasis improve with sunlight has led to the development of various methods to deliver UV light artificially.

- UV treatment is used for extensive and widespread moderate to severe plaque psoriasis that is not responding to topical treatment and is often combined with topical treatments.
- Phototherapy works by reducing epidermal hyperproliferation, reducing angiogenesis, and acting as an immunosuppressor.
- The two forms of UV light that are used clinically are **UVB** and **UVA**.

Broadband UVB
- Broadband UVB therapy uses light with wavelengths of 290 to 320 nm (visible light range—400 to 700 nm).
- UVB is one of the safest and most effective treatments for psoriasis.

Narrowband UVB
- Narrowband UVB is now more widely used. It uses a fluorescent bulb with a narrow emission spectrum that peaks at 311 nm (UVB spectrum, 290 to 320 nm).
- The selective and relatively longer wavelength is more effective, clears psoriasis faster, produces longer remissions than broadband UVB, and has less risk of burning than broadband UVB.

continued on page 244

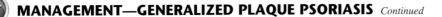
- There is no evidence of increased risk of skin cancer from UVB treatment for psoriasis.
- Narrowband UVB is an alternative to treatment with oral psoralen plus topical UVA (PUVA; see section on UVA treatment below) and is safer over the long term.

Excimer Laser UVB
- This laser device delivers high-dose light at 308 nm via a hand piece with a spot size that is less than 2 cm^2 and is best used for localized plaques.
- A single excimer treatment can induce a moderately long remission.

UVA
- UVA irradiation uses light with wavelengths of 320 to 400 nm.
- PUVA is the administration of UVA with psoralen, a photosensitizing agent. The combination results in enhanced phototoxicity and is more effective than either component alone.
- The most commonly used psoralen is 8-MOP (methoxsalen) which can be administered orally or topically.
- PUVA interferes with DNA synthesis, decreases cellular proliferation, and induces apoptosis of cutaneous lymphocytes, leading to localized immunosuppression.
- Studies have indicated a link between PUVA therapy and the development of squamous cell and basal cell carcinomas and possibly malignant melanoma.
- Adverse effects of PUVA therapy include nausea (from oral psoralens), pruritus, and a burning sensation.

Advantages
- Regular UVB phototherapy has been shown to induce disease remission in more than 80% of patients.
- Unlike biologics and oral immunosuppressants, phototherapy lacks serious systemic risks such as nephrotoxicity, hepatotoxicity, tuberculosis, and malignancy.
- Both PUVA and UVB can be combined with oral retinoid derivatives (RePUVA or ReUVB) to decrease the cumulative dose of UV radiation to the skin as well as the dosage of retinoid.
- Home UVB units are available that allow for treatments in patient's own home.
- The excimer laser is selectively directed toward lesional skin sparing the surrounding normal skin from unnecessary radiation exposure.

Disadvantages
- Time commitment required for treatments is 2 to 3 visits per week.
- May be expensive (if not covered by patient's insurance).

- Lack of accessibility of phototherapy equipment.
- An increased sensitivity to sunlight or sunburn may result, and there is a theoretical risk of cataracts if the eyes are left unprotected.
- An average of 30 treatments is often required to reach maximum improvement of psoriatic lesions.

Systemic Therapy
- Methotrexate, cyclosporine, oral retinoids, and biologic therapies all have helped induce and maintain remission in severe, widespread plaque psoriasis.
- Methotrexate, as well as several of the biologics (see below), is effective in treating both skin disease and joint disease.
- Biologics are often introduced while the other systemic agents are gradually tapered.

Methotrexate
- This antimetabolite inhibits dihydrofolate reductase, thereby hindering DNA synthesis and cell reproduction in tissues with high rates of turnover, such as those found in psoriatic plaques.
- Methotrexate should be considered as an option for the treatment of extensive chronic plaque psoriasis, erythrodermic psoriasis, or generalized pustular psoriasis.
- Dosage:
  - Methotrexate is often prescribed in a low-dose weekly regimen.
  - The initial adult dose is 2.5 to 7.5 mg/week PO (can also be given IM) as a single dose or administered in three doses over a 24-hour period, then titrated to a dose between 12.5 and 25 mg/week, depending on the clinical response.
  - **Folic acid** 1 mg daily should be taken on nontreatment days.

Advantages
- It may be administered orally, intramuscularly, or subcutaneously.
- It is effective for psoriatic arthritis.
- Inexpensive.

Disadvantages
- The main limitation of methotrexate is hepatotoxicity. Therefore, complete blood counts and regular liver and renal function blood tests should be monitored.
- Liver enzymes cannot be relied on to monitor liver health, because bridging necrosis can occur in the presence of normal liver enzymes.
- Liver biopsy is recommended after a total of 1.5 g of methotrexate has been taken.
- Many drug interactions are possible.

continued on page 245

- Long-term, continuous use may lead to myelosuppression and carcinogenicity.
- Side effects include nausea, abdominal pain, headache, and fatigue and more serious problems such as hepatoxicity and leukopenia.

Acitretin (Soriatane)

- Acitretin is in the retinoid family of drugs related to vitamin A. The mechanism of action in treating psoriasis is unknown, but it has antiproliferative, anti-inflammatory, and antikeratinizing effects. In addition, it inhibits neutrophil chemotaxis.
- Dosage:
  - Initial: 25 mg/day PO; then increase, if necessary
  - Maintenance: 20 to 50 mg/day PO

Advantages

- Acitretin should be considered as an option for the treatment of palmoplantar, erythrodermic, or generalized pustular psoriasis.
- Useful in combination with UVA (RePUVA) and UVB (ReUVB).

Disadvantages

- Acitretin is a teratogen and is *absolutely contraindicated* in pregnancy, in women who are likely to become pregnant, intend to become pregnant within 3 years following cessation of treatment, or in those women who cannot use reliable contraception while undergoing treatment (and for at least 3 years after discontinuation).
- Side effects are numerous:
  - Cheilitis is seen in virtually all patients taking retinoids.
  - May cause lipid elevation, muscle weakness, myalgias, hair loss, nail changes, skin fragility, premature epiphyseal closure or calcification, and ossification of ligaments and tendons.

Cyclosporine (Neoral, Sandimmune)

- Cyclosporine suppresses humoral immunity and, to a greater extent, cell-mediated immune reactions, such as delayed hypersensitivity. The drug acts by inhibiting production of interleukin 2, the cytokine responsible for inducing T-cell proliferation.
- Dosage: Initially, 2 to 5 mg/kg/day PO in divided doses.
- After control is achieved, maintenance therapy is continued at lower doses.

Advantages

- Remission is quite rapid for severe, uncontrollable psoriasis.
- Cyclosporine is mostly useful for short-term treatment of significant exacerbations.

Disadvantages

- Lesions tend to recur within days to weeks after treatment is stopped, and "rebounds" with worse symptoms than before treatment are often seen with abrupt cessation.
- Many drug interactions are possible.
- Evaluation of renal and liver functions should be performed often by measuring blood urea nitrogen, serum creatinine, serum bilirubin, and liver enzyme levels. Frequent monitoring of blood pressure is also necessary.
- Risk of myelosuppression, infection, and lymphoma may be increased.
- Side effects include nephrotoxicity and hypertension. Hirsutism and gingival hypertrophy have also been reported.

Apremilast (Otezla)

- Apremilast is a phosphodiesterase-4 inhibitor and is the latest oral medication approved for the treatment of moderate to severe plaque psoriasis or active psoriatic arthritis in patients >18 years old.
- Dosage: Start at 10 mg and increase by 10 mg daily to 30 mg twice daily.
- Lower dosage for those with renal impairment.
- Common side effects are:
  - Diarrhea
  - Nausea
  - Upper respiratory infection
  - Headache
- Other considerations and possible contraindications: pregnancy and breastfeeding, depression and suicidal ideation, and kidney problems.

Rotational Therapy

- The use of a rotational approach with the various systemic agents can minimize the toxic effects of long-term treatment with any one of them.
- For example, the use of agents such as UVB, PUVA, methotrexate, acitretin, or cyclosporine, which are reserved for more severe, extensive psoriasis, can also be rotated; for example, one treatment may be used from 12 to 24 months and then another modality may be used. On clearing of the condition, treatment is stopped until the psoriasis recurs, at which point another agent is used.

The Biologics

- Biologics are designed to target a specific cell surface receptor, cytokine or other molecule thought to be important in the pathogenesis of a particular disease.
- In recent years, there has been a surge in the development of targeted biologic therapeutic agents for psoriasis and psoriatic arthritis.

continued on page 246

- Currently, the biologic strategies to treat psoriasis are TNF-α blockade, and antagonism of IL-12/23 and IL-17.

Etanercept (Enbrel)

- Etanercept is a fusion protein containing the human TNF receptor bound to the Fc portion of human immunoglobulin G (IgG) antibody.
- It acts by binding and inhibiting TNF from binding to any cell surface receptors.
- Etanercept is administered as a subcutaneous (SC) injection and recommended dosing is 50 mg twice weekly for 3 months, then 50 mg weekly.

Advantages

- Can be given at home.
- Prevents bony erosions in patients with psoriatic arthritis.
- Leads to tuberculosis activation less commonly than infliximab and adalimumab (see below).
- Effective for generalized plaque psoriasis, recalcitrant palmoplantar psoriasis, and generalized pustular psoriasis as well as psoriatic arthritis.

Disadvantages

- May result in injection site reactions.
- Some patients will require twice-weekly dosing indefinitely to maintain satisfactory control.
- Side effects (common to all TNF-α inhibitors): increased risk of serious infections including TB and hepatitis B reactivation, exacerbation or new-onset congestive heart failure or multiple sclerosis, rarely drug-induced lupus, lymphoma has also been reported.

Adalimumab (Humira)

- Adalimumab is a recombinant fully humanized IgG1 monoclonal antibody that binds to TNF-α and can lyse cells that express TNF-α on their surface.
- Indicated for psoriasis and psoriatic arthritis.
- Adalimumab is administered as a SC injection and dosed as an 80-mg injection on day 1 followed by 40 mg SC on day 8, then 40 mg SC every other week.

Advantages

- Rapid acting/long acting

Disadvantages

- May result in injection site reactions.
- Rare reports of lupus-like symptoms and multiple sclerosis.
- Increased risk of infections including TB and hepatitis B reactivation.
- Heart failure (new or worsening).

Infliximab (Remicade)

- Infliximab is a chimeric monoclonal antibody that targets TNF-α and inhibits its activity.
- Infliximab is indicated for the treatment of psoriatic arthritis and plaque-type psoriasis. It is administered via IV infusion at specialized infusion centers.
- For psoriasis, dose is weight based and typically a dose of 5 mg/kg is given at 0, 2, and 6 weeks and then every 8 weeks thereafter.

Advantages

- Of the 3 TNF-α antagonists approved for psoriasis, infliximab has the fastest onset of action.

Disadvantages

- Administered intravenously at an infusion center.
- Requires monitoring of platelet counts and liver function studies.
- Common infusion reactions: pruritus, hives, nausea, and headache.
- Contraindications: congestive heart failure class III or IV.
- Same side effects listed under etanercept.

Ustekinumab (Stelara)

- Ustekinumab is a human monoclonal antibody that binds to IL-12 and IL-23 and neutralizes their activity.
- Ustekinumab is administered by SC injection in a physician's office at weeks 0, 4, and then every 12 weeks.
- Dosing for ustekinumab is weight based: >220 lb (100 kg) receive 90 mg, <220 lb receive 45 mg on week 0, a second injection 4 weeks later, and then one injection every 12 weeks.

Advantages

- Less frequent dosing schedule (every 12 weeks).
- Can be given to multiple sclerosis patients.

Disadvantages

- Stelara is only moderately effective for psoriatic arthritis.

Secukinumab (Cosentyx)

- Secukinumab is a fully human anti-interleukin-17A monoclonal antibody.
- Indicated for moderate-to-severe plaque psoriasis in patients who are candidates for systemic therapy.
- Administered by SC injection; 300 mg at weeks 0, 1, 2, 3, and 4; then, 300 mg monthly beginning at week 8.
- For some patients, a dose of 150 mg may be acceptable.

BASICS

- Acute guttate psoriasis refers to the sudden onset of multiple guttate (teardrop-shaped) psoriatic lesions (Fig. 14.11). It is often the initial presentation of psoriasis in children and young adults.
- Guttate psoriasis is often preceded by a group A beta-hemolytic streptococcal infection (positive throat culture or serologic evidence of antistreptolysin O).

CLINICAL MANIFESTATIONS

- The typical presentation is an acute onset of numerous small (1 to 10 mm), guttate (teardrop-shaped), thin salmon-pink papules or plaques with a fine scale.
- Lesions arise primarily on the trunk and proximal extremities, but may become generalized.
- Some cases are self-limited; however recurrences may appear with repeated streptococcal pharyngitis.
- Less often, guttate psoriasis may be chronic in nature without preceding streptococcal infection.

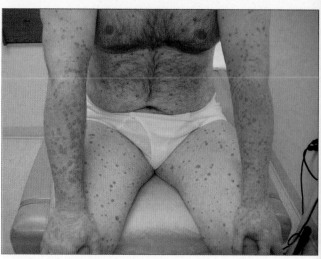

14.11 *Psoriasis (acute guttate).* This patient had a recent group A beta-hemolytic streptococcal pharyngitis.

DIFFERENTIAL DIAGNOSIS

See discussion earlier in this chapter.

Pityriasis Rosea
- *Self-limiting.*
- *Characteristic distribution.*

Drug Eruption
- *Most often morbilliform without scale.*

Parapsoriasis
- *The term "parapsoriasis" derives from the fact that the condition clinically resembles psoriasis, but in fact is a completely different entity.*

Secondary Syphilis
- *Positive serology for syphilis.*

MANAGEMENT

- Appropriate antibiotic therapy, such as penicillin, amoxicillin, or erythromycin if there is clinical, bacteriologic, or serologic evidence of infection with group A beta-hemolytic streptococcus.
- For limited plaques, a high-potency (class 1, 2, or 3) topical steroid can be used.
- For more numerous plaques, UVB phototherapy or natural sunlight exposure two to three times per week can induce remission.

Scalp Psoriasis

BASICS

- Psoriasis may involve the scalp alone, or the scalp may be affected along with other areas of the body.
- When psoriasis involves only the scalp and retroauricular areas, it is sometimes referred to as "sebopsoriasis" or "seborrhiasis."

CLINICAL MANIFESTATIONS

- Plaques on the scalp are often thick and well demarcated with overlying whitish scale (Fig. 14.12), but can range from a flaky dandruff to thick, extensive, armor-like plaques.
- Lesions are frequently hidden by hair or noted behind the ears.
- Plaques often extend beyond the hairline and become more obvious when the hair is held back or when the retroauricular area is examined (Fig. 14.13).
- Pruritus leads to scratching which may exacerbate the condition (Köbner reaction).
- Often, the external ears and ear canals are involved (Fig. 14.14).
- Plaques may be recalcitrant to treatment because hair blocks UV light as well as the application of topical psoriatic medications.

DIFFERENTIAL DIAGNOSIS

Seborrheic Dermatitis
- *Patient may have facial seborrheic dermatitis.*
- *May be indistinguishable from psoriasis of scalp.*

Atopic/Eczematous Dermatitis
- *Atopic history in patient or family.*
- *Eczema elsewhere on body.*
- *Also may be indistinguishable from psoriasis of scalp.*

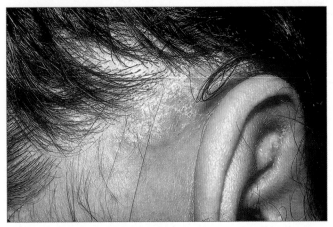

14.12 *Psoriasis of the scalp.* This discrete, scaly plaque is one of many this patient has on her scalp.

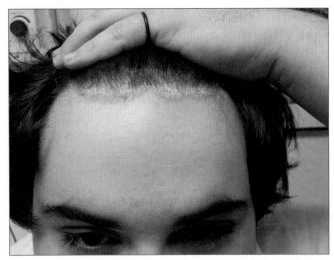

14.13 *Psoriasis of the scalp.* This is a common location on the frontal hairline.

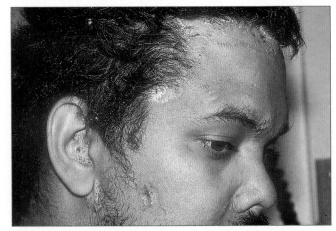

14.14 *Psoriasis of the scalp and ears.* Note the crusted excoriations behind this patient's ear and along his hairline.

MANAGEMENT

Mild Cases

- With minimal scaling and thin plaques (similar to what is seen in seborrheic dermatitis (see Chapter 13), mild scalp psoriasis can often be managed with antidandruff shampoos and a low to midpotency (class 4, 5, or 6) topical steroid, used as needed for itching.
- Over-the-counter options include shampoos that contain tar (**Zetar, T-Gel**), selenium sulfide (**Selsun Blue, Head & Shoulders**), or salicylic acid (**T-Sal**).

Topical Steroids

- A mid- or low-potency topical steroid can be used to clear thin plaques. Examples include **Fluocinolone 0.01% solution or shampoo (Capex**—class 4), and **Verdeso foam** (desonide 0.05%—class 6).
- Gel, foam, or solution preparations reach the scalp more readily than do ointments or creams.

Topical Vitamin D Derivatives

- **Dovonex Scalp Solution** or **Sorilux Foam** (both are calcipotriene 0.005%) can be applied twice daily for treatment, or once daily for maintenance or rotational therapy.

Severe Cases

- In patients with thick scales and plaques, the scale must be removed before the plaques can be treated effectively.

Scale removal is accomplished by applying either **Keralyt gel** or **Salex cream** or **lotion (salicylic acid)** one to three times per week. This regimen may be sufficient to keep scale under control, thus allowing penetration of a topical steroid.

- After the scale is removed, a medium- to high-potency (class 2, 3, or 4) topical steroid is used. For example, **fluocinonide 0.05% solution** or **gel (Lidex)** or **desoximetasone (Topicort) gel** may be applied once or twice daily as needed; or under shower cap occlusion overnight or for 3 to 4 hours during the day.
- If necessary, a superpotent (class 1) topical steroid such as **clobetasol propionate 0.05% lotion, foam, shampoo,** or **gel** can be used without occlusion. In recalcitrant situations, the superpotent topical steroid can be applied under occlusion once or twice per week.
- **Topical Vitamin D derivatives** may be applied as maintenance or rotational therapy.
- Injections of **intralesional triamcinolone** (3 to 5 mg/mL) in a limited amount (1 to 2 mL or less per treatment) every 4 to 8 weeks are used to target particularly recalcitrant or very itchy areas and may establish longer remissions.

 SEE PATIENT HANDOUT, "Scalp Psoriasis: Scale Removal" IN THE COMPANION eBOOK EDITION.

Inverse Psoriasis

BASICS

- Psoriasis noted in intertriginous areas such as the axillae (Fig. 14.15), inframammary folds (Fig. 14.16), perineal and perianal areas, scrotum, glans penis, and inguinal creases (Figs. 14.17–14.19) is referred to as *inverse psoriasis*.

CLINICAL MANIFESTATIONS

- Typically, lesions are red, glistening, well-demarcated plaques that generally lack scale.
- The absence of scale is seen when two apposing surfaces of skin rub together, such as under the breasts, in the groin, and in the axillae. Such constant rubbing does not allow scale to build up.
- Fissures may occur in these areas.

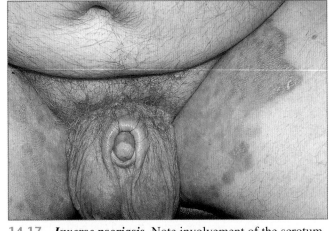

14.17   *Inverse psoriasis.* Note involvement of the scrotum, foreskin, and glans, often misdiagnosed as cutaneous candidiasis or tinea cruris.

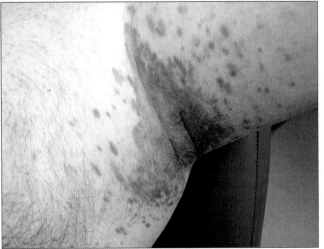

14.15   *Inverse psoriasis.* Axillary involvement is shown here. Both axillary psoriasis and inframammary psoriasis are often misdiagnosed as cutaneous candidiasis.

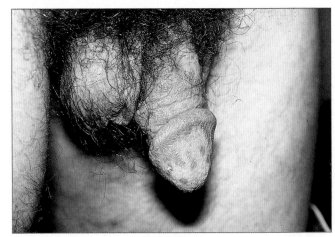

14.18   *Inverse psoriasis.* Typical psoriatic plaques on the penis.

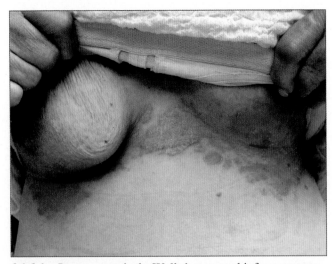

14.16   *Inverse psoriasis.* Well-demarcated inframammary lesions. This is also frequently misdiagnosed as cutaneous candidiasis.

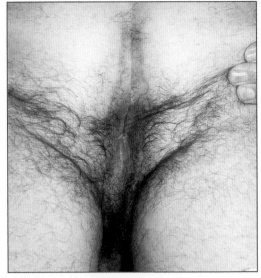

14.19   *Inverse psoriasis.* Intragluteal involvement. Note symmetry of lesion.

DIFFERENTIAL DIAGNOSIS

Irritant Intertrigo
- *Common inflammatory condition of skin folds that occurs when apposing skin surfaces rub against each other, such as seen in diaper dermatitis or irritation by antiperspirants, or shaving products.*

Common features include the following:
- *Induction or aggravation by heat, hyperhidrosis, moisture, maceration, and friction.*
- *Location in the axillae, inguinal, and intragluteal creases; often occurs under pendulous breasts and abdominal folds and as a complication of obesity.*
- *Possible colonization by secondary infection such as Candida albicans, particularly in patients with diabetes.*

Intertriginous Tinea (e.g., Tinea Cruris/Axillaris)
- *Lesions typically have a scalloped, "active border".*
- *Generally spares the scrotum and penis.*
- *Positive KOH examination and fungal culture for dermatophytes.*

Intertriginous Cutaneous Candidiasis
- *Lesions are "beefy red" in color.*
- *Satellite pustules often noted beyond the border of the plaques.*
- *Positive KOH examination for budding yeast.*
- *Positive culture for Candida species.*

Intertriginous Atopic Dermatitis
- *Eczematous lesions may be seen elsewhere on the body.*
- *Patients often have an atopic history.*

Intertriginous Seborrheic Dermatitis
- *May be indistinguishable from inverse psoriasis.*

Other Considerations
- *When lesions are present on the glans penis, **nonspecific balanitis** (more commonly seen in elderly men) and candida balanitis should be considered in the differential diagnosis.*
- ***Pruritus ani** also may be confused with inverse psoriasis.*
- *Secondary overgrowth with Candida species and tinea must also be considered.*

MANAGEMENT

- The lowest-potency, nonfluorinated, topical steroids are used to avoid atrophy and striae.
- To achieve rapid improvement, treatment may be initiated with a higher-potency (class 3 to 5) steroid for several days and then changed to a lower-potency (class 6 or 7) agent.
- **Vectical ointment** may be used alone for treatment, or in rotation with a low-potency topical steroid.
- Tacrolimus (**Protopic**) **ointment** 0.03% or 0.1% can be applied once or twice daily.
- Pimecrolimus (**Elidel**) **cream** 1% may be used once or twice daily.

HELPFUL HINTS

- Intertriginous areas are moist and naturally occluded; therefore, the penetration and efficacy of topical agents are increased in these regions; consequently, topical steroids are more likely to produce striae (linear atrophy) in these locations.
- Inverse psoriasis is commonly misdiagnosed by non-dermatologists as tinea or candidiasis. Consequently, it is often incorrectly treated with topical antifungal agents.

BASICS

- Psoriasis may affect the palms and soles alone or the palms and soles may be affected as part of more extensive psoriasis on the body.
- Psoriasis that manifests on the palms and soles presents a difficult therapeutic challenge.

CLINICAL MANIFESTATIONS

There are two variants:

HYPERKERATOTIC

- Similar to its counterparts elsewhere, this form of psoriasis is characterized by well-demarcated, scaly plaques (Figs. 14.20 and 14.21).

- Hyperkeratotic psoriatic plaques on the palms and soles may present additional problems such as pain, impairment of function, fissuring, bleeding, and social embarrassment.

PUSTULAR

- This rare form of psoriasis is most commonly seen in adults and historically, has had many clinical descriptions and eponyms (i.e., *pustulosis of the palms and soles and palmoplantar pustulosis*).
- Lesions present as small pinpoint pustules admixed with yellow-brown macules and papules or scaly erythematous plaques and tends to be bilaterally symmetric.
- It favors the insteps of the feet, the heels, and the palms, and the thenar and hypothenar eminences of the hands (Figs. 14.22 and 14.23).

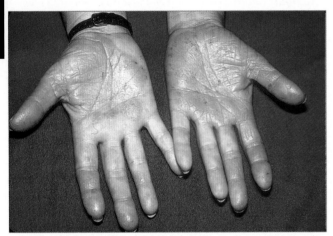

14.20   *Psoriasis.* This patient's palmar lesions are symmetric and well demarcated.

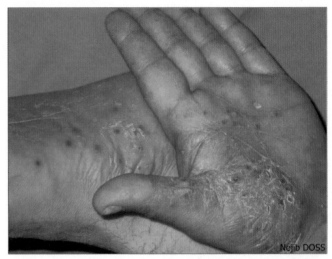

14.22   *Pustular psoriasis/palmoplantar pustulosis.* This is the pustular variant of psoriasis. (Image courtesy of Nejib Doss, MD, Tunisia.)

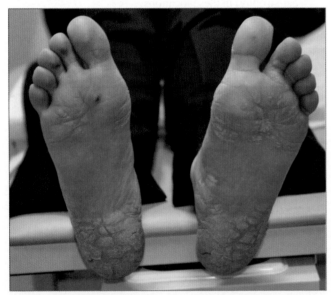

14.21   *Psoriasis of soles.* Note the clear demarcation between involved and uninvolved skin. Similar lesions were present on this patient's palms.

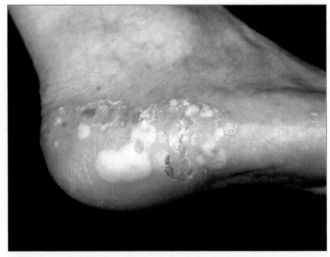

14.23   *Pustular psoriasis /palmoplantar pustulosis.* Large "lakes of pus" overlying an erythematous plaque. (From Craft N, Fox LP. *Visual Dx: Essential Adult Dermatology.* Philadelphia, PA: Lippincott Williams & Wilkins; 2010.)

DIFFERENTIAL DIAGNOSIS

Contact Dermatitis
- *Suspected, particularly if the eruption is on the dorsum of the hands or feet.*
- *The patient has a history of exposure to a suspected contactant.*

Hand Eczema or Dyshidrotic Eczema
- *"Sago-grain" vesicles may be present.*
- *Pruritus.*
- *The patient may have evidence of eczema elsewhere on the body or a personal or family history of atopy.*
- *May be indistinguishable from palmoplantar psoriasis.*

Tinea Manuum and Pedis
- *A "two-feet, one-hand" presentation is noted.*
- *The KOH examination or fungal culture is positive.*

 MANAGEMENT

- Topical treatment is the first line of therapy.
- Because of their thick stratum corneum, the palms and soles present the greatest barrier to cutaneous penetration; consequently, potent topical steroids are used, often under occlusion.

Options include the following:

- Superpotent (class 1) topical steroids, such as **clobetasol propionate**, are first prescribed without occlusion, but occlusion (under vinyl or rubber gloves) may be used if necessary
- Salicylic acid preparations such as **Keralyt gel** or **Salex cream** or **lotion** can be used to remove scale, if necessary
- **Calcipotriene (Dovonex) cream** or **Vectical** ointment

When a patient is not responding to topical therapies, treatment options can include the following:

- **PUVA** (see earlier discussion): **topical PUVA** therapy using a "hand–foot box"
- **Oral retinoids**, such as **Soriatane** (etretinate) are often quite effective
- The excimer laser, if available, is also highly effective
- **RePUVA** (low-dose etretinate combined with PUVA)
- **Oral methotrexate**
- **Oral cyclosporine**
- **Biologics** (see earlier discussion)

BASICS

- Involvement of nails is very common in patients with psoriasis (also discussed in Chapter 22). It is often mistaken for, and treated incorrectly as, a nail fungus infection (onychomycosis).
- Psoriatic nail dystrophy is a chronic, primarily cosmetic condition; however, in some instances, thickened psoriatic toenails can become painful, and psoriatic fingernail deformities may be embarrassing and interfere with function.
- Severe nail dystrophy is more commonly noted in patients who have psoriatic arthritis.

CLINICAL MANIFESTATIONS

- **Pitting** is the most characteristic nail finding in psoriasis. Pitting presents as tiny punctate depressions on the nail plate and arises from psoriasis in the nail matrix (nail root) (Fig. 14.24).
- **Onycholysis** represents a separation of the nail plate from the underlying pink nail bed. The separated portion is white or yellow-white and opaque, in contrast to the pink translucence of the attached portion (Fig. 14.25).
- **"Oil spots"/"**oil drops" are orange-brown colorations that appear under the nail plate. They are the result of psoriasis of the nail bed (Fig. 14.26).
- Thickening, or **subungual hyperkeratosis,** refers to a buildup of scale beneath the nail plate. It resembles onychomycosis, with which it is often confused and may coexist, particularly in toenails (Fig. 14.27).

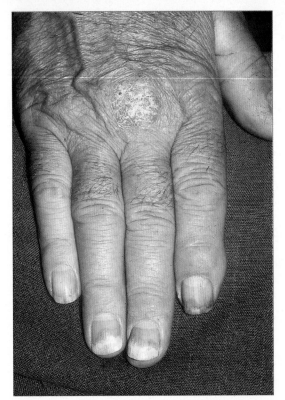

14.25 *Nail psoriasis (onycholysis).* Several nail plates have separated from the underlying pink nail bed. The separated portion is white or yellow-white and opaque, in contrast to the pink translucence of the attached portion. Note the typical psoriatic plaque on this patient's knuckle.

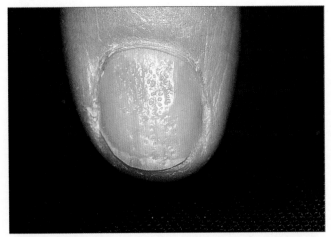

14.24 *Nail psoriasis (pitting).* The result of tiny punctate lesions that arise from the nail matrix, pitting appears on the nail plate as it grows.

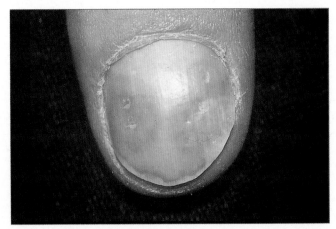

14.26 *Nail psoriasis ("oil spots" or "drops").* Orange-brown coloration appears under the nail plate, presumably the result of psoriasis of the nail bed. Onycholysis is also evident.

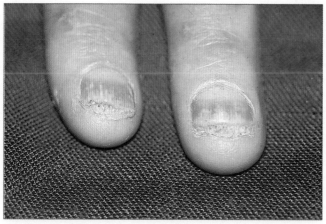

14.27 *Nail psoriasis (subungual hyperkeratosis).* A buildup of scale beneath the nail plate resembles onychomycosis. Also note in this figure "oil spots" and onycholysis. This often confused with *onychomycosis.*

DIFFERENTIAL DIAGNOSIS

Onychomycosis
• *The KOH examination or fungal culture is positive.*

Eczematous Dermatitis with Secondary Nail Dystrophy
• *Lacks subungual hyperkeratosis. Eczema is noted in the area of the proximal nail fold.*

MANAGEMENT

• Treatment is challenging and generally unrewarding, but measures listed below may be helpful.
• Careful trimming and paring of the nails.
• A superpotent (class 1, e.g., **clobetasol** 0.05% ointment) topical steroid applied daily to the proximal nail folds, followed by covering with a plastic wrap or glove. Alternatively **Cordran tape** may be used.
• **Taclonex ointment** (combination of topical steroid and vitamin D analog) applied daily to the proximal nail fold with or without occlusion.
• **Tazarotene (Tazorac) 0.1% gel** applied daily to the proximal nail fold.
• **Intralesional corticosteroids** injected into the nail matrix every 4 to 6 weeks. The proximal and/or lateral nail fold is first sprayed with a refrigerant spray (e.g., **Gebauer's ethyl chloride**) for anesthesia, and 2.5 mg/mL is injected with a 30-gauge needle.
• At present, the systemic medications most commonly used to treat nail psoriasis are **methotrexate, retinoids**, and **cyclosporine**. All have potential serious side effects and toxicities, and, in most cases, the psoriatic nail disease recurs after the systemic therapy is stopped.
• The **biologics** (e.g., **infliximab, adalimumab, etanercept**) are often used for intractable cases, particularly when psoriatic arthritis is also present.

Psoriatic Arthritis

BASICS

- Although psoriatic arthritis can be seen at any age, it most often begins between the ages of 35 and 45 years and occurs in 5% to 30% of patients with psoriasis.
- Psoriatic arthritis can develop before, but most often develops after the skin manifestations of psoriasis.
- Overexpression of TNF-α is thought to play a key role and multiple human leukocyte antigen associations are known.
- An earlier onset of psoriatic arthritis in adulthood can portend a worse prognosis that may include destructive arthropathy.

CLINICAL MANIFESTATIONS

- More likely seen in patients with severe cutaneous disease.
- Concurrent psoriatic nail disease is more frequently noted.
- Peripheral psoriatic arthritis may be indistinguishable from reactive arthritis (formerly known as Reiter syndrome).

There are **five clinical patterns** of psoriatic arthritis:

- **Asymmetric involvement of one or several small- or medium- sized joints**—the most common initial presentation of psoriatic arthritis. Typically, the proximal or distal interphalangeal joints are affected and the result is sometimes referred to as a "sausage finger deformity" (Fig. 14.28).
- **Mild involvement of the distal interphalangeal joints**—the classic form of psoriatic arthritis. Often accompanied by concomitant nail findings.
- **Symmetric joint involvement**—difficult to distinguish from rheumatoid arthritis. However, the serologic test for rheumatoid factor is usually negative.
- **Involvement of the joints in the axial skeleton**—resembles, and may overlap with, ankylosing spondylitis.
- **Mutilating, grossly deforming, arthritis of the hands** (arthritis mutilans) (Fig. 14.29)—the least common presentation of psoriatic arthritis.

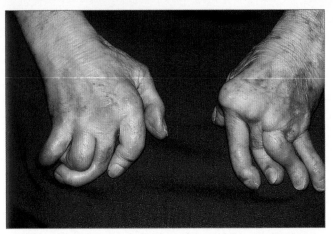

14.29 *Psoriatic arthritis ("arthritis mutilans").* This patient has severe psoriatic arthritis with marked deformities and subluxations of the small bones of the hands. Note also the characteristic onycholysis on the nails.

 MANAGEMENT

- Goals of treatment are to decrease pain and prevent disease progression to maintain joint function.
- Treatment consists of analgesics, primarily non-steroidal anti-inflammatory drugs, and systemic disease-modifying antirheumatic drugs (DMARDs).
- DMARDs that have shown efficacy for psoriatic arthritis include methotrexate, sulfasalazine, cyclosporine, anti–TNF-α agents (e.g., **infliximab, adalimumab, etanercept, golimumab**, and **certolizumab**), and the anti-IL 12/23 antibody **ustekinumab**.

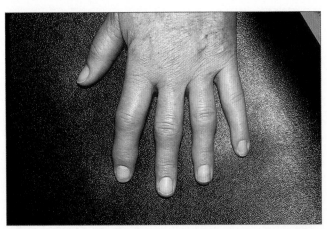

14.28 *Psoriatic arthritis.* "Sausage finger deformity" of the distal interphalangeal joint.

BASICS

- Rarely, a psoriatic patient may develop a sudden or subacute appearance of generalized scaling and/or erythema (Fig. 14.30) which is referred to as *exfoliative dermatitis* (ED) or *erythroderma* (in the United Kingdom) and *l'homme rouge* (in France).
- In adults, psoriasis is the most frequently associated underlying cause of ED.
- ED can be the presenting symptom of psoriasis or a subsequent complication of psoriatic disease (for a more comprehensive discussion of ED, see Chapter 34).
- Other triggers that have been reported to result in ED include the administration of systemic corticosteroids in patients with pre-existing psoriasis, a severe contact dermatitis, high levels of emotional stress, a medical procedure (e.g., surgery), or severe infections.

CLINICAL MANIFESTATIONS

- Appears suddenly or gradually, may become generalized, occasionally accompanied by fever, chills, and lymphadenopathy.
- ED may be a stage in the natural history of severe psoriasis.
- Marked **generalized erythema** is followed by scaling (see Figs. 14.30 and 14.31).
- There is edema and increased warmth of the skin.

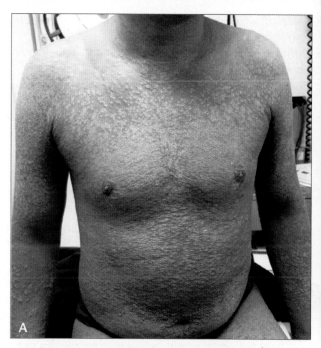

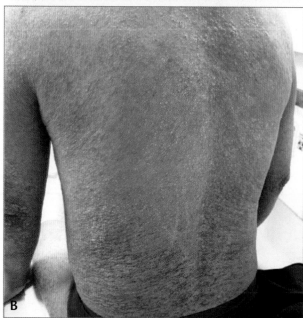

14.31 *Psoriasis–exfoliative dermatitis.* Front (**A**) and back (**B**). This patient has severe, extensive psoriasis with marked scaling.

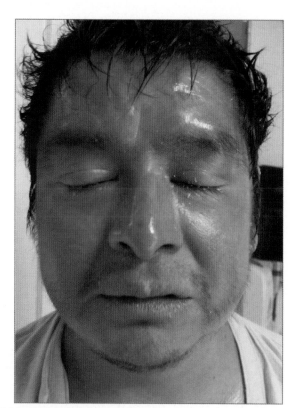

14.30 *Psoriasis.* Erythrodermic variant of exfoliative dermatitis. This patient has generalized erythema (l'homme rouge, "red man syndrome").

- Lymphadenopathy, usually a reactive type (*dermatopathic lymphadenopathy*), is often present.
- Thermoregulatory disturbances are manifested by fever or, more frequently, hypothermia.
- Protein loss secondary to a massive shedding of scale may occur, with resultant hypoalbuminemia.
- Rarely, high-output cardiac failure may develop, particularly in patients with a history of cardiac disease.

DIAGNOSIS

- The diagnosis of ED due to psoriasis is made on a clinical basis.
- Clinical findings, such as the characteristic nail pitting, or a history that suggests psoriasis, may be found.

 DIFFERENTIAL DIAGNOSIS

Toxic Epidermal Necrolysis
- *A potentially fatal condition that involves the skin and mucous membranes.*
- *Marked erythema is quickly followed by sloughing of the skin. This condition is often the result of a severe drug reaction (also discussed in Chapters 25 and 33).*

Stevens–Johnson Syndrome (Erythema Multiforme Major)
- *Widespread skin involvement.*
- *Targetoid lesions.*
- *Significant mucous membrane involvement, constitutional symptoms, and sloughing of the skin.*

 MANAGEMENT

- **Bed rest, cool compresses, lubrication** with emollients, antipruritic therapy with **oral antihistamines**, and **low- to intermediate-strength topical steroids** are used.
- Hospitalization for supportive care in extreme cases.
- Possible precipitating factors (e.g., UV exposure) or drugs that are suspected to provoke ED (e.g., antimalarials) should be avoided.
- **Systemic** and **topical steroids** are helpful, except that they may worsen psoriasis and have been known to precipitate ED or an acute fulminant form of pustular psoriasis, known as *pustular psoriasis of Von Zumbusch*. This worsening of psoriasis tends to occur after steroid withdrawal.
- If conservative therapy fails, **methotrexate, cyclosporine,** and **retinoids** (e.g., acitretin) are additional therapeutic options.
- Phototherapy, photopheresis, and photochemotherapy, as well as biologics such as infliximab (**Remicade**) and adalimumab (**Humira**), are also effective.

Inflammatory Eruptions of Unknown Cause

OVERVIEW

Pityriasis rosea, granuloma annulare, and lichen planus are unique inflammatory conditions of unknown etiology. Each has various clinical presentations and distinctive patterns of distribution. Most often the diagnosis can be readily made clinically based upon the typical signs and symptoms of these rather curious dermatoses.

There are conflicting reports about the association of these entities with certain infectious and metabolic conditions. For example, pityriasis rosea is thought to represent a viral exanthem caused by a herpesvirus. An association has been noted between lichen planus and hepatitis C, chronic active hepatitis, and primary biliary cirrhosis; and widespread granuloma annulare is considered by some investigators to be associated with diabetes mellitus.

Pityriasis Rosea

BASICS

- Pityriasis rosea (PR), which means "fine pink scale," is an acute, benign, self-limiting eruption with a characteristic clinical course.
- PR may occur at any age or season, but it tends to occur in older children and young adults in the spring and fall.

PATHOGENESIS

- The cause is unknown; but a viral etiology with human herpes virus 6 or 7 has been suggested but not confirmed.
- The occasional clustering of cases, seasonal appearances and the fact that a single outbreak tends to elicit lifelong immunity supports an infectious, transmissible origin. Repeat episodes are rare, but have been reported.
- Despite the prevailing opinion that PR is caused by an infectious agent, it does not appear to be contagious; since household contacts and schoolmates usually do not develop the eruption.

CLINICAL MANIFESTATIONS

- The typical course of PR often begins with the larger **herald patch** (Fig. 15.1), a 2- to 5-cm, solitary, pink or skin colored scaly patch or thin plaque that may exhibit central clearing and therefore may mimic, and often be confused with, tinea corporis. The herald patch is followed in several days to 2 weeks by numerous characteristic oval or elliptical, "football-shaped" (Fig. 15.2), erythematous thin papules or plaques with fine scale on the trunk, neck, arms, and legs in an "old-fashioned bathing suit" distribution. Individual lesions often develop a thin, circular, collarette of scale surrounding the perimeter of individual patches or within patches in a characteristic "trail of scale" (Fig. 15.3).
- Lesions in very dark-skinned patients may lack the typical pink color of PR and may appear darker than the surrounding

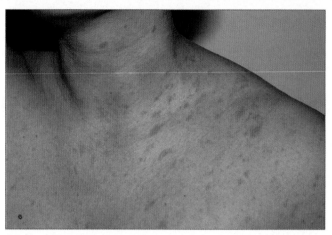

15.2 *Pityriasis rosea.* Note the characteristic elliptical ("football") shape of lesions.

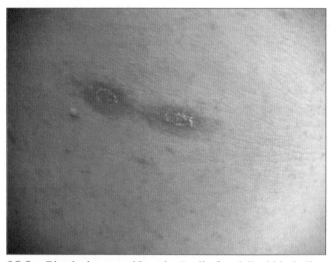

15.3 *Pityriasis rosea.* Note the "trail of scale" within individual lesions. (From Goodheart HP. *Goodheart's Same-Site Differential Diagnosis*. Philadelphia, PA: Lippincott Williams & Wilkins, 2011.)

skin. Itching is usually absent or mild but may be severe in a minority of patients.
- The eruption usually lasts for 6 to 8 weeks but may occasionally persist for several months.
- On resolution, postinflammatory pigmentary changes (hyper or hypopigmentation) may appear, particularly in dark-skinned people (Fig. 15.4).

DISTRIBUTION OF LESIONS

- The herald patch is most commonly observed on the trunk, neck, or extremities. The absence of the herald patch does not necessarily rule out the diagnosis; it may be absent or hidden in an obscure location such as the scalp or groin.
- The long axis of the lesions runs parallel to skin tension lines. This gives a so-called "Christmas tree" pattern on the trunk (Figs. 15.4 and 15.5).

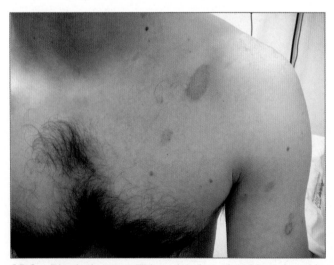

15.1 *Pityriasis rosea.* This patient has a herald patch on his left lateral clavicular area. In addition, typical, smaller, elliptical lesions of PR can be seen.

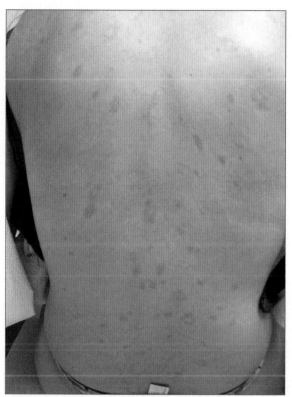

15.4 *Pityriasis rosea.* Here the lesions are less exuberant. The "Christmas tree" pattern is evident. (From Goodheart HP. *Goodheart's Same-Site Differential Diagnosis.* Philadelphia, PA: Lippincott Williams & Wilkins, 2011.)

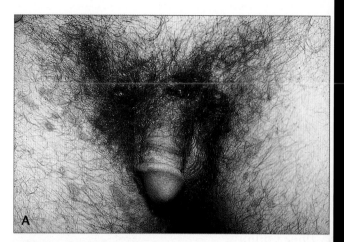

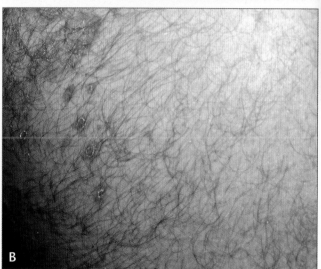

15.6 *Pityriasis rosea.* *Atypical (inguinal or inverse).*
A: The larger herald patch is present in the left inguinal area.
B: *Pityriasis rosea.* *Atypical (inverse).* Close up of **15.6A.** Note "Trail of scale."

DIAGNOSIS

- The diagnosis is made clinically in most cases.
- In general, laboratory tests are not necessary or helpful, with the following exceptions:
  1. Early in disease course when only a herald patch is present, a potassium hydroxide (KOH) examination may be helpful to rule in or rule out tinea corporis; later, in disease when numerous lesions are present a KOH may be used to distinguish tinea versicolor (see Chapter 18) from PR.
  2. If there is a high degree of suspicion for secondary syphilis, a rapid plasma reagin (RPR) or venereal disease research laboratory (VDRL) test should be performed.
  3. A skin biopsy may be performed when the eruption is atypical, the diagnosis is uncertain, or the disease has not resolved after 3 to 4 months.

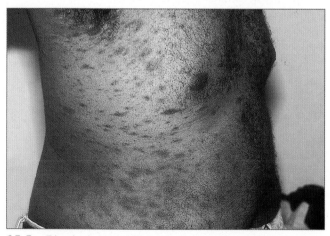

15.5 *Pityriasis rosea.* Note the hyperpigmented lesions in this African-American patient.

CLINICAL VARIANTS

- PR can occur with less typical presentations such as those in which the herald patch is not noted by the patient or clinician.
- In dark-skinned patients, the lesions may be vesicular and uncharacteristically pruritic.
- The eruption may be limited in its distribution, or it may present in an inverse fashion involving the groin (Fig. 15.6A,B) axillae, or distal extremities (*inverse PR*).

DIFFERENTIAL DIAGNOSIS

Guttate Psoriasis

- *Small, droplike, 1 to 10 mm in diameter, salmon-pink papules, usually with a thicker scale than PR.*

Secondary Syphilis

- *Positive serology for syphilis.*

Tinea Versicolor

- *Lesions have fine, furfuraceous scale.*
- *The potassium hydroxide (KOH) examination is positive.*

Tinea Corporis

- *Lesions are typically annular ("ringlike"), round, and clear in the center.*
- *The potassium hydroxide (KOH) examination or fungal culture is positive.*

Drug Eruption

- *Infrequently, drug eruptions secondary to barbiturates, bismuth, captopril, clonidine, diphtheria toxoid, gold, isotretinoin, ketotifen, levamisole, metronidazole, and D-penicillamine can resemble PR.*

Viral Exanthem

- *Symptoms of viral infection.*
- *Most often morbilliform without scale.*

Nummular Eczema

- *Coin-shaped itchy lesions.*

Parapsoriasis

- *Chronic skin condition characterized by round or oval, red, slightly scaly patches on limbs and trunk.*
- *Mostly affects adults.*
- *Patches often exhibit cigarette paper-like wrinkling.*

 ## MANAGEMENT

- Treatment is often unnecessary, because PR is a self-limiting, asymptomatic condition that resolves with no sequelae.
- Patients should be educated about the usual course of the rash and its noncontagious nature.
- Exposure to sunlight or administration of ultraviolet B by a dermatologist may speed resolution of the eruption.
- Follow-up or referral to a dermatologist should be made if the rash persists more than 8 weeks.
- In cases of severe pruritus, oral antihistamines or mid potency topical steroids such as **triamcinolone 0.1% cream** may help alleviate the itching.
- On occasion, systemic steroids (prednisone, 0.5 to 1 mg/kg/day for 7 days) may be used in patients with severe pruritus.
- Oral **erythromycin** or **azithromycin** has been reported to shorten the course of the eruption in some cases.

POINTS TO REMEMBER

- Lesions characteristically appear "from the neck to the knees," in a "Christmas tree" distribution.
- PR is observed in otherwise healthy people, most frequently in children and young adults.
- Patients should be told that PR is a benign condition that will resolve without treatment.
- Secondary syphilis should be considered in the differential diagnosis, especially when lesions are also present on the palms and soles.

BASICS

- Granuloma annulare (GA) is an idiopathic, generally asymptomatic, ring-shaped grouping of dermal papules which are often misdiagnosed as "ringworm."
- In very young children, GA is often self-limiting but in adults, GA tends to be more of a chronic condition and occurs in women more often than men (2.5:1).
- In several case series, GA (usually generalized or chronic) has been associated with diabetes mellitus.

PATHOGENESIS

- The cause of GA is unknown. It has been postulated that GA represents a delayed-type hypersensitivity reaction to an unknown antigen and trauma, insect bites, viral infections, and sun have all been proposed as possible triggering factors.
- Familial cases of GA in identical twins and siblings suggest the possibility of a hereditary component.

CLINICAL MANIFESTATIONS

- Lesions are skin-colored or red firm dermal papules, with no epidermal change (scale).
- Lesions may be individual isolated papules or they may be joined in annular or semiannular (arciform) plaques with central clearing (Figs. 15.7–15.9). The centers of lesions may be slightly hyperpigmented and depressed relative to their borders.
- GA is generally asymptomatic and is primarily a cosmetic issue, although many patients tend to find its unexpected appearance somewhat alarming.
- When localized, GA is usually self-limiting, but it may be persistent when disseminated.

DISTRIBUTION OF LESIONS

- Although any part of the cutaneous surface may be involved, lesions most often arise symmetrically on the dorsal surfaces of hands, fingers, and feet (acral areas).
- In adults, lesions may also be found around the elbows (Fig. 15.10) and on the trunk (Fig. 15.11).
- Occasionally, GA presents as subcutaneous nodules on the arms and legs (*deep* or *subcutaneous* GA).

DIAGNOSIS

- Most often made clinically.
- Skin biopsy will show the characteristic histopathologic features, consisting of foci of altered collagen and mucin surrounded by granulomatous inflammation with histiocytes and lymphocytes. The degenerative collagen is referred to as *necrobiosis*.

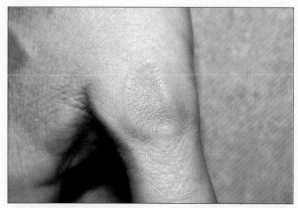

15.7 *Granuloma annulare.* These dermal plaques are typical ringlike lesions.

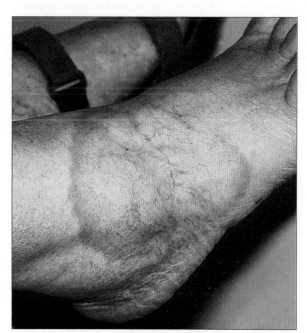

15.8 *Granuloma annulare.* An annular plaque of the dorsal foot.

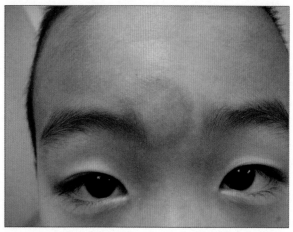

15.9 *Granuloma annulare.* An annular plaque of the forehead.

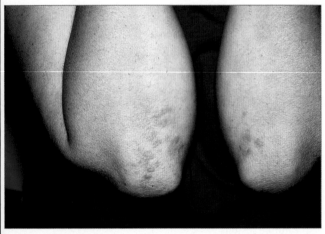

15.10 *Granuloma annulare.* Intradermal papules of granuloma annulare are located below the elbows in this middle-aged woman.

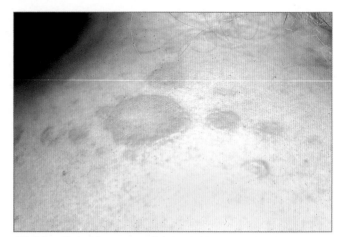

15.11 *Granuloma annulare.* Multiple annular dermal plaques on the upper back.

DIFFERENTIAL DIAGNOSIS

Tinea Corporis (see Chapter 18)
- *Often pruritic.*
- *Lesions have epidermal change (i.e., scale).*
- *The potassium hydroxide (KOH) examination or fungal culture is positive.*

Erythema Migrans (Rash of Lyme Disease, see Chapter 29)
- *Annular erythematous lesion(s).*
- *The lesion measures from 4 to 70 cm in diameter, generally with central clearing.*
- *The center of the lesion may become darker, vesicular, hemorrhagic, or necrotic.*
- *Lesions may be confluent (not annular), and concentric rings may form.*

Cutaneous Sarcoidosis (see Chapter 34)
- *Annular sarcoidosis may be indistinguishable from GA.*
- *Lesions often appear around orifices (e.g., the mouth, nose, ocular orbits) or develop in scars.*

MANAGEMENT

- The patient should be reassured of the benign nature of this condition but advised that it may be a harbinger of diabetes mellitus particularly in cases of disseminated GA.
- Because GA is usually benign and self-limited, treatment may consist of clinical observation, especially if lesions are localized, asymptomatic and on nonvisible skin.
- If symptomatic or of cosmetic concern, treatment with topical steroids such as class 2, high-potency **fluocinonide 0.5% cream (Lidex)** or super-potent class 1 clobetasol 0.05% cream may be applied. Occlusion may improve penetration. **Cordran tape** is another option (see "Introduction: Topical Therapy").
- Intralesional **triamcinolone acetonide (Kenalog)**, in a dose of 2.5 to 5 mg/mL, can also be injected directly into the elevated border of the lesions with a 30-gauge needle.
- Other treatments include UVA1 phototherapy, cryotherapy, and surgical excision (for localized disease).
- In recalcitrant or disseminated GA, anecdotal therapeutic successes have been reported with dapsone, pentoxifylline, PUVA, adalimumab **(Humira)**, SSKI, and narrow band UV.

POINT TO REMEMBER

- GA is very often misdiagnosed and treated as "ringworm" by nondermatologists.

Lichen Planus

BASICS

- Lichen planus (LP) is a relatively uncommon cutaneous inflammatory disorder.
- "Classic" LP is a pruritic, idiopathic eruption with characteristic shiny, flat-topped (*planus is Latin for* "flat") papules on the skin and mucous membranes.
- The papules are characterized by their violaceous color, polygonal shape, and, sometimes, fine scale and are most commonly found on the extremities, genitalia, and mucous membranes. Less commonly, lesions can also involve the hair and nails.
- LP is seen predominantly in adults—greater than two-thirds of patients are between 30 and 60 years of age—but it can occur at any age.
- Women are more commonly affected than men.

PATHOPHYSIOLOGY

- LP is a cell-mediated immune response of unknown origin. An association has been noted between LP and hepatitis C infection, chronic active hepatitis, and primary biliary cirrhosis.

CLINICAL MANIFESTATIONS

The "Seven Ps":

- Lesions are often **pruritic**, but can be asymptomatic.
- Lesions are typically **purple** (can be red to violet).
- Lesions tend to be **planar** (flat-topped) (Figs. 15.12 and 15.13).
- Lesions form **papules** or **plaques**.
- Lesions are often **polygonal** (Fig. 15.12).
- Lesions are frequently **polymorphic** (Fig. 15.13) in shape and configuration—that is, oval, annular, linear, confluent (plaque-like), large, and small, even on the same person.
- Lesions tend to heal with residual **postinflammatory hyperpigmentation,** leaving darkly pigmented macules in their wake (Fig. 15.14).

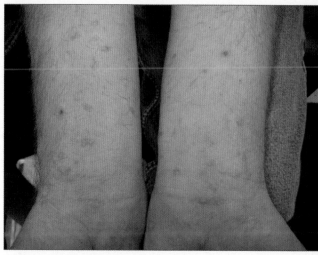

15.13　*Lichen planus.* Planar (flat-topped), violaceous, polygonal papules on the flexor wrists.

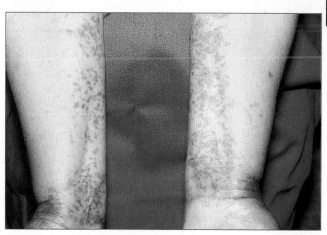

15.14　*Lichen planus.* Postinflammatory hyperpigmentation in a characteristic distribution.

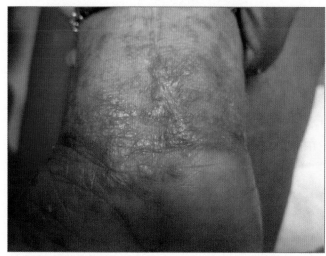

15.12　*Lichen planus.* Violaceous, polygonal papules on the flexor wrists.

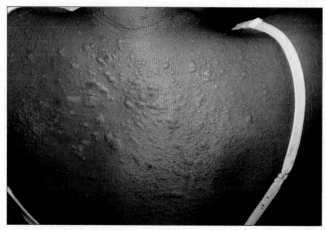

15.15　*Lichen planus.* Generalized lesions are noted on this patient.

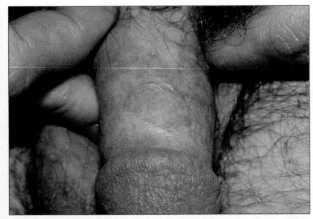

15.16 *Lichen planus.* Annular plaque on the penile shaft.

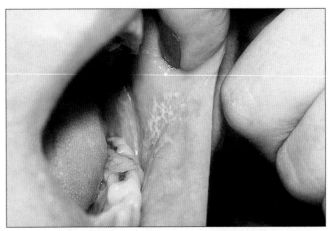

15.19 *Lichen planus.* Oral lesions, with a white, lacy, reticulated, pattern on the buccal mucosa.

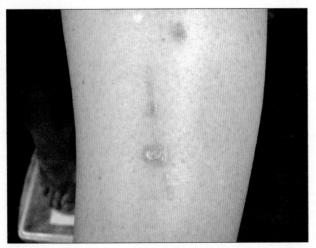

15.17 *Lichen planus.* The Köebner phenomenon (isomorphic response) results from scratching. Note linear spread of lesions.

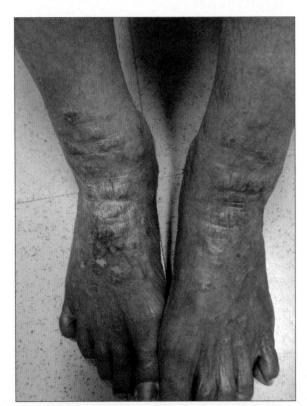

15.20 *Lichen planus, hypertrophic.* Thick, hypertropic plaques on the lower legs and dorsal feet.

DISTRIBUTION OF LESIONS

- The flexor areas such as the wrists, forearms, dorsal hands and feet, pretibial shafts, scalp, trunk, sacrum, glans penis, and labia minora are most often affected.
- Hypertrophic (verrucous) lesions tend to occur on the lower legs.
- Lesions may also become generalized (Fig. 15.15).
- Mucous membrane involvement is common and may be found without skin involvement. Lesions typically seen on the tongue and buccal mucosa but may also be noted on the gingiva, palate, or lips.

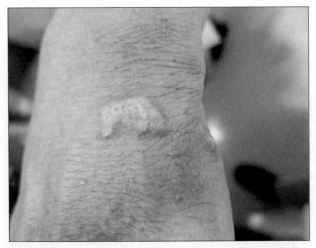

15.18 *Lichen planus.* Wickham striae are characteristic white, lacelike streaks that are best visualized on the surfaces of lesions after mineral oil application. This finding is virtually pathognomonic of LP.

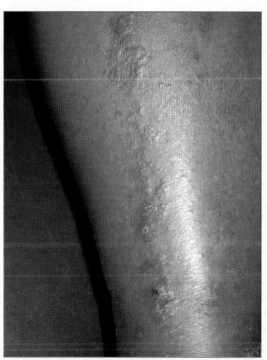

15.21 *Lichen planus, linear.* Linear variant of lichen planus.

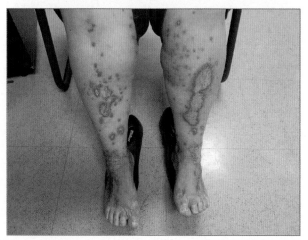

15.22 *Lichen planus, atrophic.* Atrophy resulted from resolved lesions in this patient. Note polymorphism of the resolved lesions.

- Mucous membrane involvement may become erosive and painful, particularly if ulcers are present. Rarely, malignant transformation to squamous cell carcinoma has been documented.
- Genital involvement is common in men with cutaneous disease. Typically, an annular configuration of papules is seen on the glans penis (Fig. 15.16). Less commonly, linear white streaks (Wickham striae) can be seen on male genitalia. Vulvar involvement can range from reticulate papules to severe erosions.
- Vulvar lesions can result in dyspareunia, burning, and pruritus.
- Nail lesions may exhibit symptoms ranging from a mild dystrophy to a total loss or absence of the nails (*twenty-nail dystrophy of childhood*).
- Scalp lesions result in a permanent, patchy, scarring follicular alopecia (*lichen planopilaris;* see Chapter 19).

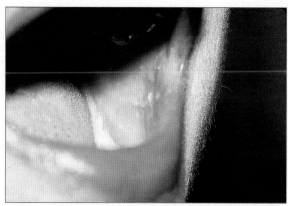

15.23 *Normal bite line.* This is a common finding on the buccal mucosa that is often confused with oral lichen planus (see Fig. 15.19). (From Goodheart HP. *Goodheart's Same-Site Differential Diagnosis*. Philadelphia, PA: Lippincott Williams & Wilkins, 2011.)

- The course of LP is unpredictable. The onset may be abrupt or gradual. The lesions may resolve spontaneously, recur intermittently, or persist for many years. Chronicity is especially likely when hypertrophic lesions appear.

ASSOCIATED CLINICAL FEATURES

- New lesions may be noted at sites of minor trauma such as scratches or burns (the Köebner reaction [isomorphic response]) (Fig. 15.17).
- Wickham striae are characteristic white, lacelike streaks that are best visualized on the surfaces of lesions after mineral oil is applied. If present, they are virtually pathognomonic of LP (Fig. 15.18).
- Mucous membrane lesions may be characterized by white lacy streaks in a netlike pattern (Fig. 15.19) or by atrophic erosions or ulcers.
- Pruritus, which may be severe, and the cosmetic appearance of lesions are the major concerns to patients.

CLINICAL VARIANTS

Variations in LP include the following:

- **Hypertrophic:** These extremely pruritic lesions are most often found on the extensor surfaces of the lower extremities (Fig. 15.20), especially around the ankles. Hypertrophic lesions are often chronic; and residual pigmentation and scarring can occur after lesions clear.
- **Linear:** Most often arise on extremities (Fig. 15.21).
- **Atrophic (rare):** Atrophic LP is most often the result of resolved lesions (Fig. 15.22).
- **Erosive:** These lesions are found on the mucosal surfaces.
- **Follicular:** Also called *lichen planopilaris;* typically seen on the scalp, can lead to scarring alopecia
- **Bullous** (rare): Intense inflammation in the dermis leads to blistering of epidermis.

DIAGNOSIS

- Despite its range of clinical presentations, LP is often diagnosed by its characteristic clinical appearance including the presence of Wickham striae, the Köebner reaction, and the characteristic oral lesions.
- Skin biopsy may be necessary if clinical presentation is atypical.

DIFFERENTIAL DIAGNOSIS

Classic Lichen Planus:
Lichen Simplex Chronicus and Other Variants of Eczematous Dermatitis (see Chapter 13)
- *Lichenification may be present.*
- *Possible atopic history.*

Pityriasis Rosea (see discussion earlier in this chapter)
Drug Eruption
Guttate Psoriasis
Lichen Nitidus
Lichenoid reactions associated with graft-versus-host disease
Drug-Induced or Chemically Induced Lichenoid ("Lichen Planus-like") Eruptions
- *Causal drugs include thiazides, furosemide, beta-blockers, sulfonylureas, antimalarials, penicillamine, gold salts, and angiotensin-converting enzyme inhibitors. Rarely, dental materials and tattoo pigments are involved.*

LP of the oral mucous membranes (also discussed in Chapter 21):
Normal bite line (Fig. 15.23)

Leukoplakia
Oral hairy leukoplakia
Candidiasis
Squamous cell carcinoma (particularly in ulcerative lesions)
Aphthous ulcers
Herpetic stomatitis
Primary bullous disease (e.g., pemphigus vulgaris)
Systemic lupus erythematosus

LP of the genital mucous membranes:
Psoriasis (penis and labia)
Lichen sclerosis
Fixed drug eruption (glans penis)
Candidiasis (penis and labia)

LP of the hair and scalp (lichen planopilaris):
Other causes of scarring alopecia such as discoid lupus erythematosus

---

MANAGEMENT

- The first-line treatment for mild cases of cutaneous LP is **potent topical steroids**. Patients with more severe cases, especially those with scalp, nail, and mucous membrane involvement, may require systemic therapy.
- High-potency (class 2) or super-potent (class 1) topical steroids may be used alone, with polyethylene occlusion, or with **Cordran tape** (see "Introduction: Topical Therapy").
- **Intralesional triamcinolone** acetonide (2.5 to 10 mg/mL) can also be used and is especially effective for hypertrophic LP.
- Narrow band UVB and PUVA can be effective treatments for LP that is often tried before systemic therapies are considered.

- **Systemic steroids** (e.g., prednisone beginning at 0.5 to 1 mg/kg daily) in short (2 to 6 weeks), tapering courses may be necessary for symptom control in severe, acute cases.
- Acitretin (**Soriatane**) has shown good efficacy for widespread LP.
- **Griseofulvin, hydroxychloroquine and sulfasalazine** have also been used successfully in recalcitrant cases.
- There are also reports of recalcitrant LP improving with the systemic immunosuppressants methotrexate, cyclosporine and mycophenolate mofetil.
- For symptomatic LP of the oral mucosa, topical steroids are usually tried first. Alternatively, topical tacrolimus 0.1% ointment (**Protopic**) has been used with some success.

HELPFUL HINTS

- Several studies have reported that oral **metronidazole** might be effective in some patients with idiopathic LP.
- Take a thorough drug history and consider drug-induced LP before starting on therapy.

POINTS TO REMEMBER

- Serial oral or genital examinations are indicated for erosive/ulcerative lesions to rule out squamous cell carcinoma.
- Hepatitis C should be considered in patients with widespread or unusual presentations of lichen planus.

Superficial Bacterial Infections, Folliculitis, and Hidradenitis Suppurativa

OVERVIEW

The gram-positive cocci, *Staphylococcus aureus* and *Streptococcus pyogenes* (also known as group A β-hemolytic streptococcus) are not generally considered normal skin inhabitants but are temporary invaders and account for the vast majority of cutaneous bacterial infections. Methicillin-resistant *Staphylococcus aureus* (MRSA), a type of *S. aureus* that is resistant to the penicillins, is now increasingly recognized as a cause of skin infections and most often presents as recurrent furunculosis.

S. aureus can be part of the normal skin flora in some people, typically inhabiting the anterior nares, hands, and perineum, and this carriage imparts an increased risk of developing impetigo or other staphylococcal infections such as those that result from surgical or traumatic wounds. Eczematous dermatitis, a disorder in which the barrier of the skin is defective, often allows for **secondary impetiginization** with *S. aureus* (see Chapter 13).

Folliculitis refers to inflammation of the hair follicle, particularly its upper portion, and is characterized by perifollicular papules and/or pustules with or without obvious emerging hairs. Folliculitis can be the result of an infection (with bacteria, or less often viruses and fungi), inflammatory skin conditions (e.g., follicular eczema), drugs or physical irritation. Furuncles ("boils") and carbuncles represent a deeper, more extensive progression of a bacterial folliculitis.

Hidradenitis suppurativa is not a primary bacterial infection, but it is included in this chapter because of the presence of furuncle-like lesions and the frequent occurrence of secondary infection with *S. aureus*.

IN THIS CHAPTER...

➤ **IMPETIGO (also discussed in Chapter 5)**

- Secondary Impetigo (Impetiginization)

➤ **BACTERIAL FOLLICULITIS**

- Staphylococcal folliculitis
- *Pseudomonas aeruginosa* folliculitis (hot tub folliculitis)

➤ **FOLLICULITIS: OTHER TYPES**

- Irritant, frictional, or chemical folliculitis
- Steroid-induced acne and rosacea (also discussed in Chapter 12)
- Eosinophilic pustular folliculitis (also discussed in Chapters 2 and 33)
- Fungal folliculitis
- Majocchi granuloma (also discussed in Chapter 18)

➤ **FURUNCULOSIS ("BOILS")**

➤ **HIDRADENITIS SUPPURATIVA (ACNE INVERSA)**

Impetigo

BASICS

- Impetigo is a common, highly contagious bacterial infection of the superficial layers of the epidermis that is most often caused by *Staphylococcus aureus* and less often by *Streptococcus pyogenes*.
- Traditionally, impetigo has been divided into two forms—*bullous* and nonbullous (*impetigo contagiosa*). Sometimes, these are clinically indistinguishable; therefore, it is probably less confusing to use the term impetigo to describe both of them.
- Impetigo is transmitted from person to person, or from an infected fomite and can spread via autoinoculation.

CLINICAL MANIFESTATIONS

- Impetigo begins as a thin-roofed fragile vesicle or pustule that soon ruptures and leaves a peripheral collarette of scale or the flaccid remains of a bulla (Figs. 16.1–16.2).
- Oozing serum dries and gives rise to the classic golden-yellow, "honey-colored," crusted lesions that seem to be stuck on the skin (Fig. 16.3). After rupturing and desiccating they may appear "varnish-like" (Fig. 16.4).
- Lesions often start at the site of a minor skin injury such as an abrasion, an arthropod bite reaction, or eczema that has been excoriated.
- Lesions are usually asymptomatic, but occasionally itch.
- Whether pustular or bullous, impetigo is a self-limited process and heals without scarring in 2 to 6 weeks even without treatment. Postinflammatory hyperpigmentation may occur, especially in dark-skinned persons.
- ***Ecthyma*** is a deeper, dermal presentation of impetigo, often caused by group A beta-hemolytic streptococci, and is characterized by thick, often blackened adherent crusts over ulcers. Unlike impetigo, which only affects the stratum corneum, ecthyma extends into the dermis. Ecthyma occurs most often on the lower extremities and can heal with scarring (Fig. 16.5).

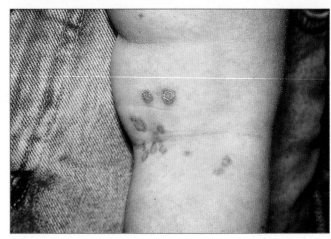

16.2 *Impetigo.* Here intact blisters are not present; only the flaccid remains (scaly collarettes) of bullae are seen.

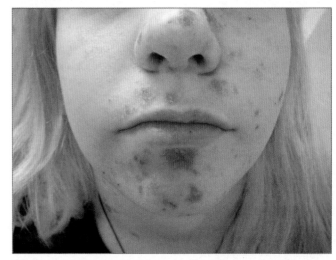

16.3 *Impetigo.* Oozing honey-colored, crusted lesions in a typical location.

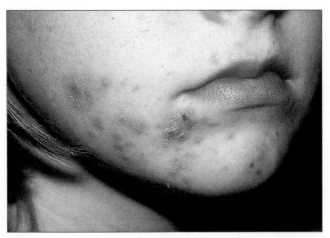

16.1 *Impetigo.* This child has a mixture of intact bullae and drying crusts.

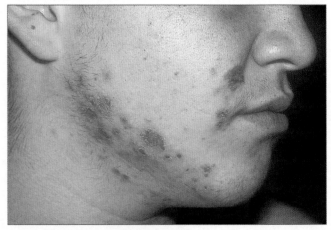

16.4 *Impetigo gladiatorum.* This is a college wrestler (see also discussion of herpes gladiatorum in Chapter 17).

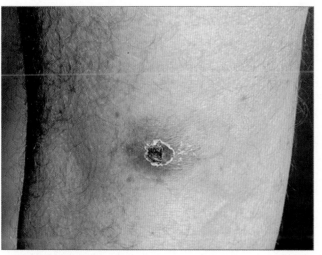

16.5 ***Ecthyma.*** The blackened crust resulted from an infected insect bite.

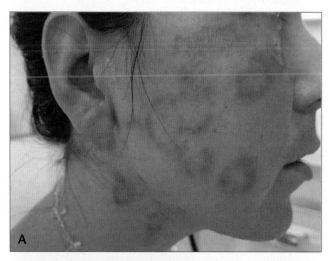

A

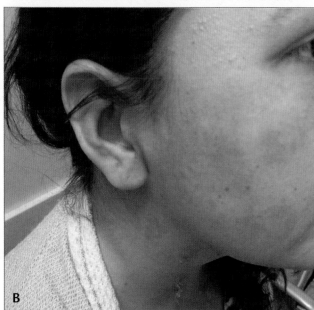

B

16.6 ***Impetigo.*** **A:** Multiple annular, crusted lesions. **B:** One week after oral dicloxacillin therapy.

DISTRIBUTION OF LESIONS

- In adults, lesions may occur anywhere on the body; however, they arise most often on exposed areas such as on the hands and face (Fig. 16.6A,B) or in skin folds particularly the axillae (Fig. 16.7).
- In children, the face (particularly in and around the nose and mouth) and the exposed parts of the body (e.g., arms, legs) are the typical sites of involvement.

SECONDARY IMPETIGO (IMPETIGINIZATION)

- Impetigo can, and often does, emerge as a secondary infection of a pre-existing skin disease (Fig. 16.8) or traumatized skin; it is then referred to as *secondary impetiginization.*

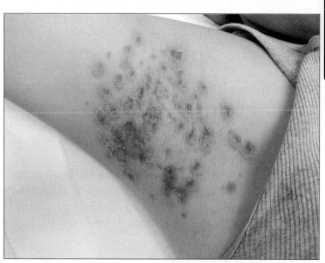

16.7 ***Impetigo of axilla.*** Multiple annular lesions; only the flaccid remains (scaly collarettes) of bullae are seen.

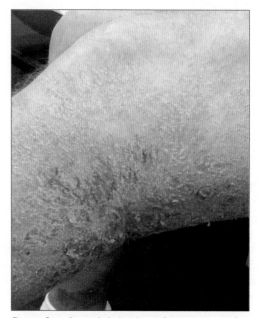

16.8 ***Secondary impetiginization of eczematous dermatitis.*** Note honey-colored areas overlying area of eczema.

- Conditions that may lead to secondary impetiginization include the following:
  - Atopic dermatitis
  - Stasis dermatitis
  - Herpes simplex and varicella infections
  - Scabies and insect bites
  - Lacerations and burns

CLINICAL SEQUELAE

- Rarely progresses to systemic infection; poststreptococcal glomerulonephritis is a rare complication of impetigo caused by *S. pyogenes*.
- Rarely, cellulitis, lymphangitis, scarlet fever, erysipelas, bacteremia with subsequent pneumonitis, septic arthritis, septicemia, and bacterial endocarditis may develop.
- Staphylococcal scalded skin syndrome can develop in younger children or immunocompromised adults with bullous impetigo.

DIAGNOSIS

- Generally made on clinical grounds.
- Bacterial culture and sensitivity testing are recommended prior to treatment especially if standard topical or oral treatment does not result in improvement.
- Recurrent or persistent impetigo may indicate a carrier state in the patient or the patient's family. A bacterial culture of the nares may be obtained to determine whether a patient is a carrier of *S. aureus*.

 DIFFERENTIAL DIAGNOSIS

Tinea Corporis
- *The potassium hydroxide examination or fungal culture is positive.*
- *Central clearing of lesions is noted and may be similar to impetigo.*

Eczematous Dermatitis
- *Ill-defined pink, thin scaly plaques.*
- *Lack honey colored crusting, unless secondarily impetiginized.*

Herpes Simplex Viral Infection
- *Tense vesicles on an erythematous base.*
- *Lesions are usually painful or tender.*

Primary Bullous Diseases (i.e., Bullous Dermatosis of Childhood and Bullous Pemphigoid)
- *Bullae are more tense and may have surrounding erythema.*

 MANAGEMENT

- Antibacterial soaps such as povidone-iodine (**Betadine**) or chlorhexidine (**Hibiclens**).
- Mupirocin 2% (**Bactroban**) ointment or cream applied three times daily may be used alone to treat very limited cases of impetigo. Retapamulin 1% ointment (**Altabax**) is another effective option. These agents are applied until all lesions are cleared. Topical application of these preparations has been shown to be as effective as oral antibiotics.
- For widespread involvement, an oral staphylocidal penicillinase-resistant antibiotic, such as a **first-generation cephalosporin, dicloxacillin**, or **erythromycin**, may be used alone or in conjunction with topical antibiotics.
- If bacterial cultures reveal MRSA, **tetracyclines, trimethoprim/sulfamethoxazole (Bactrim), clindamycin**, or **linezolid** are effective oral antibiotics.
- In patients with recurrent impetigo who are chronic nasal carriers, mupirocin 2% cream or ointment applied intranasally three times daily for 5 days each month for 3 months can reduce or eliminate bacterial colonization.

 HELPFUL HINTS

- Chronic or recurrent impetigo should alert the clinician to the possibility of a carrier state or impaired immune status.
- Regular "bleach baths" (see Chapter 13 and Patient Handout "Bleach baths" IN THE COMPANION eBOOK EDITION) help reduce the bacterial load on the skin and can lead to quicker resolution and prevent secondary impetiginization in some skin diseases.
- Consider MRSA if impetigo is not improving with first-line treatments and perform culture to determine antibiotic sensitivity.

 POINTS TO REMEMBER

- Rarely, poststreptococcal glomerulonephritis (but not rheumatic fever) has been reported to follow impetigo caused by certain strains of *Streptococci*.
- Family members should be evaluated as potential nasal carriers of *S. aureus* and treated, if necessary.

BASICS

- Folliculitis, in its broadest sense, may be defined as a superficial or deep infection or inflammation of the hair follicles.
- Folliculitis has multiple causes: bacterial or viral infections, physical or chemical irritation (i.e., excessive sweating), occlusive dressings or clothing (i.e., tight jeans), repeated trauma (such as waxing, plucking, and shaving of the face, scalp, legs, and pubic areas), and the use of topical or systemic steroids.
- Bacterial folliculitis may occur as a secondary infection in conditions such as eczema, scabies, excoriated insect bites particularly in patients who are diabetic, obese, or immunocompromised.
- Less commonly, viral folliculitis may appear in patients with herpes simplex infections, especially in patients with human immunodeficiency virus (HIV) infection.

STAPHYLOCOCCAL FOLLICULITIS

CLINICAL MANIFESTATIONS

- Bacterial folliculitis is most often caused by infection with coagulase-positive *S. aureus.*
- Lesions typically elicit mild discomfort or tenderness and occasionally itch.
- The primary lesion is an erythematous pustule or papule with a central hair (Figs. 16.9–16.10). The central hair shaft may not always be visible.
- Follicular lesions tend to manifest a grid-like pattern on hair-bearing areas of the body.
- Lesions are often polymorphic, displaying a mixture of papules and pustules, or they may be monomorphic and consist solely of papules.
- In darkly pigmented patients, hyperpigmented macules or papules arranged in a follicular pattern may be all that is clinically apparent.

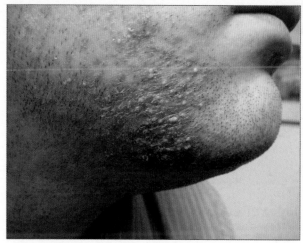

16.10 *Facial folliculitis.* Intact follicular pustules and crusted papules. Note emerging hairs from several pustules.

DISTRIBUTION OF LESIONS

- Lesions occur on hair-bearing areas—the face, scalp, thighs, and body folds.
- The axillae, groin, and legs are particularly prone to folliculitis when they are regularly shaved.

CLINICAL VARIANTS

- Tender, painful, folliculitis involving an eyelash is called a *hordeolum* or "stye."
- Similarly, folliculitis may affect a single nasal hair follicle and may produce a tender erythematous papule or pustule in or on the distal nose or near the tip of the nose (Fig. 16.11).

DIAGNOSIS

- Bacterial folliculitis is generally diagnosed by clinical findings. In cases that are resistant to treatment, the following procedures may be performed:
  - Gram stain: typically demonstrates gram-positive cocci.
  - Bacterial culture: grows *S. aureus.*

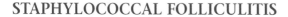

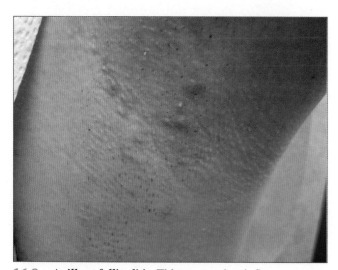

16.9 *Axillary folliculitis.* This woman has inflammatory papules and pustules secondary to shaving.

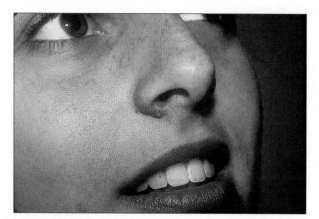

16.11 *Folliculitis.* This young woman has a tender papule that originated in a nasal hair follicle.

DIFFERENTIAL DIAGNOSIS

Acne Vulgaris/Acne-like Conditions
- *Acneform papules and pustules may be indistinguishable from folliculitis.*

Keratosis Pilaris
- *Because this condition involves the hair follicles, it manifests in a grid-like pattern, similar to that of folliculitis.*
- *Central punctum is keratotic rather than pustular.*

Insect Bite Reactions
- *Lesions are grouped in a nonfollicular pattern (see Chapter 29).*

MANAGEMENT

Initial Episode
- Mild cases of bacterial folliculitis can sometimes be prevented or controlled with antibacterial soaps such as **benzoyl peroxide** or **Hibiclens.**
- In addition, topical antibiotics, such as **erythromycin** 2% topical solution or clindamycin (**Cleocin**) 1% solution, may be applied once or twice a day to the affected areas.
- For more widespread or severe cases, systemic antibiotics such as dicloxacillin (250 to 500 mg four times a day) or a **cephalosporin**, such as **cephalexin** (1 to 4 g/day in two doses) are generally the first choices.

Chronic and Recurrent Cases
- If staphylococcal colonization is present, mupirocin 2% (**Bactroban**) ointment should be applied to the nasal vestibule twice a day for 5 days monthly × 3 months to eliminate the *S. aureus* carrier state.
- Family members may be treated similarly, if necessary. **Rifampin** (600 mg/day for 10 to 14 days) may also help eliminate the carrier state.

POINTS TO REMEMBER

- Bacterial cultures should be considered for cases that are resistant to therapy.
- Culturing and treating of family members should be considered in cases of chronic bacterial folliculitis.

PSEUDOMONAS FOLLICULITIS ("HOT TUB FOLLICULITIS")

- *Pseudomonas* folliculitis, often acquired from communal hot tubs, is caused by *Pseudomonas aeruginosa* infection.
- Jacuzzis, therapeutic whirlpools ("whirlpool folliculitis"), public swimming pools, wax hair depilation, and the use of loofah sponges can also be sources of *Pseudomonas* infection.

CLINICAL MANIFESTATIONS
- Pruritic lesions occur 1 to 3 days after bathing in a hot tub, whirlpool, or public swimming pool.
- Lesions of hot tub folliculitis consist of intensely pruritic or tender follicular papules or pustules that are most often found on the trunk, particularly on areas covered by a bathing suit (Fig. 16.12).

DIAGNOSIS
- The diagnosis is based on clinical appearance and a history of exposure.
- *Pseudomonas* organisms may be isolated in patients with this condition.

MANAGEMENT

- Hot tub folliculitis usually resolves spontaneously, but it may persist if it is very extensive or symptomatic.
- If necessary, oral **ciprofloxacin** (500 mg twice a day for 5 days) will lead to resolution.

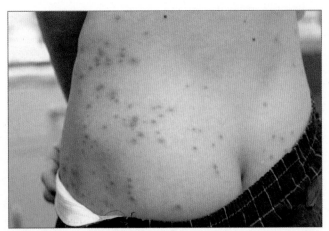

16.12 *Hot tub folliculitis ("hot tub buns").* Multiple pruritic follicular papules and pustules occurred on the buttocks of this young man 3 days after he had bathed in a hot tub. Bacterial culture grew *Pseudomonas aeruginosa.*

IRRITANT, FRICTIONAL, OR CHEMICAL FOLLICULITIS

- Nonbacterial, or sterile, folliculitis can arise from physical or chemical irritation.
- Irritants include hair removal methods such as leg waxing, shaving, electrolysis, plucking or chemical depilatories, occlusive dressings, wearing tight clothing, and excessive sweating.
- Nonbacterial folliculitis may also be related to working conditions, such as the use of greases or oils, and to the application of various cosmetics. Occasionally, secondary bacterial infection may occur.

STEROID-INDUCED ACNE AND ROSACEA (ALSO DISCUSSED IN CHAPTER 12)

- Topical or systemic steroid treatment may lead to steroid-induced acne, which is actually a form of folliculitis.
- Diagnosis of these conditions is aided by a history of potent topical or systemic steroid use (Fig. 16.13).

EOSINOPHILIC PUSTULAR FOLLICULITIS (ALSO DISCUSSED IN CHAPTERS 2 AND 33)

- Eosinophilic pustular folliculitis (EPF), another form of sterile folliculitis, is typically intensely pruritic.
- Presents in three clinical forms: (1) EPF in adults also called Ofuji disease, (2) AIDS-associated EPF, and (3) EPF of infancy which presents as recurrent grouped papulopustules most often noted on the scalp.
- Lesions appear as recurrent crops of erythematous papules and papulopustules on "sebaceous" areas of skin and spontaneously resolve over 7 to 10 days (Fig. 16.14). Recurrences may occur every 3 to 4 weeks.

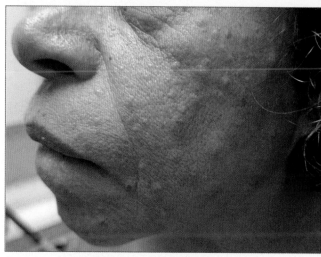

16.14 *Eosinophilic pustular folliculitis.* This patient has HIV/AIDS. The lesions are intensely pruritic.

- In all three forms there may be peripheral eosinophilia and histology will show eosinophils around the follicular infundibulum.

FUNGAL FOLLICULITIS

PITYROSPORUM FOLLICULITIS

- This acne-like eruption is usually seen on the trunk and is caused by *Malassezia furfur,* a lipophilic yeast.
- Lesions are chronic, erythematous, pruritic papules and pustules that appear on the back and chest of young adults in a follicular pattern.
- Seen more frequently in the summer months.
- *Pityrosporum* folliculitis should be considered as a diagnosis when folliculitis resists typical anti-acne antibiotic treatment.

MAJOCCHI GRANULOMA (ALSO DISCUSSED IN CHAPTER 18)

- Tinea corporis of the lower legs may produce tinea folliculitis in women who shave their legs. The organism is introduced into the hair follicle by shaving.

 POINTS TO REMEMBER

- Bacterial, fungal, or viral cultures should be considered in cases that are resistant to therapy.
- In HIV-positive patients, a skin biopsy should be performed for suspected cases of eosinophilic pustular folliculitis.

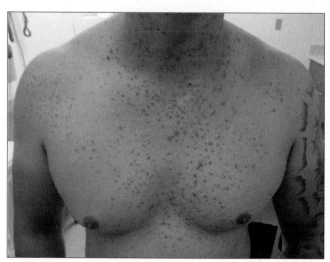

16.13 *Systemic steroid-induced folliculitis.* This patient is taking long-term prednisone for sarcoidosis.

Furunculosis ("Boils")

BASICS

- Folliculitis may evolve into a furuncle ("boil"), which is a deeper infection. The term *carbuncle* refers to an aggregation of furuncles.
- Furuncles are painful nodules or abscesses (walled-off collections of pus) that began in an infected hair follicle; they are more common in boys and young adults.
- *S. aureus* is the usual etiologic agent although MRSA is also now a frequent cause.
- As with folliculitis, furunculosis is more common in diabetic patients and in obese persons.

CLINICAL MANIFESTATIONS

- Throbbing pain and tenderness.
- A furuncle is a tender, painful subcutaneous nodule with overlying erythema (Fig. 16.15).
- Untreated, it may rupture and drain spontaneously (Fig. 16.16) or as it further evolves, a fluctuant abscess may form (Fig. 16.17).

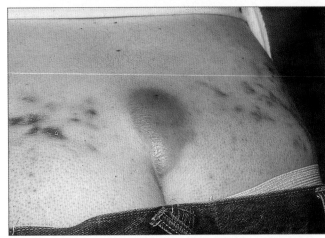

16.17 *Abscess.* This patient has the **follicular occlusion triad** ("tetrad" in this case), which consists of hidradenitis suppurativa, acne conglobata, and dissecting cellulitis of the scalp. This walled-off lesion began as a pilonidal sinus that later developed into an abscess. Note the older violaceous scars from previous furuncles and cystic acne lesions.

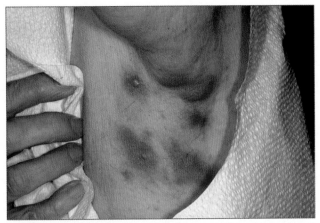

16.15 *Furunculosis.* This woman has multiple tender "boils" located in her axilla.

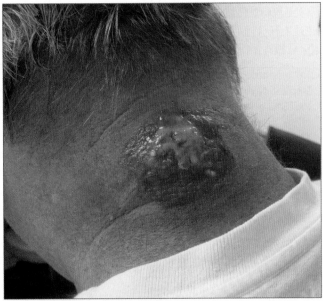

16.18 *Carbuncle.* Note the contiguous cluster of purulent furuncles on the posterior neck in this patient.

DISTRIBUTION OF LESIONS

- Can arise anywhere but most often seen in the axillae, inguinal area, posterior neck, thighs, and buttocks (hair-bearing areas and body folds).
- A contiguous cluster of furuncles, most often arising on the occipital scalp, is referred to as a *carbuncle* (Fig. 16.18 see also Fig. 5.8).

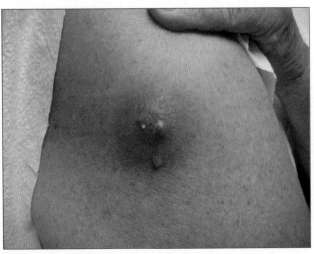

16.16 *Furuncle.* Draining purulent lesion.

DIAGNOSIS

- Based on the clinical presentation.
- Gram stain generally reveals gram-positive cocci; culture often grows *S. aureus*.

DIFFERENTIAL DIAGNOSIS

Hidradenitis Suppurativa (see below)
- Furuncles and linear cord-like lesions may be apparent.
- Often involves axillae, inguinal folds, and suprapubic skin.

MANAGEMENT

- Warm compresses can help furuncles come to a "head" and drain spontaneously which will lead to eventual resolution.
- Larger and deeper furuncles may need to be incised (with a large bore needle or no. 11 blade) and drained. Lesions should be fluctuant before attempting to incise and drain.
- Systemic staphylocidal antibiotics such as **dicloxacillin, erythromycin,** or **cephalosporin** are used (in addition to incision and drainage) for furuncles located in difficult to drain areas, for lesions that are very tender or have a lot of surrounding erythema, multiple recurrent lesions or in patients who are immunocompromised or have comorbidities. If MRSA is suspected, **minocycline** or **trimethoprim-sulfamethoxazole (Bactrim)** can be used.
- The daily coating of the distal nasal mucosa with **mupirocin** should be considered in carriers or recurrent cases.

Hidradenitis Suppurativa (Acne Inversa)

BASICS

- Hidradenitis suppurativa (HS) should not be classified as a primary infection; rather, it is a chronic, recurrent, scarring, inflammatory disease that affects the regions of the skin where apocrine sweat glands are present: the axillae, inguinal folds, suprapubic area, anogenital area, buttocks, areola, and under the female breasts.
- HS appears after puberty, usually during the second or third decades of life.
- It is seen mostly in young women and only rarely before puberty. HS in African-American women tends to be more severe.

PATHOPHYSIOLOGY

- The exact cause of HS is unknown. An autosomal-dominant inheritance has been described.
- Traditionally, it had been considered a primary inflammatory disorder of the apocrine glands (and was sometimes referred to as *apocrinitis* or *apocrine acne*).
- Currently, it is believed that primary event is poral occlusion of the hair follicle that leads to retention of secretory products, dilation, and subsequent rupture triggering inflammation. In fact, in most biopsy specimens the apocrine glands are intact and unaffected, and follicular occlusion (acne-like findings) are the constant finding. Inflammation of the apocrine glands and bacterial infection are apparently secondary events.
- As noted in acne vulgaris, HS is influenced by hormonal fluctuations and symptoms often improve during the estrogen-elevation phases of the menstrual cycle and during pregnancy, and often flare during the postpartum period.

CLINICAL MANIFESTATIONS

- Initially HS presents with nodules and abscesses that may be indistinguishable from furunculosis or common "boils" (Fig. 16.19).
- Chronic HS is indicated by the appearance of sinus tracts, fistula formation, ulcerations, and, eventually, hypertrophic, rope-like linear bands of scars and dermal contractures (Fig. 16.20).
- Characteristic multiple open comedones ("blackheads") develop in long-standing cases.

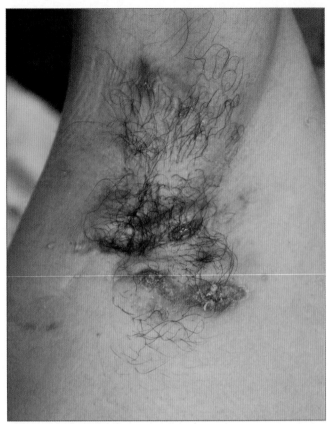

16.19 *Acute hidradenitis suppurativa.* Lesions are draining and show marked activity.

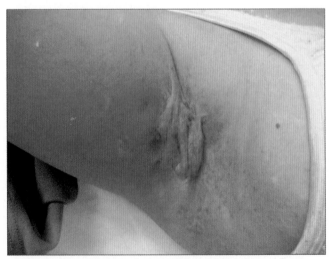

16.20 *Chronic hidradenitis suppurativa.* This patient has band-like hypertrophic scars from chronically draining abscesses.

- Lesions recur, new lesions crop up, and old lesions scar in a frustrating, unrelenting process.
- HS lesions are painful and tender and often become secondarily infected.
- Menstrual flares are common.
- Lesions may exude a serosanguineous or foul-smelling purulent material that may stain clothing.
- Often HS is a cause of embarrassment and social isolation.

DISTRIBUTION OF LESIONS

- The most common area of involvement is the axillary area and groin and tends to be symmetric.
- Lesions may also be seen on the perineum, infra-mammary areas, the buttocks, and, rarely, the neck and scalp.

DIAGNOSIS

- When multiple lesions are present with scars and sinus tracts, HS is easily distinguishable from other conditions.

PROGNOSIS

- The course of HS varies.
- Some patients only have very mild disease that may be indistinguishable from chronic furunculosis.
- There may be improvement with age or as more scar tissue develops. Spontaneous improvement has been reported after menopause.
- Total spontaneous resolution is rare.

DIFFERENTIAL DIAGNOSIS

Recurrent Folliculitis/Furunculosis (see earlier discussion)
- *An early solitary lesion of HS can resemble a* **furuncle, lymphadenitis**, *or an infected epidermoid cyst.*

Infected Bartholin Cyst
- *Present in vaginal mucosa whereas HS is present on skin.*

MANAGEMENT

- HS is a difficult, frustrating condition to control. The goal of treatment is to alleviate symptoms and induce prolonged disease-free periods.
- Actively draining lesions should be cultured.
- Antibiotics are the mainstay of treatment, especially for the early stages of the disease. Long-term oral antibiotics such as **doxycycline** (50 to 100 mg twice daily) or **minocycline** (50–100 mg twice daily) may prevent disease activation.
- Large cysts should be incised and drained. Smaller cysts respond to intralesional injections of triamcinolone acetonide (**Kenalog**, 2.5 to 10 mg/mL) and are used to treat limited acute exacerbations.

Preventive Measures During Remissions
- Weight loss helps reduce the activity and severity of HS
- Wearing of ventilated cotton clothing
- Use of absorbent powders and bacteriostatic soaps

Topical Therapy
- Limited and very early disease may be helped somewhat by the daily use of topical antibiotics such as clindamycin 1% solution (gel or lotion) and antibacterial soaps.

Systemic Therapy
- **Prednisone** can be used in short courses, particularly if inflammation is severe. A short course of prednisone,

40 to 60 mg daily, to be tapered over 2 to 3 weeks is often quite effective.
- Prednisone may be given alone or, most often, in combination with oral antibiotics, such as **minocycline, ciprofloxacin, cephalosporins**, or **semisynthetic penicillin**, given in the usual doses used for soft tissue infections. For example, **minocycline**, in doses ranging from 50 to 100 mg twice a day, may be used on an episodic basis for weeks or, if necessary, months at a time and then tapered to the lowest dosage that relieves symptoms. Long-term administration of an antibiotic, such as minocycline, can also be used to prevent episodic flares. The efficacy of minocycline seems to be attributable to its anti-inflammatory action rather than its antibiotic effect.
- Alternative antibiotics that can be helpful include **ciprofloxacin, cephalexin**, and **dicloxacillin**.
- Certain oral contraceptives have been reported to be helpful in cases that flare with menses.
- The combination of **rifampin** and **cyclosporine** and the tumor necrosis factor alpha inhibitors (infliximab [**Remicade**] and adalimumab [**Humira**]), may induce remission in patients with moderate-to-severe HS.
- Systemic retinoids, such as oral **isotretinoin**, have been used with limited benefit in early disease that has not yet produced significant scarring.

continued on page 280

MANAGEMENT *Continued*

Surgical Measures

- **Incision and drainage** are performed only on fluctuant lesions. This approach affords short-term relief of troublesome, painful abscesses. Repeated incision and drainage may lead to more scarring and sinus tract formation.
- A **narrow excision** of inflamed areas may help temporarily; however, this method has a high recurrence rate.

- **Unroofing** is a tissue-saving technique, where the "roof" of an abscess, cyst, or sinus tract is electrosurgically removed.
- **Ablation techniques** using a carbon dioxide laser that spares normal tissue have been tried successfully. These techniques may become the standard of surgical treatment.
- **Surgical removal.** Severe refractory HS that is localized is best treated with wide, complete **surgical excision** of the involved area, which may produce a definitive cure.

 POINTS TO REMEMBER

- Recurrent tender furuncles or sterile abscesses in the axillae, groin, on the buttocks, or the inframammary area suggest the diagnosis of HS.
- Many cases, especially when only localized to the thighs and vulva, are mild and misdiagnosed as recurrent furunculosis.

- Chronic disease is indicated by the presence of old scars, sinus tracts, and open comedones.

Mucocutaneous Manifestations of Viral Infections

OVERVIEW

Viruses are capable of causing a wide variety of disorders of the skin and mucous membranes. Viral-induced skin lesions include vesicles, pustules, papules, ulcers, and tumors. Cutaneous reaction patterns to viral infections most commonly appear as vesicles and bullae (herpes simplex and zoster virus infections), papulosquamous lesions (pityriasis rosea), or viral exanthems (discussed in Chapter 7).

Certain viral infections, such as warts vary greatly in their gross clinical appearance despite all being caused by different subtypes of the same human papillomavirus (HPV). For example, warts may be papillomatous (common warts), threadlike (filiform warts), flat (planar warts), exuberant moist papules (condyloma acuminata), or develop into tumors (*giant condyloma acuminatum of Buschke–Löwenstein*). In contrast, lesions of molluscum contagiosum tend to be quite monomorphic and uniform in appearance and vary primarily by size.

The virus of varicella-zoster (VZV) may produce the clinical syndrome of either chickenpox or herpes zoster. Herpes simplex virus (HSV) may manifest as a local recurrence of vesicles on the skin or rarely, it can produce a more widespread illness such as herpetic encephalitis or *Kaposi varicelliform eruption*.

IN THIS CHAPTER...

➤ **WARTS (NONGENITAL)**

➤ **MOLLUSCUM CONTAGIOSUM**

➤ **HERPES SIMPLEX (NONGENITAL)**

- Primary orolabial herpes simplex
- Recurrent orolabial herpes simplex
- Clinical variants of herpes simplex infections

➤ **HERPES ZOSTER**

Warts (Nongenital)

BASICS

- Warts are a common cutaneous viral infection and although they are much more prevalent in children and adolescents, they are also a common reason an adult may seek medical attention.
- Immunocompromised patients, patients with atopic dermatitis, especially those with hand dermatitis, are more prone to acquire a wart.
- In addition, butchers, construction workers, mechanics, housekeepers, janitors, and patients with occupations where the hands are exposed to mechanical trauma and harsh chemicals that can impair the skin barrier may develop a wart more easily.
- Chapter 6 discusses the pathogenesis, clinical variants, and treatment of warts in detail. In this chapter, representative clinical images, the differential diagnoses and treatments to consider in adults with warts will be presented.

CLINICAL VARIANTS

COMMON WARTS (AKA VERRUCA VULGARIS)

- Hyperkeratotic, exophytic papules that can be found anywhere on body but most often seen on the hands and feet (Figs. 17.1–17.5).

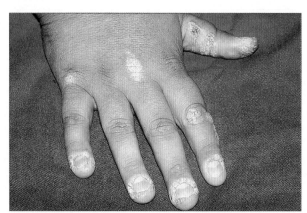

17.1 *Common warts (verruca vulgaris).* This young boy has multiple warts.

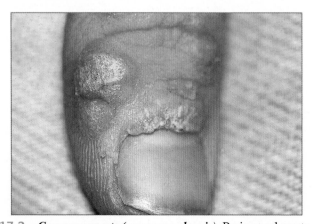

17.2 *Common warts (verruca vulgaris).* Periungual warts.

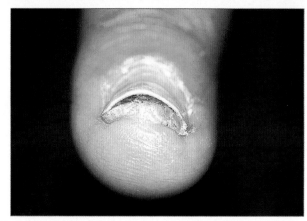

17.3 *Common wart (verruca vulgaris).* This subungual lesion could easily be mistaken for onychomycosis.

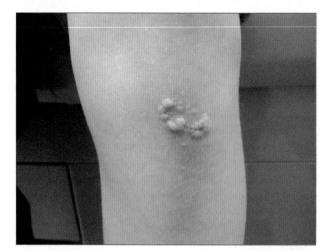

17.4 *Common wart (verruca vulgaris).* Multiple warts on knee.

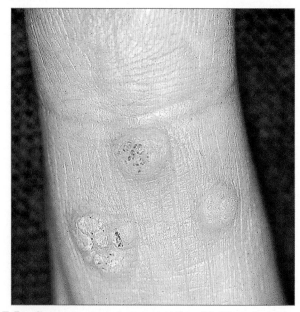

17.5 *Common warts (verruca vulgaris).* These lesions demonstrate loss of normal skin markings and "black dots" (thrombosed capillaries) that are pathognomonic for warts.

PLANTAR WARTS

- Hyperkeratotic papules that can coalesce into larger plaques called *mosaic warts* on the sole of the foot (Figs. 17.6–17.8).

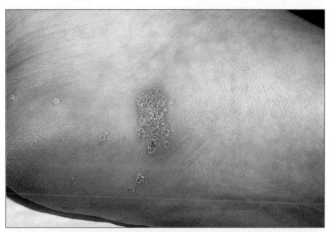

17.6   *Mosaic plantar warts.* Characteristic "black dots" are seen in this cluster of plantar warts.

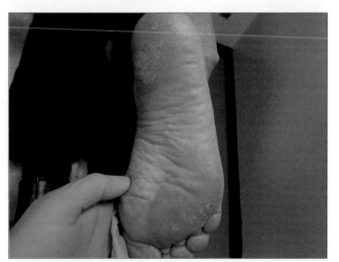

17.7   *Mosaic plantar warts.* Note clusters of warts located at pressure points on soles of feet.

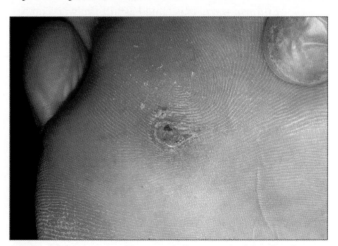

17.8   *Plantar wart.* Characteristic punctate bleeding is present after paring. Note the loss of skin markings.

FLAT WARTS

- Skin colored to tan flat-topped papules that usually occur in clusters. Often spread by scratching or shaving (Figs. 17.9–17.12).

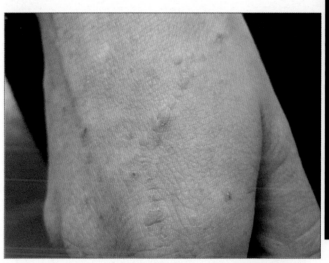

17.9   *Flat warts (verruca planae).* Lesions are slightly elevated flesh-colored papules. Note the linear configuration resulting from viral autoinoculation.

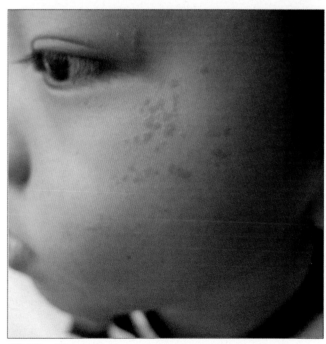

17.10   *Flat warts (verruca planae).* Tan-brownish flat-topped papules.

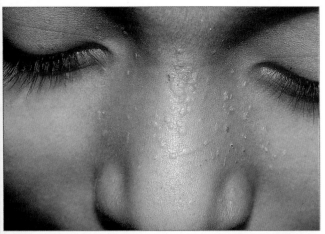

17.11 *Flat warts (verruca planae).* Lesions are slightly elevated papules that are the color of the patient's skin. Autoinoculation is apparent.

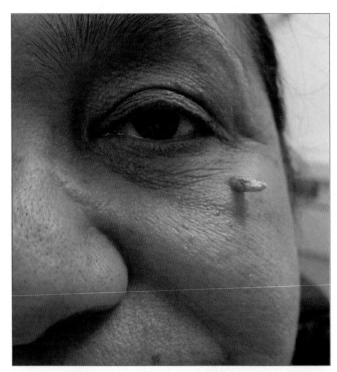

17.13 *Filiform wart.* Filiform wart in an adult.

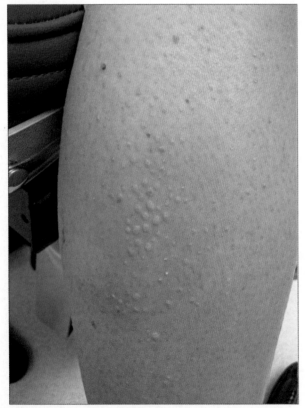

17.12 *Flat warts (verruca planae).* The warts were spread by leg shaving.

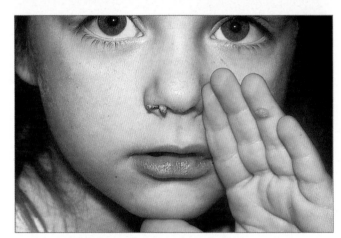

17.14 *Filiform wart.* This child has filiform warts on her nose and a common wart on her finger.

FILIFORM WARTS

- Thin, exophytic papule usually located on the face (Figs. 17.13–17.15).

GENITAL WARTS (*CONDYLOMA ACUMINATA*)

- Located on or in close proximity to genital skin; may be large and cauliflower-like, or they may consist of small papules (discussed in Chapter 28).

DIAGNOSIS

- Warts are usually diagnosed clinically.
- A biopsy should be performed if the diagnosis is in doubt or if the wart is not responding to conventional treatment, especially if a squamous cell carcinoma is suspected.

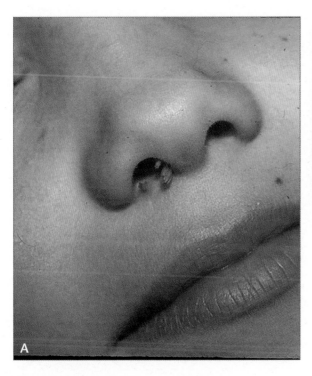

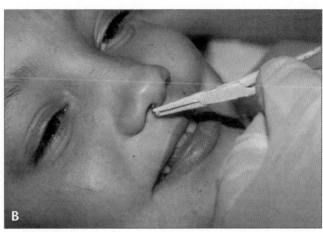

17.15 A and B: *Filiform wart treatment.* A relatively painless method is to dip a mosquito hemostat into LN$_2$ for 10 seconds and then gently grasp the wart for about 4 to 5 seconds. This treatment is repeated four to five times during each visit as tolerated.

 DIFFERENTIAL DIAGNOSIS

Common Warts
Molluscum Contagiosum
* *Dome-shaped shiny papules, central umbilication (see below).*

Seborrheic Keratosis
* *"Stuck-on" appearance.*
* *May be clinically indistinguishable from verrucae.*

Acrochordon (Skin Tag)
* *Smooth (not verrucous), small papules.*
* *May be clinically indistinguishable from verrucae.*

Solar Keratosis and Cutaneous Horn
* *Rough-textured papules in sun-exposed areas.*

Squamous Cell Carcinoma
* *Rough-textured papule, nodules, or ulcers in sun-exposed areas.*
* *A solitary squamous cell carcinoma under the nail may **easily be misdiagnosed as a subungual wart.***

Plantar Warts
Calluses
* *Broad-based hyperkeratotic plaques commonly found on the soles.*
* *Distinguished from plantar warts because they reveal an accentuation rather than interruption of skin markings.*

Corns (Clavi)
* *Similar to calluses, corns are thickened areas of the skin that develop in response to excessive pressure and friction. Like warts, corns interrupt skin markings.*

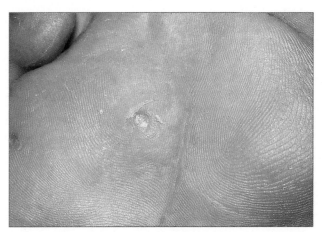

17.16 *Corn (clavus).* After paring, the circular central translucent core resembles a kernel of corn.

* *Can be distinguished by the lack of "black dots" and punctate bleeding after paring.*
* *Corns are circular and hard, and when pared down, will exhibit a polished or central translucent core, similar to a kernel of corn from which they take their name (Fig. 17.16).*

Flat Warts
Molluscum Contagiosum
Disseminated **cryptococcosis, toxoplasmosis**, and **histoplasmosis**
* *Noted especially in immunocompromised patients.*

MANAGEMENT OF WARTS
(Discussed in Chapter 6)

General Principles
- Warts often prove to be persistent and difficult to eradicate in many adults and in immunocompromised patients.
- The management of warts is challenging and there is no ideal treatment. The abundance of therapeutic modalities described in Chapter 6 is a reflection of the fact that none of them is uniformly effective.
- Adults often opt for more definitive treatment options such as electrocautery and curettage or excision.
- Before choosing a treatment, consider the patient's pain threshold, the type and size of the wart, the location of the lesion, and its cosmetic or psychological considerations.

IMPORTANT INFORMATION ABOUT PLANTAR WARTS
- **Melanoma** can mimic a plantar wart.
- **Verrucous carcinoma**, a slow-growing, locally invasive, well-differentiated squamous cell carcinoma, may also be easily mistaken for a plantar wart.

 SEE PATIENT HANDOUT "Warts" IN THE COMPANION eBOOK EDITION.

POINTS TO REMEMBER

- Freezing and other destructive treatment modalities do not kill the virus but merely destroy the "host" cells that harbor HPV.
- How to avoid getting warts? *Never shake hands. Never kiss anyone. Never walk barefoot. Never share towels. Live in a bubble...and there's still a good chance you'll get one.* HPV is highly prevalent.
- Shaving over warts in the beard area or on the legs with a razor blade tends to spread the lesions.
- A clinical "cure" is achieved when the skin lines are restored to a normal pattern and there is no recurrence.

BASICS

- Molluscum contagiosum (MC) is a common superficial viral infection of the epidermis that is most commonly seen in school-aged children.
- In adults, MC occurs in patients who are immunocompromised due to HIV or immunosuppressive medications (chemotherapy or other) or in sexually active young adults as a sexually transmitted disease.
- Although often a concern for parents of infected children, MC is rarely seen in immunocompetent adults.
- The clinical presentations of MC in adults are discussed here. Detailed pathogenesis, clinical manifestations, and management of MC are presented in Chapter 6.

CLINICAL MANIFESTATIONS

- MC lesions are dome-shaped, "waxy" or "pearly" appearing papules with a central white core or umbilication and most often appear on the face and eyelids (Figs. 17.17 and 17.18), the trunk, the axillae, the extremities (Fig. 17.19), and the genitalia. Number of lesions varies from one to hundreds.
- Lesions spread by sexual contact are often seen on the external genitalia (Fig. 17.20), lower abdominal wall, inner thighs, and pubic area. When seen in these locations in young children, MC may be a sign of sexual abuse.
- Immunocompromised patients present with "giant molluscum" consisting of coalescent double or triple lesions (Fig. 17.21). More than 100 lesions may be seen and are most commonly present on the face where they are spread by shaving. Such lesions are often chronic and are difficult to eradicate (discussed in Chapter 33).

DIAGNOSIS

- A shave biopsy is performed, if clinical appearance is not typical.
- A short application of liquid nitrogen often accentuates the central core (Figs. 17.22A,B).

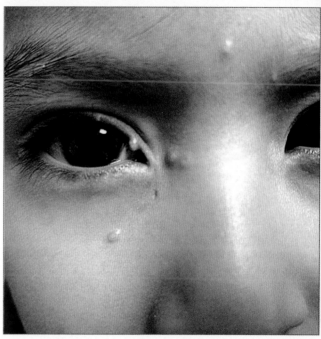

17.18 *Molluscum contagiosum.* This is a typical distribution of lesions on a child's face. Note lesions present on eyelid.

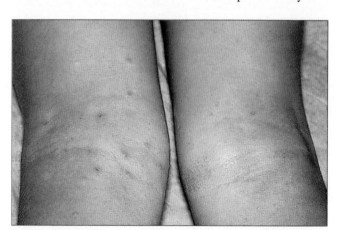

17.19 *Molluscum contagiosum.* Lesions are present on a background of atopic dermatitis of the flexural creases.

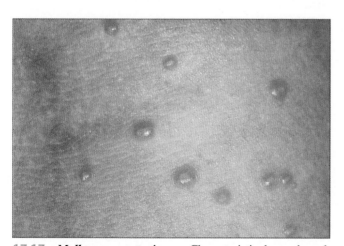

17.17 *Molluscum contagiosum.* Characteristic dome-shaped, shiny, waxy papules that have a central umbilicated core.

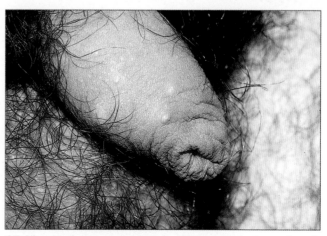

17.20 *Molluscum contagiosum.* Characteristic dome-shaped, shiny, waxy papules are present on the penis.

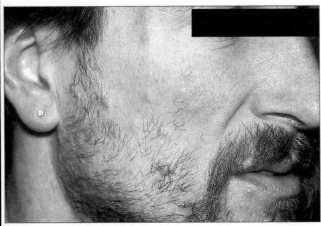

17.21 *Molluscum contagiosum.* Note the double and "giant lesions" on the face of a patient with acquired immunodeficiency syndrome.

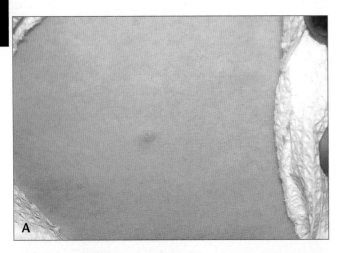

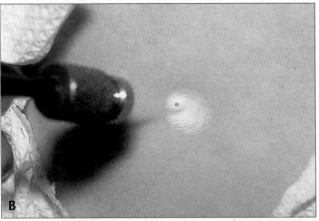

17.22 *Molluscum contagiosum.* **A:** Short application of liquid nitrogen (LN_2). **B:** LN_2 accentuates the central core.

DIFFERENTIAL DIAGNOSIS

Warts
- *Flat warts or genital warts can sometimes mimic molluscum.*
- *Close inspection will show lack of a central umbilication.*

Disseminated Cryptococcosis, Toxoplasmosis, and Histoplasmosis in Immunocompromised Patients

MANAGEMENT (Discussed in Chapter 6)

- Adults often prefer definitive treatment with curettage and electrodessication.
- Immunocompromised patients may be more challenging and require a multitude of treatments.
- Improving immune status with highly active antiretroviral therapy in HIV patients or reduction of immunosuppressive medications has been very effective in reducing the incidence and burden of MC.

HELPFUL HINTS

- Adults can often tolerate light electrodessication (at 1 to 2 W) and/or curettage without anesthesia.
- The application of a topical anesthetic cream under occlusion for 30 to 40 minutes can provide adequate anesthesia prior to removal.

POINTS TO REMEMBER

- MC rarely occurs in immunocompetent adults.
- When molluscum is present as a sexually transmitted disease consider testing for other STDs.

 SEE PATIENT HANDOUT "Molluscum Contagiosum" IN THE COMPANION eBOOK EDITION.

BASICS

- Herpes simplex virus (HSV) infections are caused by two virus types: HSV-1 and HSV-2. HSV-1 causes most nongenital skin infections.
- Nongenital HSV infection is extremely common. In fact, herpes-specific antibody (for type 1 and, less commonly, type 2) can be found in the serum of many adults who have never had clinical evidence of HSV. Asymptomatic shedding probably accounts for the widespread transmission of this ubiquitous virus.
- Patients who have HIV/AIDS or those who are under treatment with immunosuppressants for organ transplantation or cancer chemotherapy are at greatest risk for contracting severe recalcitrant HSV infections.
- Most primary HSV infections occur in childhood and are asymptomatic or subclinical. The clinical presentations and management of HSV infections in children are presented in Chapter 6.

PATHOGENESIS

- These highly contagious viruses are spread by direct contact with the skin or mucous membranes of an individual who is actively shedding the virus during an active outbreak or with body fluids containing the virus.
- After initial acute infection, HSV, a double-stranded DNA virus, establishes latent infection in the local nerve ganglia.
- The virus remains latent until precipitating factors or triggers, such as sunlight exposure, menses, fever, common colds, immunosuppression, or stress reactivate it.

CLINICAL MANIFESTATIONS

- Symptomatic primary HSV infections tend to be more severe than those of recurrent disease; findings may include gingivostomatitis, fever, sore throat, as well as submandibular or cervical lymphadenopathy.
- Encephalitis and aseptic meningitis are rare complications of primary infections.
- Distinguishing primary HSV infection from severe cases of recurrent HSV can be difficult.
- The following sequence of events describes the easily recognizable evolution of HSV infection:
  - A single vesicle or a group of vesicles overlies an erythematous base (Fig. 17.23). Vesicles may sag in the center (umbilicate).
  - Vesicles may become pustules, or they may dry and become crusts or erosions (Figs. 17.24 and 17.25).
  - Lesions generally heal without scarring.

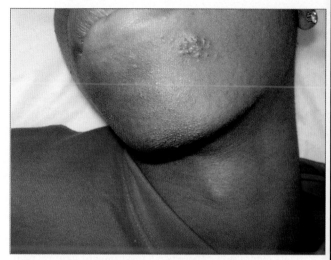

17.23 *Herpes simplex virus.* In this typical grouping, umbilicated vesicles overlie an erythematous base.

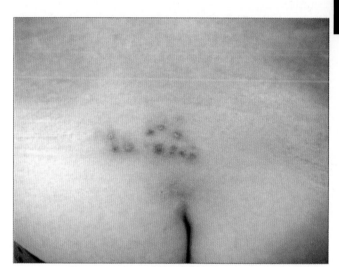

17.24 *Herpes simplex virus.* Collapsing vesicles overlie an erythematous base.

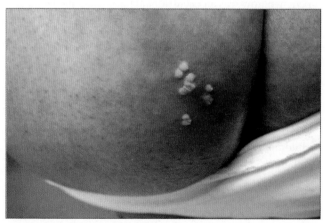

17.25 *Herpes simplex virus.* Vesicles have evolved into pustules.

CLINICAL VARIANTS

PRIMARY OROLABIAL HERPES SIMPLEX (DISCUSSED IN CHAPTER 6)

- Primary HSV-1 infection most commonly affects the lips (herpes labialis), oral mucosa, or pharynx (Fig. 17.26).
- Painful vesicles on an erythematous base may develop on the lips, gingiva, buccal mucosa, palate, or tongue and are often associated with erythema and edema. Lesions tend to ulcerate and heal within 2 to 3 weeks.

RECURRENT OROLABIAL HERPES SIMPLEX

- Symptoms are generally milder and the number of lesions fewer than those associated with primary HSV infection.
- Patients commonly experience a prodrome of itching, pain, or numbness.
- The recurrent vesicular lesions eventually erode and form crusts.
- Infrequently, regional lymphadenopathy occurs.
- Over time, recurrences decrease in frequency and often stop altogether.
- Persistent ulcerative or verrucous vegetative lesions may be seen in immunocompromised patients.
- Most cases of recurrent erythema multiforme appear to be triggered by recurrent (both clinical and subclinical) HSV episodes (discussed in Chapter 27).
- Lesions tend to recur at, or near, the same location within the distribution of a sensory nerve.
- Such recurrences are most often seen on or near the vermilion border of the lip (herpes labialis) (Fig. 17.27).

HERPETIC WHITLOW

- Painful herpetic whitlow results from the direct inoculation of the virus onto the skin of the fingertip (Fig. 17.28).
- Before the current stringent infection control measures and the widespread use of gloves by health care providers, herpetic whitlow was an occupational hazard among dental and medical health care personnel whose fingertips came in contact with infected oral or respiratory excretions.

ECZEMA HERPETICUM

- Also known as Kaposi varicelliform eruption, eczema herpeticum (Fig. 17.29) is an uncommon disseminated form of HSV infection caused by HSV-1. It occurs mainly in children who have severe atopic dermatitis, burns, or other inflammatory skin conditions (discussed in Chapter 6).

HERPES GLADIATORUM

- Herpes gladiatorum is caused by HSV-1 and is seen as a papular or vesicular eruption on the torsos of athletes in sports involving close physical contact (e.g., wrestling).

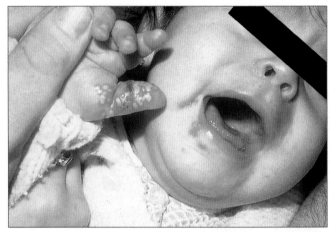

17.26 Primary herpes simplex virus infection. This infant has multiple vesicles and pustules as well as gingivostomatitis.

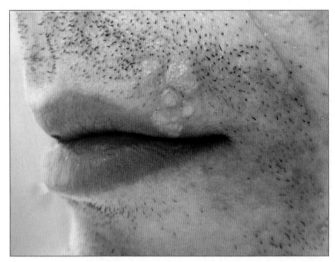

17.27 Recurrent herpes simplex virus infection (herpes labialis). Lesions are evident on the vermilion border of the lip and beyond.

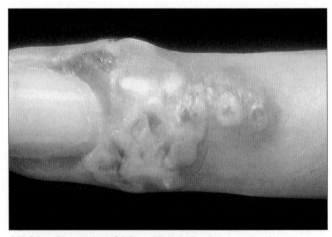

17.28 Herpetic whitlow. This infection in a health care worker was caused by a needle puncture.

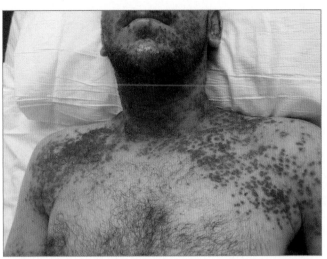

17.29 *Eczema herpeticum (Kaposi varicelliform eruption).* This patient has a disseminated form of HSV infection. The patient has underlying atopic dermatitis.

DISSEMINATED HERPES SIMPLEX

• Widespread and extensive herpes simplex infection can occur in individuals who are immunocompromised (i.e., hematologic malignancy, bone marrow or organ transplant recipients, or HIV infection).
• HSV infection in immunocompromised patients, may present with atypical signs and symptoms of HSV infection such as larger lesions in atypical locations and a more widespread distribution. Ulcers may be pustular, necrotic, or verrucous and tend to be more persistent.

HERPETIC SYCOSIS

• Herpetic sycosis presents as a vesiculopustular eruption, in a perifollicular distribution in the beard area of men.
• Often results from autoinoculation after shaving.

OCULAR HERPES SIMPLEX

• Herpes conjunctivitis, keratitis, uveitis, optic neuritis, and retinitis are possible sequelae of HSV infection of the eye.

DIAGNOSIS

• The diagnosis of HSV is usually based on clinical appearance and history.
• The following tests performed on "fresh" lesions, may help to confirm the diagnosis:
  • A Tzanck preparation is a bedside test that can rapidly determine the presence of HSV or VZV by showing multinucleated giant cells (Fig. 17.30). (See the description of the Tzanck procedure in the sidebar.)
  • Viral culture can detect and type HSV but can take 2 to 5 days. Specimen should be obtained from the base of an intact vesicle; ideally early in the course of the infection. The false-negative rate increases after 48 hours of lesion onset.
  • Direct fluorescent antibody (DFA) testing can be performed on cells obtained from the base of an intact vesicle smeared

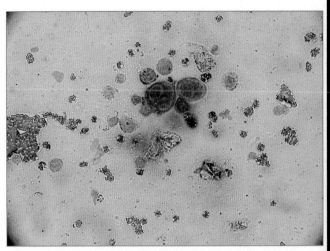

17.30 *Positive Tzanck preparation.* Note the multinucleated giant cells with large nuclei and the presence of normal sized keratinocytes which are closer to the size of neutrophils.

on a slide (similar to the specimen obtained for a Tzanck preparation). When available, it is the preferred diagnostic test because of its high sensitivity, rapid turnaround time (<24 hours), and its ability to distinguish between HSV and VZV.
• Polymerase chain reaction (PCR) is now increasingly being used as a quick, sensitive, and specific method to detect HSV DNA in specimens from the skin.
• Serologic tests for HSV are generally not very useful because the majority of the general adult population has antibodies to herpes simplex; however, primary HSV infection can be documented by demonstration of seroconversion, high titers, or rising titers.

TZANCK PREPARATION

Positive Tzanck Preparation. This test does not distinguish between herpes simplex and herpes zoster.

A Tzanck preparation is used to aid in the diagnosis of HSV, herpes zoster, and VZV. This technique furnishes an inexpensive, efficient provisional diagnosis, but it does not enable one to distinguish HSV from VZV.

1. For best results, a fresh, intact vesicle or bulla usually present for less than 24 hours is preferred.
2. After the lesion is swabbed with an alcohol preparation, the blister is unroofed by piercing it with a no. 11 blade or a large bore needle, followed by blotting with gauze.
3. The underlying moist base of the lesion is then scraped with a no. 15 scalpel blade, and a thin layer of material is spread onto a glass slide.
4. The specimen is then air-dried and stained with a supravital stain such as Giemsa, Wright, or methylene blue, which is left on for 1 minute.
5. The specimen is then gently flooded with tap water for 15 seconds to remove any remaining stain.
6. Examination, initially under 40-power magnification and then 100-power oil immersion, helps identify the characteristic multinucleated giant cells.

DIFFERENTIAL DIAGNOSIS

Aphthous Stomatitis

- *Lesions of aphthous stomatitis are small, punched-out erosions that occur on the tongue and on the buccal, labial, and gingival mucosa (see Chapter 21).*
- *Typically consist of painful, shallow, gray or yellow 2- to 3-mm erosions.*

Hand-Foot-and-Mouth Disease (HFMD)

- *Lesions are generally asymptomatic in adults.*
- *Oval erythematous erosions are most often seen on the soft palate and uvula (see Chapter 7). May also appear on the hands and feet.*
- *HFMD often presents with a mild prodrome of fever and malaise prior to mucosal and skin eruption.*

- *The enterovirus, coxsackievirus A type 16 is the etiologic agent involved in most cases of HFMD, but the illness is also associated with other enteroviruses, such as enterovirus 71 (EV-71).*

Extraorolabial Herpes Simplex
Herpes Zoster

- *Lesions of herpes zoster are unilateral, dermatomal in distribution, and often painful (see the discussion of herpes zoster below).*
- *Lesions are also grouped but tend to vary in size.*
- *May be clinically indistinguishable from HSV when lesions are located in a single focus.*

MANAGEMENT

Topical Therapy

- Skin symptoms may be eased by soaking in **Burow solution** (aluminum acetate) two to three times daily. Alternatively, soaks with water or saline may help dry the eruption and may prevent secondary infection.
- Patients can lessen the discomfort of oral HSV lesions by applying viscous lidocaine applications or OTC "caine" products, taking oral analgesics, or sucking on ice cubes for intraoral lesions.
- Patients in whom sun exposure incites recurrent HSV of the lips may apply an opaque sun-blocking agent before sun exposure.
- Topical acyclovir 5% ointment (**Zovirax**), penciclovir 1% cream (**Denavir**), and docosanol 10% cream (**Abreva**) are not very effective treatments, but they may help reduce healing time.

Systemic Therapy

- Pharmacologic agents used for the treatment of HSV include acyclovir, valacyclovir, and famciclovir. Valacyclovir is rapidly converted to acyclovir, and its bioavailability is greater than that of acyclovir. Similarly, famciclovir is converted to the more bioavailable penciclovir.
- Dose reduction is recommended for patients who have renal impairment.
- The use of valacyclovir should be given cautiously in renal and bone marrow transplant recipients and in those infected with HIV because of reports of thrombotic thrombocytopenic purpura and hemolytic uremic syndrome.

Primary Herpes Simplex

- Valacyclovir (**Valtrex**), 1 g twice daily for 7 to 10 days.
- Famciclovir (**Famvir**), 250 mg three times daily for 7 to 10 days.

- **Acyclovir**, 200 mg five times daily, or 400 mg three times daily for 10 days.

Recurrent Herpes Simplex

Treatment should be initiated at the first sign of prodrome, because it can often abort the lesions. The following are treatment options:

- Valacyclovir (**Valtrex**), 2 g twice daily for 1 day taken about 12 hours apart. This is a shorter, more economical course.
- Famciclovir (**Famvir**), single-day therapy: 1,000 mg in the morning and 1,000 mg in the evening, or 125 mg twice daily for 5 days. In HIV-positive patients, 500 mg twice a day is given for 7 days.
- **Acyclovir**, 200 mg 5 times/day; or 400 mg three times daily; or 800 mg twice daily for 5 days.
- For frequent recurrences (more than six recurrences per year), persistent HSV, severe disease, or recurrent erythema multiforme, **long-term suppressive oral therapy** may be used.
- Treatment options for long-term suppressive therapy include the following:
  - Valacyclovir, 1 g daily for 6 to 12 months; attempt to taper dose to 500 mg or to discontinue after 6 to 12 months.
  - Famciclovir, 250 mg twice daily for 12 months.
  - Acyclovir, 400 mg twice daily for 12 months.
- After 1 year of treatment with these agents, the need for daily suppressive therapy should be reassessed.
- Immunocompromised hosts with severe infection, patients with Kaposi varicelliform eruption, or with HSV encephalitis often require intravenous acyclovir therapy.

 SEE PATIENT HANDOUT "Herpes Simplex" IN THE COMPANION eBOOK EDITION.

HELPFUL HINTS

- Recurrent aphthous stomatitis (canker sores) has no known viral association but has a clinical appearance and course similar to recurrent herpes labialis, and is often misdiagnosed as such. Recurrent HSV lesions however, infrequently occur *inside the mouth*.
- HSV lesions can be seen inside the mouth in a primary infection, or in immunocompromised patients.
- Although HSV infections may occur anywhere on the body, 70% to 90% of HSV-1 infections occur above the umbilicus.
- In contrast, 70% to 90% of HSV-2 infections occur below the umbilicus (discussed in Chapter 28).
- Pregnant women with active genital HSV may need a cesarean section to prevent neonatal HSV, a potentially fatal disease.

POINTS TO REMEMBER

- Intraoral ulcers in immunocompetent patients are most likely canker sores (aphthous stomatitis).
- Recurrent HSV attacks can be aborted by short-term treatment with oral antivirals administered during the prodromal stage.
- Frequent recurrences can be suppressed with daily oral antivirals.

Herpes Zoster

BASICS

- Herpes zoster ("shingles") is caused by the same herpesvirus that causes varicella, the varicella-zoster virus (VZV). Primary infection with VZV manifests as varicella, commonly referred to as "chickenpox" (discussed in Chapter 7), an illness that has dramatically decreased in incidence since the introduction of the VZV vaccine. After the initial infection, the virus remains latent in the sensory ganglia. Reactivation of the latent VZV results in herpes zoster.
- The VZV vaccine is a live attenuated vaccine, thus herpes zoster can still result after vaccination.

PATHOGENESIS

- Reactivation—into dermatomal "shingles"—may be caused by severe illness or infection with HIV, but most often it occurs spontaneously, without an obvious precipitating cause and is most likely a sign that immunity to VZV, which most people acquire in childhood, has decreased.
- Reactivated VZV results in the anterograde migration of virions from the dorsal root ganglia to the skin resulting in a local vesicobullous eruption in a single, or less often multiple adjacent, sensory dermatomes.
- The risk of herpes zoster increases with age and is 8 to 10 times more likely to develop in people 60 years of age or older. The disease also frequently develops in immunocompromised patients, such as transplant recipients and those with HIV infection or malignancy, particularly lymphoproliferative malignancies (e.g., Hodgkin disease).
- The infectious course of herpes zoster infection, or VZV infection, is similar to that of HSV infection (see above).

CLINICAL MANIFESTATIONS

- Several days to weeks before the cutaneous eruption, patients may experience the following focal (dermatomal) symptoms: pain, numbness, pruritus, paresthesia, and skin tenderness or sensitivity (tactile allodynia).
- The pain associated with herpes zoster is neuropathic in origin and has been described as "burning," "crushing," or "stabbing." Occasionally, patients presenting with such pain have been thought to have a myocardial infarction or pleurisy, until the characteristic eruption of herpes zoster establishes the diagnosis.
- Pain may be severe and debilitating in patients older than 50 but in children, herpes zoster is often asymptomatic.
- The following sequence of events describes the evolution of herpes zoster:
  - Lesions begin as edematous, erythematous, urticaria-like papules that rapidly mature into clustered vesicles (blisters) or bullae overlying the erythematous base. Lesions tend to vary more in size than do the lesions of HSV (Figs. 17.31 and 17.32).

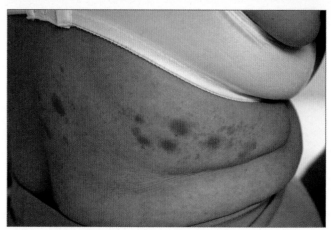

17.31 *Herpes zoster.* "Juicy," erythematous, urticaria-like papules. The patient complained of acute burning pain in a "zosteriform" distribution.

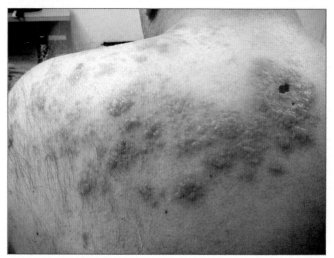

17.32 *Herpes zoster.* Multiple vesicles and bullae of various sizes are grouped on an erythematous base. (From Goodheart HP. *Goodheart's Same-Site Differential Diagnosis.* Philadelphia, PA: Lippincott Williams & Wilkins; 2011.)

- Successive crops continue to appear for 6 to 8 days. The blisters sometimes umbilicate (sag in the middle); and occasionally become pustular and/or hemorrhagic (Fig. 17.33).
- In time, the vesicles dry into crusts or erosions that may heal and disappear completely; or resolve with postinflammatory hyperpigmentation or hypopigmentation and, possibly, scarring.
- Lesions of herpes zoster in HIV-infected or other immunocompromised patients tend to be more verrucous and ulcerative, and often heal with scars.
- Infrequently, zoster may present with dermatomal pain that is accompanied or followed by nonbullous or urticaria-like lesions. Rarely, skin lesions are absent ("zoster sine herpete"). Such cases can be difficult to identify because of the absence of a characteristic eruption.

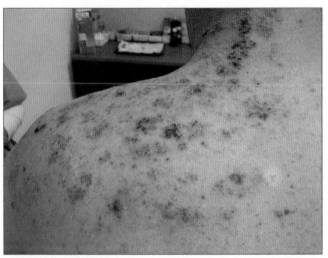

17.33 *Herpes zoster.* Drying hemorrhagic crusts appear in a "zosteriform" distribution.

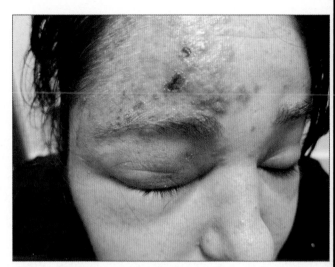

17.34 *Herpes zoster ophthalmicus.* This condition affects the first branch of the fifth cranial nerve.

DISTRIBUTION OF LESIONS

- Lesions of herpes zoster occur in a characteristic unilateral dermatomal ("zosteriform") distribution.
- Occasionally, lesions can involve contiguous dermatomes, extend beyond the midline, or occur bilaterally.
- Although it can affect any dermatome, herpes zoster is most commonly found on the thoracic, trigeminal, lumbosacral, or cervical dermatomes.
- Immunocompromised patients have a greater risk of multi-dermatomal zoster, recurrent zoster, and dissemination beyond the skin (e.g., into the eyes or the lungs).

COMPLICATIONS

- Elderly persons and immunocompromised patients also tend to have more severe disease, with complications such as postherpetic neuralgia (PHN), disseminated zoster, and chronic herpes zoster.
- **PHN** is defined as pain persisting for more than 1 month after the initial eruption of herpes zoster. The pain may also develop after a pain-free interval. The incidence of PHN increases with increasing age and lowered immune status.
- In many elderly patients, PHN can cause chronic depression, anxiety, and social isolation.
- Zoster that occurs in the ophthalmic division of the trigeminal nerve (V1 of cranial nerve V) is called **herpes zoster ophthalmicus** (Fig. 17.34). Eye involvement can present as conjunctivitis, acute retinal necrosis, uveitis, and/or retinal arteritis and can lead to blindness. Ophthalmic zoster warrants an immediate ophthalmologic consultation.
- Zoster involvement of the geniculate ganglion of the facial nerve (cranial nerve VII) is referred to as the **Ramsay Hunt syndrome** and can result in facial nerve paralysis, loss of taste in the anterior two-thirds of the tongue, and

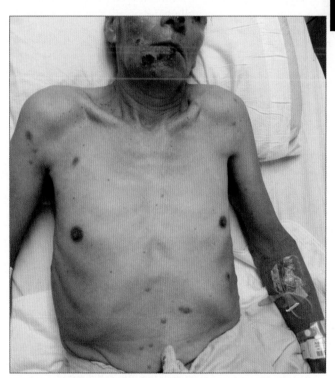

17.35 *Herpes zoster (disseminated).* Scattered hemorrhagic bullae and crusted lesions in a multidermatomal distribution in an immunocompromised patient.

dryness of the eyes and mouth. If the eighth cranial nerve is also involved tinnitus, hearing loss and/or vertigo can occur.

- **Disseminated Herpes Zoster** (Fig. 17.35) is the occurrence of >20 lesions outside the primary dermatome and usually occurs in immunocompromised patients. This condition can become chronic and indistinguishable from varicella.

- VZV infection occasionally occurs in pregnant women. A primary VZV infection (varicella) may result in severe fetal abnormalities; however, the development of herpes zoster during pregnancy does not appear to harm the developing fetus.

DIAGNOSIS

- Most straightforward cases of herpes zoster are diagnosed on the basis of clinical appearance of the lesions accompanied by pain, in a dermatomal distribution.
- If necessary, in atypical presentations, a Tzanck smear should be obtained from the base of a fresh lesion (see the discussion of Tzanck preparation earlier in this chapter). A positive result suggests either HSV or VZV infection.
- A viral culture, or direct fluorescence antibody (DFA) testing, may be necessary to establish the diagnosis. DFA testing is more sensitive than conventional viral cultures because of the lability of varicella-zoster virus (VZV).
- A skin biopsy is generally unnecessary, but it can help to confirm the diagnosis.

 DIFFERENTIAL DIAGNOSIS

Herpes Simplex Virus Infection

- *When HSV presents in a semidermatomal or linear distribution within a dermatome, it may be clinically indistinguishable from herpes zoster.*
- *The vesicles of herpes simplex, however, tend to be more uniform in size and are usually less painful than those seen in herpes zoster.*
- *Recurrence at the same site strongly suggests HSV infection.*

Poison Ivy or Allergic Contact Dermatitis

- *Poison ivy dermatitis or other allergic contact dermatitis (ACD) can occur in a linear array of blisters within a dermatome and suggest a dermatomal distribution.*
- *Poison ivy dermatitis (or other ACD), however, is pruritic and painless and most patients offer a history of contact with poison ivy or poison oak.*

 MANAGEMENT

Topical Therapy

For the acute episode of herpes zoster, the following treatments are available without a prescription:

- **Burow solution.** Wet dressings with Burow solution (aluminum acetate) are soothing and drying; so are moist soaks with water or saline.
- **Topical anesthetic "caines"** such as benzocaine may be helpful.

Systemic Therapy

Pain control is generally the paramount concern in herpes zoster.

- Oral analgesics, such as **acetaminophen, aspirin**, and other **nonsteroidal anti-inflammatory drugs**, as well as mild **narcotics**, are helpful in mild, self-limited cases.
- Both **valacyclovir** and **famciclovir** are most effective when they are given within 72 hours of the appearance of the zoster eruption. They are equally effective in accelerating cutaneous healing, shortening the duration of the acute episode, and in decreasing the incidence of PHN.
- Valacyclovir is less expensive than famciclovir; however, it should be given cautiously in immunocompromised patients and in reduced dosages in those with chronic renal disease. Both valacyclovir and famciclovir

are superior to acyclovir, which is reserved for use in children and for intravenous administration.

Treatment regimens for immunocompetent adult patients with herpes zoster include the following:

- Valacyclovir (**Valtrex**), 1 g, three times daily for 7 days. Famciclovir (Famvir), 500 mg, three times daily for 7 days. **Acyclovir**, 800 mg, five times daily for 7 days.
- Immunocompromised patients may require intravenous acyclovir. **Intravenous foscarnet** is used for acyclovir-resistant VZV infection.

Adjunctive Corticosteroids

- The use of a short course of systemic corticosteroids in combination with oral acyclovir, valacyclovir, or famciclovir to decrease nerve inflammation has been controversial. Although the combination can reduce acute pain, there is no difference in the incidence or severity of postherpetic neuralgia when compared to monotherapy with antivirals.
- It should be kept in mind that elderly patients, in whom PHN is more common, are more likely to experience significant adverse side effects from systemic corticosteroids than are younger patients.

continued on page 297

MANAGEMENT *Continued*

Treatment of Postherpetic Neuralgia (PHN)

- Treatment of PHN is problematic. The following treatments have had varying degrees of success and none appears to be totally satisfactory. Optimally, the acute episode of herpes zoster should be treated as quickly as possible after onset to decrease the risk of PHN.
- **Lidoderm** (lidocaine 5% patch) is the only lidocaine-based, topical medicine approved by the United States Food and Drug Association (FDA) for the treatment of PHN.
- Capsaicin (**Zostrix**) contains the active molecule in red hot chili peppers, capsaicin, that helps to deplete substance P, a pain impulse transmitter. It is available OTC and is applied three to five times daily. Unfortunately, many patients cannot tolerate the burning sensation that occurs after application.
- Also FDA approved for PHN, **Qutenza** (capsaicin 8% patch) is now available by prescription only.
- Low-dose tricyclic antidepressants (e.g., **amitriptyline**) may be helpful. Higher doses of tricyclic antidepressants—used alone or in combination with **phenothiazines** may also be tried.
- Serotonin and norepinephrine reuptake inhibitors such as duloxetine (**Cymbalta**) and venlafaxine (**Effexor**) can be helpful.
- Gabapentin (**Neurontin**), an antiseizure drug, has been helpful in reducing pain in patients with acute and chronic herpes zoster. A week of oral antiviral therapy combined with 4 to 8 weeks of gabapentin has been reported as having 77% reduction in the postherpetic neuralgia rate in patients with herpes zoster.

- **Neurosurgical procedures** include nerve blocks with local anesthetics. Epidural injections of anesthetic medications and corticosteroids have been shown to be of benefit to some patients.
- **Intralesional corticosteroids** may be given as subcutaneous injections.
- Botulinum toxin (**Botox**) injections into the affected area have had some success.
- **Transcutaneous electrical nerve stimulation** may be useful.
- **Acupuncture** and **biofeedback** may be helpful.

Prevention

- The **Zostavax** vaccine has been shown to reduce the risk of developing herpes zoster and postherpetic neuralgia in adults older than 60 years of age.
- Zostavax contains the same live attenuated virus as the varicella vaccine but is far more potent and the preventive effect is thought to be a result of boosting cell-mediated immunity to VZV.
- Since 2006, vaccination with a single dose of the vaccine is recommended for immunocompetent individuals aged 60 or older whether or not they have had chickenpox or a previous episode of herpes zoster.
- Zoster vaccination is contraindicated in people with active, untreated tuberculosis, pregnant women, and immunocompromised individuals.

 SEE PATIENT HANDOUT "Herpes Zoster" IN THE COMPANION eBOOK EDITION.

HELPFUL HINT

- Second episodes of herpes zoster in immunocompetent people are unusual, probably because of the immunologic "boosting" effect of the initial zoster episode.

POINTS TO REMEMBER

- Herpes zoster, particularly if recurrent or disseminated, may be an early indicator of an immunosuppressive disorder or a lymphoproliferative disease.
- An evolving herpes zoster eruption should be treated with antiviral drugs as early as possible.
- Patients with herpes zoster can transmit the virus as chickenpox to persons who have not already been infected with this virus.

Superficial Fungal Infections

OVERVIEW

Superficial fungi are capable of germinating on the dead outer horny layer of skin by producing enzymes (keratinases) that allow them to digest keratin, resulting in an accumulation of epidermal scale and an inflammatory response. Cutaneous fungal infections are named for the location on the body and include tinea pedis, tinea cruris, tinea capitis (discussed in Chapter 9), tinea corporis, and tinea unguium (onychomycosis). Yeast infections such as cutaneous candidiasis and tinea versicolor are also discussed in this chapter. (N.B.Despite having "tinea" in its name, tinea versicolor is actually a yeast.)

Fungal infections may be acquired by person-to-person contact, animal contact, especially with kittens and puppies, as well as contact with inanimate objects such as shared towels and contaminated exercise machines. Additional risk factors include a family history of tinea infections, a lowered immune status as seen in patients with acquired immunodeficiency syndrome (HIV/AIDS), diabetes, collagen vascular diseases, or those on long-term systemic steroid therapy. Infections typically occur in the warm, moist, occluded cutaneous environments found in the groin, axillae, and feet.

MAKING THE DIAGNOSIS

- A presumptive diagnosis is often made on clinical grounds; however, a direct potassium hydroxide (KOH) examination or a fungal culture is necessary to make a definitive diagnosis.
- If necessary, a Periodic acid-Schiff (PAS) stain on biopsy specimens can be helpful.
- Wood lamp examination may be useful in some cases of suspected tinea capitis and tinea versicolor.

IN THIS CHAPTER...

➤ **DERMATOPHYTE INFECTIONS**

- Tinea pedis
- Tinea cruris
- Tinea corporis (Ringworm)
- Onychomycosis (Tinea unguium)

➤ **YEAST INFECTIONS**

- Cutaneous candidiasis
- Tinea versicolor (Pityriasis versicolor)

- Most dermatophyte infections in North America are caused by *Trichophyton rubrum, Trichophyton mentagrophytes, Trichophyton tonsurans,* or *Microsporum canis,* a zoophilic fungus that is most often spread by contact from cats or dogs.
- Infections with a dermatophyte are termed *tinea* and are then further classified according to the location of the infection on the body as in tinea capitis, a dermatophyte infection of the scalp.
- In some patients, dermatophyte infections may penetrate the hair follicle and involve the dermis, a condition termed Majocchi granuloma.
- It is well known that tinea pedis, tinea manuum, tinea cruris, tinea corporis, or tinea capitis can induce *autoeczematization* (also known as an "id" or dermatophytid reaction), a secondary pruritic, dermatitis that occurs distant from the site of infection (see Chapter 13). The pathogenesis may involve an immunologic reaction to circulating immune complexes to fungal antigens.

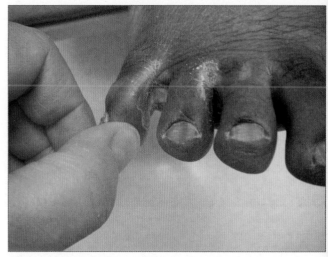

18.1 *Interdigital tinea pedis (toe web infection).* Note maceration.

TINEA PEDIS ("ATHLETE'S FOOT")

BASICS

- Tinea pedis is an extremely common problem seen mainly in young men. Ubiquitous media advertisements for athlete's foot sprays and creams are testimony to the commonplace occurrence of this annoying dermatosis.
- Most cases are caused by *T. rubrum,* which evokes a minimal inflammatory response and less often by *T. mentagrophytes,* which may produce vesicles and bullae. Much less frequently, *Epidermophyton floccosum* may be the causative agent.
- There are three distinguishable clinical forms: type 1: interdigital; type 2: chronic plantar; and type 3: acute vesicular.

CLINICAL VARIANTS

Type 1: Interdigital Tinea Pedis

- The most common type of tinea pedis is seen predominantly in men between the ages of 18 and 40 years and is unusual in children.
- Often asymptomatic; however, may itch intensely.
- Scale, maceration, and fissures are characteristic (Fig. 18.1).
- Toe web involvement especially between the third and fourth and the fourth and fifth toes; however, any web space may be involved (Fig. 18.2).
- Marked inflammation and fissures suggest secondary bacterial superinfection.

Type 2: Chronic Plantar Tinea Pedis

- Chronic plantar tinea pedis is also called the "moccasin" type of tinea pedis.
- Symptoms are absent or minimal (e.g., itching); however, painful fissures may occur.
- Patients are often not aware of this, and if untreated it usually persists indefinitely.

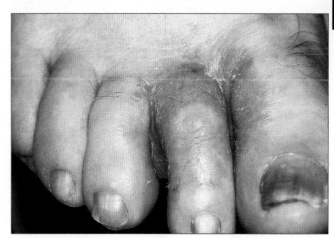

18.2 *Interdigital tinea pedis.* Here the lesions are more inflammatory.

- Lesions consist of diffuse or focal, asymptomatic scaling of the soles that are often considered to be "dry skin" by patients.
- Over time, the entire plantar surface of the foot becomes involved.
- Borders are distinct along the sides of the feet ("moccasin" distribution) (Figs. 18.3 and 18.4).
- There is often nail involvement.

"Two Feet, One Hand" (Palmar/Plantar) Tinea Pedis

- Tinea can present on one or both palms (*tinea manuum*). Not infrequently, it appears in a "two feet, one hand" distribution. This is pathognomonic for tinea (Fig. 18.5). Nail dystrophy (onychomycosis) is also often present.
- Management is similar to that for chronic tinea pedis.

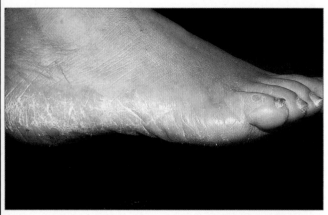

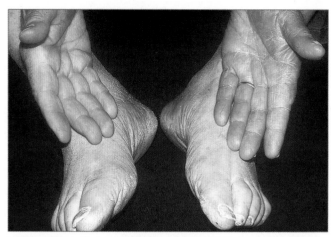

18.3 *Tinea pedis.* Chronic scaly infection of the plantar surface of the foot in a "moccasin" distribution.

18.5 *"Two feet, one hand" variant of tinea pedis.* The scale is present on one hand only. These findings are pathognomonic. Note the toenail involvement.

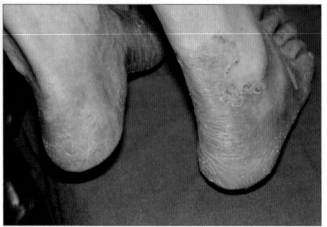

18.4 *Tinea pedis.* Chronic tinea extending to the Achilles area in this patient. (From Goodheart HP. *Goodheart's Same-Site Differential Diagnosis.* Philadelphia, PA: Lippincott Williams & Wilkins, 2011.)

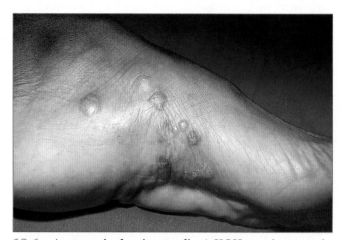

18.6 *Acute vesicular tinea pedis.* A KOH or culture specimen is obtained from under the roof of a vesicle.

Type 3: Acute Vesicular Tinea Pedis
- This is the least common clinical variant of tinea pedis.
- Tends to be quite pruritic.
- Vesicles and bullae generally occur on the sole, great toe, and instep of the foot (Fig. 18.6).

DIAGNOSIS
- A positive KOH examination or fungal culture is diagnostic.
- In acute vesicular tinea pedis, specimens taken for KOH or culture should be obtained from the inner part of the blister roof.

 DIFFERENTIAL DIAGNOSIS

Atopic Dermatitis
- *May be clinically indistinguishable from tinea pedis.*
- *KOH examination negative; fungal culture no growth.*
- *An atopic predisposition or other atopic symptoms may be present.*

Contact Dermatitis
- *Occurs most often on the dorsum of the feet.*

Palmoplantar Psoriasis
- *Scale tends to be quite thick.*
- *Psoriasis may be present elsewhere on the body.*

Dyshidrotic Eczema
- *May mimic acute vesicular tinea pedis.*
- *KOH examination negative; fungal culture no growth.*
- *Is usually very itchy.*

MANAGEMENT

Type 1: Interdigital

- For acute oozing and maceration, **Burow solution** (1% aluminum acetate or 5% aluminum subacetate) wet dressing compresses applied for 20 minutes, two to three times daily may be helpful.
- Broad-spectrum topical antifungal creams such as ketoconazole 2% (**Nizoral**), ciclopirox (**Loprox**), or clotrimazole 1% (**Lotrimin**) are applied to affected areas especially in the interdigital web spaces once or twice daily. (See Table 18.1.)

Type 2: Chronic Plantar

- Chronic tinea pedis is the most difficult type of tinea pedis to cure, because topical agents do not effectively penetrate the thickened epidermis.
- Treatment generally requires oral antifungal agents such as the following:
  - Terbinafine (**Lamisil**) 250 mg once daily for 30 days or longer, if necessary.
  - Itraconazole (**Sporanox**) 200 mg once daily for 30 days or longer, if necessary.
  - Fluconazole (**Diflucan**) 150 to 200 mg once daily for 4 to 6 weeks, if necessary.

Type 3: Acute Vesicular

- Treatment is similar to that of type 1, although **systemic** as well as **topical antifungals** may be necessary.

Infection

- Secondary infection may be treated with "bleach baths", topical antibiotics, or, if necessary, oral antibiotics.

Prevention

- **Prevention** consists of maintaining dryness and decreasing friction and maceration in the area by
  - using a hairdryer set on "cool" after bathing to dry the feet and interdigital web spaces.
  - daily application of an OTC absorbent powder, such as **Zeasorb-AF** that contains miconazole as an active antifungal ingredient applied after the eruption clears to prevent recurrence.

 SEE PATIENT HANDOUTS "Athlete's Foot (Tinea Pedis)" and "Burow solution" IN THE COMPANION eBOOK EDITION.

Table 18.1 TOPICAL ANTIFUNGAL DRUG FORMULARY

AGENT	APPLICATION	AVAILABILITY	COMMENTS
Over-the-counter			
Terbinafine 1% (**Lamisil**)	1–4 wks, twice daily	Cream, solution, spray	Tinea (not indicated for *Candida*)
Clotrimazole 1% (**Lotrimin**)	Twice daily	Cream, lotion, solution	Tinea, *Candida,* tinea versicolor
Miconazole 2% (**Micatin**)	Twice daily	Cream, lotion, spray	Tinea, *Candida,* tinea versicolor
Tolnaftate 1% (**Tinactin**)	Twice daily	Cream	Tinea
Selenium sulfide 1% (**Selsun Blue**)	Apply daily to wide area for 10 min, followed by a shower	Shampoo	Tinea versicolor
Miconazole 2% (**Zeasorb**)	As needed	Powder	Tinea, *Candida,* tinea versicolor; antifungal, antifriction/drying agent
Prescription			
Ketoconazole 2% (**Nizoral**)	Once daily	Cream	Tinea, *Candida,* tinea versicolor
Econazole 1% (**Spectazole**)	4 wks, once daily	Cream	Tinea, *Candida,* tinea versicolor, Gram-positive bacteria
Ciclopirox 0.77% (**Loprox**)	4 wks, as needed	Cream, lotion, shampoo	Lotion preferred for nail penetration
Naftifine 1% (**Naftin**)	Once daily	Cream, gel	Tinea; has anti-inflammatory activity
Sulconazole (**Exelderm**)	4 wks, twice daily	Cream, solution	Tinea, *Candida,* tinea versicolor
Miconazole (**Monistat-Derm**)	4 wks, twice daily	Cream	Tinea, *Candida,* tinea versicolor
Oxiconazole 1% (**Oxistat**)	4 wks, twice daily	Cream, lotion	Tinea, *Candida,* tinea versicolor

(*continued*)

continued on page 302

MANAGEMENT *Continued*

Table 18.1 SYSTEMIC ANTIFUNGAL DRUG FORMULARY *(Continued)*

AGENT	APPLICATION	AVAILABILITY	COMMENTS
Griseofulvin (**Fulvicin, Grisactin, Gris-PEG**)		Microsized: 250-, 500-mg tablets; ultramicrosized: 125-, 250-, 333-mg tablets. Pediatric: Microsized: 125-mg/tsp pediatric suspension	Effective only against dermatophytes Contraindicated in pregnancy Fungistatic Take with fatty meals Alcohol should be avoided Occasional headache Gastrointestinal upset Photosensitivity Elevation of liver function tests Significant drug interactions (phenobarbital, warfarin, other drugs metabolized in liver)
Terbinafine (**Lamisil**)		250-mg tablets 125-mg oral granules 187.5-mg oral granules	Side effects minimal; include rare hepatotoxicity, reversible taste loss Fewer drug interactions than itraconazole **Severe hepatotoxicity including liver failure** reported in patients with no pre-existing liver disease. A baseline hepatic profile (alanine and aspartate aminotransferase) levels is recommended and monitored in patients receiving continuous treatment >1 mo or those who develop evidence suggestive of liver disease.
Itraconazole (**Sporanox**)		100-mg capsules Oral solution (10 mg/mL)	Side effects minimal; rare hepatotoxicity Significant drug interactions and contraindications: drugs not to be taken with itraconazole include astemizole, cisapride, terfenadine, triazolam, midazolam, lovastatin, and simvastatin **Potential risk for developing congestive heart failure** (CHF). Should not be used in the treatment of onychomycosis in patients with ventricular dysfunction such as CHF or a history of CHF.
Fluconazole (**Diflucan**)		50-, 100-, 150-, 200-mg tablets; oral solution 10 mg/mL, 40 mg/mL	Side effects minimal; rare hepatotoxicity Liver toxicity must be monitored if used long term Not to be taken with cisapride

HELPFUL HINTS

- A KOH examination of the scale should be performed to confirm the diagnosis of tinea pedis and to rule out its clinical mimickers dyshidrotic eczema, foot eczema, or plantar psoriasis.
- When there is a scaly rash on the palms, the feet should *always* be examined.
- If a child younger than 12 years of age has what appears clinically to be tinea pedis, it is more likely to be another skin condition, such as eczema.
- When the diagnosis at initial presentation is in doubt, a potent topical steroid may be applied—for a week or so—to relieve the acute itch and burning. The resultant anti-inflammatory effect of the topical steroid also helps to increase the yield of obtaining organisms on KOH examination or culture.
- To increase positive yields, KOH examination or fungal cultures should be obtained only after the patient has not applied any topical corticosteroid or antifungal therapy for at least 24 to 48 hours.

POINTS TO REMEMBER

- A common error is to automatically assume that every scaly rash on the feet is fungal in origin and mistakenly treat with topical antifungal preparations alone or in combination with topical steroids as a "shotgun" approach. Careful observation and a positive KOH examination or culture reveal the true nature of the problem. This caveat also applies to tinea cruris (see the following section).
- Dyshidrotic eczema and acute vesicular tinea pedis can look exactly alike. The diagnosis should be confirmed by KOH examination of scrapings from the lesions.

 SEE PATIENT HANDOUTS "Athlete's Foot (Tinea Pedis)" and "Burow solution" IN THE COMPANION eBOOK EDITION.

TINEA CRURIS ("JOCK ITCH")

BASICS

- Tinea cruris is a common infection of the upper inner thighs that most often occurs in postpubertal males.
- It is generally caused by the dermatophytes *T. rubrum* and *E. floccosum.*
- In contrast to candidiasis (see later) and lichen simplex chronicus, it generally spares the scrotum.

PATHOGENESIS

- Tinea cruris often begins after repeated vigorous physical activity that results in excessive sweating.
- The infecting fungus is usually the patient's own tinea pedis or other fungal infection.
- Obesity, diabetes, and immunodeficient states predispose to tinea cruris.

CLINICAL MANIFESTATIONS

- Lesions are typically bilateral, fan-shaped, annular, or semiannular scaly patches with central clearing and a slightly elevated scaly "active border" (Fig. 18.7).
- Lesions may involve the upper thighs, the crural folds, and possibly extend to the pubic area and buttocks.
- Characteristically, spares the scrotum and penis.
- Typically lesions are pruritic, or can cause "burning," or be irritating.
- Frequently, the patient also has tinea pedis.

DIAGNOSIS

- A positive KOH examination or fungal culture is found most easily by sampling from the "active" border of lesions.

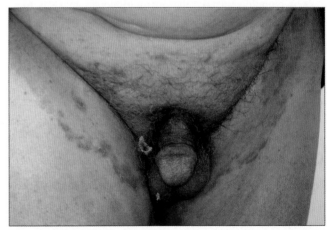

18.7 *Tinea cruris.* Note the scalloped shape with an "active border."

DIFFERENTIAL DIAGNOSIS

All the following are KOH negative and will have no growth on fungal culture.

Lichen Simplex Chronicus (Eczematous Dermatitis)
- *Lichenification is present.*
- *Often involves the scrotum.*

Inverse Psoriasis
- *Scrotal and inguinal involvement.*
- *Lesions are confluent (no central clearing).*
- *Although not always present, the identification of lesions consistent with psoriasis in other locations is useful.*

Candidiasis (see below in this chapter)
- *"Beefy" red appearance.*
- *Often involves the scrotum.*
- *Satellite pustules may be apparent.*
- *KOH positive for budding yeast; positive candidal culture.*

Also consider:

Intertrigo

Irritant Dermatitis (e.g., Diaper Dermatitis in Adults)

Erythrasma

Rarely, Extramammary Paget Disease

HELPFUL HINT

- A common mistake that many clinicians make is to prescribe combination antifungal corticosteroid products (e.g., **Lotrisone**) for the treatment of common fungal skin infections without confirming the diagnosis. Steroid atrophy may result from the potent corticosteroid in this product.

POINT TO REMEMBER

- In males, tinea cruris spares the scrotum, distinguishing it from candidal intertrigo which often involves scrotal skin.

 SEE PATIENT HANDOUT "Tinea Cruris (Jock Itch)" IN THE COMPANION eBOOK EDITION.

MANAGEMENT

- Topical antifungal creams, applied once or twice daily, are often effective in controlling, and sometimes curing, uncomplicated localized infections. Over-the-counter (OTC) preparations of miconazole (**Micatin**), terbinafine (**Lamisil**), and clotrimazole (**Lotrimin**) are readily available (see Table 18.1).
- For severe inflammation and itching, a mild OTC **hydrocortisone 1%** preparation or a moderate-strength prescription topical steroid such as hydrocortisone valerate 0.2% (**Westcort**) may be used for 4 to 5 days for symptomatic relief.
- Systemic antifungal therapy may be necessary in cases that do not respond to topical therapy and in cases of chronic recurrent tinea cruris, particularly in immunocompromised patients.
- **Prevention** is aimed toward decreasing wetness, friction, and maceration by
  - using an absorbent powder such as **Zeasorb-ANTIFUNGAL**.
  - Drying the area with a hairdryer after bathing.
  - Wearing loose clothing, that is, briefs are less frictional than boxer shorts.

TINEA CORPORIS ("RINGWORM")

BASICS

- Tinea corporis is commonly referred to as "ringworm," by laypersons and many in the health care community to describe practically any annular or ringlike eruption on the body. In fact, there are many nonfungal conditions that assume an annular "ringworm-like" configuration such as granuloma annulare, erythema multiforme, erythema migrans (seen in acute Lyme disease), and figurate erythemas such as urticaria.
- Referred to as *tinea faciale* when located on the face, tinea corporis is most often acquired by contact with an infected animal, usually kittens and occasionally dogs. It may also spread from other infected humans, or it may be autoinoculated from areas of the body that are infected with tinea such as tinea pedis or tinea capitis.
- Due to close skin-to-skin contact, wrestlers can frequently transmit tinea corporis; when this occurs it is called *tinea gladiatorum.*
- *M. canis, T. rubrum,* and *T. mentagrophytes* are the usual pathogens.

CLINICAL MANIFESTATIONS

- Lesions are generally annular or semi-annular with progressive peripheral centrifugal enlargement and central clearing. Odd gyrate or concentric rings may appear (Figs. 18.8–18.10).
- The scaly, "active border" may sometimes be pustular or vesicular.
- Lesions are single or multiple and may be pruritic or asymptomatic.
- **Majocchi granuloma** is a follicular, deep form of tinea corporis. It may result from inappropriate therapy, such as topical steroids, or from shaving that can drive the fungi into hair follicles.
- If multiple lesions are present, their distribution is typically asymmetric.
- Lesions are found most often on the extremities, face, and trunk.

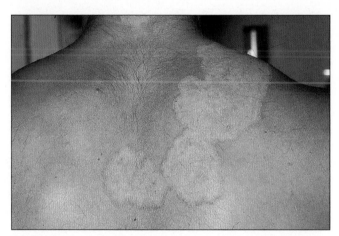

18.8 *Tinea corporis.* Annular plaque with peripheral scale on border.

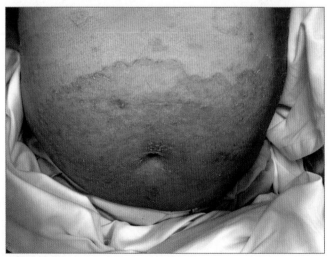

18.9 *Extensive tinea corporis.* This patient has widespread involvement.

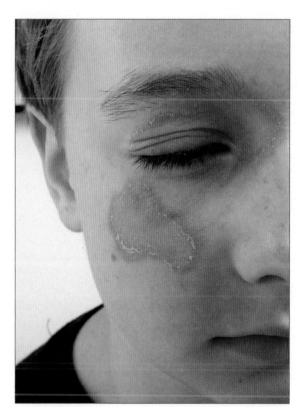

18.10 *Tinea faciale.* Two erythematous, scaly, annular lesions are noted on this child's face.

DIAGNOSIS

- Diagnosis is confirmed by a positive KOH (see Figs. 18.11 and 18.12) examination from the leading edge of a lesion or a fungal culture (it is especially easy to find hyphae in those patients who have been previously treated with topical steroids).
- A history of a newly adopted kitten or contact with an infected person may provide very helpful information.

DIFFERENTIAL DIAGNOSIS OF ANNULAR LESIONS

Urticaria
- *Unlike tinea corporis, scale is absent.*
- *Lesions are evanescent and migratory, lasting less than 24 hours.*

Granuloma Annulare.
- *Scale is absent.*

Acute Lyme Disease (Erythema Migrans)
- *Target-like appearance.*
- *Erythema with no scale.*
- *Self-limiting.*

Atopic Dermatitis
- *Scale is often dry and is present uniformly on the entire surface of the lesions.*
- *Lichenification may be present.*

Psoriasis
- *Scale is silvery white and is present uniformly on the entire lesion.*
- *Lesions are well-demarcated and symmetrical in distribution.*

Erythema Annulare Centrifugum
- *A trailing rim of scale is often evident in the superficial variant of this disorder.*

Also consider:

Subacute Lupus Erythematosus

Mycosis Fungoides (Cutaneous T-cell Lymphoma)

Erythema Multiforme

MANAGEMENT

- First-line treatment is with a topical antifungal agent that is applied to the affected areas twice daily until the eruption has resolved (see Table 18.1).
- Systemic antifungal agents (see the earlier discussion of tinea cruris) are sometimes necessary when multiple lesions are present or if infection is present in areas that are repeatedly shaved, such as men's beards (*tinea barbae*) or, especially, women's legs, in which granulomatous lesions (*Majocchi's granuloma*) may appear.
- If pets appear to be the source of infection, they may also need antifungal treatment after evaluation by a veterinarian.

POSITIVE KOH EXAMINATION

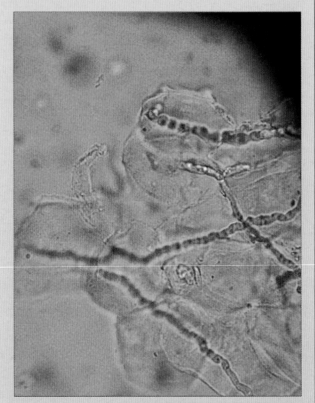

18.11 *Positive KOH examination. Dermatophyte.* Note the wavy-branched hyphae with uniform widths coursing over cell borders.

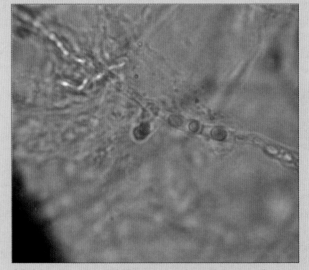

18.12 *Positive KOH examination. Dermatophyte. Close-up.* Septae and spores are visible.

HELPFUL HINTS

- Tinea corporis is very often misdiagnosed and treated with topical steroids which results in a masking of the typical clinical features and is appropriately called "tinea incognito" (Fig. 18.13).
- Tinea incognito is less red and scaly and oftentimes pustular. A high index of suspicion and thorough history is required to make the diagnosis. A KOH and fungal culture will be positive.

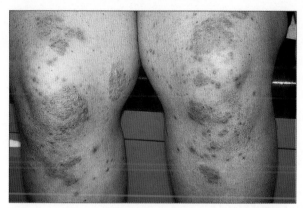

18.13   Tinea corporis (tinea incognito). This patient was treated with topical steroids for several months until the correct diagnosis was made. The topical steroids modified the typical clinical appearance of tinea corporis; in fact, her lesions initially looked more like psoriasis.

POINTS TO REMEMBER

- Inquire about sports activities, such as wrestling.
- Not all rings are "ringworm."

ONYCHOMYCOSIS (TINEA UNGUIUM)

BASICS

- The term *onychomycosis* refers to an infection of the fingernails or toenails caused by various fungi, yeasts, and molds.

In contrast, the term *tinea unguium* refers specifically to nail infections caused by dermatophytes.

- Onychomycosis is uncommon in children, but its prevalence increases dramatically with advancing age, with prevalence rates as high as 30% in those of 70 years and older.
- Many patients who have toenail onychomycosis will also have chronic tinea pedis.
- The major causes of onychomycosis are as follows:
  - Dermatophytes: *E. floccosum, T. rubrum,* and *T. mentagrophytes*
  - Yeasts, mainly Candida albicans
  - Molds, such as Aspergillus, Fusarium, and Scopulariopsis species

CLINICAL VARIANTS

- **Distal subungual onychomycosis** (Fig. 18.14) accounts for more than 90% of all cases of onychomycosis. It is usually characterized by the following:
  1. Nail thickening and subungual hyperkeratosis (scale buildup under the nail)
  2. Nail discoloration (yellow, yellow-green, white, or brown)
  3. Nail dystrophy
  4. Onycholysis (nail plate elevation from the nail bed)
- Distal subungual onychomycosis is frequently associated with chronic palmoplantar tinea (i.e., "two feet, one hand" variant of tinea [see above in this chapter]).
- In **superficial white onychomycosis** (Fig. 18.15), the fungus is superficial.
- **Proximal white subungual onychomycosis** (Fig. 18.16) may be seen in persons with human immunodeficiency virus (HIV) infection.
- Aside from footwear causing occasional physical discomfort and the psychosocial liability of unsightly nails, onychomycosis is usually asymptomatic.

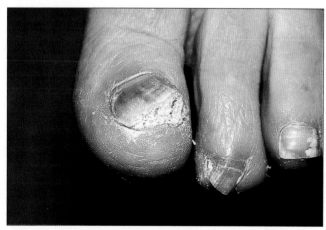

18.14   Distal subungual onychomycosis. The nail is dystrophic and discolored, and there is a buildup of keratin underneath it (subungual hyperkeratosis).

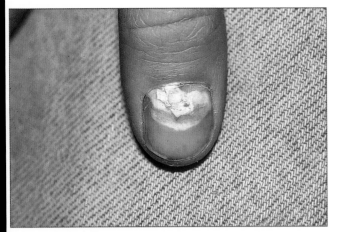

18.15 *Superficial white onychomycosis.* A KOH specimen was easily obtained from the surface of this lesion.

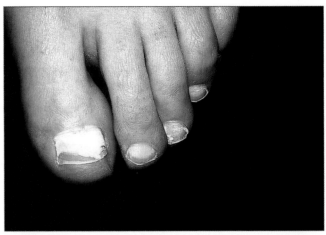

18.16 *Proximal white subungual onychomycosis.* HIV infection should be suspected in this patient.

• Onychomycotic nails may infrequently act as a portal of entry for more serious bacterial infections of the lower leg, particularly in patients with diabetes.

DIAGNOSIS

• A positive KOH examination or growth of dermatophyte, yeast, or mold on culture is diagnostic.

 DIFFERENTIAL DIAGNOSIS (also see Discussion in Chapter 22)

Psoriasis of the Nails
• *May be indistinguishable from, or coexist with, onychomycosis.*
• *Usually evidence of psoriasis is found elsewhere on the body.*
• *KOH examination is generally, but not always, negative.*
• *Characteristic nail pitting and a yellowish brown discoloration, known as "oil spots," may be present.*

Chronic Paronychia
• *Seen in patients with an altered immune status (e.g., diabetic patients) and in people whose hands are constantly in water.*

• *Erythema and edema of the proximal nail fold are noted.*
• *Absence of cuticle.*

Pseudomonas Infection of the Nail (Green Nail Syndrome)
• *Onycholysis with secondary bacterial (pseudomonas) colonization.*
• *A distinctive green coloration is apparent.*
• *Usually found in women with long fingernails.*

 MANAGEMENT

• Media attention has brought scores of patients to their health care providers to have their unsightly nails treated with the oral antifungal agent terbinafine (**Lamisil**). Lamisil is now the first-line treatment for onychomycosis, replacing griseofulvin, which is less effective and is associated with a high recurrence rate (Table 18.1).

Oral Therapy
Important factors to consider before starting oral therapy:
• Diagnostic confirmation by KOH examination or fungal culture

• Patient motivation and compliance
• Family history of onychomycosis
• Patient's age and health
• Drug cost
• Possible drug interactions and side effects (see Table 18.1)

Terbinafine (Lamisil) Tablets
• It is fungicidal, especially against dermatophytes.
• Long-term cure rate is probably no greater than 40% to 50%.

continued on page 309

MANAGEMENT *Continued*

- Side effects are infrequent. However, baseline liver function tests are performed, and the tests are repeated in 4 to 6 weeks.
- Terbinafine is an inhibitor of the CYP450 2D6 isozyme. Drugs predominantly metabolized by the CYP450 2D6 isozyme include the following drug classes: tricyclic antidepressants, selective serotonin reuptake inhibitors, beta blockers, certain antiarrhythmics, and monoamine oxidase inhibitors. Careful monitoring is necessary in patients who are also taking these medications and may require a reduction in dose of terbinafine.
- This drug has a reservoir effect. Because it persists in the nail for up to 4 to 5 months, there is no need to wait until the nail appears clinically normal as there is continued clearing even after cessation of therapy.

Dosage
- Adults: 250 mg/day for 6 weeks for fingernails; 250 mg/day for 12 weeks for toenails.
- Alternatively, pulse dosing with 250 mg/day for 1 week monthly for 4 months.
- Children: weight 20 to 40 kg: 125 mg/day; weight more than 40 kg: 250 mg/day for 6 to 12 weeks.

Itraconazole (Sporanox) Capsules
- Less common treatment option for onychomycosis.
- This is a broad-spectrum fungistatic agent.
- The primary drawback to the use of this drug is the risk for significant drug interactions.
- Long-term cure rate is probably no greater than 40% to 50%.
- Side effects are infrequent. However, liver function tests should be performed at baseline and repeated in 4 to 6 weeks.
- This drug also has a reservoir effect.

Dosage
- 200 mg/day for 6 weeks for fingernails; 12 weeks for toenails.

- Alternatively, pulse dosing with 200 mg twice daily, taken with full meals, for 7 days of each month (3 months for fingernails, 4 months for toenails).

Fluconazole (Diflucan) Tablets
- This is a broad-spectrum fungistatic agent.
- It is more extensively used in patients with HIV infection.
- It has fewer drug interactions than itraconazole.
- Side effects are minimal. Liver toxicity must be monitored if the drug is used long term.

Dosage
- 50 to 400 mg daily for 1 to 4 weeks or 150 mg once per week for 9 to 10 months

Other Treatment Methods
- **Surgical ablation** of nails is rarely indicated and is generally ineffective.
- **Laser treatment** of onychomycosis can require extensive debridement but may be effective in those who choose not to have oral therapy.
- **Carmol 40 Gel**, containing 40% urea, a keratolytic agent, is applied once daily to thickened nails and used in conjunction with topical antifungal agents to aid penetration.
- **Penlac Nail Lacquer Topical Solution** (ciclopirox 8%) is a nail lacquer often used in conjunction with oral antifungal agent or alone for the prevention of recurrent infection.
- **Amorolfine nail lacquer** is approved for sale in Australia and the United Kingdom, but not in the United States or Canada.
- Newer FDA approved topical agents such as efinaconazole 10% solution (**Jublia**) and tavaborole 5% solution (**Kerydin**) may prove to be viable alternatives to oral treatment for onychomycosis. Both require daily used for 48 weeks.

 HELPFUL HINTS

- The following important questions must be answered before oral therapy is prescribed:
  1. Patient's age and health status.
  2. How much does the nail disease affect the quality of life of the patient?
- Risk versus benefit should be evaluated before treating a condition that is often primarily cosmetic in nature.

 POINTS TO REMEMBER

- Onychomycosis should be confirmed with a positive KOH test or culture before initiating oral therapy.
- Treatment with the newer systemic antifungal agents is expensive and not always curative.
- Fingernail onychomycosis should prompt inspection of toenails and feet.
- A patient with a family history of onychomycosis is less likely to have a successful treatment outcome than a person without such a history.

Yeast Infections

- Most cutaneous yeast infections are caused by *Candida albicans* and are referred to as cutaneous candidiasis.
- Yeasts are unicellular fungi that typically reproduce by budding, a process that entails a progeny that pinches off of the mother cell.
- *C. albicans,* is an oval yeast, 2 to 6 μm in diameter that has the ability to exist in both hyphal and yeast forms (termed dimorphism). If pinched cells do not separate, a chain of cells is produced and is termed *pseudohyphae.*
- *Candidal* onychomycosis is rare and is found in only those who are immunocompromised.

CUTANEOUS CANDIDIASIS

BASICS

- Cutaneous candidiasis is a superficial fungal infection of the skin and mucous membranes. The organism, *C. albicans* thrives in moist, occluded sites, and is most likely to proliferate in:
  1. Those who continually expose their hands to water (e.g., dishwashers, health care workers, florists).
  2. Patients taking long-term systemic steroid therapy.
  3. Obese persons/patients with HIV/AIDS/patients with polyendocrinopathies
  4. Infants (see discussion in Chapter 2).

CLINICAL MANIFESTATIONS

- Cutaneous candidiasis is characterized by a beefy red color, itching, and/or burning.
- Appearance of lesions varies according to the location.

CLINICAL VARIANTS

Candidal Intertrigo
- Most often arises in intertriginous areas, such as under pendulous breasts (Fig. 18.17), in the axillae, groin, intergluteal fold, perineal region including the scrotum (Fig. 18.18) and at the corners of the mouth (perlèche).
- Initially, pustules appear, followed by well-demarcated erythematous plaques with small papular and pustular lesions at the periphery ("satellite pustules").
- Erythematous areas later become eroded and "beefy red."
- Lesions are not annular (they have no central clearing), as seen in tinea infections.

Other Variants
- **"Erosio interdigitalis blastomycetes."** Superficial interdigital scaly, erythematous erosions or fissures occur in the web spaces of the fingers (Fig. 18.19).
- **Candidal diaper dermatitis** occurs in the area occluded under diapers (see Chapter 2).
- **Candidal folliculitis** is characterized by follicular pustules.
- **Candidal balanitis** (Fig. 18.20) and **balanoposthitis** are seen in men with diabetes. Various clinical findings such as erythema, edema, papules, pustules, and moist curd-like

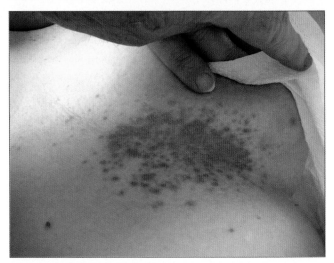

18.17   *Cutaneous candidiasis (inframammary).* This patient with pendulous breasts has rheumatoid arthritis and is on immunosuppressive therapy. Note the "beefy red" plaque and satellite pustules.

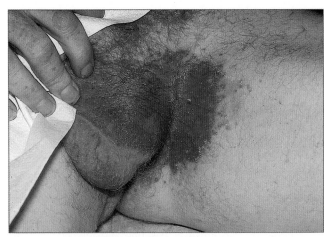

18.18   *Cutaneous candidiasis of the groin.* The characteristic "beefy red" plaque and satellite pustules are seen here.

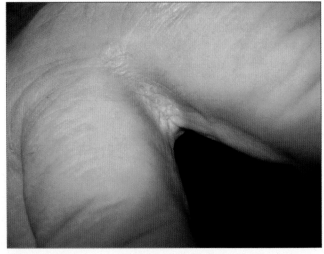

18.19   *Cutaneous candidiasis (web spaces).* "Erosio interdigitalis blastomycetes" in a diabetic person.

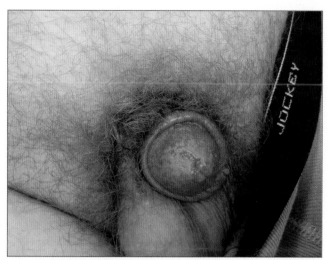

18.20 *Cutaneous candidiasis (glans penis).* This patient is also diabetic.

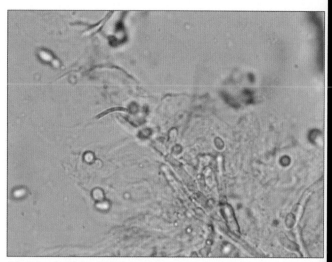

18.22 *Positive KOH examination. Candida.* Spores and pseudohyphae (lack septae).

accumulations may appear with fissuring, erosions, and ulceration of the glans and foreskin.

- **Candidal vulvitis/vulvovaginitis** consists of itchy, erosions, pustules, and erythematous plaques.
- **Candidal paronychia** is characterized by edema, erythema, and purulence of the proximal nail fold with secondary nail dystrophy (discussed in Chapter 22).
- **Oral candidiasis ("thrush")** is distinguished by white (Fig. 18.21), creamy exudate or plaques, which, when removed, appears eroded and beefy red. Oral candidiasis appears in infants ("thrush") and in the clinical settings of immunosuppression and diabetes (see Chapters 2 and 33).

DIAGNOSIS

- KOH positive for pseudohyphae, budding yeast, or mycelia (Fig. 18.22) (also see Chapter 35).
- Fungal culture on Sabouraud's media reveals creamy, dull-white colonies.

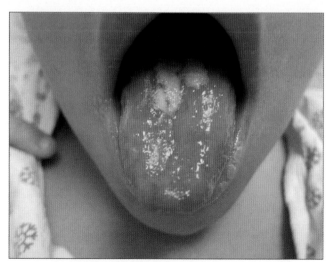

18.21 *Cutaneous candidiasis (thrush).* Oral candidiasis in an immunocompromised child.

DIFFERENTIAL DIAGNOSIS

Inverse Psoriasis
- *Psoriasis may be present elsewhere on the body.*
- *Negative KOH examination and fungal culture.*

Tinea Infections (see above in this chapter)
- *May be indistinguishable from cutaneous candidiasis.*
- *Positive KOH and fungal culture for dermatophyte.*
- *Lesions typically have a scalloped, "active border."*
- *Generally spares the scrotum and penis.*

Also consider:

Atopic Dermatitis

Intertrigo

Seborrheic Dermatitis

MANAGEMENT

- **Burow solution** in cool wet soaks, two to three times daily, applied to decrease moisture and maceration (see Table 18.1).
- The intertriginous area should be kept dry with powders, such as miconazole (**Zeasorb-AF**) powder, and by drying with a hairdryer on a "cool" setting after bathing.
- Topical broad-spectrum antifungal creams, such as prescription ketoconazole 2% (**Nizoral**) cream or the over-the-counter preparations of clotrimazole (**Lotrimin**) and miconazole (**Micatin**), applied twice daily are often effective.
- Systemic antifungal agents, such as **ketoconazole**, itraconazole, or **fluconazole**, are used for widespread involvement or recalcitrant infections.

HELPFUL HINT

- Nystatin is effective for cutaneous candidal infections, but not for the treatment of dermatophytes.

POINTS TO REMEMBER

- Cutaneous candidiasis is frequently confused with inverse psoriasis and irritant intertrigo; thus, documentation of candidal organisms should be made.
- Candidal infections may be early markers of diabetes.

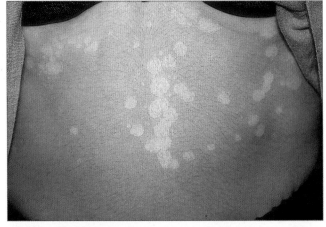

18.23 *Tinea Versicolor.* Lesions are white and resemble vitiligo.

TINEA VERSICOLOR

BASICS

- Tinea versicolor (TV), referred to as *pityriasis versicolor* by many authors, is a very common superficial yeast infection caused by the hyphal form of *Pityrosporum ovale.* The organism is also known as *P. orbiculare* and *Malassezia furfur.*
- TV is seen mostly in young adults and is unusual in the very young and elderly.
- The term "versicolor" refers to the varied coloration that TV can display, even on the same individual. The color of the lesions may vary from whitish to pink to tan or brown (Figs. 18.23–18.25). It tends to be a chronic relapsing condition because the causative fungus is part of the skin's normal flora.

CLINICAL MANIFESTATIONS

- Primary lesions are well-defined round or oval patches with an overlay of fine, *furfuraceous* scales; lesions often coalesce to form larger patches.
- Lesions most commonly appear on the trunk, upper arms, and neck and are less often seen on the face.
- Primarily of cosmetic concern.
- Common and persistent in consistently hot, tropical and subtropical climates.
- Recurs during the summer in more temperate zones.
- Usually asymptomatic, but may itch in hot weather or when patient is sweating.

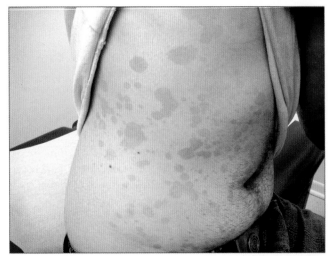

18.24 *Tinea Versicolor.* Lesions are light tan (faun-colored).

DIAGNOSIS

- If scale is present, KOH examination is positive, and the typical "spaghetti and meatball" hyphae are abundant and easily found (Figs. 18.26 and 18.27).
- Lesions of TV will fluoresce an orange-mustard color when the Wood's light is held close to the skin in a dark room. Examination with a Wood light can be used to demonstrate the extent of the infection and help confirm the diagnosis.

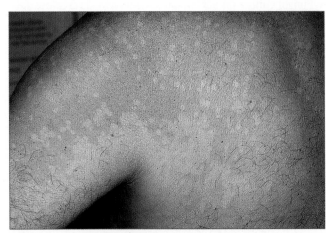

18.25 *Tinea Versicolor.* Here lesions are dark brown and confluent.

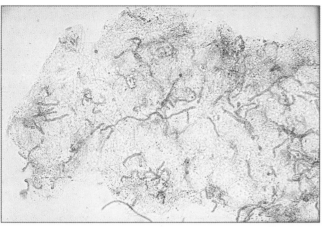

18.26 *Positive KOH examination. Tinea Versicolor.* Note the wavy hyphae (spaghetti) and the clusters of spores (meatballs).

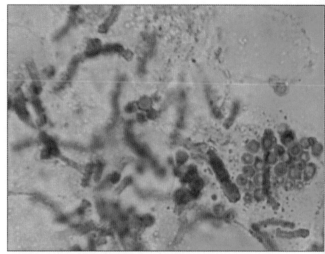

18.27 *Positive KOH examination. Tinea Versicolor (close up).* Here the hyphae and spores look more like "sausages and grapes."

 DIFFERENTIAL DIAGNOSIS

Vitiligo
- *There is depigmentation of the skin without scale.*

Pityriasis Rosea (see Chapter 15)
- *History of a herald patch.*
- *KOH is negative.*
- *Christmas tree–like distribution.*
- *Self-limited.*

Confluent and reticulated papillomatosis (CARP) of Gougerot and Carteaud
- *Closely resembles darkly pigmented tinea versicolor.*
- *KOH negative.*
- *Typically located on the trunk.*
- *Rough textured on palpation.*

Pityriasis Alba
- *Ill-defined hypopigmented slightly scaly patches usually located on the face.*

 MANAGEMENT

Topical Agents
- For mild, limited tinea versicolor, topical therapy may be applied in the shower. Daily applications of selenium sulfide (**Selsun Blue**) shampoo, pyrithione zinc (**Head & Shoulders**) shampoo, and ketoconazole 1% (**Nizoral**) cream or shampoo are inexpensive OTC methods that often clear the eruption (see Table 18.2).
- In addition, application of OTC topical antifungals such as miconazole cream or spray (**Micatin**), clotrimazole cream (**Lotrimin**), or terbinafine cream or spray (**Lamisil**) applied twice daily can result in clearance of the eruption. Sprays allow for easy application on the back.
- Alternatively, topical **ciclopirox (Loprox) gel** or **shampoo**, or **ketoconazole 2% cream (Nizoral)**, which is available only by prescription, may be applied.
- This treatment regimen may be continued for 3 or 4 weeks. It is also a good idea to repeat this regimen before the next warm season or before a tropical vacation.

Systemic Therapy
- For stubborn or widespread disease, systemic therapy with oral **ketoconazole, fluconazole (Diflucan)**, or **itraconazole** may be prescribed (see formulary in Table 18.2).
- Although administered for a very short term (3 to 5 days), systemic therapy should not be routinely used for this essentially cosmetic problem.

continued on page 314

MANAGEMENT *Continued*

Table 18.2 FORMULARY FOR TINEA VERSICOLOR

AGENT	INSTRUCTIONS
Topical agents: Over-the-counter	
Selenium sulfide 1% (**Selsun Blue**) shampoo	Apply daily to wide area for 10 min, followed by a shower
Selenium sulfide 1%, zinc pyrithione (**Head & Shoulders**) shampoo	Apply daily to wide area for 10 min, followed by a shower
Miconazole 2% (**Micatin**) spray	Spray on once daily for 2 wks
Clotrimazole (**Lotrimin**) 1% cream	Apply once daily for 2 wks
Terbinafine (**Lamisil**) 1% cream	Apply twice daily for 1–4 wks
Topical agents: Prescription required	
Ketoconazole 2% gel (**Xolegel**), 2% foam (**Extina**)	Apply twice daily for 1–4 wks
Ketoconazole 2% shampoo (**Nizoral**)	Apply daily to wide area for 10 min, followed by a shower
Selenium sulfide 2.5% shampoo (**Selsun 2.5%**)	Apply daily to wide area for 10 min, followed by a shower
Ciclopirox shampoo	Apply daily to wide area for 10 min, followed by a shower
Ciclopirox (**Loprox**) gel	Apply twice daily for 1–4 weeks
Systemic agents	
Itraconazole (**Sporanox**)	100 mg for 5 days
Fluconazole (**Diflucan**)	150 mg for 5 days

 POINTS TO REMEMBER

- The hypopigmented variety of tinea versicolor is often mistaken for vitiligo.
- Patients should be advised that the uneven coloration of the skin may take several months to disappear after the fungus has been successfully eliminated.
- Recurrences are very common, especially in warm weather.

HELPFUL HINTS

- Prophylactic application of ketoconazole cream or shampoo once or twice weekly may prevent recurrences.
- Topical therapy can be repeated 1 week before the next exposure to warm weather.

 SEE PATIENT HANDOUT "Tinea Versicolor" IN THE COMPANION eBOOK EDITION.

SUPERFICIAL FUNGAL INFECTIONS

CHAPTER 19

Hair and Scalp Disorders Resulting in Hair Loss

OVERVIEW

Hair has great social and cultural significance in all human societies. It is found on most areas of the human body, except on the palms and soles and the mucous membranes.

TYPES OF HAIR

- **Lanugo:** The fine hair that covers nearly the entire body of fetuses.
- **Vellus:** The short, fine, "peach fuzz" body hair that grows in most places on the body. Vellus hairs are soft and short and can be seen in areas of male-pattern baldness.
- **Terminal:** The mature, fully developed hair, which is generally longer, coarser, thicker, and darker than vellus hair.

HAIR TEXTURE AND SHAPE

- Hair texture and shape is genetically determined to be straight, curly, or wavy, and it can change over time. It can also be affected by hair styling practices such as chemical straighteners, braiding, or curlers.
- The shape of the follicle itself and the direction in which each strand grows out of its follicle determine whether hair is curly or straight. For example, curly hair is shaped like an elongated oval and grows at a sharp angle to the scalp.

CYCLES OF HAIR GROWTH

- Hair grows in long cycles composed of three phases: (1) the anagen, or growth phase, that can last several years, (2) the catagen or degenerative phase that is short-lived, and (3) the telogen or resting phase, during which time the hair is shed. At any given time, about 90% of scalp hairs are in anagen, 5% to 10% are in telogen, and the remainder are in the catagen stage (see Illus. 19.1).

IN THIS CHAPTER...

- ➤ **ANDROGENIC ALOPECIA**
- ➤ **ALOPECIA AREATA**
- ➤ **DIFFUSE ALOPECIA**
  - Telogen effluvium
  - Anagen effluvium
  - Senescent alopecia
- ➤ **SCARRING ALOPECIA**
  - Chronic cutaneous lupus erythematosus
  - Lichen planopilaris
  - Central centrifugal cicatricial alopecia
  - Traction alopecia
  - Cutaneous sarcoidosis
  - Folliculitis decalvans
- ➤ **PSEUDOFOLLICULITIS BARBAE AND ACNE KELOIDALIS NUCHAE**
  - Pseudofolliculitis barbae (PFB)
  - Acne keloidalis nuchae

HAIR LOSS

- Some degree of scalp hair loss or thinning generally accompanies aging in both sexes, and it is estimated that half of all men are affected by male-pattern baldness by the time they are 50 years of age.
- Drugs used in cancer chemotherapy frequently cause a temporary loss of hair, because they affect all rapidly dividing cells, not just the malignant ones. Trauma, as well as certain diseases can cause temporary or permanent loss of hair (e.g., systemic lupus erythematosus, thyroid disease).

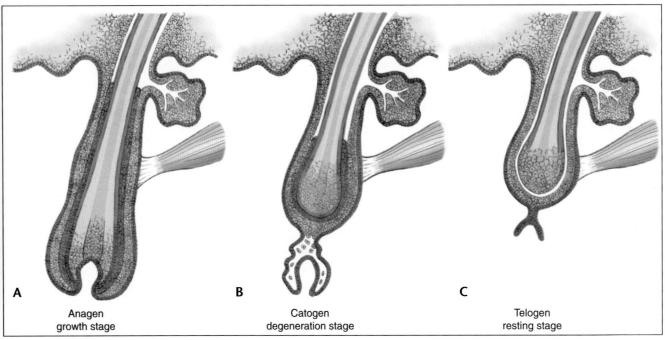

119.1 **_Cycles of hair growth._** (Modified from Sams WM Jr, Lynch PJ, eds. Structure and function of the skin. In: *Principles and Practice of Dermatology*. New York: Churchill Livingstone, 1990:8, with permission.)

Androgenic Alopecia

BASICS

- Androgenic alopecia (AGA), also known as common baldness or male- or female-pattern baldness, is an extremely common, noninflammatory type of alopecia that results from the action of androgens on the hair follicle.
- AGA is an inherited physical trait whose incidence increases greatly with advancing age.
- In most, if not all, cultures, hair plays a powerful role in a person's psychosexual identity and self-image. It is not surprising that in our youth- and image-driven society, hair replacement and retention methods have taken on almost the status of a subspecialty in health care.
- AGA is seen more frequently in men than in women because women's hair loss tends to be less apparent, less extensive, and generally begins at a later age than in men.
- The condition is genetically determined (autosomal dominant with variable penetrance). The incidence and severity of AGA tends to be highest in white men, followed by white women; it is second highest in Asians and African-Americans and lowest in Native Americans and Eskimos.

PATHOGENESIS

- AGA results from the action of dihydrotestosterone (DHT) on the hair follicle that results in a shortened anagen phase of the hair cycle, thus producing thinner, shorter hairs with each cycle.
- Gradually, terminal hairs are converted into indeterminate hairs and finally into short, wispy, nonpigmented vellus hairs in a process known as *miniaturization.*
- In women, estrogen may protect against androgen-mediated miniaturization, which explains the more gradual onset, less severe disease course and the increased incidence after menopause.

CLINICAL MANIFESTATIONS

Androgenic alopecia produces two typical patterns of hair loss:

- **In men**, AGA usually begins in late adolescence or young adulthood, with hair loss often starting at the parietal hairline.
- Hair loss may progress to an M-shaped pattern on the front and later involve the vertex of the scalp (male-pattern baldness; Fig. 19.1).
- **In women,** the loss of hair is more subtle and tends to begin at an older age. AGA in women, also termed female-pattern hair loss (FPHL), is typically characterized by a thinning of the hair at the crown of the scalp in a "Christmas-tree," midparietal pattern with preservation of the frontal hairline (Figs. 19.2 and 19.3).
- Hair loss may progress in both sexes but is more extensive in men.
- In end-stage AGA, many men have only a fringe of remaining hair usually at the occipital scalp, whereas women tend to maintain the frontal hairline and do not become frankly bald.
- Hair density on the occipital scalp remains unaffected.

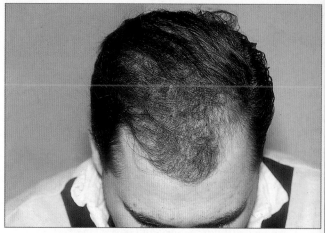

19.1 *Male-pattern alopecia.* This is characterized by an M-shaped pattern of hair loss on the front and vertex of the head.

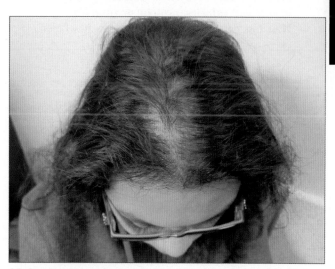

19.2 *Female-pattern alopecia.* A midparietal pattern of decreasing hair loss is noted here. The integrity of the frontal hairline is maintained.

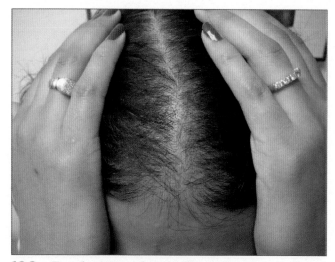

19.3 *Female-pattern alopecia.* The characteristic "widened part" in a "Christmas-tree" pattern toward the vertex is seen in this patient.

DIAGNOSIS

- The diagnosis of AGA is generally based on the clinical pattern of baldness coupled with an absence of clues pointing to a specific disease that may cause hair loss.

DIFFERENTIAL DIAGNOSIS

- It should be kept in mind that the following conditions are not only independent causes of hair loss but may coexist and exacerbate AGA; they are discussed later in this chapter:
  - **Telogen effluvium** (*shedding of resting hairs*)
  - **Anagen effluvium** (*shedding of growing hairs*)
  - **Hair loss from thyroid disease**
  - **Hair loss caused by iron-deficiency anemia** and **insufficient calories, protein,** or **vitamins**
  - **Hair loss caused by androgen excess** in women

HELPFUL HINTS

- Blood tests and other laboratory studies are necessary only when the diagnosis is in doubt, or if investigation into other causes of alopecia is warranted by the history or physical examination (see later section, "Diffuse Alopecia").
- Women with symptoms or signs of virilization should undergo a careful evaluation including hormone studies for an androgen-excess syndrome. These patients may need referral to an endocrinologist.
- Healthcare providers should take a patient's hair loss–related anxiety seriously. Hair loss should not simply be "brushed off" as an insignificant cosmetic complaint. The time spent listening to the patient may be helpful in uncovering other emotional or physical problems.

POINT TO REMEMBER

- AGA is very common; therefore, it may coexist with other forms of hair loss. Consequently, a search for treatable causes (e.g., anemia, hypothyroidism), especially in patients with an abrupt onset or a rapid progression of their disease, is indicated (see discussion below in this chapter).

 SEE PATIENT HANDOUT "Hair Loss" IN THE COMPANION eBOOK EDITION.

MANAGEMENT

Women

- **Minoxidil 2%** or **5% solution (Rogaine)**, applied twice daily, may reduce shedding and possibly contribute to some regrowth.
- A 5% solution of minoxidil in a foam formula **(Women's Rogaine)** is applied once daily.
- Regrowth is more pronounced at the vertex than in the frontal areas and may not be noted for at least 4 months.
- The mechanism of action is unknown; however, minoxidil appears to lengthen the duration of the anagen phase, and it may increase the blood supply to the hair follicle.
- Continued use is necessary indefinitely because discontinuation of treatment produces a rapid reversion to the pretreatment balding pattern.
- Women with a recent onset of AGA and small areas of hair loss respond best to minoxidil.
- Women with excess androgen may benefit from **systemic antiandrogen therapy** with agents such as **spironolactone, flutamide**, or **oral contraceptives** that decrease ovarian and adrenal androgen production, especially agents that contain a nonandrogenic progestin.

Men

- **Minoxidil 5%** solution **(Rogaine)**, applied twice daily, may reduce shedding and contribute to some regrowth.
- Finasteride **(Propecia)**, 1 mg/day, is an oral antiandrogen that acts by inhibiting type II 5-alpha reductase, the enzyme that converts testosterone to dihydrotestosterone. It is very effective in reducing further hair loss and increasing hair density.
- Recognized side effects include erectile dysfunction and, less often, gynecomastia.
- Finasteride is teratogenic and has **not been approved** for the treatment of AGA in women.

Men and Women

- **HairMax LaserComb** is a medical laser device for home use that has been FDA cleared for the treatment of AGA in men and women. Several studies have shown increase in hair thickness and density with regular use.
- **Hair transplantation** is performed by harvesting intact healthy hair follicles from donor sites, usually the occipital scalp, and inserting them into the areas of hair loss.
- Hair transplantation using a micrografting technique in which a small incision is used to insert one or more donor hairs, is particularly effective in women, because unlike men, women rarely become completely bald.

BASICS

- Alopecia areata (AA) is a common, idiopathic disorder characterized by well-circumscribed round or oval areas of nonscarring hair loss that presents with varying degrees of severity.
- **Alopecia totalis** refers to a loss of all or almost all scalp hair and eyebrows and **alopecia universalis** refers to a total loss of all scalp and body hair.
- AA most commonly affects young adults and children. Occasionally, a family history of AA exists.
- Often, onset is attributed to recent emotional or physiologic stress.

PATHOGENESIS

- AA is generally considered an autoimmune condition.
- Biopsy findings demonstrate T-cell infiltrates surrounding the hair follicles.
- AA is sometimes associated with other autoimmune disorders, such as vitiligo, thyroid disease (Hashimoto thyroiditis), pernicious anemia, and celiac disease.

CLINICAL MANIFESTATIONS

- AA most commonly presents as oval, round, or geometric patches of alopecia (Fig. 19.4).
- Lesions are most often found on the scalp, eyebrows, eyelashes, and areas of the face that bear hair, such as the beard (Fig. 19.5) or mustache on men.
- On occasion, a hand lens may reveal tiny "exclamation mark" hairs at the periphery of lesions.
- Increased friction or "stickiness" (not the expected smoothness) is felt on palpation of lesional skin because of the loss of vellus hairs (Fig. 19.6).
- Rarely, the entire scalp is involved (*alopecia totalis*), or even the entire body including pubic, axillary, and nasal hair is affected (*alopecia universalis*) (Fig. 19.7A,B).
- Infrequently, nails may demonstrate a characteristic pitting ("railroad tracks").
- Early on there is usually asymptomatic shedding of hair, which is often discovered by the patient's hairdresser or a family member.
- Frequently, hair spontaneously regrows; however, a recurrence of hair loss may be seen in 30% of patients who had experienced regrowth. Regrowing hair is initially thin and sometimes white (vitiliginous) (Fig. 19.8).
- Extensive scalp involvement, an atopic history and chronicity have a poorer prognosis. Also AA that occurs as bands along the hairline margins termed the "*ophiasis pattern*" is more difficult to treat (Fig. 19.9).

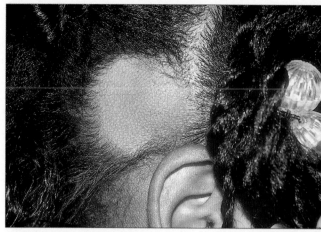

19.4 *Alopecia areata.* The hair is lost in a round patch. Note the absence of scales or inflammation.

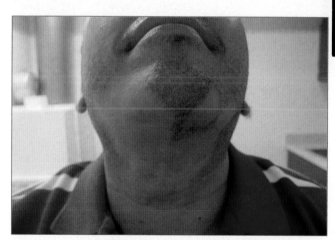

19.5 *Alopecia areata.* This man's AA is limited to his beard.

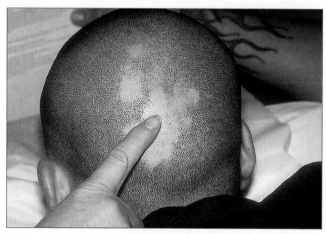

19.6 *Alopecia areata.* Increased friction ("stickiness") is noted on palpation of lesional skin as a result of the loss of vellus hairs.

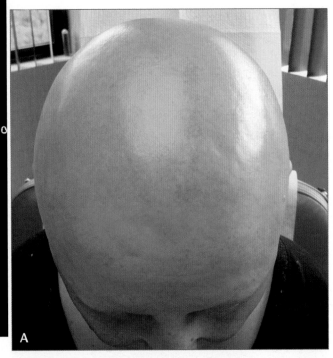

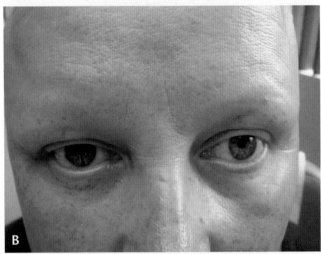

19.7 *Alopecia areata, alopecia universalis.* **A** and **B:** This patient has lost all of his hair. He has no eyelashes, intranasal, pubic or axillary hair; he also has no hair on his extremities.

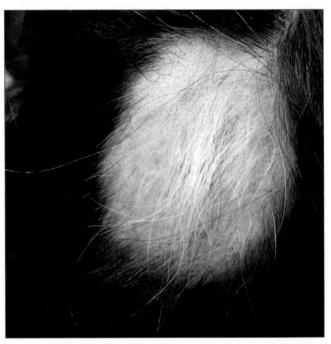

19.8 *Alopecia areata, regrowing hair.* In this patient with AA, clusters of hair regrew after intralesional triamcinolone acetonide injections. Some of the regrown hairs are white (vitiliginous).

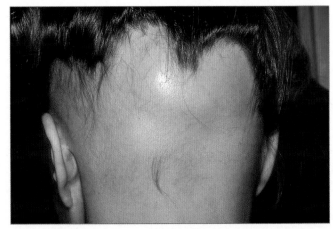

19.9 *Alopecia areata, ophiasis pattern.* A band of alopecia occurs along the hairline margins encircling the head.

DIAGNOSIS

- The diagnosis of AA is generally based on its clinical appearance; however, a scalp biopsy may be performed if the diagnosis is in doubt.

DIFFERENTIAL DIAGNOSIS

Tinea Capitis (Discussed in Chapter 9)

- *Seen most frequently in African-American children and uncommonly in African-American adults.*
- *The scalp is often scaly, itchy, and inflamed and black dots, representing broken hairs may be seen within the alopecic patches.*
- *The diagnosis is confirmed when the KOH examination is positive for hyphae and/or spores or when a fungus grows on Sabouraud medium.*

Telogen Effluvium (see below)

- *Hair loss is diffuse.*
- *Often there is a history of antecedent illness or childbirth.*

Trichotillomania (Compulsive Hair Pulling)

- *Seen most often in young girls (Fig. 19.10).*
- *Hairs tend to be broken at different lengths.*
- *A unilateral asymmetric loss of scalp hair may be noted (see also Fig. 9.7).*

Secondary Syphilis

- *Secondary syphilis should always be considered in cases of unexplained patchy hair loss.*
- *The hair loss is referred to as appearing "moth-eaten."*

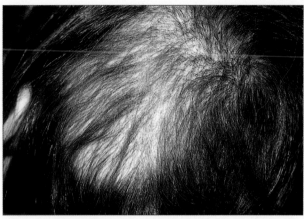

19.10 *Trichotillomania.* This condition is seen most often in young girls. Hairs tend to be broken at different lengths. The areas of alopecia are not completely devoid of hair.

Also consider:

Traction Alopecia and Hot-Comb Alopecia (Discussed below)

MANAGEMENT

- Because mild cases of AA often show spontaneous regrowth, therapy is often unnecessary.
- Both alopecia universalis and alopecia totalis are generally refractory to therapy and usually last a lifetime; spontaneous regrowth is rare.
- The daily application of a potent or superpotent **topical steroid**, such as **Lidex** (fluocinonide 0.05% ointment) or **clobetasol 0.05%, ointment** may speed hair regrowth. To increase drug penetration, the topical steroid may be applied followed by occlusion with a plastic shower cap, and left on overnight.
- If necessary, **intralesional injections** with triamcinolone acetonide (5 mg/cc) administered into the alopecic patches every 4 to 6 weeks is a very effective treatment option.

Further Treatment Modalities

- The numerous and varied treatment modalities used for severe extensive AA reflect the fact that few are very effective. The success rates associated with the following measures have ranged from no response to varying degrees of partial success:
- **Irritant therapy** involves using a topical anthralin (a coal tar derivative) preparation to the alopecic areas in order to induce an inflammatory response which may drive away the perifollicular T cells.
- **Immunotherapy** works similarly using chemical compounds such as squaric acid or diphenylcyclopropenone (DPCP) to induce a contact dermatitis.
- The following modalities have been utilized with varying degrees of success. **Topical minoxidil** in a 2% to 5% concentration, scalp massage, heat, aloe vera, vitamins, hypnotherapy, oral psoralens combined with exposure to ultraviolet light in the A range (PUVA), narrow band UVB, Excimer laser, and oral immunosuppressants including cyclosporine, methotrexate, and prednisone.

HELPFUL HINTS

- Alopecia totalis and universalis, the most severe forms of AA, generally spark great emotional problems in patients and their families.
- The most important part of widespread AA management is providing emotional support to the patient.
- The National Alopecia Areata Foundation is an excellent resource for information and can direct patients to AA support groups and information about wigs, for example. It can be reached at: National Alopecia Areata Foundation, 14 Mitchell Boulevard, San Rafael, CA 94903; phone number: 415.472.3780; web site: http://www.naaf.org/default2.asp.

 POINT TO REMEMBER

- Consider workup for other autoimmune diseases (e.g., thyroid disease) especially if there is an associated family history or if suggested by the review of systems or the physical examination.

 SEE PATIENT HANDOUT "Alopecia Areata" IN THE COMPANION eBOOK EDITION.

BASICS

- Diffuse alopecia is defined as a uniform, generally nonscarring reduction in hair density over all portions of the scalp. In contrast, AGA or alopecia caused by androgen excess presents in a characteristic pattern of hair loss.
- The vast majority of patients with diffuse hair loss are women.
- Unfortunately, the explanation for such hair loss frequently presents a confusing and frustrating challenge for primary care providers as well as for dermatologists.
- In many cases, the hair loss may not be apparent to the examiner and at times the cause may be difficult, if not impossible, to determine. The most frequent causes of diffuse alopecia are telogen effluvium, anagen effluvium, and senescent alopecia.

TELOGEN EFFLUVIUM

BASICS

- Telogen effluvium refers to the sudden onset of increased shedding of hair in response to an emotional, physiologic, or external trigger and can be acute or chronic.

PATHOGENESIS

- At baseline, about 10% to 15% of scalp hairs are in the telogen (shedding) phase (see Illus. 19.1).
- A telogen effluvium occurs when, in response to a trigger, a large number of hairs (greater than 15%) enter the telogen phase at one time, which results in a sudden and increased number of shedding hairs.
- The precipitating event usually precedes the hair loss by 6 to 16 weeks, which is the time required for a catagen hair to become a telogen hair.

CLINICAL MANIFESTATIONS

Acute Telogen Effluvium

- In acute telogen effluvium, hair shedding is typically sudden, rather than a gradual thinning. The patient may state that the shedding hair may be seen on pillows, on combs and brushes, and in the bathtub, and she or he may bring in a plastic bag full of hair as proof of the dramatic alopecia (Fig. 19.11).
- The acute type typically lasts for 3 to 6 months.
- Possible triggers of acute telogen effluvium include medications, major illness, fever, physical trauma, surgery, general anesthesia, significant weight loss such as that caused by "crash" dieting, or severe emotional stress. The patient may describe a recent history of such an event that typically occurred 3 to 4 months before the onset of alopecia.
- The medications that are most often implicated in acute telogen effluvium are anticoagulants, antimalarials, beta blockers, cholesterol-lowering medications, antidepressants, angiotensin-converting enzyme inhibitors, lithium, L dopa, propylthiouracil (which induces hypothyroidism), carbamazepine, oral retinoids, and immunizations.
- When an acute telogen effluvium occurs in women during childbearing years, it may be associated with giving birth

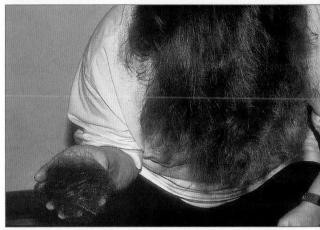

19.11 *Telogen effluvium, acute.* This patient presented with a plastic bag full of hair that had been shed over the course of 1 month.

(**postpartum effluvium** and **post-breastfeeding effluvium**), aborted pregnancy, or the discontinuation of oral contraceptives.

Chronic Telogen Effluvium

- The evidence of hair loss tends to be more subtle than in acute telogen effluvium.
- The chronic type lasts for more than 6 months.
- The diffuse (nonpatterned) hair shedding involves the entire scalp and is usually not obvious to the clinician. Scarring and inflammation of the scalp are not seen.
- It may be caused by the persistent presence of a trigger (such as medications) or by a rapid succession of several acute telogen effluviums. Chronic telogen effluvium may also have metabolic causes, such as iron or zinc deficiency, or result from low-protein diets, thyroid disease, or chronic systemic illnesses such as systemic lupus erythematosus or syphilis.
- The patient may complain of both increased shedding, albeit less severe than in acute telogen effluvium, and hair thinning that ultimately manifests as more visible scalp.
- Occasionally, patients state that the scalp hair simply feels less dense, that more of the scalp seems to be visible (Fig. 19.12), and that the hair has changed in texture. Complete alopecia is not seen.
- If the precipitating event is removed, it usually takes about 1 year to completely return to the pre-effluvium hair volume, but hair may not grow back completely and rather a new baseline hair density is set.

DIAGNOSIS

- The diagnosis is often based on history with patients reporting the loss of 400 or more hairs per day (normal shedding is 40 to 100 hairs a day).
- A gentle hair pull (of approximately 20 hairs) often yields more than four telogen hairs per pull. Telogen hairs can be identified by having a small white "bulb" at their proximal ends.

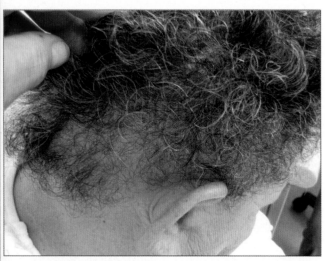

19.12 *Diffuse alopecia.* Extensive, widespread hair loss due to a beta blocker.

- If the diagnosis is in doubt, a scalp biopsy will show an increased telogen-to-anagen ratio (>15%) and an absence of inflammation and/or scarring.

LABORATORY TESTS

- When the cause of telogen effluvium is not clinically apparent, the following laboratory tests should be assessed when warranted by the history or physical examination:
  - Baseline chemistries and liver function tests
  - A complete blood count, sexually transmitted disease testing, and antinuclear antibody tests
  - Thyroid-stimulating hormone level
  - Serum ferritin and erythrocyte sedimentation rate (ESR) levels (a ferritin value >50 µg/L is optimal)
  - Serum dehydroepiandrosterone-sulfate (DHEA-S), free testosterone, prolactin, and morning cortisol levels (especially if virilization is evident)

 MANAGEMENT

- The patient should be reassured that, most often, in acute telogen effluvium the hair tends to grow back normally once the trigger has been corrected.
- Management includes identification, and elimination of the underlying cause (e.g., responsible drug) and simply to wait for the hair to grow back.
- Consultation with a dietitian may sometimes be necessary to ensure adequate caloric, vitamin, iron, zinc, and protein intake.
- Iron supplementation and correction may reverse the chronic telogen effluvium caused by this deficiency.
- However, correction of thyroid function unfortunately does not always result in a reversal of the effluvium.

 DIFFERENTIAL DIAGNOSIS

Androgenic Alopecia
- *Has a patterned distribution.*

Anagen Effluvium Secondary to Drugs
- *Cancer chemotherapy and immunotherapy drugs are causes.*
- *Hair loss is more diffuse and more rapid than telogen effluvium.*

 HELPFUL HINT

- The average normal scalp contains approximately a 100,000 hairs, and about 10% to 15% of follicles are in the telogen phase. Hence, it is normal to shed about 100 hairs per day.

 POINTS TO REMEMBER

- A careful history should assess for an antecedent illness, recent childbirth, ingestion of drugs, or a trauma 3 to 4 months before the onset of the sudden shedding.
- In women with AGA, there is usually a positive family history of patterned alopecia.
- AGA is quite prevalent and telogen effluvium may coexist with AGA.

ANAGEN EFFLUVIUM

BASICS

- Compared to telogen effluvium, anagen effluvium, the shedding of anagen hairs, produces a more extensive, more rapid, and dramatic loss of hair.
- At any given time, 80% to 90% of hair follicles on the scalp are in the anagen stage; hence a tremendous amount of shedding may occur.

PATHOGENESIS

- Anagen effluvium is usually precipitated by a toxic event, such as a reaction to certain drugs. However, an acute and severe systemic illness such as systemic lupus erythematosus (SLE) may also result in an anagen effluvium. The dramatic hair loss usually starts 1 to 2 weeks after the precipitating event.
- Among the agents that have been commonly associated with anagen hair loss are:
  - Drugs used for cancer chemotherapy (e.g., doxorubicin, nitrosoureas, cyclophosphamide).

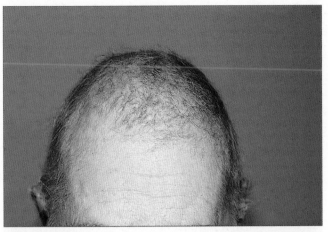

19.13 *Anagen effluvium.* This patient's alopecia resulted from chemotherapy for lung cancer. Her hair loss was diffuse, and her hair is now regrowing.

- Immunotherapeutic medications (cyclosporine, methotrexate, colchicine).
- Intoxication with thallium or mercury.
- Radiation therapy.

CLINICAL MANIFESTATIONS

- Anagen effluvium presents as a diffuse, nonscarring, noninflammatory type of hair loss (Fig. 19.13).

DIAGNOSIS

- The diagnosis tends to be straightforward because of an obvious triggering event, such as chemotherapy.
- A **hair pull test** wherein a lock of hair is grasped to determine how many can be extracted with a firm pull will be positive with at least four anagen hairs (elongated or tapered end hairs) per pull.

 MANAGEMENT

- Management of anagen effluvium simply involves the identification and removal, if feasible, of the precipitating cause.
- Local cooling of the scalp has been proposed to prevent hair loss during chemotherapy.

Prognosis
- Anagen effluvium is entirely reversible, and patients should be reassured that the hair loss is temporary. New hair growth starts a few weeks after the termination of treatment. However, the color and texture of the new hair may be different.

SENESCENT ALOPECIA

BASICS

- Aging results in a gradual decrease of scalp hair density. Whereas a newborn has about 1,100 hairs per square centimeter, by age 30 this has decreased to about 600 hairs per square centimeter, and by age 50 this has further decreased to about 500 hairs per square centimeter.
- This type of alopecia affects men and women equally and is seen in patients 50 years and older.

CLINICAL MANIFESTATIONS

- Patients generally complain of a thinning of scalp hair and do not report increased shedding.
- Senescent alopecia is a diffuse, nonscarring, noninflammatory type of hair loss. It represents a diagnosis of exclusion.

 POINTS TO REMEMBER

- The evaluation of diffuse hair loss, which is more often seen in women, should be a careful, thoughtful, and sympathetic process.
- Excessive hair loss should not be dismissed as simply a cosmetic issue.
- History taking should include questions about the patient's physical and mental health status, antecedent illnesses, medications, traumatic events (e.g., loss of a loved one), hairstyling techniques, and family history.
- In addition, masculinizing signs or symptoms should be noted.

Scarring Alopecia

BASICS

- Scarring alopecia, also known as **cicatricial alopecia**, comprises a large group of heterogeneous disorders. They can be divided into inflammatory and noninflammatory categories based on their underlying pathogenesis. The inflammatory scarring alopecias can be further grouped into either infectious (see Chapter 9) or noninfectious.
- This section will focus on the scarring alopecias that are caused by inflammatory noninfectious processes: chronic cutaneous lupus erythematosus, lichen planopilaris, central centrifugal cicatricial alopecia, cutaneous sarcoidosis, folliculitis decalvans, pseudofolliculitis barbae, and acne nuchae keloidalis.
- Scarring alopecias affect all ethnic groups and races; however, certain types of scarring alopecias are more prevalent in African-American and Afro-Caribbean women.

PATHOGENESIS

- In scarring alopecia, perifollicular inflammation (from autoimmune phenomena, superantigen response of cytokines, or infection) leads to the replacement of the hair follicle by scar tissue resulting in permanent loss of the hair follicle.
- In addition direct trauma to the hair follicle from burns, radiation dermatitis, cutaneous malignancies, cutaneous sarcoidosis, or certain hairstyling practices can result in damage and permanent destruction of the hair follicles.

CLINICAL MANIFESTATIONS

- In its early stages, there is no obvious hair loss or scarring noted and the diagnosis is often missed. The patient may present with scaling and itching and is often diagnosed as having "excessive dandruff" or "seborrheic dermatitis." The patient may then be advised to shampoo more often with an antidandruff shampoo which often results in exacerbation of symptoms.
- As the disease progresses, the hair loss becomes more apparent. The loss of follicular orifices (ostia or pores) is a key feature of scarring alopecia (Fig. 19.14), differentiating it from alopecia areata, a nonscarring inflammatory alopecia in which the follicular orifices remain intact.
- The process can further evolve and coalesce into larger areas.
- The skin within the areas of hair loss may have a thin, shiny, atrophic appearance and may spread centrifugally, with an area of central scarring surrounded by an expanding periphery of erythema.

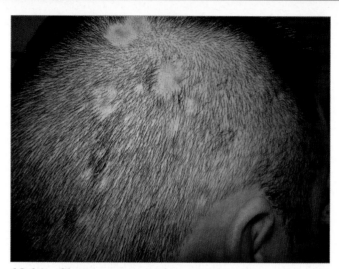

19.14 *Chronic cutaneous lupus erythematosus.* Note lack of ostia (follicular orifices).

CHRONIC CUTANEOUS LUPUS ERYTHEMATOSUS (SEE ALSO CHAPTER 34)

BASICS

- Chronic cutaneous lupus erythematosus (CCLE) accounts for about one-third of cases of cicatricial alopecia. It occurs more frequently in African-American women.
- Evidence of systemic lupus erythematosus (SLE) or other cutaneous signs of lupus may or may not be present.
- Discoid lupus erythematosus—so-named for its discoid, or disk-shaped, lesions—is by far the most common form of CCLE.
- SLE, unlike CCLE, may lead to telogen effluvium, which typically presents as a diffuse nonscarring type of hair loss (see earlier discussion); occasionally, the scarring alopecia of CCLE may also be seen in a patient with SLE.

CLINICAL MANIFESTATIONS

- Typically, the patient with CCLE initially presents with patches of alopecia on the scalp that are red, atrophic, and with mottled pigmentation (areas of hypo- and hyperpigmentation) (Fig. 19.15A,B).
- Lesions may be quite pruritic.
- Other similar lesions may be observed on the conchae of the external ears or elsewhere on the body (see detail in Fig. 19.15B).

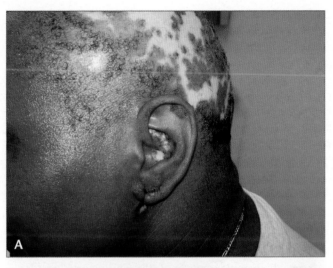

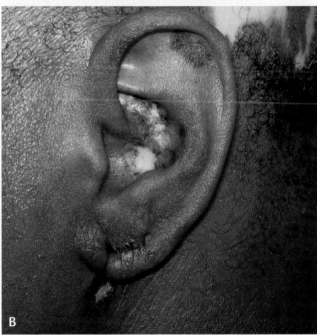

19.15 *Chronic cutaneous lupus erythematosus.*
A: Extensive scarring alopecia, as well as typical discoid lesions. **B:** Detail. Note characteristic lesions located on ear conchae.

DIAGNOSIS

- A scalp biopsy and direct immunofluorescence helps to make the diagnosis.
- Serologic studies can be useful to rule out SLE; however, the vast majority of CCLE cases may be isolated phenomena and do not demonstrate the presence of antinuclear antibodies.

 DIFFERENTIAL DIAGNOSIS

- **Other causes of scarring alopecias:** central centrifugal cicatricial alopecia (see below), tinea capitis, cutaneous sarcoidosis, and traction alopecia.

 MANAGEMENT

- **Superpotent topical corticosteroids** or **intralesional corticosteroid injections** are the first-line therapy for CCLE.
- In more extensive or recalcitrant cases, **hydroxychloroquine** (200 to 400 mg/day) is often effective.
- Other therapies that have been used include **dapsone, isotretinoin**, and **thalidomide**. The goal of treatment is to alleviate scalp pruritus or discomfort, decrease inflammation, and prevent further destruction of the hair follicles.

 HELPFUL HINTS

- When faced with a scarring alopecia in a woman of color, it is very important to rule out cutaneous sarcoidosis or, less commonly, a fungal infection of the scalp (tinea capitis), both of which can lead to a scarring alopecia.
- Glucose-6-phosphate dehydrogenase (G6PD) deficiency screening is required prior to treatment with dapsone because patients with G6PD deficiency are more prone to the hematologic side effects of this drug.
- Patients taking hydroxychloroquine need to be monitored for anemia and require retinal examination prior to and during treatment because of the potential for retinopathy.

LICHEN PLANOPILARIS

BASICS

- Lichen planopilaris (LPP) accounts for approximately another third of cases of scarring alopecia and is sometimes associated with lichen planus-like lesions on the skin, nails, and mucous membranes (see Chapter 15).

PATHOGENESIS

- Like lichen planus, LPP is thought to result from a cell-mediated immune response to an unknown trigger.

CLINICAL MANIFESTATIONS

- Patients with LPP initially complain of erythema and burning that is then followed by the development of patchy alopecia, most commonly on the vertex of the scalp.
- Typically, there is *perifollicular erythema* and scale (Fig. 19.16).
- Tufting or polytrichia, which are clumps of hairs caused by surrounding scarring, is often seen.
- There is great variability in the severity of LPP.
- LPP tends to be progressive but tends to "burn out" after several years.
- **Frontal fibrosing alopecia**, is a clinical variant of LPP which affects the frontal area of the scalp and is most often seen in elderly Caucasian women (Fig. 19.17). Frontal fibrosing alopecia is not associated with on the skin.

DIAGNOSIS

- A scalp biopsy is often necessary to make the diagnosis.
- Serologic studies to help exclude connective tissue disease are recommended.

DIFFERENTIAL DIAGNOSIS

- **Other causes of scarring alopecias:** central centrifugal cicatricial alopecia (see below), tinea capitis, cutaneous sarcoidosis, and traction alopecia.

MANAGEMENT

- **Superpotent topical** or **intralesional corticosteroids** are the first line of therapy for LPP.
- **Doxycycline** or **minocycline** (100 to 200 mg/day) is often effective in mild cases of LPP.
- Other therapies that have been used include **cyclosporine, methotrexate, hydroxychloroquine, dapsone, pioglitazone** (a PPAR-γ agonist), and **oral isotretinoin**.

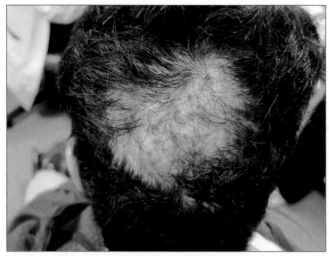

19.16 *Lichen planopilaris (LPP).* This woman has a large area of cicatricial alopecia. There is perifollicular erythema characteristic of LPP.

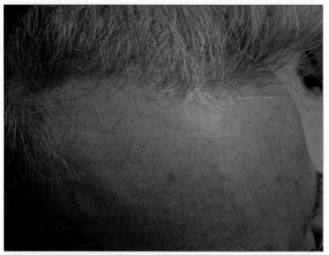

19.17 *Frontal fibrosing alopecia.* A variant of LPP which affects the frontal area of the scalp.

CENTRAL CENTRIFUGAL CICATRICIAL ALOPECIA

BASICS

- Central centrifugal cicatricial alopecia (CCCA) is the current term used to describe a type of scarring alopecia that is mostly seen in African-American women believed to be triggered by caustic hair treatment chemicals and/or heat from hot combs in a susceptible person. Previously, the traditional terms *hot-comb alopecia* and *follicular degeneration syndrome* were coined to describe this condition.

PATHOGENESIS

- It is now known that patients who develop CCCA have hair follicles that show premature desquamation of the inner root sheath even before clinical symptoms are seen.
- This abnormality predisposes the affected follicles to injury or inflammation in response to chemicals found in commercial styling products and relaxers or excessive heat from hot combs.

CLINICAL MANIFESTATIONS

- As the name implies, CCCA presents with patches of scarring alopecia on the central vertex of the scalp, and progresses centrifugally outward (Fig. 19.18).
- Early hair loss is usually asymptomatic and gradual. Most patients report only mild, occasional pruritus or pain.
- Pustules, itching, and crusting may occur in rapidly progressive disease.
- Hypopigmentation and hyperpigmentation may be seen in affected scarred scalp areas.
- Tufting or polytrichia within the alopecic area can also be noted.

DIAGNOSIS

Diagnosis is based on the following:

- Clinical appearance.
- History of hair reshaping techniques.
- Scalp biopsy, if necessary.

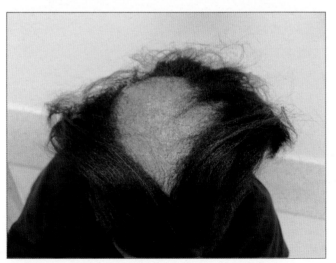

19.18 *Central centrifugal cicatricial alopecia.* The continuous use of chemical relaxers resulted in permanent hair loss at the vertex of this woman's scalp.

 DIFFERENTIAL DIAGNOSIS

- **Other causes of scarring alopecias:** chronic cutaneous lupus erythematosus (see above), lichen planopilaris (see above), tinea capitis, cutaneous sarcoidosis, and traction alopecia.

 MANAGEMENT

- Management of CCCA consists of removing, changing, or eliminating the damaging hairstyle practices as well as reducing the inflammation. Encouraging the patient to change hairstyle practices requires sensitivity as well as a good understanding of the different hairstyles and practices of black women.
- Ideally, natural hairstyles that do not place traction on the hair shaft are recommended.
- Use of mild, lye-free chemical relaxants once every 2 months is suggested, and the use of heat-relaxing devices such as hot combs and hood dryers should be discouraged.
- Anti-inflammatory therapy with **minocycline** or **doxycycline**, as well as **topical** or **intralesional corticosteroids** are helpful in the initial phases.
- Once the inflammation is completely resolved, hair transplantation into scarred areas can be used to improve cosmesis.

HELPFUL HINTS

- Although a great majority of black women are using or have used chemical and thermal relaxers, a diagnosis of CCCA should not be made presumptively. A scalp biopsy for H/E staining and direct immunofluorescence, a negative PAS stain, as well as negative or nonreactive connective tissue serologies, helps to rule out other causes of scarring alopecias.
- The importance of early diagnosis and prompt initiation of treatment for a scarring alopecia is of the utmost importance. Once the follicle is replaced by scar tissue, the hair loss is irreversible.

TRACTION ALOPECIA

BASICS

- Traction alopecia is seen almost exclusively in African-American and African-Caribbean women of all ages, who are more likely to braid their hair.
- The condition results from the prolonged and repeated trauma to the hair follicle by hairstyles such as cornrows, braiding, and tight ponytails.
- The persistent physical stress of traction injury caused by tight rollers, tight braiding, or ponytails causes hair loss.

CLINICAL MANIFESTATIONS

- Traction alopecia is manifested by a symmetric pattern of hair loss, with broken hairs.
- A characteristic border of residual hairs is often at the distal margin of the hair loss (Figs. 19.19A,B).
- Traction pattern: alopecia is evident at the temples and along the frontal hairline. Hair loss later extends to the vertex and occipital areas.
- A combination of these patterns may be seen if both traction and hot combs or chemicals are used.

DIAGNOSIS

- The clinical presentation and history are usually sufficient to make the diagnosis.

 DIFFERENTIAL DIAGNOSIS

Chemical or Heat Induced Traumatic Alopecia
- *History of chemical or heat applications.*
- *Hair loss is more irregular (less symmetric) and reflects the areas where the chemicals or hot comb were applied.*

 MANAGEMENT

- Early intervention and discontinuation of the damaging hairstyles are the mainstays of therapy, because delay may result in irreversible hair loss.

 HELPFUL HINT

- A rim of residual hair is often present. They are short hairs that cannot be "grabbed" by rollers.

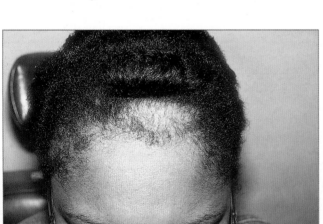 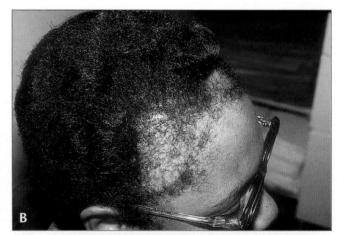

19.19   **A** and **B:** *Traction alopecia.* **A:** This woman's alopecia is the result of the use of tight curlers. Note the symmetric loss of hair in a frontotemporal distribution and the "relaxed" curl that was chemically straightened. **B:** Note the fringe of residual hairs at the distal margin of alopecia. These hairs were too short to be "grabbed" by the hair curlers.

CUTANEOUS SARCOIDOSIS (SEE CHAPTER 34)

BASICS

- Hair loss due to cutaneous sarcoidosis may closely resemble that of other scarring alopecias discussed in this chapter.
- Sarcoidosis of the scalp is most commonly noted in African-American women and in patients who have cutaneous or noncutaneous involvement elsewhere, such as pulmonary sarcoidosis.

CLINICAL MANIFESTATIONS

- Scalp lesions may present with a variety of morphologies, including alopecic papules, nodules, plaques, and infiltrated scars.

DIAGNOSIS

- A scalp biopsy demonstrating noncaseating granulomas may be necessary to distinguish sarcoidosis from other causes of scarring alopecia.
- Evidence of cutaneous sarcoidosis elsewhere on the body or systemic involvement can support the diagnosis.
- Serologic studies to exclude connective tissue diseases are recommended.

MANAGEMENT (see Chapter 34 for Other Treatment Modalities)

- **Potent topical, intralesional**, or **oral corticosteroids** may be used to control sarcoidosis of the scalp.

FOLLICULITIS DECALVANS

BASICS

- Folliculitis decalvans presents as a scarring patch of alopecia surrounded by follicular pustules.
- This condition does not merely represent a bacterial folliculitis; rather, an abnormal immune response to possible staphylococcal antigens may be involved.

CLINICAL MANIFESTATIONS

- Successive crops of peripheral pustules result in an expanding patch or patches of scarring alopecia (Fig. 19.20).

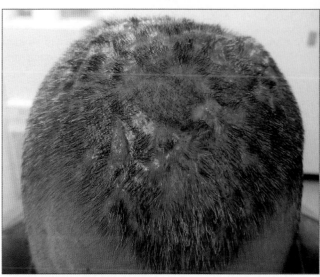

19.20 *Folliculitis decalvans.* Extensive inflammation, pustules, and scarring are present.

DIAGNOSIS

- Bacterial cultures from the follicular pustules often grow *Staphylococcus aureus.*
- A scalp biopsy for H/E staining demonstrates a scarring alopecia with a neutrophilic infiltrate.

DIFFERENTIAL DIAGNOSIS

- Although rare in adults, it is important to rule out **tinea capitis,** which can also present as a pustular scarring alopecia.

MANAGEMENT

- Prolonged antistaphylococcal treatment with **mono-therapy (dicloxacillin, minocycline, cephalexin)** or **combination therapy (rifampin** plus **clindamycin** or **cephalexin).**
- **Topical antibiotic agents,** and **topical and intralesional corticosteroids** may be used in conjunction with systemic therapy.

BASICS

- Hair follicle problems are very common in men and women of African-American, African-Caribbean, and Hispanic origin who have tightly curled hair.
- Postadolescent African-American men, in particular, experience "shaving bumps" (pseudofolliculitis barbae) and a characteristic scarring, acne-like condition located on the occiput referred to as acne nuchae keloidalis.

PSEUDOFOLLICULITIS BARBAE (PFB)

PATHOGENESIS

- Tightly coiled hairs emerge from curved hair follicles (Illus. 19.2).
- When shaved, the hair becomes a sharp tip that curves downward as it grows and reenters the epidermis; or, the sharpened hair may grow parallel to the skin and penetrate it resulting in an inflammatory foreign body-like reaction.
- Furthermore, newly erupting hairs from below may pierce and aggravate areas that are already inflamed.

CLINICAL MANIFESTATIONS

- Lesions consist of inflammatory papules and pustules typically found on the beard, neck, and submental areas (Fig. 19.21).
- Ultimately, persistent flesh-colored papules that represent hypertrophic scars and postinflammatory pigmented lesions become prominent clinical features.
- On close inspection, tight, curly hairs can be seen penetrating the skin (Fig. 19.22).

DIAGNOSIS

- Diagnosis is apparent on clinical examination.

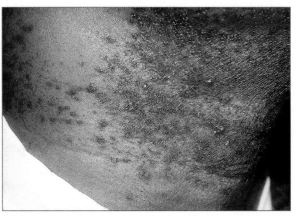

19.21   *Pseudofolliculitis barbae.* Tight, curly hairs that have been sharpened by shaving penetrate the skin resulting in inflammatory papules and pustules and scars.

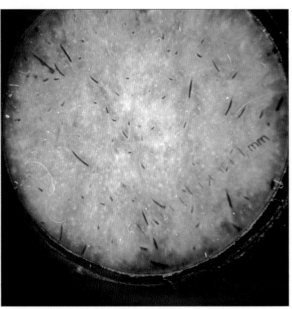

19.22   *Pseudofolliculitis barbae.* Magnified dermascopic view showing reentry of hairs.

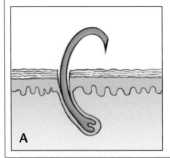
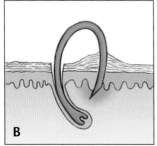
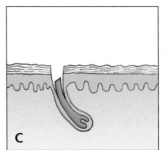
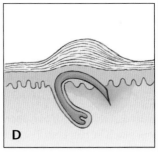

I19.2   *Pseudofolliculitis barbae, or "razor bumps," showing extrafollicular and transfollicular penetration.* **A:** A curly hair grows from a sharply curved hair root. When shaved, the hair is left with a sharp point. As this hair grows, the sharp tip curves back and pierces the skin. **B:** The sharpened hair penetrates the skin. **C and D:** When hairs are cut too closely, they can penetrate the side of the hair root. Both types of follicular reentry cause a foreign body-like reaction (papule). (Modified from Crutchfield CE III. Patient handout: Treatment of razor bumps, 1996. Available at: http://www.crutchfielddermatology.com/treatments/pseudofolliculitisbarbae/1.htm.)

DIFFERENTIAL DIAGNOSIS

Acne Vulgaris
- *Lesions are usually not confined to the neck; however, the distinction from PFB may be difficult.*

Bacterial Folliculitis
- *As with acne, folliculitis may look exactly like PFB.*

 MANAGEMENT

Preventive Measures
- Discontinuance of shaving is helpful; however, this is generally not a choice desired by most patients.
- Patients may avoid close shaving by using a guarded razor (e.g., **PFB Bump Fighter**). This razor is covered with a plastic coating that prevents the razor from contacting the skin directly. The use of an electric razor is another method that reduces the closeness of the shave.
- Hairs may be lifted with a fine needle or a toothpick before they penetrate the skin (Fig. 19.23).
- Patients should be advised not to pluck hairs because new hairs will again grow from below and penetrate a site that is already inflamed.

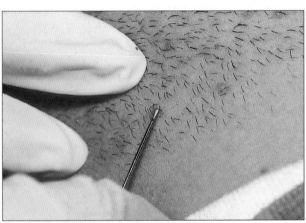

19.23 *Pseudofolliculitis barbae.* A curled hair is lifted with a fine needle after it had penetrated the skin.

Treatment
- Treatment is difficult.
- **Nonfluorinated, class 5 or 6 topical steroids** are used for inflammation and itching.
- Topical antibiotics such as **Benzamycin, BenzaClin, or Duac gel** (these combine clindamycin and benzoyl peroxide) applied once daily to the affected areas often reduces inflammation.
- Systemic antibiotics such as **minocycline** or **doxycycline** are helpful when marked inflammation and pustulation are present.
- Chemical depilatories such as **Magic Shave** and **Royal Crown powders** are effective in removing and softening hairs; the main disadvantages are that they are irritating and they have an unpleasant odor.
- Hair destruction using an **extended-pulse width laser** has been shown to be effective.
- Eflornithine hydrochloride 13.9% (**Vaniqa**) is an enzyme inhibitor that slows hair growth (discussed in Chapter 20).
- **Electrolysis** is difficult to use on inflammatory foci as well as on curly hair, but it can be partially effective as an adjunctive treatment method.

 SEE PATIENT HANDOUT "Pseudofolliculitis Barbae (Razor Bumps)" IN THE COMPANION eBOOK EDITION.

ACNE KELOIDALIS NUCHAE

BASICS
- The name **acne keloidalis nuchae (AKN)** is actually a misnomer. AKN has nothing to do with acne but is actually a type of folliculitis similar to PFB.
- The pathogenesis of acne keloidalis is similar to that of pseudofolliculitis barbae (see previous section), in which coiled hairs pierce the skin resulting in an inflammatory reaction.

CLINICAL MANIFESTATIONS
- Initially, inflammatory acneiform papules and pustules are noted.
- Ultimately, hypertrophic scarring occurs, characterized by flesh-colored to pink firm papules (Fig. 19.24) and possibly extensive keloid formation (Fig. 19.25).
- This condition is characteristically seen in the lower occipital area, but it can extend to the adjacent scalp or cover the entire scalp and thus may be indistinguishable from folliculitis decalvans.

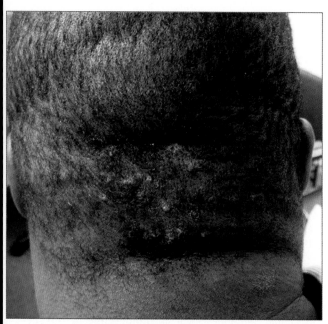

19.24 *Acne keloidalis nuchae.* Hypertrophic scarring and flesh-colored papules are seen in this patient.

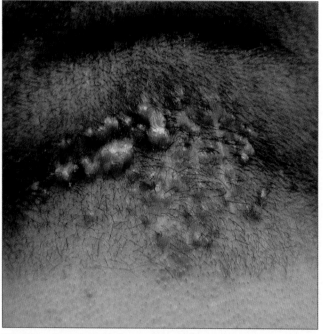

19.25 *Acne keloidalis nuchae.* Keloids are present in this female patient.

DIFFERENTIAL DIAGNOSIS

- As with PFB with which it may coexist, **acne vulgaris** and **folliculitis** may be difficult to distinguish from AKN.

MANAGEMENT

- **Potent topical** or **intralesional steroids** (5 to 10 mg/mL) help decrease itching and inflammation.
- **Topical antibiotics** are used when papules and pustules are present.
- A systemic antibiotic such as **minocycline** or **doxycycline** are helpful because of their anti-inflammatory effect.
- Surgical treatment is not without risk. It is reserved for extreme cases and may result in worse scarring.

HELPFUL HINTS

- When bacterial folliculitis is present, it is usually the result of secondary, not primary, pathogens.
- Prevention of these disorders also depends on avoidance of close "clipper" shaves and haircuts.

CHAPTER 20 Hirsutism

OVERVIEW

Hirsutism is defined as the excessive growth of thick, dark hair in women in locations where hair growth is normally minimal or absent. Such male-pattern growth of terminal body hair usually occurs in androgen-sensitive locations, such as the face, chest, and areolae.

Although the terms hirsutism and hypertrichosis are often used interchangeably, hypertrichosis actually refers to excess hair (terminal or vellus) in areas that are not predominantly androgen dependent. Whether a given patient is hirsute is often difficult to judge because hair growth varies among individual women and across ethnic groups. What is considered hirsutism in one culture may be considered normal in another. For example, women from the Mediterranean and Indian subcontinents have more facial and body hair than do women from Asia, sub-Saharan Africa, and Northern Europe. Dark-haired, darkly pigmented individuals of either sex tend to be more hirsute than blonde or fair-skinned persons.

Most of the time hirsutism is a benign, genetically determined condition that is a cosmetic nuisance for women, however it is important to evaluate for an underlying endocrinopathy in certain situations.

IN THIS CHAPTER...

> **HIRSUTISM**

- Familial hirsutism
- Ovarian hirsutism
- Adrenal hirsutism
- Drug-induced hirsutism
- Idiopathic hirsutism

Hirsutism

BASICS

- Hirsutism is often a benign condition primarily of cosmetic concern. When hirsutism is accompanied by masculinizing signs or symptoms, particularly after puberty, it may be a manifestation of a more serious underlying disorder, such as an ovarian or adrenal neoplasm. Fortunately, such disorders are rare.
- Hirsutism exceeding culturally normal levels can be as distressing an emotional problem as the loss of scalp hair.

PATHOGENESIS

- The physiologic mechanism for androgenic activity consists of three stages: (1) production of androgens by the adrenals and ovaries, (2) androgen transport in the blood on carrier proteins (principally sex hormone–binding globulin [SHBG]), and (3) intracellular modification and binding to the androgen receptor.
- Hirsutism can be caused by overproduction of androgens (from the ovaries or adrenal glands), increased peripheral conversion of androgen, decreased metabolism, and enhanced receptor binding (hair follicles that are more sensitive to normal androgen levels).
- The amount of free testosterone and its byproduct dihydrotestosterone, is regulated by SHBG. Lower levels of SHBG increase the availability of free testosterone.
- SHBG decreases in response to the following: exogenous androgens, certain disorders that affect androgen levels, such as polycystic ovary syndrome, congenital or delayed-onset adrenal hyperplasia, Cushing syndrome, obesity, hyperinsulinemia, hyperprolactinemia, excess growth hormone, hypothyroidism.
- Conversely, SHBG increases with higher estrogen levels, such as those that occur during oral contraceptive therapy. The resulting increased SHBG levels lower the activity of circulating testosterone.
- Increased circulating androgens result in an increased hair follicle size, hair fiber diameter, and duration of time hair follicles spend in the anagen (growth) phase. In addition to a change in hair quality and volume, oilier skin and hair may result from excess androgen.
- For circulating testosterone to exert its stimulatory effects on the hair follicle, first it must be converted into its more potent follicle-active metabolite, dihydrotestosterone, by 5-α-reductase, an enzyme found in the hair follicle.
- The severity of hirsutism does not correlate with the level of increased circulating androgens because of individual differences in conversion to 5-α-reductase and androgen sensitivity of hair follicles.
- Increased androgens will result in hirsutism in androgen-sensitive regions of the body but leads to thinning of scalp hair.

CLINICAL MANIFESTATIONS

- Hirsutism presents with excess terminal hair in a masculine pattern. Sites include the face (particularly the moustache, beard, and temple areas), the chest, areolae, linea alba, upper back, lower back, buttocks, inner thighs, and external genitalia.

CLINICAL VARIANTS

- Hirsutism is often classified according to the source of the excess circulating androgen which leads to a specific clinical pattern.

FAMILIAL HIRSUTISM

- Often appears during puberty as excess facial hair and prolongation of the preauricular hair line and is not associated with androgen excess.
- Familial hirsutism is both typical and natural in certain populations, such as in some women of Mediterranean or Middle Eastern ancestry (Fig. 20.1).

OVARIAN HIRSUTISM

- Ovarian hirsutism leads to excess hair growth on the lateral face and around the areolae and is often accompanied by obesity, severe acne, and seborrheic dermatitis.
- **Polycystic ovary syndrome (PCOS)** is the most common cause of androgen excess–related hirsutism.
  - In PCOS, virilization is minimal and hirsutism is often prominent.
  - Characteristic features include menstrual irregularities, dysmenorrhea, occasional glucose intolerance and hyperinsulinemia, and, often, obesity.
  - The hyperinsulinemia is believed to hyperstimulate the ovaries into producing excess androgens.

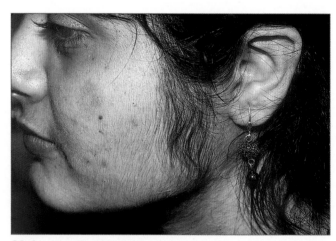

20.1 *Familial hirsutism.* As seen in this Pakistani woman, familial hirsutism is both typical and natural in certain populations.

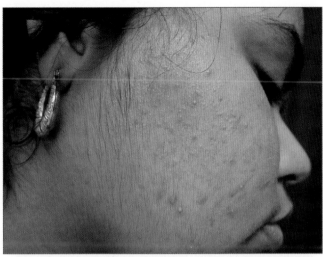

20.2 Hirsutism. This patient has the polycystic ovary syndrome. This is the most common cause of androgen excess and hirsutism. Note the lesions of acne.

- Women with PCOS may show other cutaneous manifestations of androgen excess in addition to hirsutism, such as recalcitrant acne (Fig. 20.2), acanthosis nigricans, and alopecia on the crown area of the scalp (a pattern that contrasts with the bitemporal and vertex androgenic alopecia seen in men).
- **Other ovarian causes** are usually associated with virilization and include luteoma of pregnancy, arrhenoblastomas, Leydig cell tumors, hilar cell tumors, theca cell tumors.
- Excess growth of facial hair is seen in elderly postmenopausal women and may be caused by unopposed androgen that occurs after menopause.

ADRENAL HIRSUTISM

- Adrenal hirsutism results in excess hair in a "central" distribution on the anterior neck, abdomen, and suprapubic area.
- Children with **congenital adrenal hyperplasia (CAH)**, the classic form of adrenal hyperplasia, may exhibit hirsutism. Such children may be born with ambiguous genitalia and symptoms of salt wasting, failure to thrive, and develop masculine features.
- **Late-onset congenital adrenal hyperplasia** affects about 1% to 5% of hyperandrogenic women. Although these patients have clinical features that resemble PCOS, they manifest no salt-wasting symptoms and may not develop signs of virilization or menstrual irregularities until puberty or adulthood (Fig. 20.3).
- **Cushing syndrome** is a noncongenital form of adrenal hyperplasia. It is characterized by an excess of adrenal cortisol production. The excessive growth is predominantly vellus (nonandrogen-dependent) hair.
- **Androgen-producing adrenal tumors** are extremely rare. Hirsutism appears rather abruptly when an androgen-secreting tumor arises.

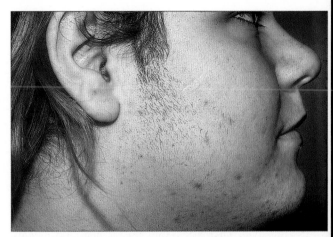

20.3 Hirsutism in late-onset congenital adrenal hyperplasia. An 18-year-old woman with clinical features that are similar to those of polycystic ovary syndrome: acne, hirsutism, menstrual irregularities, and obesity.

HYPERPROLACTINEMIC HIRSUTISM

- Hyperprolactinemic hirsutism results in excess growth both centrally and laterally and is sometimes accompanied by seborrhea, acne, oligomenorrhea, and galactorrhea.

DRUG-INDUCED HIRSUTISM

- Drugs that can induce hirsutism by their inherent androgenic effects include dehydroepiandrosterone sulfate (DHEA-S), testosterone, danazol, and anabolic steroids.
- The current low-dose oral contraceptives are less likely to cause hirsutism than were previous formulations.

IDIOPATHIC HIRSUTISM

- The few hirsute women who do not have a familial form of hirsutism or any detectable hormonal abnormality are usually given a diagnosis of idiopathic, or end-organ, hirsutism.
- Such patients have normal menses, normal-sized ovaries, no evidence of adrenal or ovarian tumors or dysfunction, and no significant elevations of plasma testosterone or androstenedione.
- Antiandrogen therapy may improve hirsutism in some idiopathic cases which suggests that this form of hirsutism may be androgen induced.
- It is believed that many of these women may have mild or early PCOS and androgen levels in the upper normal ranges.

OTHER ASSOCIATED DISORDERS

- Other less common but potentially serious disorders associated with hirsutism include anorexia nervosa, acromegaly, hypothyroidism, porphyria, and certain cancers.

DIAGNOSIS

- After familial and drug-induced causes for hirsutism have been excluded, hirsutism resulting from androgen excess should be considered.
- Initial screening for total and free testosterone and DHEA-S often determines whether further testing is necessary.
- Moderate elevations in DHEA-S suggest an adrenal origin of the hirsutism.
- Normal levels of DHEA-S accompanied by high levels of testosterone indicate that the ovaries, and not the adrenals, are producing the excess androgen.
- A tumor workup is indicated for total testosterone levels greater than 200 ng/dL (>100 ng/dL in postmenopausal women) or DHEA-S levels greater than 700 mcg/dL (400 mcg/dL in postmenopausal women).
- In PCOS, the luteinizing hormone (LH) levels are elevated and follicle-stimulating hormone (FSH) levels are depressed, which results in elevated LH/FSH ratios (>2 is common).
- If Cushing syndrome is suspected, a 24-hour urinary cortisol or an overnight dexamethasone suppression test should be performed.

 DIFFERENTIAL DIAGNOSIS

Drug-induced Hypertrichosis

- *Distinguished from drug-induced hirsutism by a uniform growth of fine hairs that appear over extensive areas of the trunk, hands, and face. Such growth is not androgen dependent.*
- *Precipitating drugs include phenytoin, minoxidil (Fig. 20.4), diazoxide, cyclosporine, penicillamine, high-dose corticosteroids, phenothiazines, acetazolamide, and hexachlorobenzene. The exact mode of action is not known, but presumably these agents also exert their effects independent of androgens.*

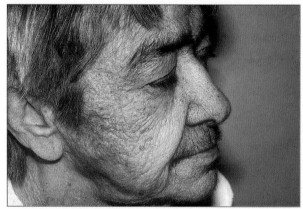

20.4 *Drug-induced hypertrichosis.* Oral minoxidil was the cause of hypertrichosis in this elderly woman.

 MANAGEMENT

General Principles

- Management depends on the underlying cause of the hirsutism.
- If circulating androgen levels are normal, then excess hair is treated primarily with physical hair removal methods if the patient is troubled by the hair growth. Treatment is unnecessary if the patient does not find the hirsutism cosmetically objectionable.
- In contrast, those patients who have excess androgen–induced hirsutism may require a combination of physical hair removal and medical antiandrogen therapy.
- As an alternative to hair removal, simple bleaching of hair is an inexpensive method that works well when hirsutism is not too excessive. Bleaches lighten the color of the hair so that it is less noticeable.

Hair Removal
Depilation

- Depilatories remove hair from the surface of the skin. Depilatory methods include ordinary shaving and the use of chemicals, such as thioglycolic acid.
- **Shaving** removes all hairs, but it is immediately followed by growth of hairs that were previously in anagen; as these hairs grow in, they produce rough stubble. There is no evidence that shaving increases the growth or coarseness of subsequent hair growth. Most women, however, prefer not to shave their facial hair.
- **Chemical depilation** may be best suited for treatment of large hairy areas in patients who are unable to afford more expensive treatments, such as electrolysis and laser epilation. Chemical depilatories separate the hair from

continued on page 339

MANAGEMENT *Continued*

its follicle by reducing the sulfide bonds that are found in abundance in hairs. Irritant reactions and folliculitis may result.

Temporary Epilation

- **Epilation** involves removal of the intact hair with its root. **Plucking or tweezing** is widely performed. This method may result in irritation, damage to the hair follicle, folliculitis, hyperpigmentation, and scarring.
- **Waxing** entails the application of hot, melted wax to the hair-bearing skin which then cools and sets and is abruptly peeled off the skin removing embedded hairs with it. This method is painful and sometimes results in folliculitis. Repetitive waxing may produce miniaturization of hairs, and, over the long run, it may permanently reduce the number of hairs.
- Certain **natural sugars**, that have been used in the Middle East for centuries, are becoming popular in place of waxes. They appear to epilate as effectively as, but less traumatically than, waxing.
- **Threading** is currently a very popular method that has been traditionally used in the Middle East and Asia. It is a technique in which cotton threads are used to pull out hairs from their roots.
- Home epilating devices that remove hair by a rotary or frictional method are available. Both methods may produce traumatic folliculitis.

Permanent Epilation

Electrolysis and Thermolysis

- Hair destruction by **electrolysis**, **thermolysis**, or a combination of both is performed with a fine, flexible electrical wire that produces an electrical current after it is introduced down the hair shaft. **Thermolysis** (diathermy) uses a high-frequency alternating current and is much faster than the traditional electrolysis method, which uses a direct galvanic current.
- Electrolysis and thermolysis are slow processes that can be used on all skin and hair colors, but multiple treatments are required.
- Electrolysis and thermolysis can be uncomfortable and may produce folliculitis, pseudofolliculitis, and postinflammatory pigmentary changes in the skin.

Laser Epilation

- Lasers that selectively target the pigment in hair leading to destruction can treat larger areas and can do so faster than electrolysis and thermolysis. They have skin-cooling

mechanisms that minimize epidermal destruction during the procedure. Skin and hair color often determine which laser should be used.

- Popular lasers used for hair removal are the 755-nm Alexandrite, 800-nm Diode, and the 1064-nm Nd:YAG.
- Lasers are most effective on dark hairs on fair-skinned people. In such patients, lighter skin does not compete with darker hairs for the laser. In dark-skinned people, lasers that deliver energy to the hairs over a longer period are safer.
- As with electrolysis and thermolysis, multiple treatments are necessary for long-term hair reduction.
- Folliculitis, pseudofolliculitis, discomfort, and pigmentary changes may result from laser therapy.
- It remains to be proved whether lasers are more effective in permanent hair removal than the more traditional methods.

Pharmacologic Treatment

- Medications (**antiandrogens**) are often administered to address the underlying etiology while cosmetic hair removal techniques are being used. These drugs must be given continuously because when they are stopped, androgens will revert to their former levels.
- Common systemic hormonal agents used singly or in combination for hirsutism include the following:
  - Ovarian suppression with **oral contraceptives**
  - Androgen receptor blockade and inhibition (**spironolactone, flutamide, and cyproterone acetate**)
  - Adrenal suppression with **oral corticosteroids**
  - 5-α-reductase inhibition with **finasteride**
- All medications listed above are absolutely contraindicated for use during pregnancy because of the risk of feminization of a male fetus.

Other Treatments

- **Eflornithine hydrochloride** 13.9% cream (**Vaniqa**) is a prescription topical cream that acts as a growth inhibitor, not a depilatory. The agent inhibits ornithine decarboxylase, an enzyme required for hair growth. It is indicated for the reduction of unwanted facial hair in women. Continued twice-daily use for at least 4 to 8 weeks is necessary before effectiveness is noted.
- **Metformin (Glucophage)** reduces insulin levels, and this change, in turn, reduces the ovarian testosterone levels by competitive inhibition of the ovarian insulin receptors. This drug is effective in treating hirsutism in women with PCOS.

HELPFUL HINTS

- Expensive hormonal laboratory tests for a woman with simple hirsutism are usually not cost-effective.
- However, if a woman shows a constellation of virilizing signs or symptoms, such as infrequent or absent menses, acne, deepening of the voice, male-pattern balding, increased muscle mass, increased libido, and clitoral hypertrophy, she should be referred to an endocrinologist.
- No direct correlation exists between the levels of testosterone and the degree of hirsutism, because hirsutism is caused by the action of dihydrotestosterone, which is the more potent testosterone metabolite.
- Elevated free serum testosterone levels (>80 ng/dL) are found in most women with anovulation and hirsutism.

 POINT TO REMEMBER

- Hirsutism that is not familial or drug-induced may be a marker for androgen excess and may occasionally signal a potentially serious underlying metabolic disorder or fatal neoplasm.

Disorders of the Oral Cavity, Lips, and Tongue

OVERVIEW

Oral mucous membrane lesions are often clues to the presence of systemic illnesses, such as acquired immunodeficiency syndrome (AIDS), syphilis, and systemic lupus erythematosus. They may also be helpful in diagnosing dermatologic conditions, including lichen planus and pemphigus vulgaris. "Canker sores" (aphthous ulcers) are often seen as isolated phenomena, but may also be an accompaniment or a precursor to a systemic disease such as Behçet disease and ulcerative colitis.

Mucous membrane lesions most frequently appear as erosions, blisters, fissures, ulcers, whitish plaques, pigmentary changes, neoplasms, cystic lesions, or as normal variants. It is often difficult to make a clinical diagnosis in the oral cavity. On the mucous membranes, leukoplakia, squamous cell carcinoma, and warts may appear indistinguishable from one another. Inflammatory oral lesions, particularly those that are vesicobullous, rarely remain intact and unruptured; instead, such lesions usually become erosions and ulcers by the time clinicians see them, adding to the difficulty of diagnosis.

IN THIS CHAPTER...

➤ **ORAL CAVITY**

- Aphthous stomatitis
- Oral lichen planus
- Systemic lupus erythematosus

➤ **TONGUE**

- Mucous patches of secondary syphilis
- Geographic tongue
- Black hairy tongue
- Pigmentation due to drugs and artifacts
- Oral leukoplakia
- Oral hairy leukoplakia
- Oral candidiasis ("thrush")

➤ **LIPS AND ORAL CAVITY**

- Perlèche (angular cheilitis)
- Actinic keratosis
- Squamous cell carcinoma
- Erythema multiforme minor
- Erythema multiforme major
- Pyogenic granuloma
- Venous lake
- Labial melanotic macule
- Oral mucous cyst (mucocele)
- Oral fibroma
- Oral warts
- Odontogenic sinus (dental sinus)

➤ **NORMAL VARIANTS**

- Fordyce spots
- Torus palatinus
- Normal bite line

APHTHOUS STOMATITIS

- Commonly referred to as "canker sores," aphthous ulcers are a common, recurrent problem consisting of shallow erosions of the mucous membranes.
- They are seen in children and adults and appear to be more common in women than men.
- Aphthous stomatitis has no known cause, but an immune mechanism is considered the most likely contributory factor.
- Patients often ascribe recurrences to psychological stress or local trauma.
- Women may correlate them with their menstrual cycle.

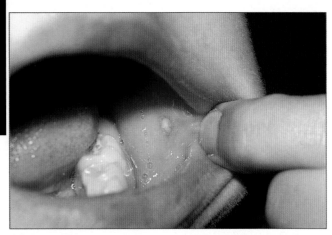

21.1 *Aphthous stomatitis.* A small punched-out erosion has a bright red margin.

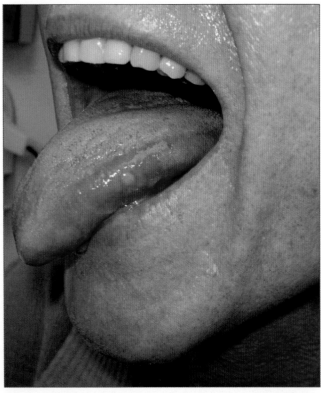

21.2 *Aphthous stomatitis.* Typical canker sore on the tongue with a yellowish center.

CLINICAL MANIFESTATIONS

- Lesions of aphthous stomatitis are small (2 to 5 mm), shallow, well-demarcated, punched-out erosions.
- Typically aphthae have a ring of erythema with a gray or yellowish center (Figs. 21.1–21.3).
- Lesions are painful and tend to heal in 4 to 14 days, a duration similar to that of HSV lesions.
- Patients with human immunodeficiency virus (HIV) or Behçet disease may develop aphthous stomatitis lesions that tend to be larger more persistent, painful, and extensive (Fig. 21.4).
- Most episodes heal spontaneously, only to recur unexpectedly.
- Most often arise on the buccal, labial, and gingival mucosa, as well as on the tongue.

DIAGNOSIS

- The diagnosis is made clinically.

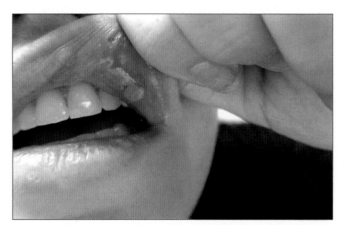

21.3 *Aphthous stomatitis.* Recurrent erosive canker sore on the lingual mucosa.

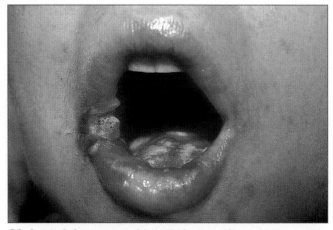

21.4 *Aphthous stomatitis in Behçet syndrome.* Large, painful erosions and extensive aphthae are evident on the lips and tongue of this woman.

DIFFERENTIAL DIAGNOSIS

Primary HSV Infection (Discussed in Chapters 6 and 17)

- *Oral erosions that are often indistinguishable from aphthous stomatitis are sometimes seen in primary herpes simplex virus (HSV) infections.*
- *Primary herpes gingivostomatitis occurs mainly in infants and young children, often subclinically, mild and unnoticed, but they can be severe, although less severe than recurrences.*
- *Fever, malaise, restlessness, and excessive drooling are common.*

Autoimmune Bullous Diseases such as Pemphigus Vulgaris and Bullous Pemphigoid

- *Chronic; bullous lesions often present elsewhere on the body.*

Cyclic Neutropenia

- *Dominantly inherited recurrent oral erosions/ulcers that occur every 3 weeks and last 3 to 6 days at a time.*
- *Ulcers result from changing rates of neutrophilic cell production by the bone marrow.*

Also consider:

Systemic Lupus Erythematosus (see below)

Behçet Disease

 MANAGEMENT

Therapeutic options include the following:
- Application of viscous lidocaine (**Xylocaine**) to lesions.
- **Vanceril** (beclomethasone dipropionate) aerosol can be sprayed directly on lesions.
- Superpotent topical steroids may be applied directly to lesions and held there by pressure with a finger in a rubber glove or applied with a cotton swab.
- **Tetracycline suspension** (250 mg/tsp); patients should "swish and swallow."
- Diphenhydramine (**Benadryl**) suspension; patients are directed to "gargle and spit."
- Tacrolimus **0.1%** ointment (**Protopic**) and pimecrolimus1% cream (**Elidel**) applied at bedtime may accelerate healing.
- **Silver nitrate**, applied with an applicator stick directly to lesions, also can promote healing (Fig. 21.5).
- **Intralesional corticosteroid injections** or a brief course of **systemic corticosteroids** are effective in reducing pain and healing lesions in patients with large, persistent, painful ulcers.

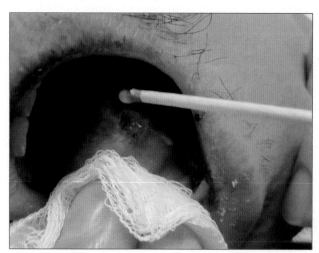

21.5 *Aphthous stomatitis.* Here silver nitrate is applied directly to a lesion.

- **Thalidomide** has been used with some success in healing large, recalcitrant, painful, persistent aphthae in persons with HIV infection.

 HELPFUL HINT

- A single, nonhealing ulcer (lasting more than 2 months) should undergo biopsy to rule out squamous cell carcinoma.

 POINT TO REMEMBER

- The vast majority of recurrent intraoral ulcers in immunocompetent patients are canker sores, not HSV lesions; recurrent HSV infection are unlikely to occur inside the mouth.

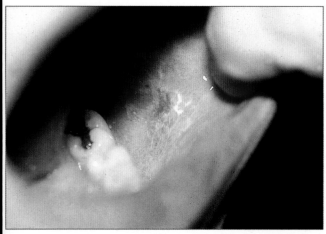

21.6 *Oral lichen planus, erosive.* A white, lacy network of lesions as well as erythematous erosions are present on the buccal mucosa.

ORAL LICHEN PLANUS (SEE ALSO CHAPTER 15)

CLINICAL MANIFESTATIONS

- A white, lacy network of lesions are present on the buccal mucosa (see Fig. 15.19), tongue, or gums.
- When erosive or ulcerative, lesions are painful and interfere with eating (Fig. 21.6).
- Evidence of lichen planus may or may not be present elsewhere on the body.

DIAGNOSIS

- Diagnosis can be made on clinical examination especially when cutaneous lesions of lichen planus are evident.
- Biopsy, if necessary.

 DIFFERENTIAL DIAGNOSIS

- *White oral lichen planus lesions are often mistaken for:*
  Oral candidiasis
  Oral leukoplakia
  Normal bite lines (see Fig. 15.23)

 MANAGEMENT

- Topically applied steroid gels or ointments to affected sites provide symptomatic relief.
- Intralesional triamcinolone into affected areas may be useful for localized disease.
- If necessary, systemic steroids such as prednisone may be prescribed for a few weeks or longer.
- Topical tacrolimus 0.1% ointment (**Protopic**) may be effective.
- Preventive dental hygiene care is also very important.

SYSTEMIC LUPUS ERYTHEMATOSUS (DISCUSSED IN CHAPTER 34)

CLINICAL MANIFESTATIONS

- Painless, shallow oral ulcers, most often occur on the hard and soft palate.
- Lesions appear as macules that later transform into irregular erosions and ulcers and often heal with scarring.
- Purpuric lesions such as ecchymoses and petechiae may occur.

MANAGEMENT

- As with oral lichen planus (described above), erosions and ulcers can be treated topically with steroid gels or ointments, topical tacrolimus ointment, intralesional steroid injections, or if necessary, systemic steroids.

MUCOUS PATCHES OF SECONDARY SYPHILIS

- The lesions of secondary syphilis on the tongue are known as *mucous patches* (Fig. 21.7); (see discussion of syphilis in Chapter 28).

CLINICAL MANIFESTATIONS

- Characterized by asymptomatic, round or oval, eroded lingual lesions or papules devoid of epithelium. Lesions "teem with spirochetes."
- **Rapid Plasma Reagin** (RPR) is positive.

GEOGRAPHIC TONGUE

- Geographic tongue, or *benign migratory glossitis,* is a common idiopathic finding (Fig. 21.8).

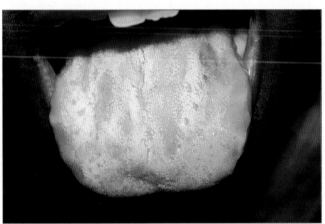

21.7 *Mucous patches of secondary syphilis.* These mucous patches result from eroded epithelium of the tongue. (See also Fig. 28.18.)

CLINICAL MANIFESTATIONS

- Lesions consist of shiny, red, patches that are devoid of papillae that resemble mucous patches. Such lesions seem to move about on the surface of the tongue and change configurations from one day to the next, thus accounting for the bizarre, shifting patterns.
- Reports have suggested an association of geographic tongue with psoriasis; however, its 2% incidence in patients with psoriasis is no greater than that would be expected in the otherwise healthy population.
- No treatment is necessary.

BLACK HAIRY TONGUE

- Black hairy tongue is more than just a pigmentary change. Actually, it represents benign, asymptomatic hyperplasia (an accumulation of keratin) or hypertrophy of the filiform papillae of the tongue. The pigmentation results from the normal pigment-producing bacterial flora that colonize the keratin.
- It has been debatably associated with smoking, excessive coffee or tea drinking, and the prolonged use of oral antibiotics.

CLINICAL MANIFESTATIONS

- A velvety, hair-like thickening of the tongue's surface is apparent (Fig. 21.9).
- Color can range from a yellowish brown or green to jet black.

 MANAGEMENT

- Brushing with a dilute hydrogen peroxide solution may bleach the pigmented tissue.
- A toothbrush can be used to scrape off the excess keratin.
- Tretinoin 0.05% gel or lotion has also been used.

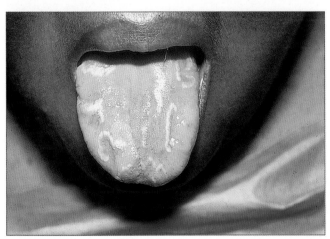

21.8 *Geographic tongue.* Shiny, red patches are devoid of papillae (note the resemblance to the mucous patches shown in Fig. 12.7).

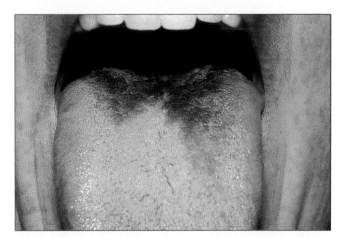

21.9 *Black hairy tongue.* A velvety, hairlike thickening of the tongue's surface is noted. The color can range from a yellowish-brown or -green to jet black.

PIGMENTATION DUE TO DRUGS AND ARTIFACTS

CLINICAL MANIFESTATIONS

- A black discoloration of the tongue should be distinguished from black hairy tongue. In these cases, there is no hyperkeratosis or hypertrophy of papillae.
- Oral mucous membrane pigmentation has been noted to result from the following agents:
  - Antimalarials (Fig. 21.10), bismuth (Fig. 21.11), chlorhexidine mouth rinses, doxorubicin, fluoxetine, inhalation of heroin smoke, ketoconazole, propranolol, risperidone, sulfonamides, terbinafine, tobacco, zidovudine, and tetracycline.

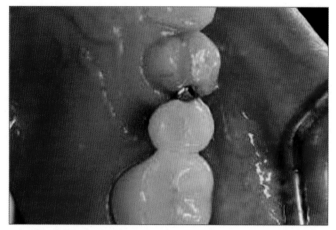

21.12 *Pigment artifact (amalgam tattoo).* Dental amalgam filling implantation into oral mucosa.

- Artifactual pigmentation has also been noted to result from iatrogenic amalgam tattoos and dental fillings caused by traumatic implantation of dental amalgam into soft tissue. Lesions are gray, blue or black macules on the oral mucous membranes (Fig. 21.12).

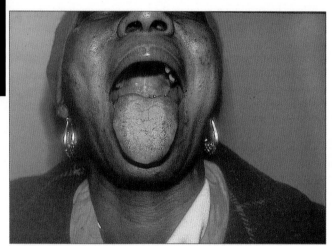

21.10 *Antimalarial hyperpigmentation.* Pigmentation of this patient's tongue is due to antimalarial therapy with hydroxychloroquine (**Plaquenil**).

ORAL LEUKOPLAKIA

- White macular or plaque-like lesions are considered precursors to squamous cell carcinoma of the mucous membranes.
- Smoking, chewing tobacco, and ethanol abuse are all contributing factors.

CLINICAL MANIFESTATIONS

- White adherent plaques are present.
- Lesions occur on the tongue (Fig. 21.13), buccal mucosa, hard palate, and gums.

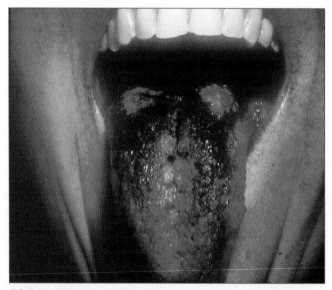

21.11 *Pigment artifact.* The black pigmentation on this patient's tongue was caused by the deposition of bismuth, the active ingredient in **Pepto-Bismol**. It was easily removed with a toothbrush.

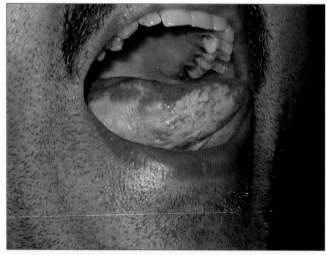

21.13 *Leukoplakia.* (Image courtesy of Ashit Marwah, MD.)

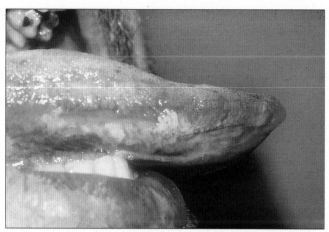

21.14 *Oral hairy leukoplakia.* This patient has HIV/AIDS. Note the filiform papules on the sides of the tongue that resemble white hairs. (From Goodheart HP. *Goodheart's Same-Site Differential Diagnosis.* Philadelphia, PA: Lippincott Williams & Wilkins, 2011.)

- Oral leukoplakia may resemble oral lichen planus, oral hairy leukoplakia, or white plaques caused by trauma.
- Less than 5% of lesions have been reported to develop into squamous cell carcinoma.

ORAL HAIRY LEUKOPLAKIA

- Oral hairy leukoplakia is associated with the Epstein–Barr virus.
- Seen in patients with HIV infection (see Chapter 24) and in transplant recipients.

CLINICAL MANIFESTATIONS

- Filiform papules that resemble white hairs are seen on the sides of the tongue (Fig. 21.14).
- Lesions are usually asymptomatic.

ORAL CANDIDIASIS ("THRUSH")

- Most oral fungal infections are caused by *Candida albicans*, a harmless commensal organism inhabiting the mouths of almost 50% of the world's population. Under suitable circumstances, it can become an opportunistic pathogen.
- In infants, acute pseudomembranous candidiasis (thrush) may be observed in healthy neonates or in people in whom antibiotics, corticosteroids, or xerostomia (dry mouth) disturb the oral microflora.
- Oral candidiasis is most prevalent in people with immunosuppressive conditions (HIV-associated oral candidiasis) and diabetes as well as those on long-term broad-spectrum antibiotics as well as systemic and aerosolized corticosteroids. Xerostomia (as in *Sjögren syndrome*) and radiotherapy to the head and neck also predisposes individuals to oral yeast infections.

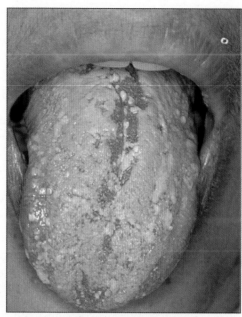

21.15 *Oral candidiasis (thrush).* Confluent white plaques on the surface of the tongue. (From Goodheart HP. *Goodheart's Same-Site Differential Diagnosis.* Philadelphia, PA: Lippincott Williams & Wilkins, 2011.)

CLINICAL MANIFESTATIONS

- White patches/plaques are present on the surface of the buccal mucosa, palate, or tongue.
- Lesions develop into confluent plaques that resemble milk curds (multiple white-fleck appearance) and can be wiped off to reveal an erythematous base (Fig. 21.15).
- Erythematous areas found generally on the dorsum of the tongue, palate, or buccal mucosa.
- Lesions may involve the tongue, the oropharynx, buccal mucosa, and the angles of mouth (*angular cheilitis* [see below]).
- Lesions on the dorsum of the tongue present as depapillated areas.

DIAGNOSIS

- A potassium hydroxide examination or fungal culture is positive.

MANAGEMENT

- Intermittent or prolonged topical or oral antifungal treatment is usually necessary.
- Nystatin suspension 500,000 U, 4 to 5 times per day or clotrimazole troches 10 mg 5 times per day.
- Oral therapy with fluconazole (**Diflucan**) 100 mg daily produces remission within approximately 1 week.

PERLÈCHE (ANGULAR CHEILITIS)

- Perlèche (derived from the French word meaning "to lick") is an erythematous eruption that occurs at the corners of the mouth. It is also known as *angular cheilitis*.
- It is sometimes seen in young patients who have atopic dermatitis (Fig. 21.16).
- Perlèche also appears in the elderly and may be caused by aging and atrophy of the muscles of facial expression that surround the mouth, which results in "pocketing" at the corners of the mouth (Fig. 21.17). These pockets become macerated and serve as a nidus for the retention of saliva, resulting in the secondary overgrowth of microorganisms such as yeasts and/or bacteria.

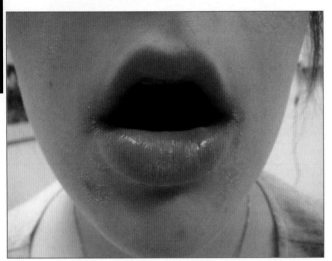

21.16 *Perlèche (angular cheilitis) and atopic cheilitis.* This child has scaling, fissuring, and crusting at the corners of her mouth, as well as eczema of her lips. She also has eczema on other areas of her skin.

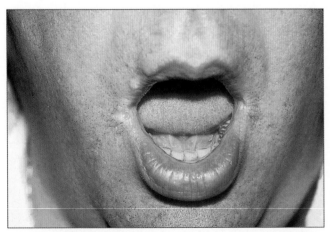

21.17 *Perlèche (angular cheilitis).* This patient's problem was believed to be caused by a problem with his dentures. (From Goodheart HP. *Goodheart's Same-Site Differential Diagnosis.* Philadelphia, PA: Lippincott Williams & Wilkins, 2011.)

- In many instances, perlèche is simply a form of intertrigo, a common inflammatory condition of skin folds that occurs when opposing moist skin surfaces are in constant contact with each other.
- Other factors such as poor-fitting dentures, malocclusion, orthodontic devices, anodontia, and bone resorption may lead to drooling or vertical shortening of the face, thus accentuating the melolabial crease.
- Lip licking, thumb sucking in children, mouth breathing, and orthodontic devices are also risk factors.
- Vitamin deficiencies such as from iron, riboflavin or vitamin B12, pyridoxine, folic acid, niacin, and zinc are often blamed but rarely proved as a cause of perlèche.

CLINICAL MANIFESTATIONS

- Redness, scaling, fissuring, and crusting occur at the corners of the mouth.
- Children and young adults may also have evidence of atopic cheilitis and/or atopic dermatitis elsewhere on the body.
- Elderly patients may have missing teeth, poor-fitting dentures, drooling, or evidence of bone resorption.

 MANAGEMENT

- A mild over-the-counter **hydrocortisone 1% ointment** often helps resolve the inflammation. If necessary, a more potent topical steroid desonide 0.05% ointment **(DesOwen)** or mometasone 0.1% ointment **(Elocon)** may be applied.
- Petrolatum or other ointments are used to protect and moisturize the area.
- If indicated, a topical anticandidal **(ketoconazole, clotrimazole, nystatin)** or an antibacterial agent **(mupirocin)**, either alone or in combination with a mild **topical hydrocortisone ointment** (as noted above), are often effective.
- For refractory cases, fluconazole tablets 100 mg daily for 1 week followed by 150 mg weekly for 6 weeks' duration may be helpful.
- Topical immunomodulators such as **Protopic 0.1% ointment** or **Elidel 1% cream** may also be prescribed.
- If necessary, a dental referral is suggested to correct potential causative factors mentioned earlier. For elderly edentulous persons, refer the patient to a dental specialist to adjust the dentures, adding vertical dimension.
- Injection of **collagen** into the responsible overlapping skin folds has been beneficial in some selected patients.

HELPFUL HINTS

- Treatment and prevention of recurrences require reduction of maceration and/or use of a barrier ointment.
- Treat concomitant oral candidiasis such as oral thrush, if present.

ACTINIC KERATOSIS (SOLAR KERATOSIS, ACTINIC CHEILITIS) (SEE CHAPTER 31)

- Seen in elderly men and women with fair complexions.

CLINICAL MANIFESTATIONS

- Generally, lesions are slow-growing, firm, rough-textured papules.
- Also may arise as a nonhealing erosion or rough papule on the vermillion border of the upper lip (Fig. 21.18).
- Actinic keratoses are also seen on the lower lip, where there is maximal sun exposure. This is referred to as *actinic cheilitis* (Fig. 21.19).

SQUAMOUS CELL CARCINOMA

- A squamous cell carcinoma may evolve from a solar keratosis in this area (Fig. 21.20), from leukoplakia or arise *de novo* inside the oral cavity (Fig. 21.21).

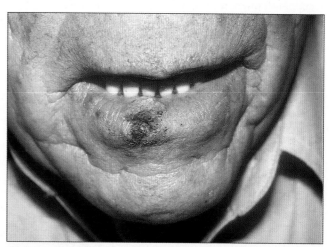

21.19 *Actinic cheilitis.* The entire sun exposed area of his lower lip has actinic damage. (Image courtesy of Benjamin Barankin, MD.) (From Goodheart HP. *Goodheart's Same-Site Differential Diagnosis.* Philadelphia, PA: Lippincott Williams & Wilkins, 2011.)

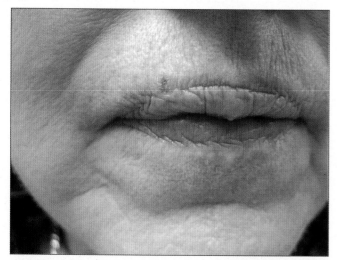

21.18 *Actinic keratosis.* Note the small hyperkeratotic papule on the vermillion border of this patient's upper lip.

21.20 *Squamous cell carcinoma.* Mucous membrane lesions such as this are more likely to metastasize. (From Goodheart HP. *Goodheart's Same-Site Differential Diagnosis.* Philadelphia, PA: Lippincott Williams & Wilkins, 2011.)

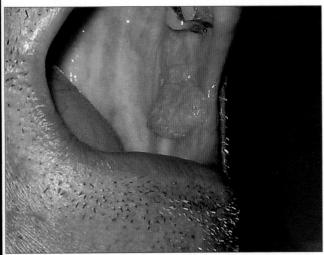

21.21 *Squamous cell carcinoma.* This patient has a nodular squamous cell carcinoma on the buccal mucosa. (Image courtesy of Ashit Marwah, MD.)

ERYTHEMA MULTIFORME MINOR (SEE CHAPTER 27)

• Erythema multiforme minor is a self-limited eruption characterized by symmetrically distributed erythematous macules or papules, which develop into the characteristic target-like lesions consisting of concentric color changes with a dusky central zone that may become bullous.

• EM minor is not a disease but a syndrome with multiple underlying causes and associations such as drug reactions, and, most often, recurrent herpes virus infection.

• EM minor is most commonly seen in late adolescence and in young adulthood.

• Most cases are idiopathic; however, the most common precipitating cause of EM minor is recurrent labial herpes simplex virus infection; recurrences of herpes progenitalis also have been reported to precede or sometimes occur simultaneously with episodes of recurrent EM minor.

CLINICAL MANIFESTATIONS

• There may be a history of an antecedent HSV infection, less likely, an active vesicular, or crusted lesion of recurrent HSV present on the vermilion border of the lip during (Fig. 21.22), or prior to, an outbreak of erythema multiforme.

ERYTHEMA MULTIFORME MAJOR (SEE CHAPTER 27)

• EM major tends to be seen more often in an older age group and when there is a known or suspected cause, a drug reaction is most often implicated.

• As in EM minor, EM major is often idiopathic.

CLINICAL MANIFESTATIONS

• This is the more serious variant of erythema multiforme. It has extensive mucous membrane involvement, systemic symptoms, and widespread lesions.

• Hemorrhagic crusts on lips and other mucous membranes are seen in addition to the extensive targetoid lesions elsewhere (Fig. 21.23).

• Erythema multiforme major is often accompanied by fever, malaise, myalgias, and severe, painful mucous membrane involvement.

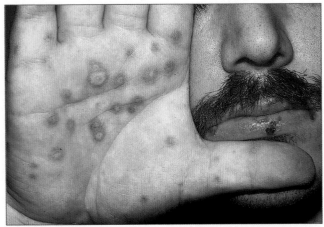

21.22 *Erythema multiforme minor caused by herpes simplex virus.* This patient has a recurrent HSV infection. Note the drying crust of the herpetic "cold sore" on his lower lip and the target-like lesions on his palm.

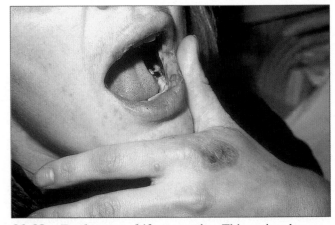

21.23 *Erythema multiforme major.* This patient has multiple intraoral erosions, target-like bullae on her hand, as well as vaginal erosions. (From Goodheart HP. *Goodheart's Same-Site Differential Diagnosis.* Philadelphia, PA: Lippincott Williams & Wilkins, 2011.)

PYOGENIC GRANULOMA (SEE CHAPTER 30)

- Pyogenic granuloma (PG) is a benign vascular hyperplasia of the skin and mucous membranes that occurs most often in children and young adults.
- PGs are also seen on the lips and gums, particularly during pregnancy (*granuloma gravidarum*; Fig. 21.24).
- Spontaneous resolution may occur after childbirth.

VENOUS LAKE

- A venous lake (*venous varix*) is a common benign vascular neoplasm; it usually occurs in patients older than 60 years of age.
- This neoplasm is generally characterized by dark blue to purple macules or papules that may be seen on the lower lip (Fig. 21.25), face, ears, and eyelids.

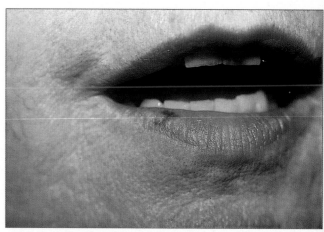

21.26   *Labial melanotic macule.* This is a common, benign, pigmented macule on the lower lip of adults. It is probably caused by sun exposure.

LABIAL MELANOTIC MACULE

- This is a common, benign, pigmented macule on the lower lip of adults.
- It is probably caused by sun exposure (Fig. 21.26), although similar lesions may be seen on the vulvae and penis and other non–sun-exposed areas.
- Typical lesions can just be observed. Suspicious lesions, including lesions showing progressive change, should be biopsied.
- If treatment is requested the macules can be frozen (cryotherapy), or removed using a laser or intense pulsed light.

ORAL MUCOUS CYST (MUCOCELE)

- A mucous cyst (*mucocele*) (Fig. 21.27) is a common, mucus-filled, blister-like lesion of the minor salivary glands in the oral cavity. Some authors prefer the term *mucocele* since most of these lesions are not true cysts because of the absence of an epithelial lining.

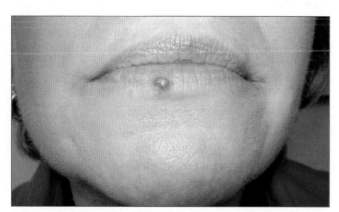

21.24   *Pyogenic granuloma.* This angiomatous-appearing lesion proved to be a pyogenic granuloma after it was biopsied.

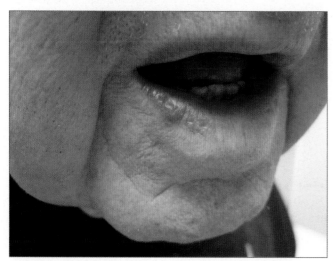

21.25   *Venous lake.* These soft, compressible blebs are common findings on the lips of the elderly.

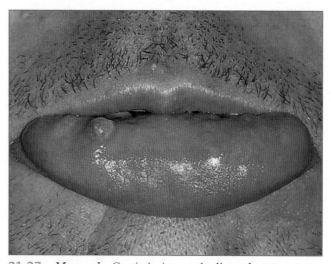

21.27   *Mucocele.* Cystic lesion on the lingual mucosa.

- The lesions are considered to be caused by trauma to the openings of salivary glands.
- This condition is seen most commonly in infants, young children, and young adults.

CLINICAL MANIFESTATIONS

- A bluish or clear papule that contains mucoid material.
- It is easily ruptured and sometimes recurrent.
- Eventually, the surface of the lesion turns irregular and whitish because of multiple cycles of rupture and healing caused by trauma or puncture.
- The most frequent locations are in the lower lip, floor of the mouth, cheek, palate, retromolar fossa, and dorsal surface of the tongue. Lesions usually spare the upper lip.
- Mucous cysts may spontaneously disappear, particularly in infants.

🔧 MANAGEMENT

- Reassurance.
- If necessary, **cryosurgery** with liquid nitrogen spray may be performed. After 4 to 7 days, a necrotic surface is observed in the treated area.
- The advantages of the procedure include simple application, minor discomfort during the procedure, and low incidence of complications (e.g., secondary infection, hemorrhage).

For repeated recurrence:
- **Argon laser treatment.**
- **Electrodesiccation.**
- **Intralesional injections** of **triamcinolone acetonide** also have been reported as effective treatments for mucous cysts.
- For deeper, recalcitrant lesions, **surgical excision may be necessary**.

ORAL FIBROMA

- Most often observed in adults, oral fibromas are the most common intraoral neoplasm.
- Lesions likely represent reactive fibrous hyperplasia caused by trauma or local irritation.
- They are seen most often on the buccal mucosa along the plane of occlusion of the maxillary and mandibular teeth.
- Oral fibromas present as asymptomatic, smooth-surfaced, firm, solitary papules (Fig. 21.28). The diameter may vary from 1 mm to 2 cm. Ulceration caused by repeated trauma may occur.

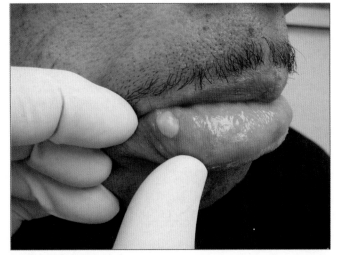

21.28 *Oral fibroma.* This firm nodule may appear on the lip, tongue, or buccal mucosa.

- The clinical differential diagnosis of a fibroma includes verruca vulgaris, giant cell fibroma, neurofibroma, peripheral giant cell granuloma, mucocele, benign and malignant salivary gland tumors, as well as squamous cell carcinoma.

ORAL WARTS (SEE CHAPTERS 6, 17, AND 28)

- Oral warts may be seen in children and adults. All are caused by the human papilloma virus (HPV) and can involve the lips (Fig. 21.29) and anywhere in the oral cavity.

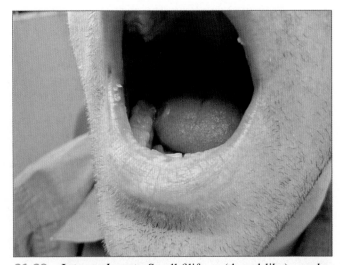

21.29 *Intraoral warts.* Small filiform (thread-like) papules in a patient with HIV/AIDS.

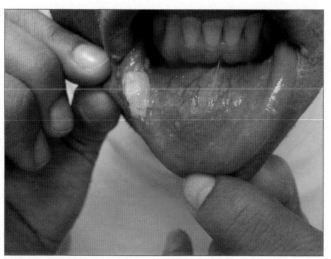

21.30 *Intraoral wart.* The white color of this lesion is due to the constant environment of moisture.

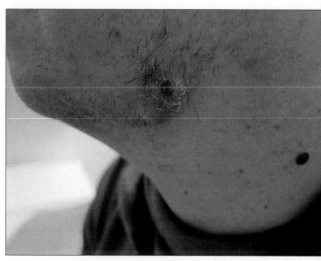

21.31 *Odontogenic sinus.* Often misdiagnosed, this lesion originated from a subjacent mandibular dental abscess.

- They are generally asymptomatic and are clinically similar in appearance to genital warts when they arise on mucous membranes.
- Their appearance varies. The soft, papules or nodules may be flat or cauliflower-like, and white or pinkish-white in color. The white color results from the perpetual moist environment and the lack of a stratum corneum in mucosa (Fig. 21.30).

ODONTOGENIC SINUS (DENTAL SINUS)

- Most often, these lesions appear on the chin or lower jaw. The lesion often has a small indentation that results from scarring (Fig. 21.31).

- The pathologic process evolves from an intraoral abscess that forms a sinus tract that dissects subcutaneously and exits through the face or neck. The patient is usually unaware of the underlying dental etiology.
- Often diagnosed incorrectly, this lesion of dental origin often resembles a furuncle, a cyst, a pyogenic granuloma, or an ulceration.

 MANAGEMENT

- Panoramic or apical radiographic examinations help to make the diagnosis.
- Treatment may require oral antibiotics, tooth extraction, and/or root canal therapy.

Normal Variants

FORDYCE SPOTS

- Fordyce spots (Fig. 21.32) are normal findings that represent ectopic sebaceous glands. They are brought to medical attention when they are noticed by the patient.
- Present as 1- to 2-mm yellow to yellow-white papules on the vermillion zone of the lips or buccal mucosa.
- The lesions are more obvious when the skin is stretched.
- They are incidental findings that require no treatment.

TORUS PALATINUS

- Tori are developmental abnormalities that result in overgrowth of mature bone (Fig. 21.33); they differ only by their location.
- These findings have been known to occur more commonly in certain ethnic groups (e.g., Native Americans, Inuit, African Americans, and certain Asian populations). In these groups, the conditions show an autosomal dominant inheritance pattern.
- Treatment is not necessary.

NORMAL BITE LINE

- Appears as a white horizontal line along the buccal mucosa at the level of the occlusal plane, which is where the posterior teeth meet (see Fig. 15.23).

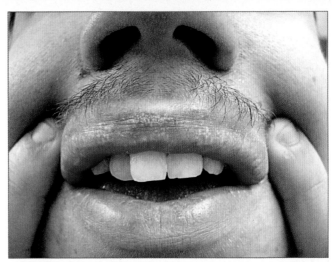

21.32   *Fordyce spots.* Yellow papules on the labial mucosa. These lesions are normal variants that become more apparent when the skin is stretched.

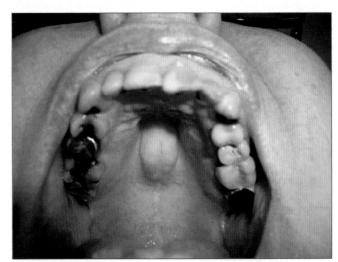

21.33   *Torus palatinus.* This woman has an asymptomatic bony hard swelling located on the midline of her hard palate. The location, clinical appearance, and texture of tori and exostoses are so characteristic that the diagnosis can be made without resorting to biopsy.

CHAPTER 22

Diseases and Abnormalities of Nails

OVERVIEW

Mammals use their nails as weapons, as primitive tools, for grooming purposes, for scratching, and for the removal of infestations. Similarly, humans use their fingernails to help pick up small objects and to scratch itchy skin. Fingernails protect vulnerable fingertips; toenails protect toes from the impact of footwear and external trauma. Nails are also important contributors to the aesthetic appearance of the hands and feet. For the health care provider, nail abnormalities may be the first signal that a systemic disease is present.

IN THIS CHAPTER...

➤ **COMMON NAIL PROBLEMS**

- Longitudinal ridging (onychorrhexis)
- Brittle nails (onychoschizia)
- Onycholysis
- Green nail syndrome

➤ **TRAUMATIC NAIL LESIONS**

- Subungual hematoma
- Median nail dystrophy

➤ **INFLAMMATORY NAIL DISORDERS**

- Psoriasis (see also Chapter 14)

➤ **INFECTIONS OF THE NAIL AND SURROUNDING TISSUES**

- Acute paronychia
- Chronic paronychia
- Onychomycosis

➤ **MISCELLANEOUS NAIL DISORDERS**

- Digital mucous (myxoid) cyst
- Leukonychia striata
- Yellow nail syndrome
- Increased transverse nail curvature (pincer nails)
- Koilonychia
- Trachyonychia (see also Chapter 9)
- Melanonychia (see also Chapter 30)
- Junctional nevus
- Subungual verruca (see also Chapter 17)
- Sarcoidosis
- Dermatomyositis (see Chapter 34)
- Terry nails
- Half-and-half nails
- Dystrophy from preformed artificial nails

Common Nail Problems

LONGITUDINAL RIDGING (ONYCHORRHEXIS)

BASICS

- Longitudinal ridging is a very common nail issue and is considered a normal variant in elderly persons.
- It consists of parallel ridges that run lengthwise along the nail plates (Fig. 22.1) and are more commonly observed in fingernails than in toenails.
- Occasionally, longitudinal ridging is seen in younger persons.
- The etiology is unknown and the condition is not indicative of any trauma, infection, or nutritional deficiency.

 MANAGEMENT

- There is no treatment available to decrease longitudinal ridging, except for filing and buffing the ridges down with a soft file.

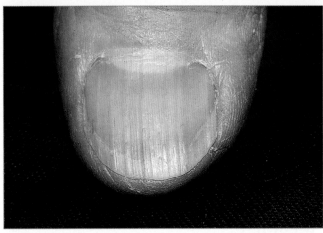

22.1 *Longitudinal ridging.* Parallel elevated ridges are characteristic of this normal variant. The ridges may have a beaded appearance.

BRITTLE NAILS (ONYCHOSCHIZIA)

BASICS

- Brittle and split nails (onychoschizia) are common in adults (Fig. 22.2). In some people, nails become fragile and easily break off at the free edge.
- Onychoschizia has traditionally been considered a sign of nail plate dehydration; however, a recent study has indicated that the water content of brittle nails is not significantly different from that of normal nails.
- Brittle nails are a common complaint in adult and elderly women and can also be observed in people with iron deficiency and thyroid disease.
- Elderly men are less apt to present with this problem. The increased incidence in women may be a result of their higher cosmetic awareness, their frequent use of nail products, menopausal status, or frequent exposure to harmful extrinsic factors (e.g., detergents and water).

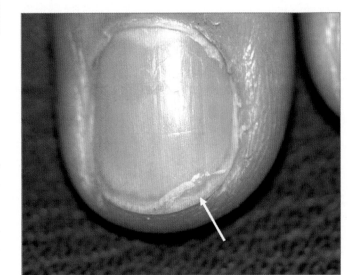

22.2 *Onychoschizia.* The distal nail splits into layers parallel to the nail's surface.

 MANAGEMENT

- Traditionally, distal nail splitting has been compared to scaly, dry skin elsewhere on the body. Thus, many treatment recommendations are similar to those for dry skin.
- Avoid excessive contact with water, soaps, and other detergents. Wear gloves when washing dishes.
- Wear gloves in cold weather.
- Apply moisturizing creams or ointments (e.g., **lactic acid creams** in 5% to 12% concentrations or **Vaseline Petroleum Jelly**) at bedtime or after bathing or washing.

- Keep the nails short and trim when they are well hydrated so they are less likely to be frayed. Use a soft file to keep the distal nail edge smooth.
- **Biotin** supplementation (2.5 to 5 mg/day) has shown some efficacy in increasing nail integrity and thickness.
- **Genadur** (12 mL), a hydrosoluble nail lacquer, is reported to protect intact or damaged nails. May be applied under nail polish and is available by Rx only.

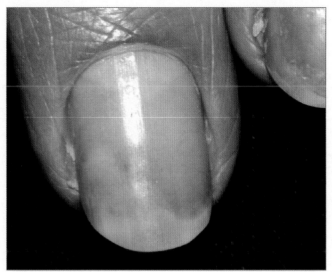

22.3 ***Onycholysis.*** The separated portion of the nail is yellowish white and opaque; the attached portion is pink and translucent.

ONYCHOLYSIS

BASICS

- Onycholysis represents a separation of the nail plate from its underlying attachment to the pink nail bed (Fig. 22.3). The separated portion is white and opaque, in contrast to the pink translucence of the attached portion. Normal *physiologic onycholysis* is seen at the distal free margin of healthy nails as they grow.
- Onycholysis is most frequently seen in women, particularly in those with long fingernails.
- Onycholysis usually starts distally and progresses proximally. When the separation progresses more proximally, the onycholysis is more obvious, becomes cosmetically objectionable, and may interfere with the routine function of the nails (e.g., picking up small objects, such as coins and paper clips).
- In some patients, the separated part of the nail takes on a green or yellow tinge (see the discussion of green nail syndrome later in the next section).

PATHOGENESIS

External Causes:

- Irritants such as nail polish, nail wraps, nail hardeners, and artificial nails.
- Frequent contact with water as seen in bartenders, hairdressers, manicurists, citrus fruit handlers, and domestic workers.
- Trauma, especially habitual finger sucking, athletic injuries to the toes, wearing of tight shoes, and the use of fingernails as a tool.

- Lack of appropriate nail care. It is often difficult for elderly patients to trim toenails frequently because of arthritis, decreased fine motor control or flexibility.
- Fungal infections such as chronic paronychia and onychomycosis (see Chapter 18).
- Certain drugs can act as phototoxic agents to induce fingernail onycholysis. Such drugs include diuretics, sulfa drugs, tetracycline, doxycycline, and, particularly, demethylchlortetracycline. Hemorrhagic onycholysis may result from taxanes, chemotherapeutic agent used in the treatment of various cancers (see Fig. 26.14).

Internal Causes:

- Psoriasis is the most common cause of onycholysis. Often there is evidence of psoriasis elsewhere on the body, or there may be other psoriatic nail findings, such as pitting, subungual hyperkeratosis, and "oil spots" (see discussion in Chapter 14).
- Inflammatory skin diseases of the nail matrix (root), such as eczematous dermatitis (see below) or lichen planus.
- Thyroid disease, pregnancy, and anemia have been reported as potential associations.

Also:

- Subungual warts and subungual neoplasms (see Chapters 17 and 31).

 MANAGEMENT

- The goal of management is to keep the newly growing nail attached by:
  - Keeping nails dry and cut closely; proper trimming (along the contour) on a regular basis can protect the nails from injury.
  - Using nail polish sparingly.
  - Avoiding unnecessary filing and manipulation of nails.
  - Treating or avoiding the underlying cause of the problem, if known.

 HELPFUL HINT

- Nails must be kept short. A long nail acts as a lever and magnifies traumatic damage.

GREEN NAIL SYNDROME

BASICS

- Green nail syndrome is a painless, blue-green discoloration under the nail that is a consequence of a *Pseudomonas* infection of an onycholytic nail and should not be confused with a subungual fungal infection.

PATHOGENESIS

- The "dead space" under the onycholytic nail serves as an excellent breeding ground for microbes.
- Infection with *Pseudomonas aeruginosa* results in a green, greenish-yellow, or green-black nail color due to the bacteria's production of pyocyanin pigment (Fig. 22.4).

 MANAGEMENT

- Soaking the affected nail twice daily in a mixture either of one part **chlorine bleach** and three parts water or equal parts **acetic acid (vinegar)** and **water** generally eliminates the discoloration.
- If possible, avoid or minimize the underlying causes (see onycholysis discussed above).

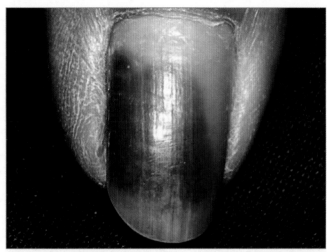

22.4 *Green nail syndrome.* The "dead space" under the nail often harbors *Pseudomonas* species. The green color is virtually pathognomonic for *Pseudomonas*.

BASICS

- Injuries to the nail root (the matrix that directly underlies the proximal nail fold) and nail bed may be caused by direct trauma. In fact, trauma is the most common cause of nail disorders.

SUBUNGUAL HEMATOMA

- A subungal hematoma results from trauma to the nail matrix or nail bed from a single substantial impact (e.g., from a hammer) or repeated minor injury (e.g., tight shoes or sports injuries).
- An acute subungual hematoma that results from rapid accumulation of blood under the nail plate can be very painful (Fig. 22.5), whereas small lesions may be painless and go unnoticed for some time.
- Chronic, painless subungual hematomas that are not clearly the result of trauma may appear similar to a melanocytic neoplasm. Because the coagulated blood remains until the nail grows out (for 6 to 12 months), the diagnosis may be in doubt for some time and sometimes requires a nail bed or nail matrix biopsy.

DIFFERENTIAL DIAGNOSIS

- **Junctional nevus** (see Fig. 22.20).
- **Acral lentiginous melanoma** should also be considered (see Fig. 22.21).

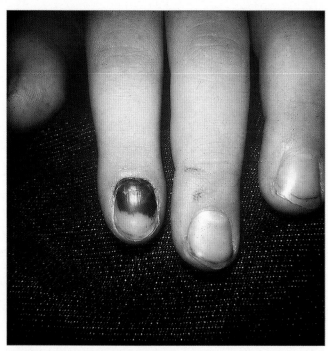

22.5 *Acute subungual hematoma.* This results from the rapid accumulation of blood.

POINT TO REMEMBER

- If there is a suspicion of melanoma, the nail bed or matrix should undergo biopsy.

MANAGEMENT

- An acute, painful, swollen subungual hematoma may be incised and drained by placing the red-hot end of a heated paper clip on the area elevated by the hematoma. The small hole created with this procedure allows the blood to drain and thus quickly relieves the pain. (Note: This technique should be performed by a health professional.)
- Twirling a 27-gauge needle to create a similar hole is an alternative method for draining the blood.

MEDIAN NAIL DYSTROPHY

- Median nail dystrophy results from a compulsive habit of repeated trauma to the proximal nail fold of the thumb, usually inflicted by the nail of the adjacent index finger (Fig. 22.6A,B).
- The resultant nail deformity is analogous to an injury to the root of a tree that deforms the growing tree trunk.

DIAGNOSIS

- The patient can sometimes be observed performing the repeated action without being aware of it. This is particularly true in children.

MANAGEMENT

- Treatment of any habit is difficult; the habit and resultant nail deformity are usually chronic by the time a patient seeks medical attention.
- It can be suggested to patients that breaking this habit may be aided by an alternative activity, such as knitting or needlepoint.
- Parents may be advised to have children keep tape or another dressing on the affected nails.

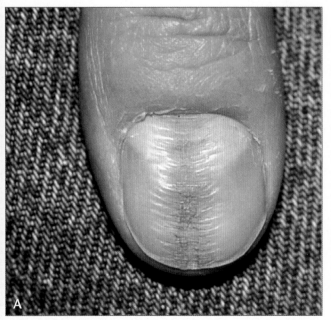
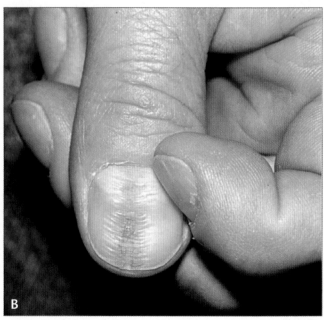

22.6 *Median nail dystrophy.* **A:** Note the vertical ridging ("washboard" appearance) in the nails caused by a habitual tic. After repeated trauma to the proximal nail fold, median nail dystrophy can result. **B:** Most often, the patient habitually presses the nail of the adjacent finger against the proximal nail fold.

Inflammatory Nail Disorders

BASICS

- Inflammatory disorders that involve the nail matrix, such as psoriasis, can result in distinctive deformities of the nails. For example, nail pitting, "oil spots," and onycholysis are commonly seen in patients with psoriasis. Other conditions, such as eczema of the proximal nail fold, result in nonspecific deformities.

PSORIASIS

- The typical nail changes are pitting, onycholysis, thickening (subungual hyperkeratosis), and "oil spots" (Fig. 22.7; see also Figs. 14.25–14.27).

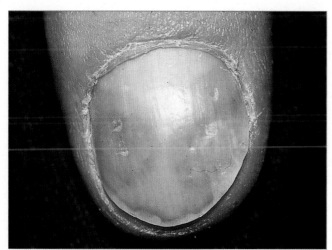

22.7 Psoriasis. Pitting, onycholysis, and "oil spots" are evident in this nail.

 MANAGEMENT (see Discussion in Chapter 14)

Eczematous Dermatitis with Secondary Nail Dystrophy

- Nail deformity secondary to eczematous dermatitis is a problem that is often overlooked in patients with severe atopic dermatitis (Fig. 22.8).
- It results when eczematous dermatitis involves the distal extensor surface of the fingers, and the associated inflammation also involves the matrix, or "root," of the nail. The inflamed matrix, which underlies the proximal nail fold, consequently gives rise to a dystrophic nail plate.
- The nails generally have a ripple-like deformity that corresponds to the time of activity of the underlying inflammatory process.

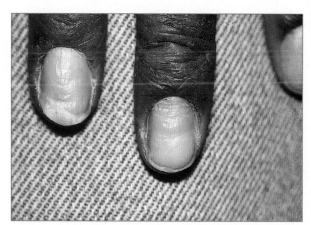

22.8 Eczematous dermatitis. The eczema of the proximal skin also affects the matrix (root) of the nail; this results in nail dystrophy and onycholysis.

 MANAGEMENT

- Improvement of the appearance of the nail plate follows control of inflammation of the proximal nailfold skin with the use of topical steroids.

DISEASES AND ABNORMALITIES OF NAILS

BASICS

- The term *paronychia* refers to inflammation of the nail fold surrounding the nail plate and can be acute or chronic.
- *Onychomycosis* refers to an infection of the fingernails or toenails caused by various fungi, yeasts, and molds. In contrast, the term *tinea unguium* refers specifically to nail infections caused by dermatophytes.

ACUTE PARONYCHIA

PATHOGENESIS

- Acute paronychia usually results from an infection caused by *Staphylococcus aureus;* less commonly by streptococci or *Pseudomonas* species.
- The condition may occur spontaneously, or it may follow trauma or manipulation, such as nail biting, a manicure, or removal of a hangnail.

CLINICAL MANIFESTATIONS

- Acute paronychia is heralded by the rapid onset of bright red swelling of the proximal or lateral nail fold behind the cuticle with no evidence of chronic nail dystrophy.
- A throbbing, tender, and intensely painful lesion often results (Fig. 22.9).
- Generally, only one nail is involved.

DIAGNOSIS

- Often made clinically; a bacterial culture may be useful to determine organism and its sensitivity to antibiotics.

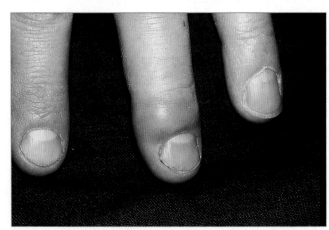

22.9 *Acute paronychia.* Acutely red, tender, unilateral involvement of the proximal nail fold. Often, pus is visible through the proximal or lateral nail fold.

 DIFFERENTIAL DIAGNOSIS

Chronic Paronychia (see Discussion below)

- *Minimal or no pain or tenderness.*
- *Absent or damaged cuticle(s).*
- *More than one nail may be involved.*
- *Nail dystrophy.*

Herpetic Whitlow

- *Acute bacterial paronychia can be easily confused with a painful herpetic whitlow.*
- *A Tzanck preparation or viral culture should be considered when the diagnosis is in doubt.*

 MANAGEMENT

- Mild cases may require only warm saline or aluminum acetate (**Domeboro 1:40**) soaks for 10 to 15 minutes two to four times daily.
- In more severe cases, simple **incision and drainage** (with a no. 11 surgical blade) usually afford rapid relief of pain.
- Occasionally, systemic therapy with anti-staphylococcal antibiotics, such as **dicloxacillin** or a **cephalosporin**, may be necessary.

CHRONIC PARONYCHIA

- Chronic paronychia results from a combination of chronic moisture, irritation, and trauma to the cuticle and proximal nail fold.
- It occurs much more often in women than in men, and it is particularly common in persons whose hands are frequently exposed to a wet environment, such as housewives, domestic workers, bartenders, janitors, bakers, dishwashers, dentists, dental hygienists, and children who habitually suck their thumbs. It is also seen more often in patients with diabetes and in persons who manicure their cuticles.

PATHOGENESIS

- The predisposing factor is usually trauma or maceration that produces a break in the barrier (cuticle) between the nail fold and nail plate. This allows moisture to accumulate and microbial colonization and inflammation of the nail matrix ensues. The result is nail plate dystrophy.

- Although *Candida* is frequently isolated from the proximal nail fold of patients with chronic paronychia, a primary pathogenesis for this organism has never been proven.
- In fact, evidence indicates that frequently this condition is not a fungal infection at all but is actually an eczematous process. For this reason, topical steroids are often a more effective therapy than topical or even systemic antifungal agents.
- *Candida* may play a primary pathogenic role in patients who are diabetic and those with primary mucocutaneous candidiasis.

CLINICAL MANIFESTATIONS

- Chronic paronychia usually develops slowly and asymptomatically.
- There is an absence or damage to the cuticle.
- Secondary nail plate changes typically occur distal to the absent or involved area of the cuticle (Fig. 22.10). Onycholysis (see earlier discussion) and a greenish or brown discoloration along the lateral borders and transverse ridging of the nails may appear.
- One or more fingers/nails may be involved.

DIAGNOSIS

- The diagnosis can generally be established based on the typical clinical appearance of the fingers and nails, as well as from the patient's history.

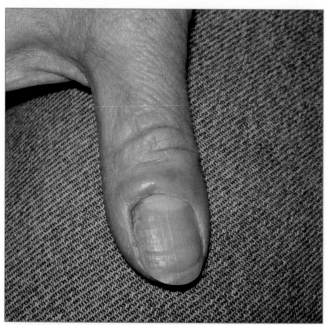

22.10 *Chronic paronychia.* Erythema and edema of the proximal nail fold, absence of the medial cuticle, and medial nail plate dystrophy.

- Various pathogens and contaminants—including *Candida* species, gram-positive or gram-negative organisms, or mixed bacterial flora—may be cultured from the pus obtained from under the proximal nail fold.

 DIFFERENTIAL DIAGNOSIS

Acute Paronychia (see Discussion above)
- *Marked pain and tenderness.*

Onychomycosis
- *Lesions are typically subungual.*
- *Positive KOH or fungal culture for dermatophyte.*

 MANAGEMENT

- Avoid frequent hand washing and manicures.
- Wear gloves (the cotton-under-vinyl variety is best) when performing tasks such as washing dishes.
- A superpotent topical steroid such as **clobetasol 0.05% cream** can be applied once or twice daily to the proximal nail fold. Alternatively, **Cordran tape** may be applied nightly to this area.
- One to two drops daily of **3% thymol in 70% ethanol** (compounded by a pharmacist) can be placed under the proximal nail fold.
- A topical broad-spectrum antifungal agent, such as **clotrimazole, ketoconazole, econazole**, or **miconazole**, is often combined with a potent topical corticosteroid to provide antifungal as well as anti-inflammatory effects.

 HELPFUL HINT

- Chronic paronychia is frequently misdiagnosed—and treated—as an acute staphylococcal paronychia or as presumptive onychomycosis (*tinea unguium*).

ONYCHOMYCOSIS

For a complete discussion, see Chapter 18.

Miscellaneous Nail Disorders

BASICS

- In addition to the disorders already described, various other conditions can affect the nails. Some of these disorders produce characteristic nail findings that may serve as clues to unrecognized systemic disease.

DIGITAL MUCOUS (MYXOID) CYST

- This is not a true cyst, because it lacks an epidermal lining. It is actually a focal collection of clear, gelatinous, viscous mucin (focal mucinosis) that occurs over the distal interphalangeal joint or, most commonly, at the base of the nail.
- Pressure from the lesion on the nail matrix (root) often results in a characteristic longitudinal groove in the nail plate (Fig. 22.11).
- When the lesion occurs more proximally, such as over the distal interphalangeal joint, there is no longitudinal groove (Fig. 22.12).

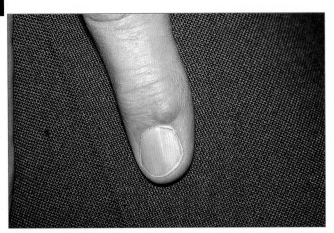

22.11 *Digital mucous (myxoid) cyst.* Note the longitudinal groove in the nail plate.

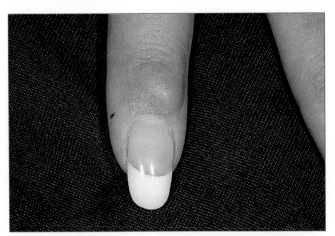

22.12 *Digital mucous (myxoid) cyst over the distal interphalangeal joint.* Note the absence of the longitudinal groove.

- This dome-shaped, rubbery lesion occurs exclusively in adults, particularly in women older than 50 years of age. Some myxoid cysts are believed to be a consequence of osteoarthritis, rather than trauma.

 MANAGEMENT

- Digital mucous cysts are benign lesions that do not require treatment particularly if it is asymptomatic.
- Firm daily compression has led to resolution in some cases.
- Incision and drainage (Fig. 22.13A,B), cryosurgery with liquid nitrogen, and intralesional triamcinolone injections may be performed, with varying results.
- Surgical excision is reserved for the occasional painful or otherwise troublesome lesion.

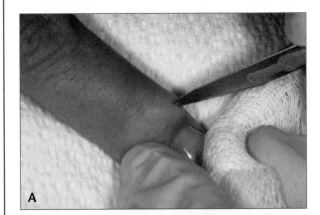

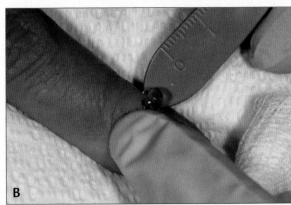

22.13 **A, B:** *Digital mucous (myxoid) cyst.* Incision and drainage. Blood-tinged, viscous, jellylike mucoid material is expressed.

LEUKONYCHIA STRIATA

- Leukonychia striata, which is also called *transverse striate leukonychia,* is often mistaken for a fungal nail infection.
- These white lines (Fig. 22.14) result from an injury to the nail matrix that may have occurred about 2 to 3 months earlier. The underlying injury is often an antecedent illness or the repeated trauma of manicuring or liquid nitrogen therapy for periungal warts.

YELLOW NAIL SYNDROME

- The nails are yellow, opaque, curved, and grow very slowly (Fig. 22.15).
- This syndrome is associated with certain respiratory disorders (e.g., bronchiectasis, chronic respiratory infections, lymphedema, pleural effusion, and ascites).
- Yellow nail discoloration also has been reported in patients with acquired immunodeficiency syndrome.

INCREASED TRANSVERSE NAIL CURVATURE (PINCER NAILS)

- Increased transverse curvature is often manifested as a pincer nail deformity (Fig. 22.16).
- In this deformity, the nails' normal transverse curvature increases along the longitudinal axis and becomes more pronounced at the distal edge, which results in "pinching" of the underlying skin. This condition can become quite painful and may predispose the patient to infections and ingrown nails.
- Pincer nails are often congenital and may be seen in persons with the yellow nail syndrome or as a normal variant. They are also seen in women who wear ill-fitted shoes.

KOILONYCHIA

- Acquired koilonychia, also known as spoon nails, may be seen in association with trauma to the cuticle and proximal nail folds, iron-deficiency anemia, hemochromatosis, or endocrine or cardiac disease (Fig. 22.17).
- Spoon-shaped or concave nails may also be seen in early infancy and may be self-limited.

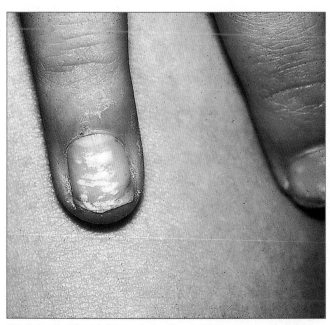

22.14 *Leukonychia striata.* These white spots caused by trauma are extremely common.

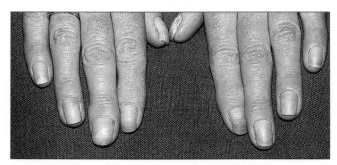

22.15 *Yellow nail syndrome.* These are thickened, slow-growing nails.

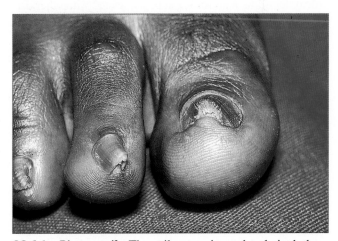

22.16 *Pincer nails.* The nails curve inward and pinch the nail bed.

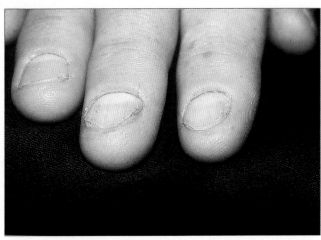

22.17 *Koilonychia.* Note the spoon-shaped curve of the nail.

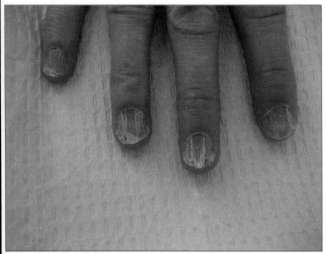

22.18 *Trachyonychia.* This child has brittle, thin nails, with longitudinal ridges.

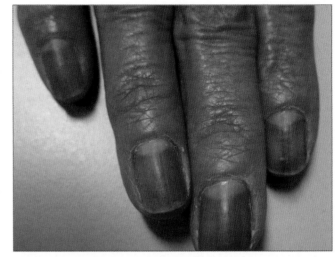

22.19 *Melanonychia.* Note multiple parallel pigmented streaks that were present in several nails.

TRACHYONYCHIA

- Trachyonychia or rough nails, may present as an idiopathic disorder of the nails, or it can be associated with other dermatologic conditions such as lichen planus (Fig. 22.18).
- Characterized by brittle, thin nails, with excessive longitudinal ridging.
- It may involve one, several or all digits. When most or all digits are involved, the term twenty-nail dystrophy is commonly used.
- In childhood, it may present as *twenty-nail dystrophy.* In most cases of childhood trachyonychia, the nail abnormalities improve spontaneously.

MELANONYCHIA

- Melanonychia is brown or black pigmentation of the nail unit. It is a common physiologic finding, noted frequently in dark-skinned individuals of all ages. White-skinned people are less commonly affected.
- It presents as a pigmented band, or multiple bands, that extend from the nail fold (cuticle) to the free edge of the nail. It may affect a single nail or be observed in multiple nails (Fig. 22.19).
- When arranged lengthwise along the nail unit, it is often referred to as *longitudinal melanonychia* or *melanonychia striata.*
- The most concerning cause of melanonychia is subungual melanoma. Other causes include trauma, inflammatory disorders, fungal infections, drugs, and benign melanocytic hyperplasias.

DIAGNOSIS

- Dermatoscopic examination of benign longitudinal melanonychia should reveal light to dark brown lines or bands that are parallel, regular in color, and regular in width as the band extends from the nail fold to the free edge. The borders should be clearly defined and usually of a width of less than 3 mm.
- Nail biopsy: Definitive exclusion of melanoma of the nail unit is obtained with a nail matrix biopsy. There should be a low threshold for biopsy especially in elderly patients where melanonychia has appeared in a single digit.

 DIFFERENTIAL DIAGNOSIS

Subungual Hematoma (see earlier in this chapter)
- *Typically preceded by trauma, although this may be unnoticed (e.g., from tight shoes).*
- *The pigment is red to purple in color.*
- *Within a few weeks, the purple patch may begin moving outward toward the free edge of the nail.*

 MANAGEMENT

- When melanonychia is attributed to a benign cause, no further treatment is necessary.

HELPFUL HINTS

- A band of brown pigment in a single nail must be examined and investigated with caution, as melanonychia may be the presenting sign of melanoma of the nail unit.
- ABCDEF's of acral lentiginous melanoma:
  A: Age >50 years old.
  B: Brown to black, blurred borders, breadth >3 mm.
  C: Changes of melanonychia or nail plate.
  D: Digit: single digit, especially thumb, big toe, and index finger.
  E: Extension of pigment into nail fold (Hutchinson sign).
  F: Family or personal history of melanoma.

POINT TO REMEMBER

- A solitary longitudinal melanonychia poses a clinical dilemma.

JUNCTIONAL NEVUS

- This evenly pigmented linear nevus emanates from nests of nevus cells in the nail matrix (Fig. 22.20).
- These lesions are quite common in blacks and may be multiple. They are much less common in whites.
- Any smudging or leaching of pigment or variation from the original black band should prompt an immediate biopsy to rule out malignant melanoma (Fig. 22.21).

SUBUNGUAL VERRUCA

- A solitary wart of the nail bed lifting the nail plate is often mistaken for a fungal infection (Fig. 22.22).
- The possibility of subungual squamous cell carcinoma, basal cell carcinoma, or other neoplasm should always be considered if only one nail or periungual area is involved.

HELPFUL HINT

- Squamous cell carcinoma usually presents in the elderly and has a male predominance.

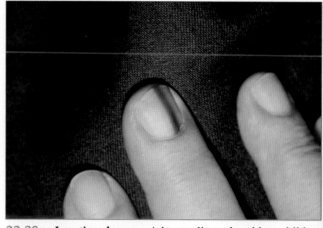
22.20 *Junctional nevus.* A brown linear band in a child.

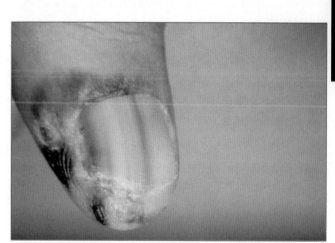
22.21 *Melanoma.* Acral lentiginous melanoma. Note spread of pigment to periungual skin (Hutchinson sign) and to the distal digit.

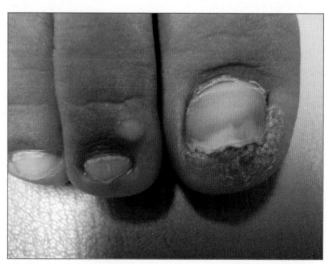
22.22 *Subungual warts.* Note distal onycholysis (lifting of nail) due to warts.

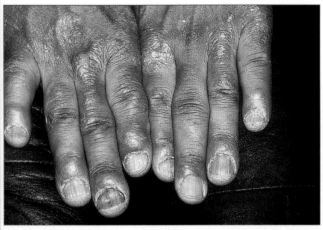

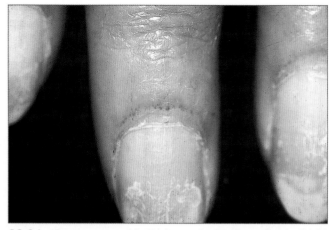

22.23 *Sarcoidosis.* Note that the dystrophic nail plate changes are seen only in the digits that have sarcoidal lesions at the proximal nail folds.

22.24 *Dermatomyositis.* Periungual telangiectasias (nailfold capillaries), thickened cuticles, as well as nail plate dystrophy are apparent.

SARCOIDOSIS

- Dystrophic, thickened nail plates result from infiltration of the proximal nail folds by sarcoidal plaques (Fig. 22.23).

DERMATOMYOSITIS

- The proximal nail fold demonstrates periungual erythema, telangiectasias, thickening of the cuticles ("ragged cuticles"), and distal nail plate thinning (Fig. 22.24).

TERRY NAILS

- Terry nails are characteristic color changes in the nail associated with cirrhosis, congestive heart failure, and adult-onset diabetes mellitus. May be seen as a normal finding associated with age.
- The patient shown in Figure 22.25 had a liver transplant for cirrhosis. His nail beds are white with a narrow zone of pink under the distal end of the plate (Fig. 22.25).

HALF-AND-HALF NAILS

- The proximal half of the nail is white and the distal portion retains the normal pink color.
- These characteristic color changes may be seen in chronic renal failure (Fig. 22.26).

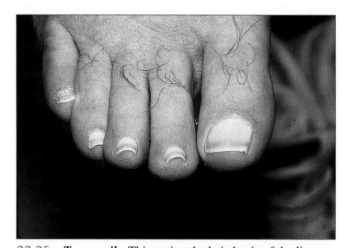

22.25 *Terry nails.* This patient had cirrhosis of the liver.

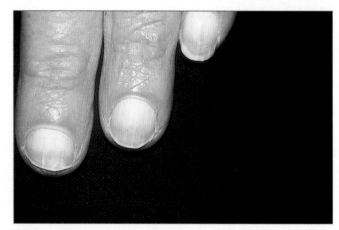

22.26 *Half-and-half nails.* Note that the proximal half is white and the distal half is pink. This patient had renal failure.

DYSTROPHY FROM PREFORMED ARTIFICIAL NAILS

- Acrylic sculptured nails and the less expensive preformed plastic artificial nails are used for nail elongation. They are attached directly to the natural nail plate, which they cover entirely. The artificial nails are glued to the natural nail plate with an acrylate-based adhesive.
- Minor upward pressure on the distal tip of the artificial nail can result in significant distal onycholysis; complete nail avulsion can even result. Any space between the natural nail plate and the artificial nail may become infected (bacterial or fungal) or deformed, and this will often not be noticed until removal of the artificial nail (Fig. 22.27).

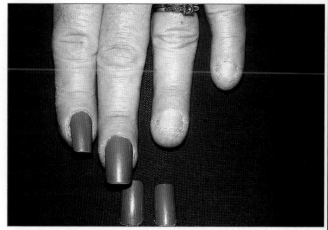

22.27 *Nail dystrophy from artificial nails.* The nail deformity, periungual erythema and scale in this woman was noticed when her artificial nails were removed.

Pigmentary Disorders

OVERVIEW

Skin color is mainly due to melanin. The amount of melanin is determined primarily by hereditary factors and by the result of exposure to ultraviolet radiation (tanning).

MELANOGENESIS

Melanocytes in the basal layer of the epidermis produce melanin. The melanin pigment is manufactured in melanosomes (intracytoplasmic organelles). Once made, the melanosomes are carried along dendrites and delivered to neighboring keratinocytes of the epidermis. Darkly pigmented skin has larger melanosomes that contain more melanin than those in light-skinned individuals.

Increase in melanin (hyperpigmentation or hypermelanosis) can be due to an increased number of melanocytes or from increased production of melanin. Reduced melanin production or a loss of melanocytes results in pale patches (hypopigmentation or hypomelanosis) or white patches (*leukoderma*). Vitiligo is a specific type of leukoderma characterized by depigmentation of the epidermis due to a partial or complete loss of melanocytes.

IN THIS CHAPTER...

➤ **DISORDERS OF HYPOPIGMENTATION**

- Vitiligo vulgaris
- Postinflammatory hypopigmentation
- Idiopathic guttate hypomelanosis
- Other types of hypomelanosis

➤ **DISORDERS OF HYPERPIGMENTATION**

- Melasma
- Postinflammatory hyperpigmentation
- Phytophotodermatitis and berloque dermatitis
- Poikiloderma of Civatte
- Confluent and reticulated papillomatosis (Gougerot–Carteaud disease)
- Acanthosis nigricans
- Carotenemia

VITILIGO VULGARIS

BASICS

- Vitiligo vulgaris (common vitiligo) is an acquired disorder of skin depigmentation that affects 1% to 2% of the world's population.
- Thirty percent of patients with vitiligo report a positive family history of the disorder.

PATHOGENESIS

- Although the cause of vitiligo vulgaris is still unknown, the condition is thought to result from an autoimmune process that prompts the loss of melanocytes.
- Vitiligo sometimes occurs in patients with other autoimmune conditions, including thyroid disease, Addison disease, alopecia areata, diabetes mellitus, and pernicious anemia, all of which suggest an autoimmune mechanism.
- Another theory proposes that vitiligo is caused by an abnormality of nerve endings adjacent to skin pigment cells.

CLINICAL MANIFESTATIONS

- Lesions are well-demarcated, depigmented, chalk-white macules or patches that develop cyclically. A rapid loss of pigment is followed by a stable period (during which some repigmentation may occur), followed by recurrence in some cases.
- Vitiliginous lesions tend to have a bilateral, symmetric distribution and typically occur on acral areas (e.g., the hands and feet), body folds, bony prominences, and external genitals.
- Lesions characteristically appear around orifices (Fig. 23.1) (e.g., the mouth, eyes, nose, and anus), but may also involve the eyebrows, eyelashes, and scalp hair, resulting in white hairs (Fig. 23.2) (*leukotrichia*).
- In severe cases, vitiligo may be more widespread (Fig. 23.3) or even total (*vitiligo universalis*).
- Some patients spontaneously experience partial repigmentation or total repigmentation.
- Patients with severe vitiligo may experience embarrassment and lowered self-esteem.
- Occasionally, lesions may have various shades of color that include islands of repigmentation (see Fig. 23.2).
- In dark-skinned individuals, pigmentary loss may be observed at any time of year, whereas in light-skinned people, lesions may be most obvious in the summer, because the tanning effects of the summer sun can accentuate the contrast between the light and dark skin.

DIAGNOSIS

- A clinical diagnosis of vitiligo is commonly based on the characteristic appearance of the skin lesions.

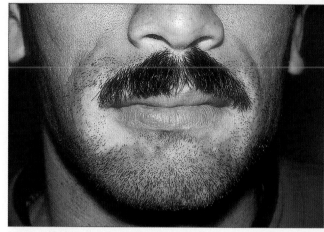

23.1 *Vitiligo.* Depigmented macules are characteristic of vitiligo vulgaris. Note the characteristic periorificial distribution in this patient.

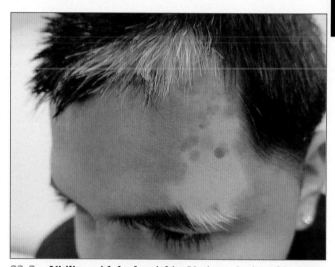

23.2 *Vitiligo with leukotrichia.* Various shades of hypopigmentation, depigmentation, and islands of spontaneous repigmentation can be seen in this patient.

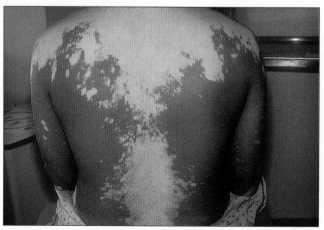

23.3 *Vitiligo.* Extensive depigmentation is evident in this patient.

• Diagnosis can be aided by Wood lamp examination, which reveals a "milk-white" fluorescence. A Wood lamp is a handheld black light that makes hypopigmented areas appear lighter and depigmented (Fig. 23.4A,B).

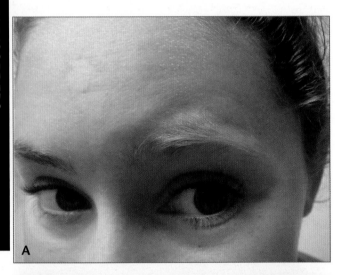

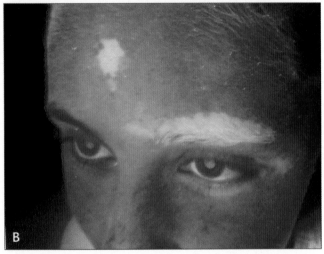

23.4 A, B: *Vitiligo*. Wood lamp examination reveals a "milk-white" fluorescence in areas depigmented by vitiligo. Note the depigmented eyebrows and eyelashes.

 DIFFERENTIAL DIAGNOSIS

Postinflammatory Hypopigmentation

• *Because the lesions of this disorder are not totally depigmented, they are generally off-white in color and borders are often indistinct.*

• *Patients often reveal a history of a pre-existing inflammatory dermatitis such as eczema or tinea versicolor.*

Hypopigmented Tinea Versicolor

• *Patients with active, untreated tinea versicolor have a whitish scale, whereas inactive or postinflammatory hypopigmented spots of tinea versicolor lack scale.*

• *In addition, under Wood lamp examination, active, scaly lesions may appear as a yellow-orange fluorescence, and skin scrapings are positive for KOH examination.*

Chemical Leukoderma

• *Develops on the hands of persons who work with germicidal detergents (especially phenolic compounds) or with certain rubber-containing compounds that destroy melanocytes thus simulating vitiligo.*

• *Diagnosis is established based on the location of the lesions (e.g., only on the hands) and a history of exposure (Fig. 23.5).*

Leprosy (Hanson Disease)

• *Cutaneous leprosy often manifests with areas of hypopigmentation. Lesions may appear as hypopigmented macules, plaques, or nodules that become insensitive to touch.*

• *Leprosy is extremely rare in the United States, but it may be seen occasionally in patients who emigrate from endemic areas, such as India or parts of South and Central America.*

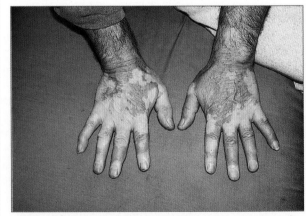

23.5 *Chemical leukoderma*. Chemically induced depigmentation is limited to this patient's hands. Exposure to a cleaning product containing phenol caused the areas of depigmentation in this patient, who routinely used the product at work.

MANAGEMENT

Topical Therapy

- Treatment options for vitiligo involve repigmentation therapies and, rarely, an effort to depigment remaining healthy skin in patients with very extensive disease.
- If administered early to patients with limited disease, **potent** (class 2) and **superpotent** (class 1) **topical corticosteroids** are occasionally helpful in promoting repigmentation.
- Tacrolimus 0.1% ointment **(Protopic)** or picrolimus 1% cream **(Elidel)** twice daily for 2 to 3 months can also induce repigmentation.
- The hands and feet respond poorly to therapy.

Phototherapy

- **Photochemotherapy**, using psoralens and natural sunlight or psoralens and ultraviolet A light (PUVA) in a phototherapy light box, is sometimes tried; however, this treatment is time-consuming and often ineffective. It should generally not be used for children younger than 9 years of age.
  - Hands and feet respond poorly to this method
- **Narrow-band UVB** and **excimer laser** therapy is an effective treatment.

Surgery

- **Surgical transplants:** The following methods may be tried for small, stable areas of vitiligo that have not repigmented with traditional therapies:
  - **Punch grafts:** Punch biopsy specimens from the patient's pigmented donor site are transplanted into depigmented sites; however, a residual, pebbled pigmentary pattern may result.
  - **Minigrafting:** Small donor grafts are inserted into incisional recipient areas of vitiligo and held in place with pressure dressings. As with punch grafting, this procedure does not result in total return of normal pigment, and a mottled pigmentation may result.

Cosmetic Cover-ups

- Special cosmetic makeup that is formulated to match the patient's normal skin color (e.g., **Dermablend** or **Covermark**) or self-tanning compounds that contain dihydroxyacetone (see below) may effectively hide the white patches.
- Sunscreens can be used to avoid exacerbating the contrast between normal skin and lesions and to protect the vitiliginous lesions which are sensitive to the sun.

Depigmentation

- If attempts at repigmentation do not produce satisfactory results, depigmentation may be attempted in selected patients. Those with extensive vitiligo (more than 50% loss of pigment) may elect to have the remaining skin "bleached" with **Benoquin** (20% monobenzyl ether of hydroquinone). The results are permanent (Fig. 23.6).

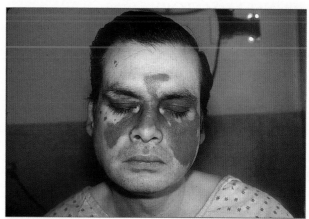

23.6 Vitiligo. Extensive depigmentation. The residual normal pigmentation was treated with Benoquin (20% monobenzyl ether of hydroquinone).

HELPFUL HINTS

- Health care professionals should resist the tendency to trivialize vitiligo by referring to it as simply a cosmetic disorder.
- Clinicians should be sensitive to patients who have emigrated from countries in which leprosy is endemic and generally dreaded. Such patients may feel particularly embarrassed and stigmatized by focal areas of lightened skin color, regardless of the cause of the hypopigmentation.
- Artificial tanning lotions such as products that contain dihydroxyacetone, a color additive that darkens skin by reacting with amino acids in the skin's surface layer, can help camouflage depigmented areas.

POINTS TO REMEMBER

- Patients should be urged to use sunscreens whenever they are exposed to the sun. By minimizing tanning, sunscreens lessen the contrast between healthy skin and lesions; sunscreens also protect the vitiliginous skin, which is sensitive to the sun.
- Patients with vitiligo should be screened for other auto-immune conditions especially if indicated by positive findings in the patient's review of systems or physical examination. The frequency of these associations is not sufficiently high to warrant routine blood tests.
- Response rates to treatments for vitiligo often are disappointing. Lesions on the backs of the hands and feet are particularly resistant to therapy.

 SEE PATIENT HANDOUT "Vitiligo" IN THE COMPANION eBOOK EDITION.

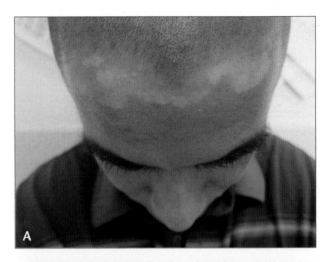

POSTINFLAMMATORY HYPOPIGMENTATION

BASICS

- Postinflammatory reactions are the most common cause of hypopigmentation.
- Localized alterations in skin color are often sequelae of many cutaneous inflammatory conditions.
- Lightening of the skin may follow nearly any inflammatory cutaneous eruption (e.g., eczema and psoriasis (Figs. 23.7 and 23.8).

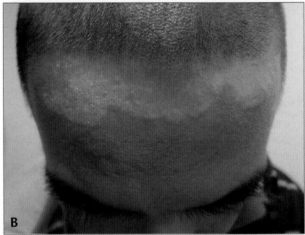

23.8 *Postinflammatory hypopigmentation.* **A** and **B:** The hypopigmented areas on this patient's frontal hairline correspond to the location of a psoriatic plaque that was present prior to treatment.

- In **pityriasis alba**, hypopigmented round spots are commonly seen on the face and other areas of the skin in children with atopic dermatitis (see discussion in Chapter 4).
- Postinflammatory hypopigmentation may also develop after an injury to the skin, such as a burn or surgical scar. The areas of hypopigmentation roughly correspond to the location and shape of the antecedent trauma.

CLINICAL MANIFESTATIONS

- Asymptomatic, ill-defined areas of hypopigmentation.
- Occasionally, a combination of light and dark patches may develop.
- Often, the pigmentary changes are self-limited requiring only time for resolution.

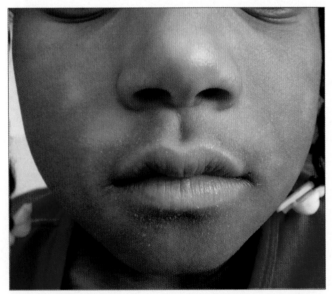

23.7 *Pityriasis alba.* Postinflammatory hypopigmented macules on this child who has atopic dermatitis.

MANAGEMENT

- In general, the pigmentary changes that follow mild inflammatory dermatoses slowly revert to normal over several months. However, those that follow more severe inflammation or injury may be permanent.
- For facial lesions (e.g., pityriasis alba), if there is any scale or erythema, treatment with a mild class 6 topical steroid such as **hydrocortisone 2.5%** cream twice daily or **tacrolimus 0.03%** or **0.1% ointment** twice daily may be helpful.
- The passage of time often improves the cosmetic abnormality.

HELPFUL HINTS

- Postinflammatory hypopigmentation is generally of greater concern to patients with darker skin.
- Pityriasis alba, atopic dermatitis, and tinea versicolor are the most common causes of postinflammatory hypopigmentation; all three are commonly misdiagnosed as vitiligo.

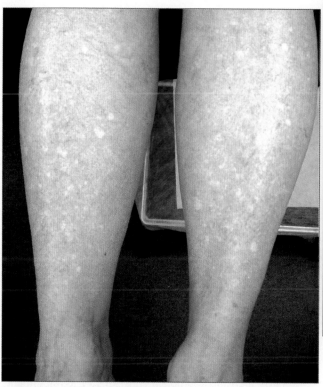

23.9 *Idiopathic guttate hypomelanosis.* Note the white spots on this elderly woman's shin.

IDIOPATHIC GUTTATE HYPOMELANOSIS

BASICS

- Idiopathic guttate hypomelanosis (IGH) refers to the small white spots that often appear on the arms and lower legs of middle-aged and elderly people.
- IGH occurs in all races, but as with vitiligo, it is more apparent in persons with darker skin. Typically, it develops first on the legs of women in early adult life (Fig. 23.9).

CLINICAL MANIFESTATIONS

- The characteristic asymptomatic, "confetti-like," discrete, angular, or circular macules are 1 to 3 mm in diameter; however, lesions may measure up to 10 mm in diameter.

- Lesions arise in areas of chronic sun damage, particularly on the anterior lower legs and less often on extensor forearms. Inexplicably, the face is not involved.
- There is no effective treatment.

OTHER TYPES OF HYPOMELANOSIS

- In the appropriate clinical or environmental context, various systemic and congenital conditions may cause hypopigmentation. They include the following:
  - Endocrine diseases, such as Addison disease and hypothyroidism
  - Genetic conditions, such as congenital vitiligo, tuberous sclerosis, and albinism
  - Infectious diseases, such as leprosy, pinta, and yaws
  - In addition, hypomelanosis may result from the use of intralesional and topical corticosteroids, as well as topical hydroquinone, and retinoids
  - Nutritional deficiencies (especially vitamin B_{12} deficiency and kwashiorkor) may also cause a loss of pigmentation

Disorders of Hyperpigmentation

MELASMA

BASICS

- Formerly known as chloasma, melasma, or the "mask of pregnancy," is an acquired form of hyperpigmentation arising most often on the face.
- It is rare before puberty and most commonly occurs in women during their reproductive years, particularly those who have darker complexions and live in sunny climates.
- Melasma is seen in Asia, the Middle East, South America, Africa, and the Indian subcontinent. In North America, it is most prevalent among Hispanics, African-Americans, and immigrants from countries in which it is common.
- It may appear during pregnancy, from oral contraceptive use, during menopause, or it may arise *de novo* for no apparent reason.
- Melasma is exacerbated by exposure to sunlight.
- When men are affected, the clinical and histologic picture is identical; however, the explanation for this condition in males is unknown.

CLINICAL MANIFESTATIONS

- Primarily a cosmetic problem consisting of asymptomatic, blotchy darkening of the facial skin.
- Lesions are found mainly on the cheeks, angles of the jaw, forehead, nose, chin, and above the upper lip (Fig. 23.10).
- The hyperpigmentation often follows the rim of the zygomatic arch and the nasolabial fold is generally spared (Fig. 23.11).
- Lesions are tan to brown, hyperpigmented macules that may coalesce into symmetric, well-demarcated patches.
- During pregnancy, the darkening of the skin often occurs in the second and third trimesters and most often spontaneously fades after termination of pregnancy.
- Melasma also tends to fade on discontinuance of oral contraceptives or avoidance of sunlight; however, it may persist indefinitely.

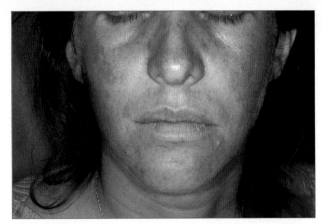

23.11 ***Melasma.*** Note sparing of nasolabial area. (From Goodheart HP. *Goodheart's Same-Site Differential Diagnosis*. Philadelphia, PA: Lippincott Williams & Wilkins, 2011.)

 DIFFERENTIAL DIAGNOSIS

Postinflammatory Hyperpigmentation (see the Discussion below)
- *Previous inflammatory eruption or injury. In general, lesions roughly correspond to the location of inflammation or injury and have less clearly defined margins than seen in melasma.*

Solar Lentigines ("Liver Spots")
- *These lesions have uniform coloration and are acquired during middle age on sun-exposed areas, such as the face and backs of the hands (see Chapter 30).*

 MANAGEMENT

- Treatment of melasma often involves a combination approach using one or more bleaching agents, cosmetic camouflage, and meticulous sun avoidance and blockage.
- Bleaching creams that contain the tyrosinase inhibitor hydroquinone are readily available and are an effective first-line treatment for melasma.
- Over-the-counter preparations such as **Ambi** and **Esoterica** contain 2% hydroquinone.
- Preparations of 3% hydroquinone (**Melanex**) and 4% hydroquinone (**Eldoquin Forte**) are available by prescription only. Some products such as **Eldopaque** also contain a sunblock; **Lustra**, a 4% hydroquinone agent, also contains vitamins C and E and glycolic acid.
- Hydroquinone preparations are applied twice daily to areas of darkening only.
- Other lightening agents include the tyrosinase inhibitor azelaic acid (**Azelex 20% cream**), which may be used in addition to hydroquinone.

continued on page 377

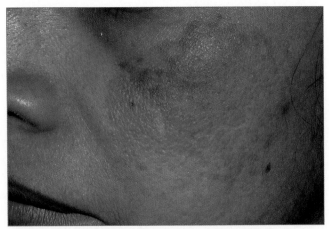

23.10 ***Melasma of cheeks.*** Melasma may result from pregnancy, oral contraceptive use, or menopause, or it may arise *de novo* for no apparent reason.

MANAGEMENT *Continued*

- Topical **tretinoin** can also be used in combination with both hydroquinone and a topical steroid (**Tri-Luma cream**).
- **Alpha-hydroxy acid** products, such as mild **glycolic acid** peels, may also be used to hasten the effect of other topical lightening agents. They should be used cautiously in darkly pigmented Hispanics, Asians, and blacks because of the risk for postinflammatory pigmentary hyperpigmentation (see the next section).
- **Kojic acid**, a tyrosinase inhibitor, is commonly used in Japan and the Middle East, and it seems to have an efficacy similar to that of hydroquinone.

HELPFUL HINTS

- Lightening agents work slowly and results may not be visible for months. Therefore patience is required.
- Without the strict avoidance of sunlight, potentially successful treatments for melasma are doomed to failure.
- Destructive modalities (e.g., cryotherapy, medium-depth chemical peels, lasers) yield unpredictable results and are associated with numerous potential adverse effects.

 SEE PATIENT HANDOUT "Melasma" IN THE COMPANION eBOOK EDITION.

POSTINFLAMMATORY HYPERPIGMENTATION

BASICS

- Darkening of the skin may occur after nearly any inflammatory eruption, such as eczema (Figs. 23.12 and 23.13), lichen planus, acne, or after an injury to the skin such as a burn. Elective skin treatments (e.g., chemical peels, laser resurfacing, or dermabrasion) may also precipitate postinflammatory hyperpigmentation.
- The hyperpigmentation stems from the melanocyte's exaggerated response to cutaneous insult, which results in an increased or abnormal distribution of the pigment melanin.
- As with melasma, postinflammatory hyperpigmentation tends to develop more often in people with dark complexions.

CLINICAL MANIFESTATIONS

- As in postinflammatory hypopigmentation (discussed above), this is an asymptomatic cosmetic issue.
- Lesions tend to conform in location and shape to the preceding eruption or injury (Fig. 23.14A,B).
- May be exacerbated by sun exposure.

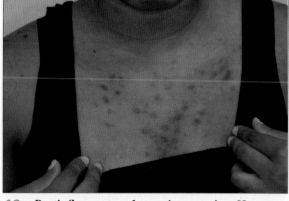

23.12 *Postinflammatory hyperpigmentation.* Hyperpigmentation that resulted from healed acne lesions.

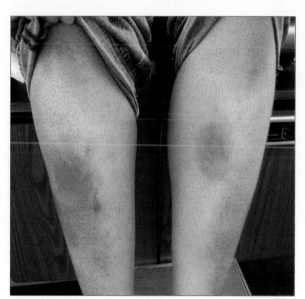

23.13 *Nummular eczema, postinflammatory hyperpigmentation.* In this patient, healing lesions resulted in hyperpigmentation.

MANAGEMENT

- Often, the passage of time, coupled with sun protection, affords a gradual lightening of darkened areas.
- Avoidance and treatment of the inciting underlying dermatosis may prevent future lesions. Treatment of acne, for example, prevents the formation of new inflammatory lesions and allows time for older pigmented lesions to fade.
- When lesions persist, many of the measures used to treat melasma (see the discussion above) may be tried. Agents such as **azelaic acid, topical retinoids** such as Tazorac 0.1% cream in addition to an agent containing a hydroquinone may be of some benefit; however, persistent postinflammatory hyperpigmentation tends to be much more recalcitrant than is melasma.
- Cosmetic cover-ups may be used.

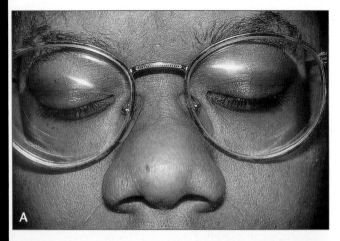

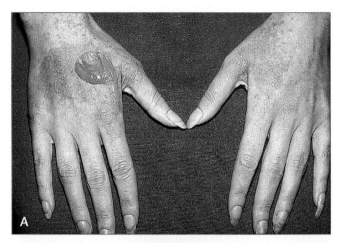

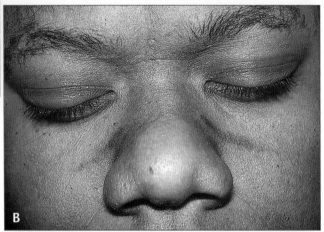

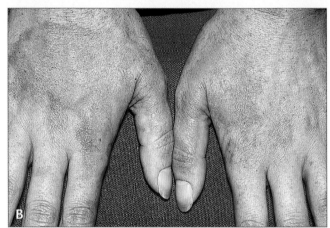

23.14 A, B: *Postinflammatory hyperpigmentation.* In this patient, the cause was contact dermatitis from his eyeglasses. Note how the lesions conform to the shape of the frames.

23.15 *Berloque dermatitis.* **A:** This woman was squeezing limes for an outdoor barbecue 2 days before this blistering, hyperpigmented eruption began. **B:** This is the same patient 2 weeks later. Note the postinflammatory hyperpigmentation.

PHYTOPHOTODERMATITIS AND BERLOQUE DERMATITIS

BASICS

- **Phytophotodermatitis** is a phototoxic reaction that results from contact with a photosensitizing agent followed by sun exposure.
- Photosensitizing chemicals are called furocoumarins and are commonly found in several citrus fruits and plants, including lemons, limes, bergamot oranges, grapefruit, celery, parsley, parsnip, and hogweed.
- The reaction is a chemically induced, nonimmunologic, acute skin reaction requiring light (usually within the UVA spectrum; i.e., 320 to 400 nm).
- A botanical cause for dermatitis is suspected when the pattern of an eruption is linear or streaky, such as noted in the contact dermatitis caused by poison ivy (see Chapter 13).
- When the phytophotodermatitis is caused by perfume or other agents such as oil from the bergamot lime (*Citrus bergamia*), an ingredient in some perfumes and fragrances, it is referred to as *berloque dermatitis*.

CLINICAL MANIFESTATIONS

- The initial skin response resembles an exaggerated sunburn which may be accompanied by blisters (Fig. 23.15A). The reaction typically begins within 24 hours of exposure and peaks at 48 to 72 hours.
- Postinflammatory hyperpigmentation that may last several weeks or longer typically ensues (Fig. 23.15B).

 HELPFUL HINTS

- Limes are a common culprit of phytophotodermatitis and characteristically appear as a stippled pattern localized to the first dorsal interosseous area of the hand(s).
- Ask the patient if he or she was squeezing lemons or limes on chicken or fish while outdoor barbequing.

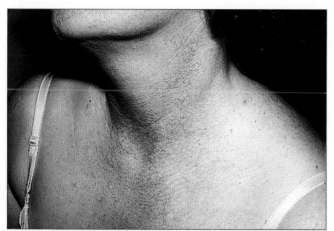

23.16 *Poikiloderma of Civatte.* The persistent erythema in this patient is characteristic. Note the sparing of the shaded areas under the chin and jawline.

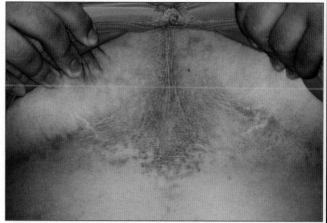

23.17 *Confluent and reticulated papillomatosis.* Darkly pigmented patches and papules coalescing centrally with peripheral reticulation on the central chest.

POIKILODERMA OF CIVATTE

BASICS

- This common condition occurs primarily in middle-aged, fair-skinned women.
- Hormonal changes related to menopause or low estrogen levels may be a causal factor.

CLINICAL MANIFESTATIONS

- Basically of cosmetic concern to patients.
- Lesions consist of erythema associated with a mottled pigmentation located on the sides of the neck and other sun-exposed areas.
- The shaded submental and submandibular areas are usually spared, supporting chronic sunlight exposure as the apparent cause of this condition (Fig. 23.16).

 MANAGEMENT

- The patient should be advised about avoidance of sun exposure and the proper use of sunscreens to prevent further skin involvement.
- The pulsed-dye laser may be used to decrease the erythema in this condition.

CONFLUENT AND RETICULATED PAPILLOMATOSIS (GOUGEROT–CARTEAUD DISEASE)

BASICS

- Confluent and reticulated papillomatosis (CARP) is an uncommon condition of unknown etiology. Causal theories include an endocrine disruption, a disorder of keratinization, and an abnormal host reaction to *Pityrosporum* organisms or bacteria.

CLINICAL MANIFESTATIONS

- CARP usually presents shortly after puberty.
- CARP is characterized by hyperkeratotic papules and plaques that coalesce to form hyperpigmented, confluent plaques centrally with a reticular pattern peripherally (Fig. 23.17).
- CARP is usually located on the trunk, back, lateral or posterior neck or the flanks (Fig. 23.18).
- Lesional skin is "rough" textured on palpation.

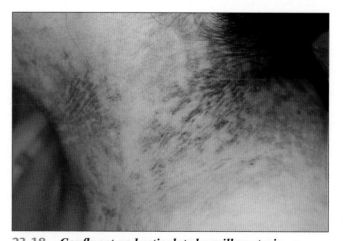

23.18 *Confluent and reticulated papillomatosis.* Characteristic, darkly pigmented, hyperkeratotic, reticulated papules and plaques on the lateral neck. Note that this patient also has evidence of acanthosis nigricans on her posterior neck.

DIAGNOSIS

- Clinical appearance is characteristic and a KOH is negative.

DIFFERENTIAL DIAGNOSIS

Acanthosis Nigricans (see the following section)
- *Indistinguishable from CARP histopathologically.*

Darkly Pigmented Tinea Versicolor
- *KOH positive, not "rough" textured on palpation.*

MANAGEMENT

- CARP responds to oral tetracyclines, such as minocycline or doxycycline 100 mg twice a day for 2 to 3 months.

HELPFUL HINT

- Many patients with CARP also have coexistent acanthosis nigricans (see below).

ACANTHOSIS NIGRICANS

BASICS

- Acanthosis nigricans (AN) has a characteristic hyperpigmented skin pattern that occurs primarily in flexural folds. The skin is thought to darken and thicken in reaction to circulating growth factors and insulin resistance.
- The majority of cases of AN, including idiopathic cases and those associated with obesity, are referred to as *benign AN.*
- Other benign forms of AN are associated with endocrine disorders, such as insulin-resistant diabetes, polycystic ovary syndrome, Cushing disease, Addison disease, pituitary tumors, pinealomas, and hyperandrogenic syndromes with insulin resistance.
- AN is sometimes related to drug use, most commonly secondary to glucocorticoids, nicotinic acid, diethylstilbestrol, or growth hormone therapy. AN may also be inherited without any disease associations.
- The rare, so-called *malignant AN* is associated with an internal malignant disease, usually an intra-abdominal adenocarcinoma. Affected patients generally have a poor prognosis. The skin condition is sometimes seen before the cancer is recognized; it can also be associated with recurrences and metastases.

CLINICAL MANIFESTATIONS

- AN generally presents with a gradual evolution of symmetric, asymptomatic, tan or brown to black, leathery or velvety plaques.
- Plaques are sometimes "warty" (papillomatous) and studded with skin tags.
- They have linear, alternating, dark and light pigmentation that becomes more apparent when the skin is stretched (Fig. 23.19).
- The most common sites of involvement are the axillae, the base of the neck, the inframammary folds, the inguinal areas, and the antecubital fossae (Fig. 23.20).
- The dorsa of the hands (especially the knuckles), the elbows, and the knees are also common locations.
- Less commonly, mucous membranes, the vermilion border of the lips, and the eyelids are involved.

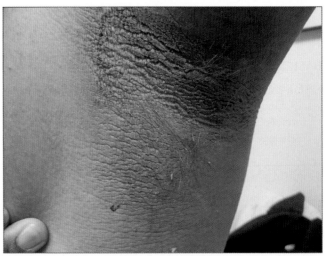

23.19 *Acanthosis nigricans.* Linear, alternating dark and light pigmentation becomes more apparent when the skin is stretched.

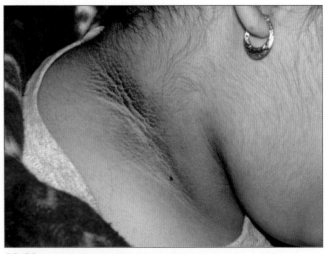

23.20 *Acanthosis nigricans.* This patient has diabetes. Note the marked hyperpigmentation.

MANAGEMENT

- The underlying etiology of AN should be investigated and addressed.
- Common interventions include correcting hyperinsulinemia through diet and medication; weight loss for obesity-associated AN; excise or treat any underlying tumor, discontinue offending medicines in drug-induced AN.
- After associated factors are addressed, AN is primarily a cosmetic concern.
- Treatments to that have been used to improve the cosmetic appearance and include topical retinoids, topical hydroquinone, dermabrasion, and laser therapy.

HELPFUL HINTS

- The vast majority of AN cases are associated with obesity.
- Despite identical histopathology, AN does not improve with oral tetracyclines, whereas CARP responds well to this treatment.

POINTS TO REMEMBER

- Besides obesity, other causes of AN may be identified by screening for insulin resistance and diabetes.
- When AN suddenly arises in a nonobese adult who has no family history of the condition, it is extremely important to perform a thorough workup for an underlying malignancy and identify a hidden tumor.

CAROTENEMIA

BASICS

- Carotenemia is characterized by yellow pigmentation of the skin caused by an increased level of beta-carotene in

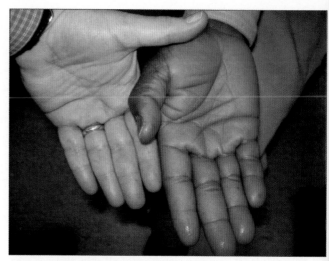

23.21 *Carotenemia.* The yellow-orange palms in this patient from West Africa were attributed to his diet, which consisted of an abundance of yams.

the blood. Most cases result from prolonged and excessive consumption of carotene-rich foods, such as carrots, squash, and yams (sweet potatoes).
- Less commonly, carotenemia has been associated with diabetes mellitus and hypothyroidism.

CLINICAL MANIFESTATIONS

- The yellow-orange pigmentation often first appears on the palms and soles (Fig. 23.21).
- The tip of the nose, the nasolabial folds, the palate, and other areas of the skin may become involved.
- The sclerae are spared, which distinguishes carotenemia from jaundice.

MANAGEMENT

- Diet-induced carotenemia is a benign condition. The yellow pigmentation generally resolves with dietary changes.

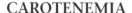

Pruritus: The "Itchy" Patient

OVERVIEW

Pruritus, the most common symptom of all skin diseases, can be simply defined as an unpleasant sensation that elicits the urge to scratch. It may present as a primary complaint, as an indication of an underlying systemic or psychiatric disorder, or as an isolated problem with no other explanation (pruritus of unknown origin).

Pruritus may result from the following:

- Common primary skin disorders such as eczema, lichen simplex chronicus, psoriasis, lichen planus, dry skin (xerosis) or, rarely, dermatitis herpetiformis.
- Exogenous causes such as drugs, cocaine abuse, contact dermatitis (e.g., poison ivy), scabies, lice, fiberglass, and aquagenic pruritus.
- Internal disorders such as chronic renal failure, acquired immunodeficiency syndrome, polycythemia vera, cholestasis, pregnancy-related disorders, primary biliary cirrhosis, diabetes mellitus, thyroid disease, and carcinoid syndrome.
- Psychogenic causes such as delusions of parasitosis, neurotic excoriations, pruritus ani, and obsessive-compulsive disorder.
- Associated malignant diseases such as Hodgkin disease, leukemia, and multiple myeloma.

IN THIS CHAPTER...

➤ **PRURITUS OF UNKNOWN ORIGIN**

➤ **NEUROTIC EXCORIATIONS/FACTITIAL DERMATITIS**

➤ **DELUSIONS OF PARASITOSIS**

➤ **CLINICAL VARIANTS OF PRURITUS**

- Aquagenic pruritus
- Notalgia paresthetica
- Brachioradial pruritus
- Pruritus from systemic disease

BASICS

- Pruritus of unknown origin (PUO) is focal or generalized itching for more than 2 to 6 weeks with no determined cause.

CLINICAL MANIFESTATIONS

- Focal or widespread linear excoriations, crusts, lichenified plaques, or wheals may be present. Postinflammatory hypo- or hyperpigmentation may also be evident (Figs. 24.1 and 24.2).
- Pruritus with no apparent lesions is quite common.
- May have secondary infection of lesions (impetiginization).
- Possible insomnia and/or depression.
- Lesions may have bizarre appearances; therefore, *facticia* or *"neurotic excoriations"* should be suspected (see below).

DIAGNOSIS

- A search for the cause of the pruritus is based on the following:
  - A careful history
  - Physical findings (linear excoriations, crusts)
- The workup for PUO includes the following:
  - Rectal and pelvic examinations, if indicated
  - Complete blood count
  - Stool examination for parasites and occult blood
  - Chest radiograph
  - Thyroid, renal, and liver function tests
  - Follow-up of the patient for as long as necessary to make a diagnosis

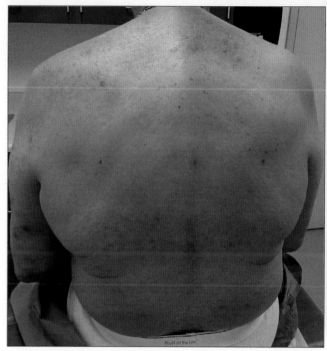

24.1   *Chronic pruritus.* The "butterfly" sign, shown here, refers to the sparing of the area on the mid-back that cannot be reached by the patient.

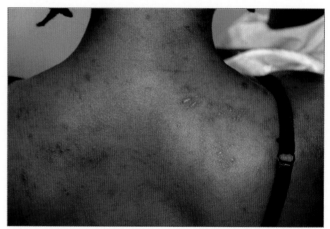

24.2   *Chronic pruritus.* Crusts and areas of linear hypopigmentation suggest chronicity on this woman's upper back.

MANAGEMENT

- Whenever possible, treatment of the underlying systemic disease that is causing the pruritus may bring relief.
- **Antihistamines** are of more benefit in the treatment of allergic conditions, urticaria, and drug reactions than they are for the treatment of itching and may be no more effective than a placebo. Despite this finding, the powerful effect of antihistamines as placebos and as soporifics should not be overlooked.
- **Topical therapy** that can be soothing and helpful in some patients includes the following:
  - Menthol, phenol, camphor, and calamine lotions (e.g., **Sarna, Prax, PrameGel**).
  - **Cold applications** of frozen vegetable packets may be helpful.
  - Topical steroids are generally not very helpful when no lesions are apparent.
- Gabapentin (**Neurontin**) and a serotonin re-uptake inhibitor such as sertraline hydrochloride (**Zoloft**) may be successful in relieving intractable pruritus.

HELPFUL HINTS

- The dosage of antihistamines should be titrated gradually upward using nonsedating agents during the daytime and sedating agents at bedtime.
- It is important not to overlook a drug reaction as the cause of PUO.
- Scabies should be considered if more than one family member itches.
- Hodgkin disease may present with PUO that precedes the diagnosis by up to 5 years.
- Topical emollients are an essential component of the therapy of pruritus when xerosis is present.

POINT TO REMEMBER

- Antihistamines often exert their antipruritic action by inducing sleep.

BASICS

- Patients with **neurotic excoriations**, compulsively pick at their skin and often, no precipitating cause can be determined.
- **Factitial dermatitis** is a self-induced condition caused by habitual scratching or picking, in which lesions tend to show a wide range of bizarre patterns uncharacteristic of any specific disease (Fig. 24.3).

CLINICAL MANIFESTATIONS

- Erosions, linear crusts, or ulcerations that suggest manipulation by the patient.
- Postinflammatory hyperpigmentation and whitish hypopigmented postinflammatory lesions indicate chronicity (see Fig. 24.2).
- Many lesions tend to be located on the upper back or ankles—areas that are easily reachable by the patient (see Figs. 24.1 and 24.2).
- Factitial lesions often present as deep ulcerations with geometric shapes (Fig. 24.4).
- The presence of factitial dermatitis may imply that the patient has severe emotional problems such as obsessive-compulsive disorder, or delusions of parasitosis (see below) that underlie the repetitive self-destructive behavior.

DIAGNOSIS

- The diagnosis is either given by the patient, who readily admits that the lesions are self-created, or the lesions themselves may be indicative of the disorder.
- Bizarre-appearing lesions and an affect of *la belle indifférence* on the part of the patient suggest factitial dermatitis as the cause.

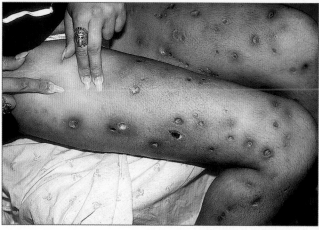

24.3 *Neurotic excoriations.* These are self-induced ulcers in a patient who was convinced that she was infested with lice.

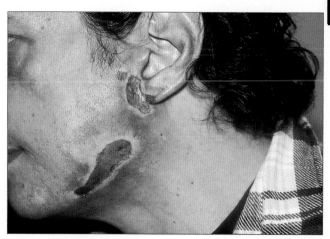

24.4 *Factitial ulcerations.* These were created by the patient. Note their geometric appearance. The patient has a severe psychiatric disorder.

 MANAGEMENT

- High-potency topical corticosteroids, topical corticosteroids under occlusion, and intralesional corticosteroids are sometimes useful, but these treatments will be ineffective if the underlying psychological cause is not addressed.
- Bedtime antihistamines are sometimes helpful.
- Psychotherapy and/or psychopharmacologic drugs should be used, if indicated.

 HELPFUL HINT

- When the diagnosis is in doubt, the lesions may be covered with a thick dressing, and the patient is then instructed not to remove it. Consequently, when the patient cannot access the lesions, they tend to heal rapidly.

Delusions of Parasitosis

BASICS

- As the name suggests, delusions of parasitosis (DOP) is a condition where an individual has the mistaken belief that they are being infested by parasites such as mites, lice, fleas, spiders, worms, bacteria, or other organisms. They have a fixed false belief that they are infested and they usually go from doctor to doctor seeking a cure.
- DOP is closely related to the so-called **Morgellons syndrome**, in which an individual believes that they have fibers coming out of their skin.
- The cause of DOP is unknown but it has been classified as a monosymptomatic hypochondrial psychosis. Apart from their DOP, patients may have an otherwise normal personality or more commonly an acceptable degree of eccentricity with a tendency toward social isolation. It can also occur as a manifestation of other psychiatric illnesses.
- DOP occurs most commonly in white middle-aged or older women, although people of all races, sex, and age may be affected.

CLINICAL MANIFESTATIONS

- People suffering from DOP often describe the infestation as being in or under the skin, just inside body openings, in sputum, inside their stomach, intestines or on their surrounding habitat such as their bed, couch, or throughout their home.
- The patient typically seeks numerous opinions from medical doctors, exterminators, and entomologists.
- The patient typically brings fragments of skin, hair, dried blood, or scabs in a container.

- Patients are often hostile or suspicious.
- Sensations of itching, burning, crawling and biting that may lead to self-mutilation.
- One or more family members sometimes share DOP (*folie à deux*).

DIAGNOSIS

- Rule out any true infestations, for example, with scabies.

MANAGEMENT

- Tactful management requires repeated visits in order to gain the patient's trust before broaching the actual existence of the infestation and noting that the problem is a psychiatric illness.
- Since patients with DOP are totally convinced of the existence and infestation of "their" parasites, they are generally reluctant to agree to seek psychiatric help.
- In most cases treatment with psychotropic medications is usually necessary.
- Depressive symptoms should be screened for and treatment of depression may be useful. **Escitalopram**, a selective serotonin reuptake inhibitor, has been reported to be effective.
- Antipsychotics such as **pimozide, risperidone**, and **olanzapine** may also be helpful.

A patient may complain of itching caused by reasons that seem totally inexplicable or bizarre. Many histories have various twists and turns, such as the following:

AQUAGENIC PRURITUS

- The person with aquagenic pruritus experiences intense itching *only* after exposure to water.

NOTALGIA PARESTHETICA

- Notalgia paresthetica is a common condition seen most often in middle-aged and elderly patients.
- It is thought to represent a sensory neuropathy that may be caused by nerve impingement from spinal arthritis.
- Notalgia paresthetica most often presents with a localized, very focal, unilateral area of recurrent itching that characteristically occurs on the lower or mid-scapula. The postinflammatory hyperpigmentation that sometimes results from the chronic rubbing and scratching reveals the diagnosis (Fig. 24.5).
- Treatment is often futile. Capsaicin (**Zostrix**) cream, which depletes nerve endings of their chemical transmitters, applied 3 to 5 times daily can improve symptoms.
- Topical corticosteroids, topical anesthetics (e.g., pramoxine, lidocaine), gabapentin, and acupuncture have all been tried with variable results.
- There have been case reports of successful treatment with **botulinum toxin type A** for this condition.

BRACHIORADIAL PRURITUS

- Brachioradial pruritus (BRP) is an intense itching sensation of the arm, usually between the shoulder and elbow of one or both arms.
- There is ongoing debate regarding whether BRP is caused by a nerve entrapment in the cervical spine or a prolonged exposure to sunlight, because the outer, sun-exposed aspects of the arms are most often affected.

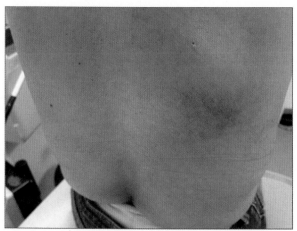

24.5 *Notalgia paresthetica.* Note the typical location on the lower scapula. The postinflammatory hyperpigmentation resulted from the chronic rubbing and scratching of this itchy area.

- Measures to treat BRP include the following:
  - **Sun protection**—wearing clothing with long sleeves is more effective than use of sunscreens alone
  - Capsaicin (**Zostrix**) cream
  - Ice packs
  - **Amitriptyline** tablets at bedtime
  - Anticonvulsant agents, including gabapentin (**Neurontin**) 300 mg three times daily
  - Electrical cutaneous nerve field stimulation

PRURITUS FROM SYSTEMIC DISEASE

- Internal disorders such as chronic renal or liver failure can result in generalized pruritus.

MANAGEMENT

For Renal Disease

- Renal pruritus occurs most often in those receiving hemodialysis.
- **Ultraviolet B (UVB) therapy** is often effective. **Narrow-band UVB** is particularly effective.
- Oral ingestion of **activated charcoal** may be helpful. It is inexpensive and generally well tolerated; therefore, it is considered a reasonable treatment when UV therapy has failed.
- Successful **kidney transplantation** is the only definitive treatment for chronic renal pruritus.

For Liver Disease

- Cholestyramine (**Questran**), a bile acid sequestrant, can be used to treat the pruritus that often occurs during liver failure because of the liver's inability to eliminate bile.
- Cholestyramine binds bile in the gastrointestinal tract to prevent its reabsorption.
- Pruritus associated with obstructive malignancy of the biliary tract (e.g., primary sclerosing cholangitis) may be relieved by placing a stent to relieve the obstruction.

For Hypothyroidism

- The pruritus of hypothyroidism is primarily secondary to xerosis and should be treated with emollients and thyroid hormone replacement.

For Hyperthyroidism

- Pruritus secondary to hyperthyroidism generally improves with correction of thyroid function.

For Hodgkin Disease

- Pruritus caused by lymphoma may precede the diagnosis.
- Systemic corticosteroids with palliative chemotherapy in late-stage Hodgkin disease often provide relief.

Xerosis: The "Dry" Patient

OVERVIEW

Xerosis, or dry skin, is a common occurrence in winter climates, particularly in conditions of cold air, low relative humidity, and indoor heating. Xerosis can affect anyone, but it tends to be more severe in certain persons, especially those with a hereditary predisposition. Modern lifestyles are also contributing factors. In Western societies, people tend to over bathe and often live and work in overheated spaces.

The word "dry" is sometimes misapplied. Skin that appears to be dry (i.e., that shows a buildup of scale) may not always be suffering from a lack of water but rather from an over adherence or hyperproliferation of scale. Over adherence of scale occurs in patients with ichthyosis (see discussion in Chapter 4). Hyperproliferation of scale is noted in atopic dermatitis, psoriasis, seborrheic dermatitis, and common dandruff.

IN THIS CHAPTER...

➤ **XEROSIS**

- Asteatotic eczema (see Chapter 13)
- Atopic dermatitis (see Chapters 4 and 13)

BASICS

- Xerosis, or dry skin, is caused by a relative loss of water from the skin through evaporation and a lack of normal desquamation and lubrication.
- Xerosis is especially prevalent in persons who are older than 65 years of age who tend to have a decrease in the production of sebum, the skin's natural lubricant and sealant.
- As skin loses moisture its surface tends to fissure.
- Xerosis tends to be most apparent on the hands and lower legs.
- Dry areas may result in dermatitis, crazy-paving appearance on the lower legs or round patches scattered over the trunk and limbs (a dry form of nummular eczema). Sometimes the dry skin is just itchy, without much of a rash ("winter itch").
- Contributing factors include hypothyroidism, cool weather, especially when windy or the humidity is low, excessive bathing, showering or swimming, especially in strongly chlorinated, hot or cold water, excessive contact with soap, detergents, and solvents.

PATHOGENESIS

- The reasons why the skin becomes, or appears to become, dry are not well understood. It has been proposed that xerosis may be secondary to diminished production of sebum (asteatosis), as well as to reduced eccrine gland activity. However, other biochemical factors related to aging skin have also been implicated.
- Popular folklore and the lay literature often blame xerosis on inadequate water ingestion, but there is no scientific basis for this claim.

CLINICAL VARIANTS

ASTEATOTIC ECZEMA

- Asteatotic eczema occurs almost exclusively in adults.
- This form of eczema is a common, sometimes pruritic, low-grade dermatitis that presents with seasonal recurrences in the winter.
- Early on, the affected skin feels and looks dry; later, an inflammatory dermatitis may evolve.
- Lesions most commonly appear on the shins, arms, hands, and trunk (see Chapter 13).
- The eruption often resembles the surface of a cracked porcelain vase and is often referred to as *erythema craquelé.* It is also likened to the appearance of a dry riverbed (Fig. 25.1).
- A clinical variant consists of small, square-shaped, rectangular, or annular, scaly plaques that are often mistaken for tinea corporis (ringworm) and are often treated as such (Fig. 25.2).

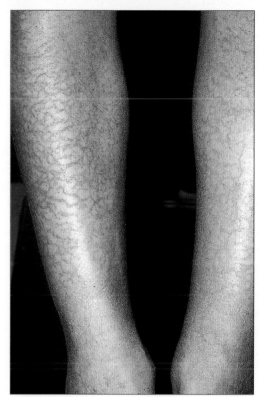

25.1 *Asteatotic eczema.* Here the skin resembles a cracked porcelain vase (erythema craquelé).

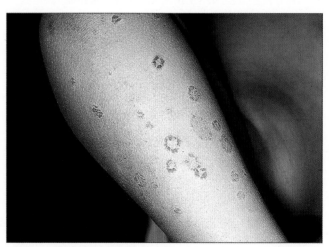

25.2 *Asteatotic eczema.* In this patient there are characteristic small, square-shaped plaques that resemble ringworm (tinea corporis).

ATOPIC DERMATITIS

- Dry, xerotic, exquisitely sensitive, itchy skin is a major feature of atopic dermatitis (see Chapters 4 and 13 for management of this condition).
- Atopic skin is characterized by decreased water content, increased water loss, and reduced water-binding capacity, as well as epidermal hyperproliferation, resulting in *lichenification* (an exaggeration of normal skin markings) and buildup of scale. Underlying causes include intrinsic defects in the epidermal barrier, alterations in the cutaneous innate, and adaptive immunity, as well as environmental triggers.
- Patients usually have a personal or family history of allergies, asthma, or hay fever.
- In both young and old, "chapped lips" is a very common problem, especially in individuals who have atopic cheilitis or an atopic predisposition (Fig. 25.3).
- In addition to scaly eczematous plaques, such patients may develop painful linear cracks or fissures from xerosis, particularly on the palms, soles, and fingertips (Figs. 25.4 and 25.5).

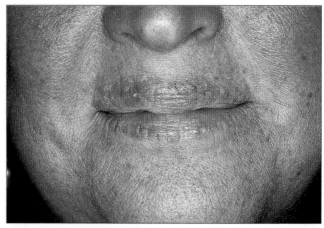

25.3 *Atopic cheilitis.* Note the multiple small fissures on this woman's dry eczematous lips.

 DIFFERENTIAL DIAGNOSIS

Ichthyosis Vulgaris (see Discussion in Chapter 4)

- *Ichthyosis vulgaris (the most common variant of ichthyosis) resembles dry skin; however, it is actually caused by over adherence of scale.*
- *Frequently associated with atopy.*
- *Skin with ichthyosis vulgaris resembles fine fish scales and tends to be most clinically obvious on the shins.*

Dry Skin That Is Not "Dry" (Exfoliation)

- *Many patients complain of "dry skin" from the use of topical retinoids such as Retin-A for the treatment of acne. Actually, the "dryness" is scaling that results from the exfoliative effect of the topical retinoid.*
- *Another common complaint is that of scaling and "dryness" from seborrheic dermatitis of the face and scalp. In such cases, the skin is not always dry and deprived of moisture; rather, the scales and flakes may derive from the inflammatory process.*

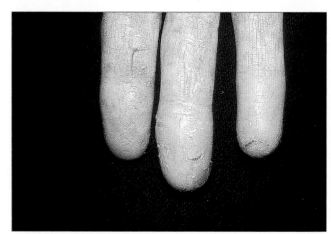

25.4 *Atopic dermatitis, hand eczema.* Dry, sensitive, itchy, lichenified skin is characteristic of this condition. This patient has painful fissures of the distal fingers.

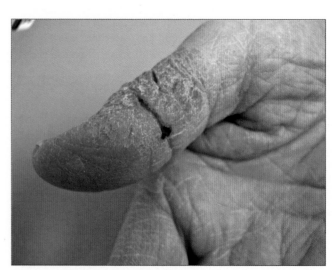

25.5 *Atopic dermatitis, hand eczema.* A deep painful fissure is present on this patient's thumb.

MANAGEMENT

Moisturizers

- Moisturizers do not add water to the skin, but they help retain or "lock in" water that is absorbed while bathing. Therefore, moisturizers should be applied while the skin is still damp.

Other Strategies

- For the dermatitis, itching, and erythema of atopic dermatitis or asteatotic eczema, low- to medium-potency (class 4 to 6) **topical corticosteroids** are valuable. In severe cases, more potent topical corticosteroids (class 1 to 3) may be applied for brief periods when necessary.
- Tepid showers and baths that are less frequent and shorter may be helpful.
- Soap avoidance (on affected areas), mild soaps (e.g., **Dove, Basis**) or a soap substitute (e.g., **Cetaphil non-soap gentle cleanser**) may be tried. However, excessive use of any soap or substitute should be avoided, especially on affected areas. **CeraVe cream** or **Eucerin Daily repair cream** are also excellent options.
- Adhesive dressings (**Band-Aids**) are effective in promoting healing of fissures.
- Lined gloves, worn while washing dishes, can keep hands dry.
- Scarves, gloves, and other apparel can help to provide adequate protection from exposure to outdoor cold.
- The use of room humidifiers and the ingestion of copious amounts of water are of questionable value.

 SEE PATIENT HANDOUT "Dry Skin (Xerosis)" IN THE COMPANION eBOOK EDITION.

Adverse Cutaneous Drug Eruptions

OVERVIEW

An adverse drug reaction is any nontherapeutic deleterious effect due to a prescribed or over-the-counter medication or vaccine. Drug eruptions can mimic almost any dermatosis. Such reactions may be allergic (immunologic) or nonallergic (toxic). **Allergic drug reactions** are not dose dependent. They are classified as one of four types of immunologic reactions:

- Type I: classic immediate hypersensitivity (urticaria, angioedema, anaphylaxis)
- Type II: cytotoxic (hemolysis, purpura)
- Type III: immune complex (vasculitis, serum sickness, urticaria, angioedema)
- Type IV: delayed hypersensitivity (contact dermatitis, exanthematous reactions, photoallergic reactions)

Nonallergic drug eruptions are more common than allergic-type eruptions; they may be dose related, idiosyncratic, localized cutaneous, or systemic. Localized cutaneous eruptions are most often secondary to topical medications such as benzoyl peroxide or topical retinoids. Systemic reactions include symptoms of vertigo secondary to high-dose minocycline. Drug reaction with eosinophilia and systemic symptoms (DRESS syndrome) and acute generalized exanthematous pustulosis (AGEP) are examples of nonallergic idiosyncratic reactions.

Allergic drug eruptions are most often due to antimicrobial agents, nonsteroidal anti-inflammatory drugs (NSAIDs), cytokines, biologics, chemotherapeutic agents, and psychotropic agents. Allergic drug reactions typically result in urticaria, angioedema, and/or potentially fatal anaphylaxis.

The spectrum of adverse cutaneous drug reactions varies widely and includes alopecia due to chemotherapeutic drugs and beta blockers, bullous reactions secondary to furosemide, pigmentary alterations due to antimalarials, thrombocytopenia and necrosis from heparin, and contact dermatitis due to topical neomycin.

IN THIS CHAPTER...

➤ **DRUG ERUPTIONS**

- Exanthematous eruptions
- Urticarial eruptions
- Photosensitive and phototoxic eruptions
- Vasculitic eruptions
- Erythroderma (exfoliative dermatitis)
- Stevens–Johnson syndrome
- Toxic epidermal necrolysis
- Erythema nodosum
- Acneiform eruptions
- Fixed drug eruptions

➤ **MISCELLANEOUS DRUG ERUPTIONS**

- Drug reaction with eosinophilia and systemic symptoms (DRESS syndrome)
- Acute generalized exanthematous pustulosis (AGEP)
- Hemorrhagic onycholysis due to taxane chemotherapeutic agents
- Hand–foot syndrome
- Cocaine/levamisole-induced vasculitis

Drug Eruptions

BASICS

- Most drug eruptions are exanthematous (red rashes) and usually fade in a few days.
- More serious reactions include Stevens–Johnson syndrome (SJS), toxic epidermal necrolysis (TEN), serum sickness, and anaphylaxis.
- The presence of urticarial lesions, mucosal involvement, palpable purpura, blisters, or an extensive eruption almost always requires discontinuation of the responsible drug; decisions regarding milder or nonlife threatening eruptions are determined on a case-by-case basis.
- Risk factors include the following:
  - Age: Drug eruptions are more commonly seen in elderly persons because they often take more drugs than younger people and they often take more than one drug at a time; consequently, they are more likely to have been previously sensitized.
  - A history of previous drug reactions.
  - A family history of drug eruptions.
  - Prolonged use of a drug.
  - Paradoxically, although human immunodeficiency virus (HIV) infection causes profound anergy to other immune stimuli, the frequency of drug hypersensitivity reactions is increased markedly compared with both immunocompetent and HIV-negative immunocompromised populations.

CLINICAL MANIFESTATIONS

- Pruritus is a cardinal feature of most drug eruptions regardless of whether a rash is present.

- Drug eruptions may be limited to the skin, or associated with systemic anaphylaxis, extensive mucocutaneous exfoliation (e.g., TEN) or multisystemic involvement (e.g., DRESS syndrome [see below]); however, most drug eruptions are mild, self-limited, and resolve after the offending agent is discontinued.
- The most common types of drug eruptions are exanthematous and urticarial.
- The various clinical presentations of drug eruptions as well as their specific regional predilections will be presented below. The most commonly implicated drugs for the different clinical types of drug reactions are listed in Table 26.1.

CLINICAL VARIANTS

EXANTHEMATOUS ERUPTIONS

- Exanthematous eruption typically appears 4 to 14 days after starting the medication.
- Lesions are morbilliform (resembling measles) and are pink, "drug red," or purple (violaceous) in color (Figs. 26.1 and 26.2).
- Lesions begin on the chest (centrally) and spread outward with areas of confluence.
- Exanthems tend to be symmetric and occasionally generalized in distribution; they are noted particularly on the trunk, thighs, upper arms, and face.

URTICARIAL ERUPTIONS

- Typically occur as wheals that may coalesce or take cyclic or gyrate forms (Fig. 26.3).

Table 26.1 COMMONLY IMPLICATED DRUGS FOR DIFFERENT DRUG REACTIONS

DRUG ERUPTION TYPE	COMMONLY IMPLICATED DRUGS
Exanthems and urticarial reactions	Sulfonamides, penicillins, hydantoins, allopurinol, quinidine, angiotensin-converting enzyme inhibitors, barbiturates, carbamazepine, isoniazid, NSAIDs, and phenothiazine, as well as thiazide diuretics, aspirin, blood products, cephalosporins, dextran, opiates, radiocontrast dye, ranitidine, and vaccines
Acneiform eruptions	Systemic steroids, topical steroids, lithium, oral contraceptives, and androgenic hormones
Photo-induced	Tetracyclines, particularly demethylchlortetracycline and doxycycline; griseofulvin; certain diuretics such as HCTZ; sulfonylurea agents used to treat diabetes; NSAIDs; and phenothiazines
Bullous eruptions	Penicillin, sulfonamides, vancomycin, captopril, iodides, gold, and furosemide
Purpura	Anticoagulants and thiazides
Vasculitic eruptions	Allopurinol, aspirin or other NSAIDs, cimetidine, gold, hydralazine, penicillin, phenytoin, propylthiouracil, quinolones, sulfonamide, tetracycline, and thiazides
Erythema nodosum	Iodides, oral contraceptives, penicillin, gold, amiodarone, sulfonamides, and opiates
Erythema multiforme major (Stevens–Johnson syndrome) and erythema multiforme minor	Sulfonamides, penicillins, tetracyclines, hydantoins, and barbiturates
Fixed drug eruptions	Tetracyclines, sulfonamides, griseofulvin, barbiturates, phenolphthalein, and NSAIDs
Contact dermatitis	Neomycin and preservatives in topical medications

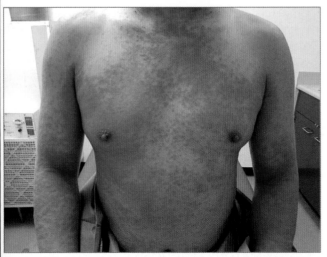

26.1 *Drug eruption.* Exanthematous reaction to a sulfa drug.

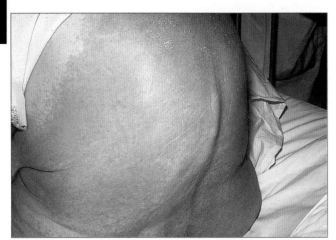

26.2 *Drug eruption.* Note the "drug red" color of this confluent eruption caused by a penicillin derivative.

- Lesions usually appear shortly after the start of drug therapy and resolve rapidly when the drug is withdrawn.
- Urticaria can be seen anywhere on the body.
- Angioedema occurs in a periorbital, labial, and perioral distribution.

PHOTOSENSITIVE AND PHOTOTOXIC ERUPTIONS

- This may appear as erythematous (an exaggerated sunburn; Fig. 26.4), eczematous, or lichenoid (resembling lichen planus) eruption.
- Lesions generally occur on sun-exposed areas such as the "V" of the neck, upper sternum, extensor forearms, and the face (Fig. 26.5).

VASCULITIC ERUPTIONS (SEE DISCUSSION IN CHAPTER 27)

- Characterized by *palpable purpura,* sometimes accompanied by fever, myalgias, arthritis, and abdominal pain.

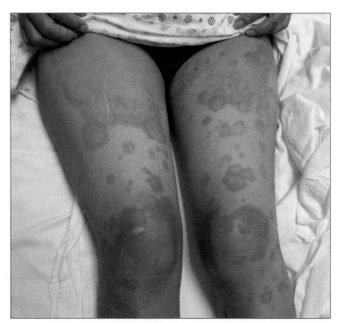

26.3 *Urticarial/figurate drug eruption.* Note the bizarre shapes of the urticarial plaques.

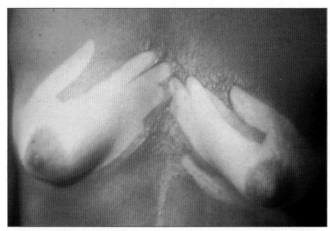

26.4 *Drug photosensitivity eruption.* Erythematous (exaggerated sunburn) reaction in a person who was taking demeclocycline (Declomycin) and fell asleep on the beach. (Courtesy of the Albert Einstein College of Medicine, Division of Dermatology, Bronx, New York.)

- Vasculitis typically begins 7 to 21 days after the onset of drug therapy and may involve other organ systems.
- Often idiopathic, palpable purpura can be a reaction to a drug; however, a systemic illness (e.g., systemic lupus erythematosus) may underlie the vasculitis.
- Histopathology reveals *leukocytoclastic vasculitis.*
- A comprehensive review of systems and laboratory evaluations to exclude internal involvement is mandatory.
- Purpura and vasculitic drug eruptions also tend to occur on the lower extremities.

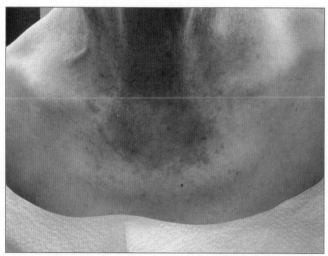

26.5 ***Phototoxic drug eruption.*** This is a phototoxic eruption caused by hydrochlorothiazide. The eruption appears in a photo distribution—the "V" of the neck. This patient also had involvement of her extensor forearms.

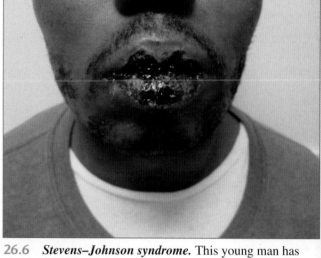

26.6 ***Stevens–Johnson syndrome.*** This young man has painful mucous membrane lesions.

ERYTHRODERMA (EXFOLIATIVE DERMATITIS)

- This is widespread inflammation of the skin (discussed in Chapter 34), and it may result from an underlying skin condition, drug eruption, internal malignancy, or immunodeficiency syndrome.
- Lymphadenopathy is often noted, and hepatosplenomegaly, leukocytosis, eosinophilia, and anemia may be present.

STEVENS–JOHNSON SYNDROME

- Stevens–Johnson syndrome (SJS) was traditionally referred to as "erythema multiforme major," but it is now clear that erythema multiforme (EM) is a distinct cutaneous disorder that is usually triggered by infections (commonly herpes simplex virus), and rarely drugs (see Chapter 27).
- SJS and toxic epidermal necrolysis (TEN) are variants on a clinical spectrum of drug reactions.
- SJS is most often due to drugs, is sometimes idiopathic, but can occasionally be caused by infection with *Mycoplasma pneumonia* and rarely, immunizations.
- SJS is characterized by dusky red macules that may or may not have blistering located on the face and trunk.
- Mucous membrane involvement may be severe and is often painful (e.g., erosions, ulcers) (Fig. 26.6).
- Constitutional symptoms are often present and can progress to TEN.
- By definition, in SJS there is <10% body surface area (BSA) with epidermal detachment (i.e., blistering or sloughing). If there is epidermal detachment of 10% to 30% of the BSA then there is an SJS–TEN overlap and TEN occurs when there is >30% BSA of epidermal detachment.

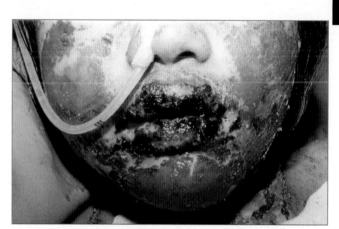

26.7 ***Toxic epidermal necrolysis.*** A child with a severe, generalized eruption with epidermal necrosis and denuded erosive areas. (Image courtesy of Ashit Marwah, MD.)

TOXIC EPIDERMAL NECROLYSIS (TEN; SEE DISCUSSION IN CHAPTER 33)

- TEN is a severe, potentially fatal skin reaction that involves a prodrome of painful skin, followed by rapid, widespread (>30% BSA), skin sloughing (Fig. 26.7).
- Most cases of TEN are the result of drugs; most commonly implicated agents include sulfonamide antibiotics, antiepileptic drugs, oxicam nonsteroidal anti-inflammatory drugs, allopurinol, nevirapine, abacavir, and lamotrigine.
- Symptoms may also include hyperpyrexia, hypotension secondary to hypovolemia, and tachycardia.
- Secondary infection and sepsis are major concerns.
- Septicemia and multisystem organ failure are the primary causes of death.

ERYTHEMA NODOSUM (SEE DISCUSSION IN CHAPTER 34)

- Characterized by tender, red, subcutaneous nodules that typically appear on the pretibial areas.
- Erythema nodosum is a reactive process often secondary to infection, but it may be caused by medications, especially oral contraceptives and sulfonamides.

ACNEIFORM ERUPTIONS (SEE DISCUSSION IN CHAPTER 12)

- Lesions generally appear on the trunk as monomorphic folliculitis-like papules and pustules.
- Generalized acneiform eruptions are usually due to systemic steroids (Fig. 26.8).
- Rosacea-like lesions may occur on the face secondary to use of topical steroids and are often clinically indistinguishable from ordinary rosacea. A history of long-term, indiscriminate misuse of a potent topical steroid on the face helps confirm the diagnosis (Fig. 26.9).
- The condition typically worsens when the topical steroids are discontinued.
- Steroid atrophy most often occurs in body folds (axillae and inguinal creases) (Fig. 26.10).

FIXED DRUG ERUPTIONS

- This is a reaction of circular red plaques or blisters that recurs at the same cutaneous site each time the drug is ingested. In other words, a rechallenge of the drug results in an identical eruption at the same site or sites.

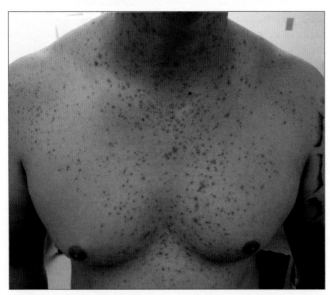

26.8 *Acneiform eruption caused by oral corticosteroids.* This patient developed multiple papules and pustules in a characteristic distribution.

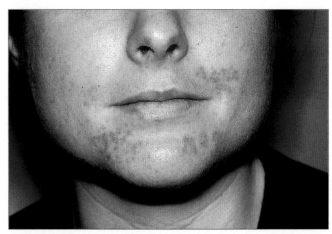

26.9 *Topical steroid-induced rosacea.* This woman has been applying a potent topical steroid to her face for many months.

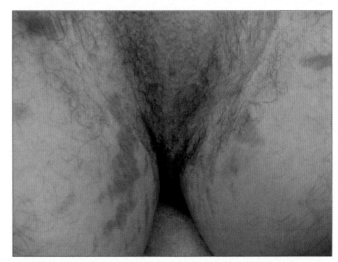

26.10 *Atrophy secondary to a potent topical steroid.* The combination product of clotrimazole and betamethasone produced severe linear, violaceous atrophic plaques in this patient.

- Lesions may be round or oval, single, or multiple (Fig. 26.11).
- Lesions initially are erythematous; later they become violaceous.
- Lesions often blister and erode.
- Lesion occurs most often on the hands, feet, and genitalia; multiple lesions may occur on the trunk and extremities. A lesion on the glans penis is not unusual (Fig. 26.12).
- The eruption often heals with characteristic postinflammatory hyperpigmentation.

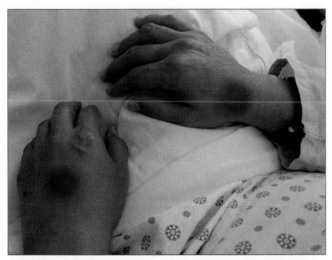

26.11 *Fixed drug eruption.* Two oval lesions occurred at the identical sites where they had occurred previously. In both episodes, the rash emerged after this patient ingested a sulfonamide antibiotic.

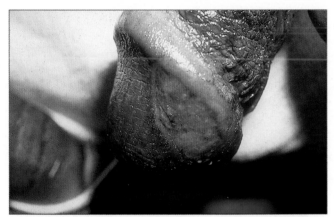

26.12 *Fixed drug eruption.* An oval erosion on the glans penis occurred in this patient who was taking minocycline. According to the patient, an identical lesion—in the same location—appeared when he was given minocycline previously.

MISCELLANEOUS DRUG ERUPTIONS

DRUG REACTION WITH EOSINOPHILIA AND SYSTEMIC SYMPTOMS (DRESS SYNDROME)

- Formally referred to as drug hypersensitivity syndrome and anticonvulsant hypersensitivity syndrome, DRESS is an uncommon potentially life-threatening complex of symptoms. The syndrome carries about a 10% mortality.
- Symptoms usually begin several weeks after exposure to the offending drug, but it has been reported to develop 3 months or later into therapy.
- Drugs that commonly induce DRESS syndrome include phenobarbital, carbamazepine, phenytoin, valproic acid, captopril, minocycline, sulfonamides, allopurinol, and dapsone.

- Patients present with a morbilliform (exanthematous rash), fever, sore throat, and lymphadenopathy. The eruption may become widespread with edema (often facial) and evolve into vesicles, bullae, targetoid lesions, and purpura.
- Thrombocytopenia, atypical lymphocytosis, and leukocytosis with eosinophilia are often noted.
- Systemic involvement may include hepatitis (phenytoin, minocycline, and dapsone), nephritis (allopurinol, carbamazepine, and dapsone), as well as pulmonary (minocycline) and cardiac (ampicillin and minocycline) symptoms.

ACUTE GENERALIZED EXANTHEMATOUS PUSTULOSIS (AGEP)

- AGEP is an uncommon skin eruption characterized by the rapid appearance of widespread areas of erythema studded with small pustules (Fig. 26.13).
- The onset of AGEP is usually within 2 days of exposure to the responsible medication.
- Typically it starts on the face or in the axillae and groin, and then becomes more widespread.
- It may be associated with a fever and malaise, but generally the patient is not very sick.
- The eruption may last for 1 to 2 weeks followed by exfoliation and resolution.

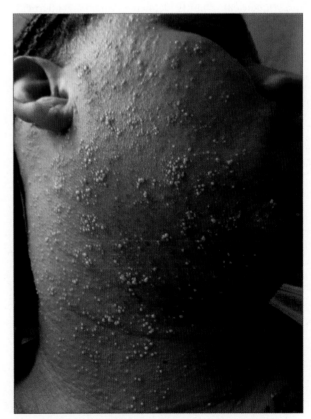

26.13 *Acute generalized exanthematous pustulosis (AGEP).* These small pustules appeared 4 days after this patient began taking a cephalosporin antibiotic for an upper respiratory infection.

- The vast majority of cases of AGEP are thought to be provoked by medications, most often beta-lactam antibiotics (penicillins) and cephalosporins. Other drugs include tetracyclines, calcium channel blockers, oral antifungals, and hydroxychloroquine.
- Viral infections with Epstein–Barr virus and cytomegalovirus have also been implicated in some cases.

HEMORRHAGIC ONYCHOLYSIS DUE TO DOCETAXEL

- Nail changes are a common side effect of docetaxel (**Taxotere**), a semisynthetic taxane, used as a chemotherapeutic agent in the treatment of various cancers including ovarian, breast, and lung cancer. Nail bed purpura, subungual hematomas (Fig. 26.14), and suppuration have been described.

HAND–FOOT SYNDROME (PALMAR–PLANTAR ERYTHRODYSESTHESIA)

- Hand–foot syndrome is a common reaction to chemotherapy drugs that occurs on palms and soles with painful erythema and swelling.
- Various chemotherapy agents such as 5-fluorouracil infusion, its oral prodrug capecitabine, and pegylated liposomal doxorubicin have been reported to cause these symptoms.
- It often begins with tingling of the palms and soles followed by symmetrical, sharply defined erythema, tenderness, a tight feeling due to edema, bullae, severe pain and difficulty walking, or using the hands.

- Initially hand–foot syndrome resolves within 1 to 5 weeks after the drug is ceased, but recurs more severely with each cycle and takes longer to resolve with subsequent chemotherapy cycles.

COCAINE/LEVAMISOLE-INDUCED VASCULITIS

- Levamisole is an adulterant in much of the US cocaine supply. There are numerous reports of patients developing agranulocytosis and a thrombotic vasculopathy from the use of levamisole-tainted cocaine. Levamisole, and not cocaine, is suspected to be the cause.
- Patients present with a retiform purpura that may appear anywhere on the body, but tend to preferentially involve the external ear (Figs. 26.15 and 26.16).
- Some patients also have positive autoantibodies, most commonly p- or c-ANCA and anticardiolipin.
- Lesions resolve spontaneously 2 to 3 weeks after cessation of levamisole.
- A skin biopsy demonstrates leukocytoclastic vasculitis with extensive intravascular fibrin thrombi.

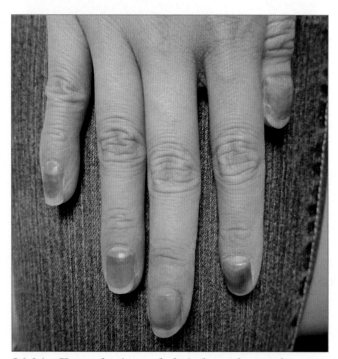

26.14   *Hemorrhagic onycholysis due to docetaxel.* Subungual hematomas, suppuration, and onycholysis are present in this patient who is being treated for breast cancer.

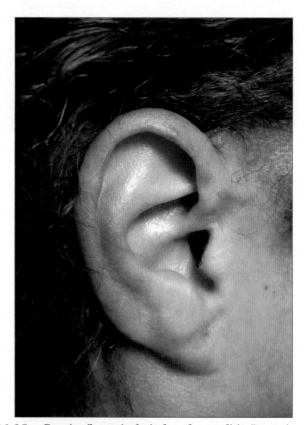

26.15   *Cocaine/levamisole-induced vasculitis.* Purpuric lesions of the earlobe of a 50-year-old cocaine user. (Image courtesy of Lauren Geller, MD.)

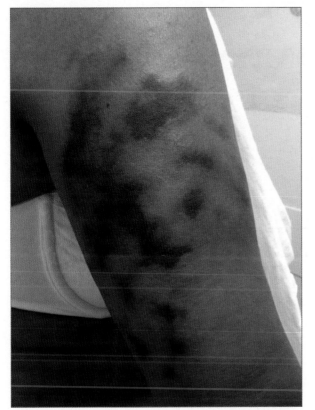

26.16 *Cocaine/levamisole-induced vasculitis.* Retiform purpuric patches on the upper arms of the patient in Figure 26.15. (Image courtesy of Lauren Geller, MD.)

DIAGNOSIS

- Obtaining a detailed, careful history from the patient or family is paramount.
- The morphology of a drug eruption can often provide clues to the most likely responsible agent.
- A handy reference to drug eruptions and interactions should always be available.
- Patients occasionally have eosinophilia.
- Skin biopsy of an exanthem showing perivascular lymphocytes and eosinophils may be helpful, but it is not diagnostic. Characteristic histopathologic changes may occur in some cases, such as leukocytoclastic vasculitis in palpable purpura and panniculitis in erythema nodosum; however, these findings are not necessarily diagnostic of a drug-related origin.

 DIFFERENTIAL DIAGNOSIS

Viral or Bacterial Exanthems
- *Generally occur with fever and other symptoms; however, they are often indistinguishable from a drug eruption.*

Acute and Chronic Urticaria (not drug induced)

- Rechallenging with a suspected drug as a diagnostic tool is generally discouraged, unless the reaction is minor or alternative agents are not available and the drug is indispensable to the patient.

 MANAGEMENT

- The drug should be discontinued, *if feasible.* However, the decision to discontinue a potentially vital drug may present a dilemma.
- If it is necessary to continue the drug (i.e., there is no alternative medication) and the adverse reaction is mild or tolerable, the difficulty may be minimized by decreasing the dosage or treating the adverse reaction.
- Oral antihistamines, such as diphenhydramine (**Benadryl**), hydroxyzine (**Atarax**), or the nonsedating agents cetirizine (**Zyrtec**) and loratadine (**Claritin**), may be helpful.
- Topical steroids are sometimes useful.
- Severe drug reactions such as SJS and TEN often require hospitalization for supportive care.

 POINT TO REMEMBER

- Persons who are immunocompromised have a greater risk of developing a drug eruption than the general population.

 HELPFUL HINTS

- Drug reactions can occur even after years of continuous therapy with the same drug.
- Drug reactions may also occur days after a drug has been discontinued.
- A drug eruption may easily be confused with a feature of the condition that it is intended to treat (e.g., a viral exanthem treated with an antibiotic).
- Patients with infectious mononucleosis are likely to develop a diffuse, nonallergic morbilliform rash, when they are given ampicillin or amoxicillin.
- Exanthematous eruptions in adults are mostly the result of medications; in children, however, they are more likely to be a result of a viral infection.
- If a patient presents with localized purpuric lesions, particularly involving the earlobes, a careful drug history should be taken and toxicology studies should be performed.

Diseases of Cutaneous Vasculature

OVERVIEW

Cutaneous manifestations of vascular disorders can range from a mild rash to urticaria, vasculitis, erythema multiforme major, or to anaphylaxis. Vasculitis includes those disorders that feature inflammation of blood vessel walls and can affect various organ systems. The vast majority of vasculitic dermatologic disorders involve the smaller blood vessels in the skin; less often, large and medium vessels may be involved. In this chapter the discussion will be limited to those vasculitides that involve the smaller blood vessels. The differential diagnosis of vasculitis is broad and includes vasculopathic disorders such as cryoglobulinemia, Waldenstrom macroglobulinemia and Churg–Strauss syndrome.

Purpuric lesions can be a sign or symptom of vascular disorders such as coagulopathies or vasculitis and can also serve as clues to systemic diseases such as systemic lupus erythematosus. Of lesser concern are the so-called "benign" variants—the benign pigmented purpuras (BPPs) that are caused by capillaritis, which allows blood to exit small vessels (extravasation) and create petechiae. As their name implies, BPPs are not associated with any systemic disease.

IN THIS CHAPTER...

> **URICARIA AND ANGIOEDEMA**

- Acute urticaria
- Chronic urticaria
- Dermatographism
- Cold urticaria
- Light-induced (solar) urticaria
- Cholinergic urticaria

> **ERYTHEMA MULTIFORME**

> **PURPURA**

- Nonpalpable purpura and capillaritis
- Palpable purpura

BASICS

- Urticaria, commonly referred to as hives, is a reaction of cutaneous blood vessels that produces a transient dermal edema consisting of papules or plaques in different shapes and sizes.
- *Angioedema* refers to edema that is deeper than urticaria that involves the dermis and subcutaneous tissue.
- A total of 10% to 20% of the population has at least one episode of urticaria or angioedema at some point in his or her lifetime.

PATHOGENESIS

- Mast cell activation causes degranulation of intracellular vesicles that contain histamine, leukotriene C_4, prostaglandin D_2, and other chemotactic mediators that recruit eosinophils and neutrophils into the dermis.
- Histamine and chemokine release lead to extravasation of fluid into the dermis (edema). Histamine effects account for many of the clinical and histologic findings of urticaria.
- As with drug reactions, urticaria may be immune-mediated or nonimmune-mediated (see discussion in Chapter 26).
- Causes of urticaria and angioedema include the following:
  - Immunologic: mediated by immunoglobulin E (IgE) includes food, drugs, and parasites.
  - Complement-mediated: includes serum sickness and whole blood transfusions.
  - Physical stimuli: non–IgE-mediated includes cold, sunlight, and pressure (e.g., dermatographism).
  - Occult infections: sinusitis, dental abscesses, and tinea pedis.

- Urticaria may be classified as acute or chronic urticaria, physical urticaria, urticarial vasculitis, and hereditary angioedema (rare).

ACUTE URTICARIA

- Acute urticaria, by definition, lasts less than 6 weeks.
- Outbreaks are often IgE-mediated.
- There may be an obvious precipitant such as drug ingestion, an acute respiratory illness, a parasitic infection, or a bee sting.
- The most common drugs that may cause acute hives are antibiotics (especially penicillin and sulfonamides). Pain medications such as aspirin, nonsteroidal anti-inflammatory drugs (NSAIDs), narcotics, radiocontrast dyes, diuretics, and opiates such as codeine, are also frequently implicated.
- The most common foods associated with acute urticaria are milk, wheat, eggs, chocolate, shellfish, nuts, fish, and straw-berries. Food additives and preservatives such as salicylates and benzoates may also be responsible.
- Systemic diseases such as lymphomas and collagen vascu-lar diseases may have an associated urticaria.
- Acute urticaria also may be caused by physical stimuli such as pressure, cold, sunlight, or exercise. Such hives are called physical urticaria (see later discussion).
- In children the most common trigger of acute urticarial is a viral illness.
- Anaphylaxis or an anaphylactoid reaction can be associated with acute urticaria.
- Episodes of acute urticaria lasts for hours to days (generally less than 30 days).

CHRONIC URTICARIA

- Chronic urticaria is, by definition, urticaria that lasts longer than 6 weeks, although this cutoff point is an arbitrary one.
- Occurs in a 2:1 female-to-male ratio.
- Seen predominantly in adults.
- Lesions generally itch.
- The cause is usually unknown or undetermined; however, chronic urticaria may, very infrequently, be a sign or symp-tom of one of the following systemic diseases: systemic lupus erythematosus (SLE), serum hepatitis, lymphoma, polycythemia, macroglobulinemia, or thyroid disease.
- Clinically presents with skin-colored or pale red wheals that are sometimes accompanied by a white halo at the periphery (Fig. 27.1).
- Papules and plaques have various shapes: annular, linear, arciform, or polycyclic; frequently they are multiple, with bizarre shapes (Figs. 27.2 and 27.3).
- Individual lesions disappear within 24 hours (evanescent wheals).
- Lesions may be accompanied by a deep swelling (angioedema) around the eyes, lips, and tongue that often looks frightening (Fig. 27.4). Fortunately, angioedema usu-ally lasts less than 24 hours.

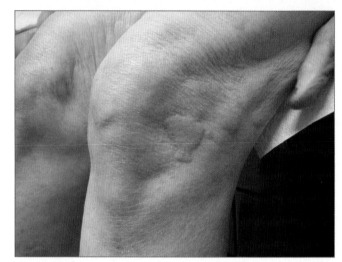

27.1 *Urticaria.* A 57-year-old woman with acute lesions secondary to penicillin.

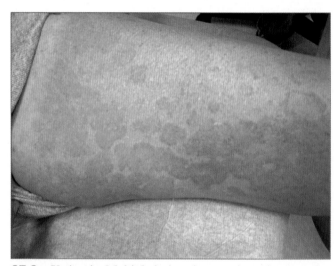

27.2 *Urticaria.* Multiple lesions have various shapes and sizes.

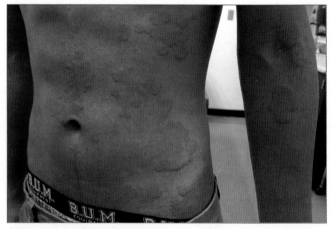

27.3 *Acute urticaria.* Lesions are annular, arciform, and polycyclic, with bizarre shapes.

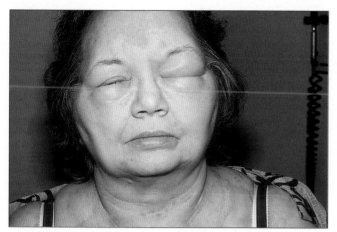

27.4 *Urticaria.* Marked periorbital angioedema.

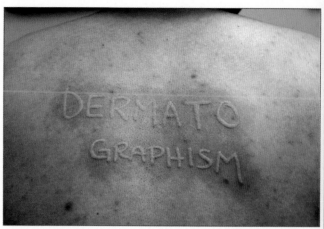

27.5 *Dermatographism ("skin writing").* These lesions occurred 3 minutes after stroking with the wooden tip of a cotton swab.

- Less often, arthralgia, fever, malaise, and other symptoms may accompany urticaria when it is the result of an underlying disorder such as hepatitis, serum sickness, or a collagen vascular disease.
- Emotional stress may trigger recurrences.
- In contrast to atopic dermatitis and many other dermatitides, scratching and rubbing of urticarial lesions generally does not produce scabs or crusts.

DERMATOGRAPHISM ("SKIN WRITING")

- Dermatographism affects more than 4% of the general population, in whom it is physiologic and asymptomatic.
- Linear erythematous wheals occur within 3 to 4 minutes after firmly stroking the skin with the wooden handle of a cotton swab; lesions fade within 30 minutes (Fig. 27.5).
- Lesions may arise under constrictive garments, such as belts and bras, or after a person scratches.
- In some patients, itching is the primary symptom.
- Episodes of dermatographism are generally self-limited but may persist for years.

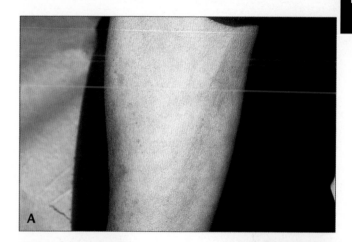

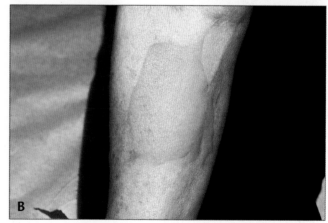

COLD URTICARIA

- Cold urticaria occurs mainly in young adults and children.
- Itchy hives occur at sites of cold exposure, such as areas exposed to cold winds or immersion in cold water.
- In the "ice cube test," a wheal arises on the skin after application of an ice cube (Fig. 27.6A,B).

LIGHT-INDUCED (SOLAR) URTICARIA

- Solar urticaria occurs in sun-exposed areas of the skin and is triggered by various wavelengths of light (Fig. 27.7A,B).

27.6 **A** and **B:** *Cold urticaria.* The "ice cube test." **(A)** Before, and **(B)** 5 minutes after application of an ice cube. A large wheal and surrounding erythema have appeared.

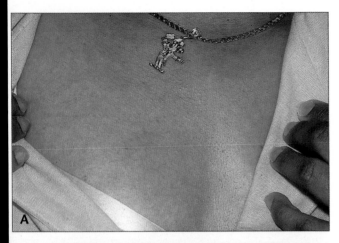

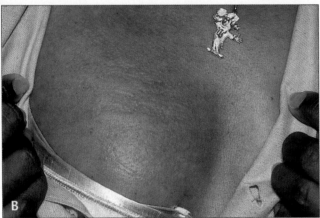

27.7 **A** and **B:** *Solar urticaria induced by ultraviolet A light.* **(A)** Before sun exposure. **(B)** After 15 minutes of sun exposure through a window. The window glass filters out UVB and allows passage of UVA which is responsible for the eruption in this patient.

CHOLINERGIC URTICARIA

- Cholinergic urticaria is induced by exercise or a hot shower.
- The patient exercises to the point of sweating, which provokes lesions and establishes the diagnosis.
- Typical lesions are multiple, small, monomorphic wheals (Fig. 27.8).

DIAGNOSIS

- The diagnosis of acute and chronic urticaria is usually based on clinical observation and history.
- A physical urticaria is diagnosed by careful history taking and challenge testing.

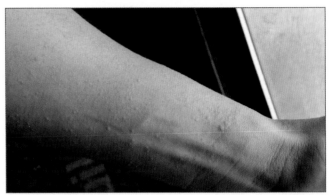

27.8 *Cholinergic urticaria induced by exercise.* After 5 minutes of vigorous exercise, note the small, subtle, itchy flesh-colored papules.

- If a complete review of systems is normal, and a physical urticaria is ruled out, it is often futile to perform multiple laboratory tests to determine a cause for chronic urticaria.
- Nonetheless, a symptom-directed search for underlying illness (e.g., SLE, thyroid disease, lymphoma, and necrotizing vasculitis) may warrant evaluations such as:
  - Complete blood count.
  - Erythrocyte sedimentation rate.
  - Fluorescent antinuclear antibody test.
  - Thyroid function studies.
  - Hepatitis-associated antigen test.
  - Assessment of the complement system.
  - Radioallergosorbent test for IgE antibodies.
  - Stool examination for ova and parasites—in the presence of eosinophilia.
- CD203c assay, an *in vitro* diagnostic test that is used to detect autoimmune urticaria and identifies antibodies that are responsible for many cases of chronic idiopathic urticaria.

DIFFERENTIAL DIAGNOSIS

Insect (Arthropod) Bite Reactions (Sometimes Referred to as *Papular Urticaria* [see Discussion in Chapter 29])

- *Reactions to insect bites may be indistinguishable from ordinary hives.*
- *Bites are generally seen on exposed areas.*
- *They may have a central punctum and crust; they may also blister.*
- *Individual lesions may last more than 24 hours.*

Erythema Multiforme Minor (see Discussion below)

- *Lesions are targetoid.*
- *Last more than 24 hours.*
- *Generally nonpruritic.*

Erythema Migrans (Acute Lyme Disease [see Discussion in Chapter 29])

- *May be indistinguishable from urticaria.*
- *Lesions are usually solitary, annular, and target-like.*

- *Lesions may last more than 24 hours.*
- *Lesions are generally nonpruritic.*

Urticarial Vasculitis

This condition is rare and is probably related to circulating immune complexes.

- *Persistent hive-like lesions last more than 24 hours.*
- *Lesions may be tender rather than itchy.*
- *Residual purpura or hyperpigmentation often ensues on resolution of lesions.*
- *Evidence of vasculitis (e.g., purpura) is occasionally seen in the lesions.*
- *The diagnosis is confirmed by skin biopsy.*
- *Patients may have hypocomplementemia and an elevated erythrocyte sedimentation rate.*
- *Urticarial vasculitis may be associated with collagen vascular diseases.*

MANAGEMENT

- If possible, the cause of the hives should be eliminated, and tight clothing and hot baths and showers should be avoided, particularly in people who have a physical urticaria.
- Salicylates, NSAIDs, and narcotics, which are all histamine-releasing agents, may aggravate both acute and chronic urticaria and should be avoided.
- In 85% to 90% of patients with chronic urticaria, the origin remains unknown.
- Anti-histamines are used to control and/or prevent hives and alleviate symptoms.
- First-generation antihistamines are histamine receptor 1 (H_1) blockers and include hydroxyzine (**Atarax**), diphenhydramine (**Benadryl**), and cyproheptadine (**Periactin**). These are usually sedating.
- H_1 and H_2 blockers may be used in combination, such as cimetidine (**Tagamet**) plus hydroxyzine.
- Nonsedating antihistamines, such as loratadine (**Claritin**) 10 mg, desloratadine (**Clarinex**) 5 mg, fexofenadine (**Allegra**) 60/180 mg, and cetirizine (**Zyrtec**) 10 mg, may be used during the day, and a more sedating H_1 blocker or a tricyclic antidepressant drug, such as doxepin (**Sinequan**), may be tried at bedtime. Doxepin can be given at much lower doses than when it is used

as an antidepressant (e.g., from 5 mg two times daily to 50 mg three times daily).
- For problems at bedtime, a sedating antihistamine such as diphenhydramine or hydroxyzine may be added.
- Patients with chronic urticaria often require much higher than the usual doses of antihistamines.
- **Systemic steroids** are sometimes used for short periods to break the cycle of chronic urticaria; however, they are not indicated for long-term use in the treatment of chronic idiopathic urticaria.
- Montelukast (**Singulair**), a leukotriene receptor antagonist used to treat asthma, has been found to be effective in some cases of CIU that are refractory to antihistamines.
- Immunotherapies using prednisone, plasmapheresis, intravenous immunoglobulin, low-dose methotrexate, oral psoralens plus ultraviolet A treatment, oral tacrolimus, azathioprine, and cyclosporine have been used in severe, recalcitrant cases.
- There have been some encouraging outcomes with the administration of the monoclonal antibody omalizumab (**Xolair**), a drug used for asthma, in the treatment of CIU.
- If all else fails, a diary of daily foods eaten may be kept, with subsequent food elimination; however, this approach is rarely successful.

HELPFUL HINTS

- **Epinephrine**, which is often administered by intramuscular or subcutaneous injection for acute urticaria, **should not** be used for routine cases of hives. It should be reserved for cases of acute anaphylaxis.
- For the treatment of anaphylaxis, an **EpiPen** is a device that contains a spring-loaded needle that penetrates the recipient's skin, to deliver a predetermined dose of epinephrine via subcutaneous or intramuscular injection.
- Patients with documented cold urticaria should be advised not to immerse themselves abruptly in cold water.
- Children with chronic urticaria occasionally have an underlying autoimmune disease; thyroid antibodies are the most common positive finding.
- Most cases of CIU resolve with or without treatment; on average: 50% are free of hives after 3 to 12 months; 20% are free of hives after 12 to 36 months, and 20% are free of hives after 36 to 60 months.
- In some patients, hives may recur for many years.

POINTS TO REMEMBER

- Except for a physical urticaria and urticaria that is obviously associated with drugs and systemic disease, determining the cause of chronic urticaria is generally a fruitless task.
- Most often, routine blood tests are of little or no value in determining the cause of acute or chronic urticaria.
- Antihistamines remain the mainstay for treating chronic urticaria; a combination of these agents may be necessary for control.
- Allergies are almost never the cause of chronic urticaria. Allergy testing is expensive and often tests that are positive for allergies have no relation to the patient's urticaria.
- When individual wheals persist for more than 24 to 36 hours, the process is unlikely to be urticaria.

 SEE PATIENT HANDOUT "Hives (Urticaria)" IN THE COMPANION eBOOK EDITION.

BASICS

- Erythema multiforme (EM) was initially described by Ferdinand von Hebra in the late 19th century as a "a self-limited eruption characterized by symmetrically distributed erythematous papules, which develop into characteristic target-like lesions consisting of concentric color changes with a dusky central zone that may become bullous" (Fig. 27.9).
- This classic description still holds true for the typical lesions of EM.
- EM minor, by definition, occurs when only typical skin lesions are present.
- EM major, traditionally referred to as Stevens–Johnson syndrome (SJS), occurs when the target lesions are accompanied by extensive mucosal involvement and systemic symptoms. SJS is currently considered to be part of the spectrum of toxic epidermal necrolysis (TEN) and distinct from EM major (see Chapters 26 and 33). Sometimes clinical distinction between the two is difficult to make.
- Both types of EM are most often seen in young adults.
- EM is most often triggered by an infection (most often HSV).
- Affected people are generally in good health.

PATHOGENESIS

- It is currently thought that EM represents a mucocutaneous immune reaction pattern in response to an infection.
- About 90% of cases are triggered by a preceding infection.
- HSV1, and less often HSV2, are the most commonly associated infectious agents.
- The most common precipitating cause of recurrent EM is recurrent herpes labialis (Fig. 27.10) and usually the herpes outbreak precedes the skin eruption by 3 to 14 days.
- Other infectious triggers include Epstein–Barr virus (EBV), *Mycoplasma pneumonia,* histoplasmosis, *Streptococcus* infection, hepatitis A and B, and coccidioidomycosis.
- Rarely, EM is precipitated by a drug or a systemic disease. Reported associated drugs include sulfonamides, penicillin, hydantoins, barbiturates, allopurinol, and NSAIDs.

CLINICAL MANIFESTATIONS

- EM presents with the acute onset of characteristic erythematous lesions with dusky centers in a symmetric distribution, with most lesions appearing within 24 hours.
- The skin lesions seen in EM can vary from erythematous patches with slightly dusky centers to the typical target, "bull's eye" lesions.

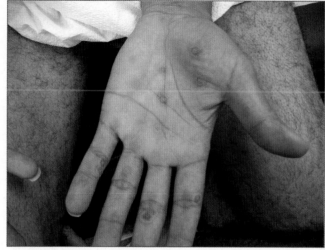

27.9 *Erythema multiforme.* Characteristic target-like lesions are noted on the palm.

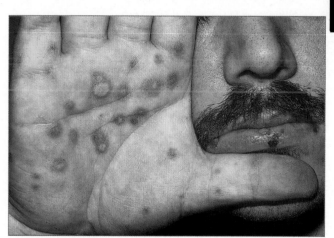

27.10 *Erythema multiforme minor.* This patient has a recurrent herpes simplex virus infection. Note the drying crust of the herpetic "cold sore" on his lower lip and the target-like lesions on his palm (see also Fig. 12.4).

- Lesions begin as round, well-demarcated, erythematous macules or patches (<3 cm).
- Some lesions evolve to form typical target lesions consisting of three distinct zones, a central dusky zone, a surrounding pale zone, and a peripheral red zone.
- Some lesions are atypical targets with dusky centers and a surrounding zone of erythema.
- The dusky center may become vesicobullous or crusted.

- Lesions persist (are "fixed") for at least 1 week.
- The eruption is bilateral and symmetric and typically occur on the palms and soles, dorsa of hands and feet, extensor forearms and legs, face, and genitalia.
- **Erythema multiforme minor** presents with the skin lesions with little to no mucosal involvement and no systemic symptoms.
- **Erythema multiforme major** presents with the typical skin lesions plus severe mucosal involvement and systemic features.
- Extensive, severe, mucous membrane lesions in EM major may be located in multiple sites, including the mouth, pharynx, eyes, and genitalia (see Fig. 26.6).
- Possible complications include keratitis, corneal ulcers, upper airway damage, and pneumonia.

DIAGNOSIS

- Typical target lesions may be present.
- Skin biopsy is performed, if necessary.

DIFFERENTIAL DIAGNOSIS

Urticaria
- *Lesions are transient, not "fixed."*
- *Lesions are pruritic.*
- *The center of annular lesions is not dusky in color.*

Primary Herpes Gingivostomatitis and Primary Bullous Diseases of the Oral Cavity
- *Clinically lesions may be indistinguishable from those of mucous membrane EM.*
- *Mucous membrane biopsy may be necessary to distinguish oral bullous EM from primary bullous diseases such as pemphigus vulgaris or bullous pemphigoid.*

MANAGEMENT

- EM is generally an acute self-limited disorder but may be recurrent in some cases.
- If known, the precipitating infectious cause should be treated.
- Suspected etiologic drugs should be discontinued.
- Wet dressings (e.g., **Burow solution**) and topical steroids may be applied to oozing lesions.
- Oral antihistamines may help alleviate associated skin symptoms.
- For recurrent EM minor due to HSV, prophylactic daily treatment with oral acyclovir, famciclovir (**Famvir**), or valacyclovir (**Valtrex**) may prevent or mitigate recurrences (see Chapter 17 for dosages).
- In cases of severe mucosal involvement, as may occur in EM major, hospitalization may be required.
- The use of systemic steroids in such severe cases is controversial, and their effectiveness has not been established.
- For severe recurrent EM azathioprine, cyclosporine and prednisone have all been used.

HELPFUL HINT

- EM will not progress to toxic epidermal necrolysis (TEN).

POINTS TO REMEMBER

- Solid evidence supports the current concept that EM is a condition distinct from SJS and TEN.
- Both EM minor and major are a reaction pattern to underlying stimuli and can present with varying degrees of severity.
- Even in the clinical absence of herpes simplex virus infection, recurrent EM minor may be suppressed with oral acyclovir, famciclovir, or valacyclovir.

BASICS

- Purpura is defined as a hemorrhage of blood into the skin or mucous membranes and is most commonly seen on dependent areas (i.e., the lower legs and ankles) (Fig. 27.11).
- Purpuric skin is purple, violaceous, or dark red in color and is nonblanchable because blood is present *outside* of vessel walls.
- In contrast, erythema is red in color and blanches on compression because blood remains *within* the vessels.
- Purpuric lesions can be a sign or symptom of an underlying vascular disorder or systemic disease or can represent a "benign" variant.
- Purpura is divided into **nonpalpable** (macular) and **palpable** (papular) categories. Nonpalpable purpuric lesions that are smaller than 3 mm in size are referred to as *petechiae;* those larger than 3 mm are called *ecchymoses.*

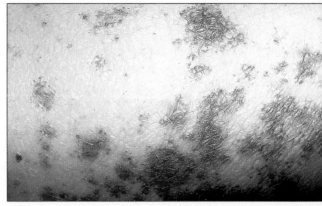

27.11 *Purpura.* Petechiae and ecchymoses combine and form areas of nonblanching purpura.

Purpura—Clinical Variants

NONPALPABLE PURPURA

- Minor trauma to the skin may precipitate purpura, particularly when a patient is taking drugs such as aspirin, clopidogrel (**Plavix**), NSAIDs, and warfarin (**Coumadin**), all of which increase clotting time.
- Long-term application of potent topical steroids on the skin of elderly patients may lead to ecchymoses.
- Blood dyscrasias and coagulopathies, such as thrombocytopenia, leukemia, and disseminated intravascular coagulopathy can also result in petechiae and purpura.
- **Actinic purpura** (formerly known as *senile purpura*) is a prevalent finding on the dorsal forearms in elderly people that are believed to result from minor trauma to an area of chronic sun exposure. Age-related thinning of skin and "fragile capillaries" are considered the cause (Fig. 27.12).
- Chronic venous insufficiency of the lower extremities can result in purpura.

BENIGN PIGMENTED PURPURAS

- The benign pigmented purpuras (BPPs) are nonpalpable purpuras that result from capillaritis, an inflammation of the superficial dermal capillaries that leads to leakage of blood (extravasation) creating petechiae.
- As their name implies, BPPs are not associated with any systemic disease.
- Patients with BPP often present to medical attention for cosmetic concerns or to be reassured that the purpura is not a sign of a serious disease.
- Lesions begin as nonblanching, red, pinpoint-sized macules (petechiae) or bruises (ecchymoses) that may coalesce.
- Lesions are generally asymptomatic, but they may be mildly pruritic.
- Lesions may persist for months to years or indefinitely.
- Older lesions become purple, then brown as hemosiderin forms.

SCHAMBERG PURPURA

- It is the most common of the BPPs and occurs primarily in adults, especially in the elderly.
- Characterized by the so-called "cayenne pepper" purpura (Figs. 27.13 and 27.14).
- Most commonly seen on the lower extremities.

MAJOCCHI PURPURA (PURPURA ANNULARIS TELANGIECTODES OF MAJOCCHI)

- Majocchi purpura is typically seen in adolescents and young adults on the trunk and proximal lower extremities but it may appear at any site.
- Lesions consist of 1 to 3 cm annular purpura and pigmentation, often with a central clearing. The purple, yellow, or

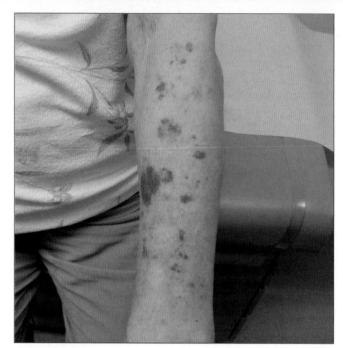

27.12 *Senile, or actinic, purpura.* Ecchymoses are present on the dorsal forearms in an elderly person.

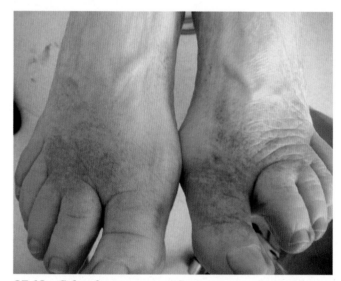

27.13 *Schamberg purpura.* "Cayenne pepper" petechiae are seen on the distal feet.

brown areas consist of telangiectasias and hemosiderin deposition (Fig. 27.15). Punctate petechiae may be seen in the borders.

DIAGNOSIS

- The diagnosis is made on clinical presentation.
- Lesions are not palpable and are nonblanching on diascopy (direct pressure).

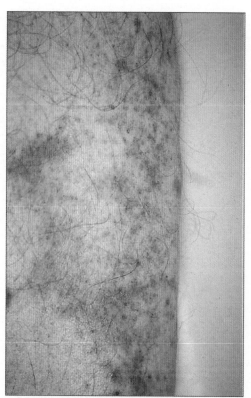

27.14 *Schamberg purpura.* In this patient, the lesions are more extensive than in Figure 27.13. Coalescence of petechiae has created large areas of nonpalpable purpura. Note the hyperpigmented macules indicating the presence of hemosiderin in the skin. (Image courtesy of Art Huntley, MD.)

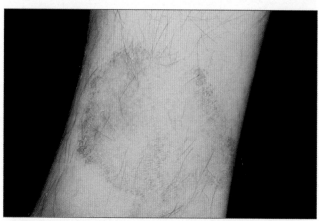

27.15 *Majocchi purpura (purpura annularis telangiectodes).* This subtle ring-shaped nonblanching purpuric lesion resembles tinea corporis and is often treated with topical antifungals. (Image courtesy of Art Huntley, MD.)

 DIFFERENTIAL DIAGNOSIS

Leukocytoclastic Vasculitis
- *Biopsy may be necessary at times to distinguish benign purpura from leukocytoclastic vasculitis, the histopathologic finding in palpable purpura (see the next section).*

 MANAGEMENT

- BPP generally requires no workup; however, if a blood dyscrasia or coagulopathy is suspected, appropriate laboratory tests should be ordered.
- Possible offending drugs should be evaluated regarding their risk-to-benefit ratio.

HELPFUL HINT

- The annular lesions of Majocchi Purpura (Purpura Annularis Telangiectodes) are often confused with those of tinea corporis.

PALPABLE PURPURA

BASICS

- The presence of palpable purpura (PP) represents a small vessel vasculitis of the skin. Cutaneous small vessel vasculitis is the result of inflammation of the blood vessels in the middle or upper dermis.
- Vasculitis can be limited to the skin or involve the skin plus other organs. The most common extracutaneous sites of involvement are the gastrointestinal tract, kidneys, central nervous system, and joints.
- Cutaneous vasculitis may be acute or chronic and the prognosis is good when no internal involvement is present.

PATHOGENESIS

- Vasculitis results from the deposition of circulating immune complexes in the postcapillary venules which leads to inflammation and destruction of the blood vessel wall, a feature that is common to all forms of vasculitis.
- In the skin, blood vessel destruction, accumulation of inflammatory cells, and the leakage of blood from the vessels result in the palpability of lesions. In other organ systems, similar damage to blood vessels can present with gastrointestinal bleeding, hematuria, or arthralgias.

- **Leukocytoclastic vasculitis** is the characteristic histopathologic finding of palpable purpura and cutaneous vasculitis. Biopsy of lesions shows characteristic neutrophilic "nuclear dust."
- In the majority of cases, the cause of the cutaneous vasculitis is unknown, or idiopathic; and it may occur in the absence of any underlying systemic disease.
- Less often it may be associated with a hypersensitivity to antigens from drugs (most often antibiotics, NSAIDs, allopurinol, thiazide diuretics, or hydantoins), malignancies, infectious diseases (such as beta-hemolytic streptococcal infection, viral hepatitis, particularly hepatitis C, and human immunodeficiency virus infection), cryoglobulinemias, and other underlying diseases such as systemic lupus erythematosus, Sjögren syndrome, rheumatoid arthritis, and inflammatory bowel diseases.

CLINICAL MANIFESTATIONS

- Lesions present as variably sized (1 mm to 3 cm) palpable purpuric or erythematous papules, urticarial lesions or vesicles.
- Lesions tend to appear in crops; are red to violaceous to purple in color and do not blanch (Fig. 27.16).
- The lesions are characteristically symmetric in distribution mostly noted in dependent areas such as the lower legs and ankles and on the buttocks in bedridden patients, but any area of the skin can be involved.
- Lesions may be asymptomatic, mildly pruritic, slightly painful, or very painful when ulcerated.
- There may be associated malaise and possible fever.
- In severe forms, lesions may become generalized.
- Infrequently, hemorrhagic vesicles or bullae may occur and develop into painful ulcerations (Fig. 27.17).
- Healing takes place within 1 to 2 weeks and may result in postinflammatory hyperpigmentation and/or scarring.
- Systemic symptoms occur in 5 to 20% of cases. In systemic vasculitis, symptoms are referable to the organ involved.
- PP may recur; however, the majority of patients have only a single episode.

DIAGNOSIS

- Laboratory investigations that are useful for identifying any underlying disease include complete blood count, a blood chemistry panel, erythrocyte sedimentation rate, urinalysis, and stool examination for occult blood. Further studies (e.g., serum complement, antinuclear antibodies) should be directed by the patient's symptoms.
- Other testing may include serum protein electrophoresis, cryoglobulins, and hepatitis C antibody for patients who have no identifiable disease.
- Biopsy of fresh lesions shows characteristic leukocytoclastic vasculitis ("nuclear dust"). A biopsy performed too early or too late in its evolution may not reveal these findings.

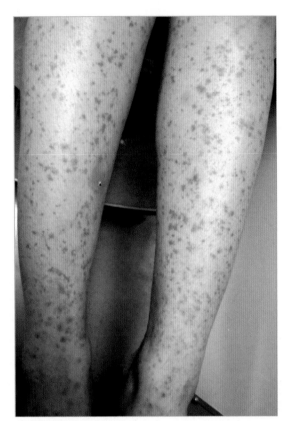

27.16 *Palpable purpura.* Nonblanching violaceous papules suggest vasculitis.

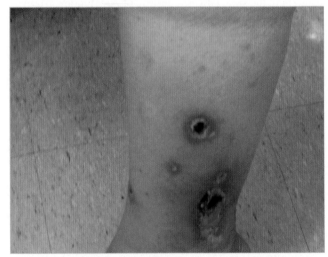

27.17 *Vasculitis.* This patient has cryoglobulinemic vasculitis. Hemorrhagic blisters have evolved into multiple ulcerations on her lower leg.

DIFFERENTIAL DIAGNOSIS

Henoch–Schönlein Purpura (see Chapter 10)
- *Henoch–Schönlein purpura (HSP) is a type of small vessel vasculitis that usually follows an upper respiratory infection, generally seen in children.*
- *Clinical and histopathologic findings are similar to those of cutaneous small vessel vasculitis in addition to perivascular IgA immunofluorescent deposition.*
- *Abdominal pain, arthralgia, hematuria, and proteinuria may also be present.*

Arthropod Bite Reactions
- *When these appear on the lower extremities, they can mimic PP.*
- *The history of exposure to bites is often obtainable.*

Septic Vasculitis
- *Palpable and nonpalpable purpura may also be seen in septic vasculitis, in which lesions are more often acral (i.e., distal on toes or fingertips) and tend to be few in number (e.g., gonococcemia).*
- *Lesions also tend to lack the characteristic symmetry of small vessel cutaneous vasculitis.*
- *Patients may also be febrile and show other signs and symptoms of their underlying infection.*

Other Vasculitides
- *It should be kept in mind that cutaneous vasculitis, and thus PP, may be seen in patients with rare diseases such as Wegener granulomatosis, polyarteritis nodosa, cryoglobulinemic vasculitis, antiphospholipid syndrome, microscopic polyangiitis, and Churg–Strauss syndrome (allergic granulomatosis).*
- *Many of these conditions involve larger vessels than are typically involved in PP.*

Atrophie Blanche (Livedoid Vasculopathy)
- *Results from vascular occlusion (vasculopathy) of the dermal blood vessels, which may be idiopathic or secondary to coagulopathies, abnormalities in fibrinolysis and platelet function, or chronic venous hypertension.*
- *Patients present with small, porcelain-white, stellate (star-shaped) scars with surrounding telangiectasias (Fig. 27.18).*
- *Initial lesions are typically painful, purpuric macules, or papules, on the malleoli and the adjacent dorsa of the feet that appear in clusters and form irregular patterns of superficial punched-out ulcers.*

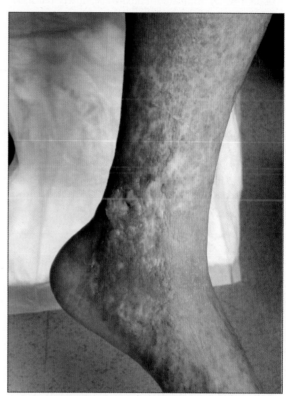

27.18 *Atrophie blanche (livedoid vasculopathy).* White-colored stellate scars as well as active ulcerations are present. Coalescence of purpuric lesions and ulceration seen here are indicative of more severe vessel involvement.

MANAGEMENT

- If known, the precipitating cause (e.g., drug) should be eliminated or the responsible underlying disease (e.g., SLE) should be treated.
- Elevation of the legs (above the level of the heart) and/or compression stockings may be useful because the disease often affects dependent areas.
- In general, no treatment is necessary for mild, self-limited episodes.
- For severe, extensive, or recalcitrant cases, **oral corticosteroids** are indicated. The dose is slowly reduced over the course of several weeks.

HELPFUL HINTS

- Vasculitis in patients with Wegener granulomatosis, polyarteritis nodosa, or Churg–Strauss syndrome can be considered a potentially fatal disease. Treatment with systemic corticosteroids and/or immunosuppressive/cytotoxic agents is generally necessary.
- Rituximab (**Rituxan**) has been reported to be helpful in some cases of vasculitis.

POINTS TO REMEMBER

- PP may be a sign of systemic vasculitis, sepsis, drug allergy, underlying disease, or an idiopathic benign reaction pattern.
- Patients with PP that primarily affects the skin, and not the internal organs, have a favorable prognosis.
- When evaluating purpura (both palpable and nonpalpable, septic and nonseptic) of the lower extremities, other, often rare, entities must also be considered as diagnostic possibilities in the proper clinical context.
- The diagnosis of BPP is generally made on clinical grounds, and the patient should be reassured about the benign nature of these lesions.

28 Sexually Transmitted Diseases

OVERVIEW

Until the 1990s, sexually transmitted diseases (STDs) were commonly known as venereal diseases. *Veneris* is the Latin form of the name Venus, the Roman goddess of love. STDs are illnesses that have a significant probability of transmission between humans by means of sexual behavior, including vaginal intercourse, anal sex, and oral sex.

Anogenital warts, the most common STD in the United States, is caused by the human papilloma virus (HPV). It is estimated that 1% of the population of the United States has clinically evident lesions of anogenital warts with possibly 15% having subclinical infection by HPV. Certain subtypes of HPV are thought to be one of the main underlying causes of cervical cancer as well as other types of cancers of the female and male reproductive systems.

Syphilis is common worldwide, and since the late 1990s, infectious early syphilis has reemerged as an important disease in Western Europe and the United States and is an important facilitator of human immunodeficiency virus (HIV) transmission.

Sexually transmitted herpes simplex virus (HSV) is an STD that presently has no cure. The incidence of HSV-2 infection is also one of the most rapidly increasing among STDs in the United States.

Chancroid is rare in the United States and Western Europe. In the United States, it is associated with the use of crack cocaine.

Lymphogranuloma venereum and granuloma inguinale are also reported rarely in the United States and Western Europe and are more frequently seen in tropical and subtropical regions.

Anogenital Warts

BASICS

- Anogenital warts, for the most part, are sexually transmitted viral warts caused by infection with specific types of HPV. Despite the generally benign nature of the proliferations, certain types of HPV can place patients at a high risk for anogenital cancers.
- Transmission of HPV is by sexual contact, oral sex, and by vertical infection (mother to baby by passing through an infected birth canal).
- In infants and small children, genital warts raise the possibility of sexual abuse, but in many cases it is due to vertical transmission or by incidental spread caused by nongenital HPV infections.
- The incubation period is variable, ranging from 3 weeks to 8 months, with a reported average, in one study, of 2.8 months.
- HPV has been identified in the skin of infected persons at a distance of up to 1 cm from the actual lesion; this feature may explain the high recurrence rate.
- HPV types 16, 18, 31 to 35, 39, 42, 48, and 51 to 54 have been identified in cervical and anogenital cancers.
- Lesions tend to be more extensive and recalcitrant to treatment in immunocompromised persons; they also tend to grow larger and more numerous during pregnancy.
- Women with HPV infection who are pregnant or who are considering pregnancy pose specific challenges. In addition to the potential for rapid proliferation, the presence of HPV infection raises concerns regarding the risk of laryngeal papillomatosis or genital HPV infections in the newborn. A cesarean section does not eliminate the risk of transmission.

RISK FACTORS

- Transmission of anogenital HPV infection occurs largely by sexual intercourse.
- Other risk factors for infection include cigarette smoking, participating in sexual activity at an early age, having a high number of sexual partners, having another STD, immunosuppression, and having an abnormal Pap smear result.

CLINICAL MANIFESTATIONS

- There are various morphologic types of anogenital warts. The appearance of warts depends on its location; for example, the condyloma acuminatum type tends to occur on moist surfaces.
- Condyloma acuminatum may resemble small cauliflowers (Fig. 28.1).
- Warts may appear as smooth, dome-shaped, papular lesions (Fig. 28.2).
- They can appear as typical lobulated verrucous papules or plaques that resemble common warts (Fig. 28.3).
- Usually asymptomatic; however, they may become pruritic, particularly the perianal and inguinal lesions. Pain and bleeding may occur if lesions are traumatized.
- They may resolve spontaneously or, rarely, progress to invasive squamous cell carcinoma.

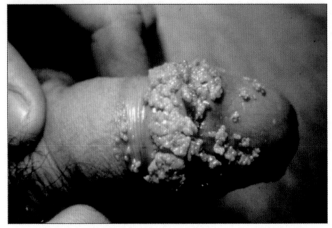

28.1 *Condyloma acuminatum.* Lesions resemble small cauliflowers.

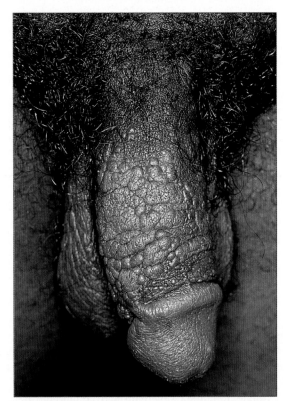

28.2 *Condyloma acuminatum.* Smooth, dome-shaped papular lesions are present. (From Edwards L, Lynch PJ. *Genital Dermatology Atlas*, 2nd ed. Philadelphia, PA: Lippincott Williams & Wilkins, 2011.)

ANOGENITAL WARTS AND CANCER

- The HPV types that cause external visible warts (HPV types 6 and 11) rarely cause cancer.
- Other HPV types (most often types 16, 18, 31, 33 and 35) are less common in visible warts but are associated with penile and vulvar intraepithelial neoplasia and squamous cell carcinoma of the genital area especially cervical

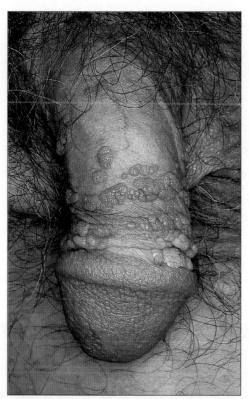

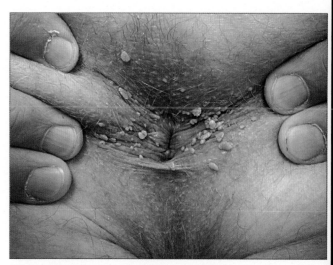

28.4 *Condyloma acuminatum.* Perianal warts are seen in this patient.

28.3 *Condyloma acuminatum.* These papules have the appearance of common warts. (From Edwards L, Lynch PJ. *Genital Dermatology Atlas.* 2nd ed. Philadelphia, PA: Lippincott Williams & Wilkins; 2011.)

cancer, and less frequently, invasive vulvar cancer and anal cancer.

DISTRIBUTION OF LESIONS

- In men, lesions occur on the penis, scrotum, mons pubis, inguinal crease, and perianal area (Fig. 28.4).
- In women, the vagina, labia (Fig. 28.5), mons pubis, perianal area, and uterine cervix.
- Intra-anal warts are seen predominantly in patients who have engaged in receptive anal intercourse.
- Warts may also be found in the peri- and intraurethral areas in men.

DIAGNOSIS

- The diagnosis of anogenital warts is generally straightforward when the patient presents with the typical cauliflower-like lesions of condyloma acuminatum or with characteristic verrucous or filiform lesions.
- However, when lesions are papular (flat-topped), pigmented, moist, or erosive, the diagnosis may not be as clinically obvious.
- Normal anatomical structures may easily be confused with AGA.

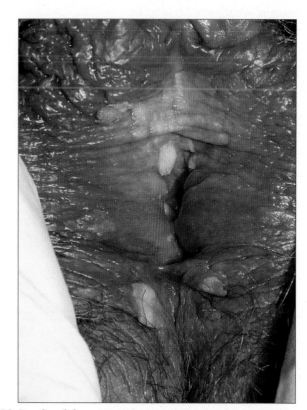

28.5 *Condyloma acuminatum.* Labial and inrtralabial lesions are seen here.

ACETOWHITE TEST ON MUCOUS MEMBRANES

- In women, colposcopy is performed using 35% acetic acid, which produces an acetowhitening of subclinical lesions on the vaginal and cervical mucosa (Fig. 28.6).
- Atypia or koilocytosis found on PAP smears represents early changes resulting from HPV infection.

BIOPSY

- A biopsy may be needed to identify confusing anogenital lesions.
- After local anesthesia with lidocaine, a curved iris scissors may be used to obtain a small specimen (snip biopsy) from the labia minora, or perianal area. A punch biopsy or a shave biopsy may be obtained from nonmucous membrane skin (see Chapter 35). If an ulcer or an indurated nodule is present—particularly if carcinoma or bowenoid papulosis is suspected—a punch or excisional biopsy should be performed.

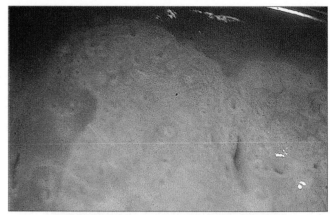

28.6 *Cervical warts.* Acetowhitening of subclinical lesions on the cervical mucosa.

DIFFERENTIAL DIAGNOSIS

Normal Anatomic Structures

- *In women, **vestibular papillae** are normal anatomic structures. Unlike warts, vestibular papillae (vulvar papillomatosis) occur near the vaginal vestibule in symmetric clusters or in a linear pattern. They often appear as monotonous, small, smooth projections that resemble cobblestones (Fig. 28.7).*
- *In men, **pearly penile papules** are frequently mistaken for warts. They are small, skin-colored to shiny, pearly papules that are located around the rim of the corona of the glans penis (Figs. 28.8 and 28.9).*

Benign Lesions

- *Common benign skin lesions, such as **skin tags, seborrheic keratoses**, and **melanocytic nevi**, may also be easily mistaken for warts.*
- ***Fordyce spots** are angiokeratomas. They occur on the medial labia minora in women and on the scrotum in men (see Figs. 30.44 and 30.45).*
- *Skin tags are smooth and may be pigmented or skin-colored. Seborrheic keratoses and melanocytic nevi often have a verrucous (keratotic) appearance and may be pigmented.*

Other Conditions
Hemorrhoids

- *Not infrequently, anal hemorrhoids are mistaken for warts. Hemorrhoids are smooth and compressible.*

Molluscum Contagiosum

- *This pox virus infection can easily be confused with, and may coexist with, genital warts. Seen most often in young children and in patients with HIV infection and in sexually active young adults (see Chapters 17 and 33).*
- *The lesions are dome-shaped, waxy or pearly white papules with a central white core, which is often revealed by inspection with a handheld magnifier.*

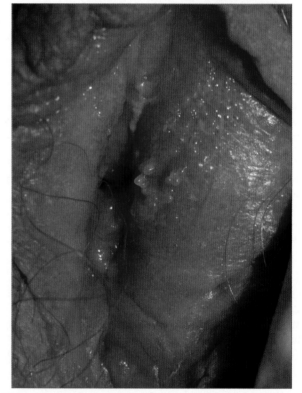

28.7 *Vestibular papillae (vulvar papillomatosis).* These normal anatomic structures occur near vaginal vestibule in symmetric clusters or in a linear pattern. They are frequently mistaken for warts. (From Edwards L, Lynch PJ. *Genital Dermatology Atlas.* 2nd ed. Philadelphia, PA: Lippincott Williams & Wilkins; 2011.)

continued on page 419

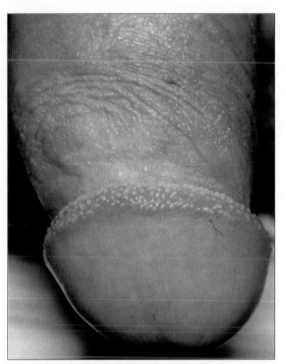

28.8 *Pearly penile papules.* These normal anatomic structures occur as shiny papules that are present around the corona of the glans penis and the frenum of the penis. They can be differentiated from warts by their location and uniform size.

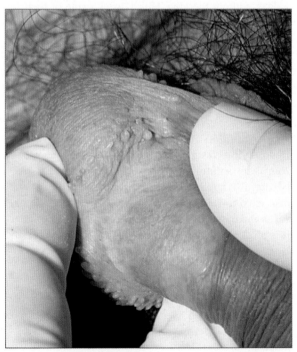

28.9 *Pearly penile papules.* These hairlike papules are sometimes referred to as "hirsutoid papules." They are also frequently misdiagnosed and treated as warts.

Condyloma Latum of Secondary Syphilis
- *Lesions are "moist," smooth-surfaced, and, usually, whitish and flat-topped. Serologic tests for syphilis are positive (see Fig. 28.20).*

Malignant Neoplasms
- *When any of the following conditions are suspected, a biopsy should be performed:*

Bowenoid Papulosis
- *These lesions are clinically similar to, and often indistinguishable from, flat or dome-shaped genital warts. They are associated with HPV type 16 or 18. Histologically, bowenoid papulosis demonstrates squamous cell carcinoma in situ; however, it follows a largely benign clinical course.*

Giant Condyloma Acuminatum
- *Also known as the Buschke–Löwenstein tumor, this lesion is a low-grade, locally invasive squamous cell carcinoma that can arise from and appear as a fungating condyloma (Fig. 28.10). It is associated with HPV types 6 and 11 and should be considered in the differential of lesions measuring greater than 1 cm in diameter. Radical surgical extirpation is considered appropriate treatment.*

Squamous Cell Carcinoma
- *These lesions are rapidly growing nodules or tumors, and they may be erosive or ulcerative.*

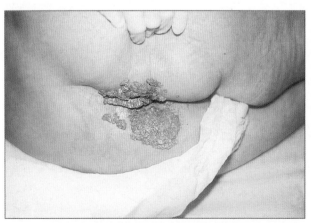

28.10 *Giant condyloma acuminatum.* This low-grade, locally invasive malignant tumor can arise from and appear as a fungating condyloma.

MANAGEMENT

Counseling

- Treatment of genital warts can be difficult and lengthy and patients should be so advised.
- Patients should also be counseled about their risk of infectivity to others, as well as their increased risk of having other STDs.
- They should also be informed about the long latency period of HPV; thus, a patient may not have contracted condyloma from his or her current partner.
- Male patients should use condoms at least 1 year after clinical infection is treated; however, condoms are not perfect protection because warts can occur on genital areas other than the penis or vagina.
- In affected women, there is a risk of malignant degeneration (cervical intraepithelial neoplasia or squamous cell carcinoma). If cervical warts are found during examination or if vulvar neoplasia is confirmed by biopsy, referral for colposcopic evaluation is indicated.
- It is recommended that anogenital warts be treated in pregnant women during the second and third trimesters and that vaginal delivery be performed if possible.
- In affected men with perianal warts, there is a risk of malignant degeneration to anal intraepithelial neoplasia or anal carcinoma.
- The U.S. Centers for Disease Control and Prevention (CDC) recommends cesarean section only when the vaginal outlet is obstructed by extensive condylomata or if vaginal delivery would cause excessive bleeding.
- Patients who have internal anal or rectal warts tend to have continual recurrences of external warts and should be referred to a rectal surgeon.
- Diagnosis of genital warts in a child requires that the clinician report suspected sexual abuse to begin an evaluation process that may or may not confirm abuse (Fig. 28.11).

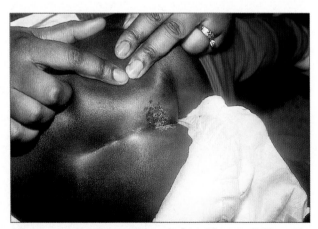

28.11 *Perianal warts in an infant.* The possibility of child abuse should always be considered in these cases.

Surgical Therapy

- **Cryosurgery with liquid nitrogen (LN2).** Cryosurgery is very effective for treating multiple, small warts (e.g., lesions on the shaft of the penis, vulva, and perianal area). LN2 is also safe for the mother and fetus when used during the second and third trimesters of pregnancy.
- **Electrodesiccation and curettage.** This is quite effective for a limited number of lesions on the shaft of the penis or vulvae.
- **Surgical excision** is useful for debulking large "cauliflower" lesions. Large, unresponsive lesions around the rectum or vulva can be treated with scissor excision of the bulk of the mass followed by electrocautery of the remaining tissue down to the skin surface.

Topical Therapy

Patient-applied Therapy

- **Imiquimod** 5% (**Aldara**) or 3.75% (**Zyclara**) cream enhances the body's immune response to the infection by increasing local interferon. **Aldara** is applied three times weekly at bedtime for up to 16 weeks; and **Zyclara** should be applied daily for 8 weeks.
- Warts seem less likely to recur compared to other treatments. It is not currently recommended during pregnancy.
- Podofilox (**Condylox**) 0.5% solution or gel is used twice daily (morning and evening) for 3 days, then followed by 4 days without therapy. This 1-week cycle of treatment may be repeated up to four times until no wart remains. Safety for use in pregnancy is not known.
- **Sinecatechins ointment (Veregen)** is an extract obtained from green tea leaves. It is applied three times daily for up to 16 weeks. It has antiviral and immune-stimulating properties.

Provider-applied Therapies

- **Podophyllin** resin 10% to 25% in tincture of benzoin is an antimitotic agent that causes local tissue. It is carefully applied to the wart surface. The patient is instructed to wash the area in 4 to 6 hours and the interval is increased for subsequent treatments, as tolerated. It is most effective on warts on moist surfaces (perianal, labial, and under the prepuce). It should not be used in pregnant women or on extensive mucosal surfaces.
- **Trichloroacetic** or **bichloracetic acid 80%** to 90% are applied after normal epithelium is coated with a protective substance such as 2% lidocaine or Vaseline petroleum jelly. These agents can cause intense burning of mucosal surfaces. They are most effective on small warts and on nonmucosal surfaces.

continued on page 421

MANAGEMENT *Continued*

HPV Vaccination

- **Gardasil** vaccine is recommended for preteen boys and girls at age 11 or 12 so they are protected before ever being exposed to the virus. HPV vaccine also produces a higher immune response in preteens than in older adolescents. Healthcare providers may give it to girls as young as 9 years. The vaccine can prevent almost 100% of disease caused by the four types of HPV (6, 11, 16, and 18) targeted by the vaccine. It may also be given to boys aged 9 to 26.

- **Cervarix is a bivalent vaccine that** helps protect females from 9 to 25 years of age against HPV 16 and 18, the subtypes that cause about 70% of cervical cancer cases. It does not treat these conditions and does not protect against all HPV types.

- Only Gardasil has been tested and licensed for use in males. Both **Gardasil** and **Cervarix** are given in a series of three shots over a 6-month period.

 HELPFUL HINT

- Cesarean delivery should not be performed solely to prevent transmission of HPV infection to the newborn; however, it is advisable to remove visible lesions during pregnancy.

 POINTS TO REMEMBER

- As with all HPV infections, the underlying viral infection may or may not persist even if the visible warts clear. Although skin warts are common in the general pediatric population, genital warts are uncommon in children. Consequently, the diagnosis of genital warts in children should alert the healthcare provider to the possibility of sexual abuse.

- Confusing condyloma lata for genital warts misses the diagnosis of highly infectious secondary syphilis and leads to inappropriate therapy and potentially disastrous sequelae for the patient.

- Confusing pearly penile papules, vestibular papillae, or Fordyce spots with genital warts result in unnecessary treatment and unwarranted psychosocial stress.

- Pearly penile papules, vestibular papillae, and other normal anatomic structures are often mistaken for condyloma acuminatum.

- Developing genital warts during a long-term relationship does not necessarily imply infidelity.

 SEE PATIENT HANDOUT "Genital Warts" IN THE COMPANION eBOOK EDITION.

Herpes Simplex Genitalis

BASICS

- Herpes simplex genitalis is a genital disease caused most commonly by HSV-2, although HSV-1 can also infect genital skin. It is most commonly, but not invariably, sexually transmitted.
- HSV is the most common cause of ulcerative genital lesions. The disease is highly contagious during its prodrome and while lesions are present.
- HSV establishes latency in the dorsal root ganglia and reappears after different triggers in individual patients (see Chapters 6 and 17). Triggers include psychologic or physiologic stress, physical trauma such as from sexual intercourse, menses, and immunosuppression.
- Affected patients may have recurrences that are infrequent or as common as once monthly. Patients who have six or more episodes per year are candidates for long-term suppressive therapy.

RISK FACTORS

- Women have higher acquisition rates and more recurrences than do men.
- People between 15 and 35 years of age have a greater chance to contract HSV-2.
- Infection with HPV and a greater number of sexual partners are also risk factors for HSV infection.

DESCRIPTION OF LESIONS

- Initially, lesions appear as grouped vesicles on an erythematous base (Fig. 28.12).
- Lesions may then become pustular, crusted, and eroded (Fig. 28.13).
- Crusting of the lesions occurs over 15 to 20 days, before reepithelialization begins.
- Chronic ulcerations or crusted or verrucous papules may develop in immunocompromised patients (see Figs. 33.3 and 33.4).

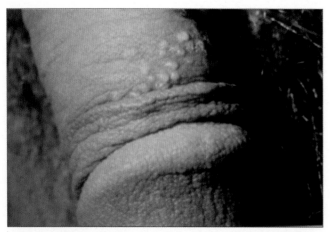

28.12   Herpes simplex genitalis. Grouped intact vesicles are evident.

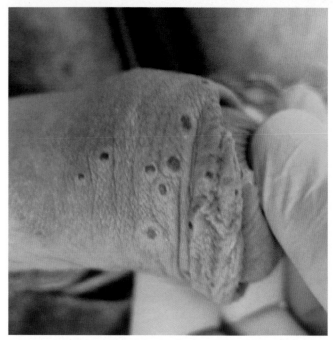

28.13   Herpes simplex genitalis. Fragile vesicles rupture quickly and become grouped crusts or erosions as seen here.

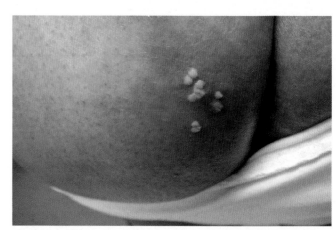

28.14   Herpes simplex. This is a common site of HSV-2 in women. These opaque vesicles appear now to be pustules after being present for several days; however, piercing the vesicles reveals serous fluid rather than thick pus.

DISTRIBUTION OF LESIONS

- In women, the vulvae, perineum, inner thighs, buttocks, and sacral area (Fig. 28.14) are the most common sites of involvement.
- In men, the penis, scrotum, thigh, and buttocks are the typical locations.

PRIMARY HERPES SIMPLEX

- As with HSV-1, this may be more severe than recurrent infections (see Chapter 6).

- The duration is generally from 10 to 14 days. Regional adenopathy may be present.
- Fever, dysuria, urinary retention, and constipation may also occur.
- Alternatively, the initial outbreak may be mild or asymptomatic, so that the patient sheds virus intermittently without realizing that he or she is infected.

RECURRENT HERPES SIMPLEX

- There is often a prodrome of itching, burning, numbness, tingling, or pain 1 to 2 days before a clinical outbreak.
- Lesions are localized and recur at the same site or in close proximity each time.
- Regional adenopathy may be present.
- Vulvar involvement may cause dysuria.
- The duration is generally from 3 to 5 days.
- Chronic ulcerative lesions are indicative of immunosuppression.
- The risk of neonatal transmission is less than 3% and is greatest in patients with primary HSV at the time of delivery.

COMPLICATIONS

- Genital ulcer disease puts the patient at an increased risk of HIV infection.
- The risk of neonatal transmission depends on when the maternal infection is acquired. The risk to the neonate is less than 1% if the maternal infection is recurrent or is acquired at the beginning of pregnancy and is 30% to 50% if the maternal infection is acquired near term.
- If maternal HSV is acquired near the time of delivery, cesarean section is usually advised.
- Patients with certain skin diseases, such as atopic dermatitis, are in danger of developing dissemination of herpes simplex, also known as Kaposi varicelliform eruption or eczema herpeticum (see Figs. 6.14 and 17.29).

DIAGNOSIS

- Most often, the diagnosis is based on the clinical appearance.
- The Tzanck preparation (see Chapter 6) may be helpful, but it lacks sensitivity.
- Viral culture is the current standard of diagnosis, but the sensitivity declines rapidly as the lesions begin to heal.
- Diagnosis in tissue culture using monoclonal antibodies or polymerase chain reaction is sensitive; however, it is very expensive and has not been approved by the U.S. Food and Drug Administration for the diagnosis of genital lesions.
- Serologic testing may be useful, according to CDC guidelines, for those with (a) recurrent genital signs and symptoms and negative cultures, (b) a clinical diagnosis of genital herpes without laboratory confirmation, and (c) a partner with genital herpes. It is not recommended for screening of the general population.

 DIFFERENTIAL DIAGNOSIS

Herpes Zoster (see Chapter 6)
- *Herpes simplex may be dermatomal and may appear clinically identical to herpes zoster.*
- *A history of recurrences strongly suggests HSV.*

Primary Syphilis (Chancre)
- *Classically, the lesion has been described as being "painless"; however, secondarily infected lesions may be painful.*
- *The border is indurated (see below).*

Chancroid
- *There are multiple painful ulcers (see below).*

 MANAGEMENT

Patient Education
- The patient should be given written educational materials and clear instructions regarding safe sexual practices.
- The use of **condoms** should be encouraged.
- The patient should be advised about asymptomatic viral shedding.
- The risk of neonatal infection should be emphasized to both female *and* male patients.

Topical Therapy
- **Topical antivirals** are of limited effectiveness and are not recommended.

- Symptomatic relief may be achieved with cold compresses, viscous lidocaine (**Xylocaine), EMLA** (eutectic mixture of lidocaine and prilocaine), or **oral analgesics.**

Systemic Antiviral Therapy
Primary Herpes Simplex
- **Acyclovir** 200 mg five times daily or 400 mg three times daily for 10 days *or*
- Famciclovir (**Famvir**) 250 mg three times daily for 10 days *or*
- Valacyclovir (**Valtrex**) 1 g twice daily for 7 to 10 days

continued on page 424

MANAGEMENT *Continued*

Recurrent Herpes Simplex: Episodic Therapy
- Treat at the first sign of the prodrome
- **Acyclovir** 400 mg three times daily for 5 days, 800 mg twice daily for 5 days, or 800 mg three times daily for 3 days, *or*
- **Famciclovir** 125 mg twice daily for 5 days or 1,000 mg twice daily for 1 day, *or*
- **Valacyclovir** 500 mg twice daily for 3 days or 1,000 mg daily for 5 days

Recurrent Herpes Simplex (with more than Six Recurrences per Year) or Chronic Recurrent Erythema Multiforme (Daily Suppressive Therapy)
- Treat as for recurrent HSV for 5 days, then continue therapy with **acyclovir** 400 mg twice daily, *or*
- **Famciclovir** 250 mg twice daily, *or*
- **Valacyclovir** 500 mg or 1,000 mg, once daily.
- After 1 year of treatment with these agents, the medication should be discontinued to determine the recurrence, and the dosage can be adjusted as needed.
- The safety of daily acyclovir has been established for a period of 6 years and for famciclovir and valacyclovir for 1 year.

Acyclovir-Resistant Herpes Simplex
- This is seen in patients with AIDS.
- Co-resistance to famciclovir and valacyclovir has been reported.

- **Foscarnet** can be given 40 mg/kg IV two to three times daily for 14 to 21 days.
- Recurrent HSV after foscarnet treatment is often acyclovir sensitive.

Herpes Simplex in Pregnant Women
- The safety and efficacy of oral antiviral therapy during pregnancy have not been established.
- Although acyclovir readily crosses the placenta, several studies did not reveal any increased risk to the developing fetus.
- Antiviral therapy is recommended for pregnant women who are experiencing a primary HSV infection.
- If vaginal delivery occurs through an infected birth canal, the neonate should be observed, and any suspicious lesions should be cultured.
- If no symptoms or signs are present during labor, vaginal delivery is recommended.
- Although the risk of neonatal infection is lower in women with recurrent HSV than it is in women with primary infection, the presence of active herpetic lesions or symptoms of vulvar pain or burning may call for cesarean delivery, regardless of the type of maternal herpetic infection.

 ## HELPFUL HINTS

- A recent study found that 500 mg Valtrex, taken once daily by people with HSV-2, decreased the risk of transmitting the infection to uninfected partners by 50%. This suggests that Valtrex can be prescribed in the so-called discordant couples—those in which one partner is infected and the other is not.
- Maternal acquisition of HSV-1 or HSV-2 during pregnancy accounts for most neonatal HSV infections, which often result in infant deaths.
- Episodic treatment of recurrent herpes requires initiation of therapy within 1 day of lesion onset or during the prodrome that precedes some outbreaks. The patient should be provided with a supply of drug or a prescription for the medication with instructions to initiate treatment **immediately** when symptoms begin.

 ## POINTS TO REMEMBER

- Asymptomatic infections are common and contribute significantly to HSV transmission because of subclinical viral shedding.
- Condoms are clearly not foolproof, because the virus spreads by contact with herpes sores and condoms may not cover all sores.

BASICS

- Syphilis is a systemic STD caused by the spirochetal bacterium *Treponema pallidum*. The likelihood of infection is enhanced in the setting of immunosuppression such as occurs with HIV.
- The disease is characterized by asymptomatic periods of varying duration, interrupted by three overlapping stages of clinical disease: primary, secondary, early latent; late latent; and tertiary stages.
- Tertiary syphilis is exceedingly rare in the modern era, presumably because most infected patients have had exposure to multiple courses of antibiotics during the course of their lives and such treatment may have prevented the infection from progressing.

PRIMARY SYPHILIS

CLINICAL MANIFESTATIONS

- A painless ulcer (chancre) arises, with a rolled, indurated border (Fig. 28.15).
- Most often presents on or near the glans penis in men and less commonly on the shaft of the penis.
- In women the labia majora or minora, the clitoris, or the posterior commissure are the sites of predilection; however, visible primary lesions are rarely reported or found.
- The lesion is usually single, but may be multiple.
- The base of the ulcer is "clean" (not purulent) unless it is superinfected.
- Regional adenopathy may be present.
- An untreated chancre heals within 3 months.
- Anal lesions may occur after receptive anal intercourse.

DIAGNOSIS

- Nontreponemal serologic tests such as Venereal Disease Research Laboratory (VDRL) and the rapid plasma reagin (RPR) tests, both of which detect antibodies to cardiolipin, are the most commonly used. Positive results can be titrated providing a tool for determining response to therapy. Such tests may not become positive until 1 or 2 weeks after the chancre

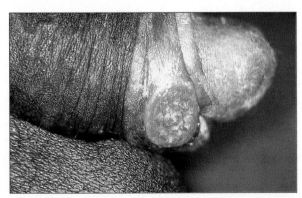

28.15 *Chancre of primary syphilis.* This ulcer has a rolled, indurated border and a base with a "clean," nonpurulent exudate.

has appeared. Other drawbacks include both false-positive as well as false-negative results. False-negative results may occur due to the *prozone phenomenon*.
- Treponemal-specific tests such as the fluorescent treponemal antibody absorption test (FTA-ABS) and other treponemal-specific tests offer nearly 99% specificity and sensitivity.
- Darkfield examination of chancre traditionally afforded the fastest way to make the diagnosis of primary syphilis; however, this test has almost completely fallen out of use due to the necessity of the presence of a darkfield microscope and the current lack of skills required to use this device.

 DIFFERENTIAL DIAGNOSIS

Herpes Simplex
- *Lesions are generally multiple and painful.*
- *Vesicles precede erosions and ulcerations.*

Chancroid
- *Chancroid is unusual in the United States.*
- *Lesions are generally multiple and painful.*

Aphthous Ulcers
- *May be similar to a chancre, but are painful and may be multiple such as noted in Behçet disease.*

 MANAGEMENT

- Test for HIV infection and re-test 3 months later if negative.

Non–Penicillin-Allergic Patients
- **Benzathine penicillin G (Bicillin L-A)** 2.4 million units IM in a single dose.

Penicillin-Allergic Nonpregnant Patients
- **Doxycycline** 100 mg PO twice daily for 2 weeks *or*
- **Tetracycline** 500 mg four times daily for 2 weeks
- **Azithromycin** 2 g as a single dose
- **Ceftriaxone** 1 g IM daily for 10 days

Penicillin-Allergic Pregnant Patients
- The CDC recommends desensitization to penicillin rather than the use of a second-line treatment with a non-penicillin antibiotic.
- Subsequent treatment with benzathine penicillin G 2.4 million units IM, with a second dose 1 week later.

HIV-Infected Patients
- **Benzathine penicillin** G 2.4 million units IM in one dose
- Some experts recommend repeated treatment

HELPFUL HINTS

- Patients should be informed of one of the possible side effects of syphilis treatment with penicillin. It is called the Jarisch–Herxheimer reaction. It frequently starts within 1 hour and lasts for 24 hours, with symptoms of fever, muscles pains, headache, and tachycardia. It is caused by cytokines released by the immune system in response to lipoproteins released from rupturing syphilis bacteria.
- Follow-up visits in patients with syphilis should be performed at 3-, 6-, and 12-month intervals. Patients with HIV infection or patients treated with a non-penicillin regimen should be monitored for life.

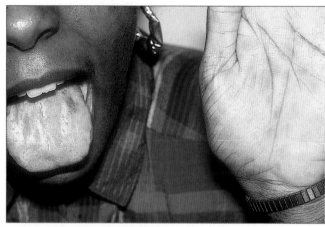

28.17 *Secondary syphilis.* Mucous patches are present on this patient's tongue. She also has palmar lesions.

SECONDARY SYPHILIS

CLINICAL MANIFESTATIONS

- Secondary lesions appear 2 to 6 months after primary infection; chancre may still be present (15% of cases).
- Scaly, erythematous, oval, papulosquamous lesions appear (Fig. 28.16).
- Lesions are generally asymptomatic, but the patient may have fever, generalized adenopathy, and mild systemic symptoms.
- Mucous patches of the tongue may be noted (Fig. 28.17). (See also Fig. 21.7.) The so-called "split papules" may also be seen at the corners of the mouth.

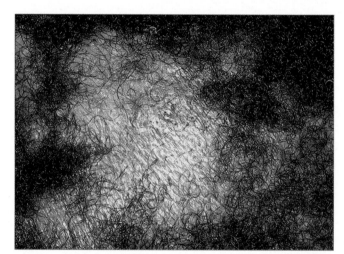

28.18 *Secondary syphilis.* Note the "moth-eaten" appearance of alopecia in this patient.

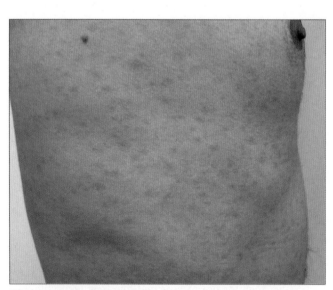

28.16 *Secondary syphilis.* Scaly, erythematous oval patches and papules are noted. Note similarity to pityriasis rosea (see Figs. 15.2 and 15.4). (Figure courtesy of Miguel R. Sanchez, M.D.)

- "Moth-eaten," diffuse alopecia (Fig. 28.18) and condyloma latum (Fig. 28.19) can also seen in secondary syphilis.
- Lesions are widespread and may include the palms (Fig. 28.20), soles, scalp, and mucous membranes.
- Secondary lesions fade within 2 to 6 weeks, after which the latent stage begins.

DIAGNOSIS (SEE DISCUSSION ABOVE FOR PRIMARY SYPHILIS)

- The diagnosis is often suggested by the clinical presentation.
- VDRL and the RPR usually at a titer greater than 1:16; treponemal-specific tests such as FTA-ABS and other treponemal-specific tests confirm the diagnosis.
- A skin biopsy with silver or immunoperoxidase stain may also confirm the diagnosis.
- Serologic titers may be negative in HIV-infected persons.

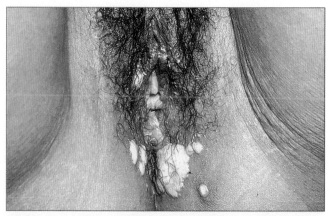

28.19 *Secondary syphilis. Condyloma latum.* These moist, wartlike papules are highly infectious. They "teem" with spirochetes.

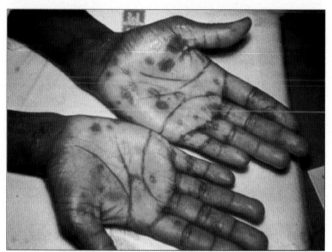

28.20 *Secondary syphilis.* Characteristic copper or "ham-colored," papulosquamous lesions are seen on this patient's palms.

LATENT SYPHILIS

- Latent syphilis is manifested by positive serologic tests for nontreponemal and treponemal antibodies in the absence of clinical manifestations. It is divided into early latent syphilis and late latent syphilis.
- Early latent syphilis is syphilis documented to be of less than 1 year in duration and is treated with the same regimen as primary and secondary infections.
- The duration of late latent syphilis is more than 1 year or is unknown. The recommended treatment is benzathine penicillin 2.4 million units intramuscularly weekly for 3 weeks.

- HIV-infected patients with latent syphilis of any duration should have a cerebrospinal fluid examination to rule out neurosyphilis before treatment.

TERTIARY SYPHILIS

- Tertiary syphilis occurs about 20 years after the onset of untreated syphilis, and it is rare in the antibiotic era.
- Treatment is the same as for late latent syphilis.

CONGENITAL SYPHILIS

- Congenital syphilis can affect infants born to mothers with: (1) untreated syphilis, or (2) syphilis treated during pregnancy with erythromycin, or (3) syphilis treated less than 1 month before delivery, or (4) syphilis treated with penicillin without a four-fold decrease in serologic titer.
- The CDC recommends that all pregnant women be tested for syphilis at least once during pregnancy and at the time of delivery in at-risk populations.

 DIFFERENTIAL DIAGNOSIS

Pityriasis Rosea
- *Usually, pityriasis rosea is confined to the skin above the knees, and usually spares the face, palms, and soles (see Figs. 15.2 and 15.4).*
- *It is prudent to check syphilis serologic tests in patients with pityriasis rosea.*

Other Diagnoses
- *Other papulosquamous eruptions such as psoriasis, lichen planus, and drug eruptions should be considered.*

 MANAGEMENT

- This is essentially the same as for primary syphilis (see above).
- After appropriate treatment, the serologic titer should fall fourfold in 6 months. If it does not, the patient should have a cerebrospinal fluid examination. If it is negative, some experts advise retreatment with benzathine penicillin 2.4 million units weekly for 3 weeks.

Chancroid

BASICS

- Chancroid is an ulcerative STD that is most common in developing countries and is rare in the United States and Western Europe. In the United States, it is associated with prostitution and with the use of crack cocaine.
- The causative organism, *Haemophilus ducreyi,* a gram-negative *Streptobacillus,* is fastidious and requires specific conditions for culture.
- Chancroid occurs as a mixed infection with syphilis or herpes simplex in 10% of cases.
- Clinical infection is more common in men than in women.

CLINICAL MANIFESTATIONS

- The location of lesions depends on the site(s) of inoculation.
- In **men**, the prepuce, balanopreputial fold, and the shaft of the penis are the typical sites.
- In **women**, lesions are noted on the labia majora, posterior commissure, or perianal area.
- Extragenital lesions have been described.
- The incubation period is 25 days.
- The earliest manifestation is a papule, which becomes a pustule and ulcerates.
- Fully developed lesions are painful, with undermined borders and peripheral erythema (Figs. 28.21 and 28.22).
- Borders are not indurated.
- There may be satellite ulcers.
- Tenderness and pain are common.
- Unilateral or bilateral inguinal adenopathy (*buboes*) may be present.

DIAGNOSIS

- The diagnosis is often made based on the clinical appearance.
- A negative darkfield examination, syphilis serologic testing, and HSV cultures help to exclude other diagnoses.
- Obtaining a culture is difficult.
- A Gram stain shows characteristic "schools of fish" or "Chinese characters."
- Polymerase chain reaction may help in making a diagnosis.

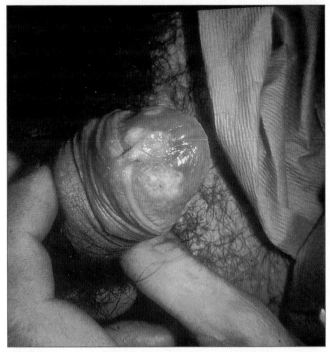

28.21 *Chancroid.* This patient has multiple painful ulcers on the glans penis.

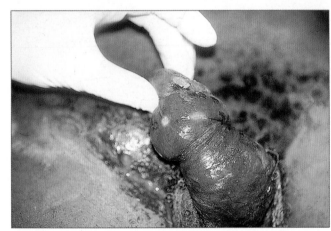

28.22 *Chancroid.* Multiple painful ulcers and a purulent, draining bubo are present.

DIFFERENTIAL DIAGNOSIS

Herpes Simplex
• *Preceded by vesicles and the borders are not undermined.*

Chronic HSV
• *In patients with HIV/AIDS may resemble chancroid.*

Primary Syphilis
• *The borders are indurated not undermined, and the lesion is generally painless.*

 ## MANAGEMENT

Drug Therapy
• **Azithromycin** 1 g PO in a single dose *or*
• **Ceftriaxone** 250 mg IM in a single dose *or*
• **Erythromycin** 500 mg PO four times daily for 7 days *or*
• **Ciprofloxacin** 500 mg PO twice daily for 3 days
• Pregnant women and HIV-infected patients should be treated with erythromycin.
• Symptomatic improvement usually occurs in 3 days; objective improvement is seen in 7 days.
• Complete healing may take more than 2 weeks.
• HIV testing should be performed on all patients and repeated 3 months later if negative.

 ## POINTS TO REMEMBER

• Chancroid is rare in the United States, but epidemics have been described in crack cocaine users.
• Always test for coinfection with HIV, syphilis, and HSV.

Lymphogranuloma Venereum

BASICS

- Lymphogranuloma venereum (LGV) is caused by *Chlamydia trachomatis* types L1, L2, and L3. It is most often sexually transmitted.
- LGV is most common in Southeast Asia, Africa, Central America, and the Caribbean. LGV accounts for 2% to 10% of genital ulcer disease in India and Africa.
- An inconspicuous cutaneous ulceration occurs at the site of inoculation, and it often heals without being noticed.

CLINICAL MANIFESTATIONS

- Evanescent papulopustule or ulceration occurs.
- The primary lesion, if present, is found on the penis, vaginal wall, cervix, or perirectally. It is rarely seen in women.
- Regional lymphadenitis is characteristic. The groin fold divides lymph nodes into upper and lower groups ("the groove sign") (Fig. 28.23). Sometimes, the adenopathy is bilateral.
- Fluctuance and sinus tracts may develop.
- LGV may be associated with malaise and joint stiffness.
- Scarring may result in genital lymphedema.
- Erythema nodosum occurs in 10% of women with LGV.
- Rectal exposure can lead to proctocolitis, which if not treated promptly may lead to chronic colorectal strictures and fistulas.

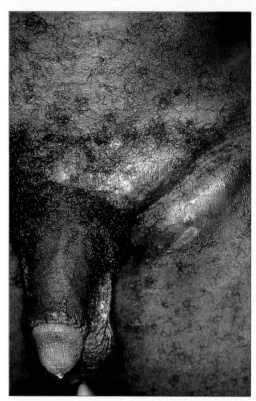

28.23 *Lymphogranuloma venereum.* Regional lymphadenitis ("the groove sign") is present.

DIAGNOSIS

- The diagnosis of LGV depends mainly on the exclusion of other causes of suppurative adenopathy and serologic testing: a complement fixation test and two immunofluorescent tests.
- Culture of the organism is also available.

 MANAGEMENT

- **Doxycycline** 100 mg PO twice daily for 3 weeks minimum.
- Alternative regimen (and in pregnant women): **erythromycin** 500 mg PO four times daily for 3 weeks minimum.
- Buboes may need to be aspirated or incised and drained.

 DIFFERENTIAL DIAGNOSIS

Cats Scratch Disease
- *Usually, there is a history of contact with cats at a site proximal to involved lymph nodes.*

Pyogenic Adenitis
- *A positive Gram stain and bacterial cultures may be found.*

Tuberculous Adenitis
- *A positive acid-fast bacillus stain and cultures and a positive purified protein derivative (PPD) test are obtained.*

Granuloma Inguinale (Donovanosis)

BASICS

- Granuloma inguinale (GI) is a chronic genital granulomatous ulcerative disease caused by the gram-negative bacillus *Klebsiella granulomatis,* an intracellular gram-negative bacterium.
- GI is thought to be sexually transmitted, with low infectivity.
- The disease occurs rarely in the United States, although it is endemic in some tropical and developing areas, including India; Papua, New Guinea; the Caribbean; central Australia; and southern Africa.
- No FDA-cleared molecular tests for the detection of *K. granulomatis* DNA exist, but such an assay might be useful when undertaken by laboratories that have conducted a CLIA verification study.

CLINICAL MANIFESTATIONS

- The initial lesion is a nonspecific papule or a nodule that ulcerates.
- GI appears in the genital, pubic, perineal, groin, or perianal areas.
- The ulcer is painless, slowly progressive, and has an undermined border.
- The lesions are highly vascular (i.e., beefy red appearance) and bleed easily on contact.
- There is no regional lymphadenopathy.
- The presence of pain or adenitis suggests superinfection.
- Subcutaneous granulomas (*pseudoboboes*) might also occur.
- Extragenital lesions occur in 3% to 6% of cases can occur with extension of infection to the pelvis, or it can disseminate to intra-abdominal organs, bones, or the mouth.

DIAGNOSIS

- The causative organism is difficult to culture.
- Smears from the edge of the lesion may show characteristic Donovan bodies (organisms within macrophages).
- The biopsy specimen should be taken from the edge of the lesion.

 DIFFERENTIAL DIAGNOSIS

Syphilis
- *Must be excluded by darkfield and serologic examinations.*
- *The borders of the ulcers are indurated and not undermined.*

 MANAGEMENT

- The treatment of choice is **doxycycline** 100 mg twice daily for 3 weeks minimum or until the ulcers have healed.
- Alternative regimens:
  - **Azithromycin** 1 g once weekly for at least 3 weeks or until the ulcers have healed *or*
  - **Ciprofloxacin** 750 mg twice daily for at least 3 weeks or until the ulcers have healed *or*
  - **Erythromycin** 500 mg four times daily for at least 3 weeks or until the ulcers have healed *or*
  - **Trimethoprim-sulfamethoxazole** one double-strength tablet twice daily for at least 3 weeks or until the ulcers have healed

29 Bites, Stings, and Infestations

OVERVIEW

In much of the world, arthropod bites commonly serve as vectors that transport diseases such as malaria, leishmaniasis, West Nile virus, filariasis, and rickettsial diseases. In modern industrial societies, most bites are more of a nuisance than a potential carrier of a life-threatening illness.

Insects such as mosquitoes, fleas, and flies have six legs. Arachnids such as spiders have eight legs, a group that also includes ticks, mites, and scorpions. In the United States, mosquitoes, fleas, biting flies as well as ticks, spiders, bed bugs, chiggers, and lice account for the majority of bites. Mosquito and fly bites occur most often from outdoor exposures, particularly in the summer months. Flea bites are most often acquired indoors, from pets. Stings are often caused by bees, wasps, hornets, and fire ants. In arid areas, including much of the Southwest and parts of California, flying insects are less common, and crawling arthropods are the primary cause of bites and stings.

There is individual variability in the human attraction of insects, possibly related to pheromones. Furthermore, the reactions to bites and stings are probably related to individual hypersensitivity. Lesions occur as a result of the body's immune response to injected foreign chemicals and proteins introduced by a bite or sting.

Discussed in this chapter are waterborne stings and seashore infestations that occur from visiting the beach and swimming in salt or freshwater which exposes people to a variety of organisms. Such encounters can result in seabather's eruption and cutaneous larva migrans. Encounters with jellyfish (e.g., sea nettle, Portuguese man-of-war, thimble jellyfish) can also cause skin reactions.

IN THIS CHAPTER...

➤ **INSECT BITE AND STING REACTIONS**

- Fleas, mosquitoes, biting flies, bees
- Bed bugs

➤ **ARACHNID BITE REACTIONS**

- Brown recluse spider bite

➤ **TICK BITES**

- Lyme disease (Lyme borreliosis)

➤ **MITE INFESTATIONS**

- Scabies

➤ **LICE INFESTATIONS (PEDICULOSIS)**

➤ **WATERBORNE STINGS AND SEASHORE INFESTATIONS**

- Jellyfish stings
- Seabather's eruption ("sea lice")
- Cutaneous larva migrans ("creeping eruption")

Insect Bite and Sting Reactions

FLEAS, MOSQUITOES, BITING FLIES, BEES

BASICS

- The development of an immediate hive-like skin lesion to a bite or sting (Fig. 29.1) reflects a type I hypersensitivity reaction (mediated by immunoglobulin E).
- Delayed pruritic papules, nodules, and vesicles usually become symptomatic within 48 hours after an insult and are manifestations of a type IV hypersensitivity reaction (cell-mediated immunity).

CLINICAL MANIFESTATIONS

- Insect bites may be a chronic, recurrent problem or simply a nuisance.
- Itching may be intense and may persist for weeks.
- Secondary bacterial infection may occur.
- Bites often go unnoticed and the lesions that arise from them may not appear for days after the bite (delayed immune-mediated hypersensitivity reaction). Consequently, a patient may seek medical advice for unexplained itchy bumps or blisters.
- Stings generally cause immediate pain and are therefore usually remembered.
- A sting can be due to a sting of a bee, wasp, hornet, or yellow jacket. Such stings can be quite painful.
- A bee sting may trigger a dangerous anaphylactic reaction.

DESCRIPTION OF LESIONS

- Bite reactions typically present as intensely pruritic erythematous papules that commonly are excoriated.
- Such reactions may be indistinguishable from ordinary hives.
- Grouping of lesions often occurs, particularly after flea bites ("breakfast, lunch, and dinner" lesions [Fig. 29. 2]).
- Lesions may have a central punctum and crust and also may become vesicobullous (Fig. 29.3).
- Insect bite reactions are also known as *papular urticaria* when lesions persist for longer than 48 hours.

DISTRIBUTION OF LESIONS

- In general, lesions are found on exposed areas, more often on nonclothed body parts such as the distal lower extremities, the forearms, and hands.

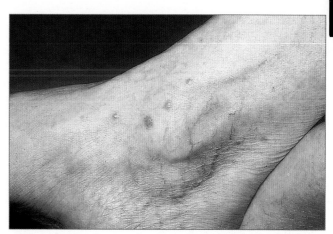

29.2 *Flea bites.* Note the arrangement of lesions in groups of three ("breakfast, lunch, and dinner"); the fourth lesion probably represents a "midnight snack."

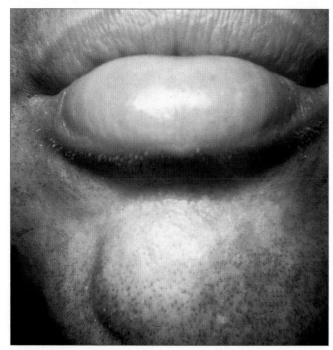

29.1 *Angioedema caused by a bee sting.* This patient developed an immediate hypersensitivity reaction after being stung on his lower lip.

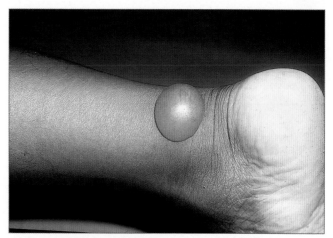

29.3 *Bullous arthropod bite reaction.* Note the tense bulla that resulted from a chigger bite.

- Flying insects tend to bite on the upper trunk or extremities, whereas crawling insects tend to bite or sting on the lower trunk or extremities.
- Axillary and anogenital areas are usually spared.

DIAGNOSIS

- The diagnosis is usually made on clinical appearance and history.
- Inquiry about household pets currently and formerly residing in one's house may be a clue to the diagnosis. For example, if the residence was formerly host to a dog or cat infested with fleas, the fleas left behind may have found new human hosts.
- A skin biopsy is not diagnostic, but it may show suggestive findings consisting of a dense lymphocytic infiltrate (resembling lymphoma) with many eosinophils. The responsible agent is rarely found in a biopsy specimen.

 DIFFERENTIAL DIAGNOSIS

Urticaria Unrelated to Insect Bites (Discussed in Chapter 27)
- *Often indistinguishable from insect bites; lacks a central punctum.*

Fiberglass Dermatitis
- *Nonspecific itching is noted.*
- *The patient has a history of exposure (e.g., works with roofing materials).*

Scabies (see Discussion later in this chapter)

 HELPFUL HINT

- Patients who seek medical help generally do not consider the "mundane" nature of insect bites to be the cause of their dermatosis or itching; rather, they seek attention because they assume that other factors caused their problem.

 POINTS TO REMEMBER

- A careful history and knowledge of the patient's environment and possible exposures should be sought.
- Symptoms may persist for weeks after the original bites.
- Other causes should be diligently sought if symptoms persist for more than 4 to 6 weeks.

 MANAGEMENT

- **Insect repellents** that contain N,N-diethyl-m-toluamide (**DEET**) help prevent bites and stings.
- The higher the concentration of DEET, the longer the protection afforded.
- Picaridin-containing insect repellents have also been shown to be effective.
- Acute reactions to stings are treated symptomatically with **topical** or **intralesional steroids** and/or **oral antihistamines**; people with severe reactions from stings may profit from desensitization therapy.
- Anaphylactic reactions require epinephrine, **systemic steroids**, and antihistamines.
- If flea infestation is suspected, pets should be evaluated by a veterinarian. If fleas are present in the home, thorough vacuuming and shampooing of flea-infested areas and sometimes even **fumigation** may be necessary.

BED BUGS

BASICS

- Bed bugs (*Cimex lectularius*) are small insects that feed on human blood. Their preferred habitat is in warm houses and especially nearby or inside of beds and bedding. They often hide in cracks in furniture, floors, or walls.
- Bed bugs are mainly active at night when people are sleeping. They usually feed on their hosts without being noticed.
- Adult bed bugs have flat rusty red–colored, flat, oval bodies and are about the size of an apple seed (Fig. 29.4).

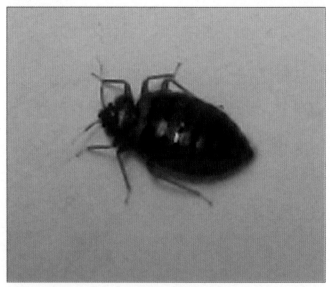

29.4 *Bed bug (Cimex lenticularis).* This adult bed bug is engorged with blood. It has a flattened, oval shape. Bed bugs have segmented abdomens that give them a banded appearance.

- When bed bugs feed, their bodies swell and become bright red. They can live for a year without feeding on a host.
- In most cases people carry bed bugs into their homes unknowingly in infested luggage, furniture, bedding, or clothing. Bed bugs may also travel between apartments through small crevices and cracks in walls and floors.

CLINICAL MANIFESTATIONS

- The bites are painless, but later turn into pruritic urticarial papules.
- Although bed bugs are a great nuisance, they are not known to cause or spread any diseases.

DIAGNOSIS

- The diagnosis is usually based upon the actual demonstration of the bugs coupled with the clinical findings that are suggestive of bites.

- Also helpful is seeing small bloodstains from crushed insects, eggs, or dark spots from their feces. White bed sheets help in this recognition.
- They are often hard to find because they hide in cracks.
- Detection aides: A bright flashlight, dry ice-baited traps, sticky traps, and detection dogs.

PREVENTION

- Clothing should be washed in hot water and dried on the highest dryer setting.
- Luggage should be inspected immediately after returning from a trip.
- Areas where bed bugs are likely to hide as well as bedding, linens, curtains, rugs, and carpets should be cleaned thoroughly.
- Commercially available mattress encasements.
- Carpets in affected areas should be vacuumed and all debris is placed in taped bags before disposal.

Arachnid Bite Reactions

BROWN RECLUSE SPIDER BITES

BASICS

- Most spiders are harmless to humans. Only the six-eyed brown recluse *Loxosceles* (discussed in this chapter) and the black widow spider have ever been associated with significant disease and very rare reports of death.
- Deaths from brown recluse spiders have been reported only in children younger than 7 years.
- Brown recluse spiders are native to the midwestern and southeastern United States. With increasing travel, individual spiders and spider bites can be found in areas where the spider is not endemic, and health care practitioners should consider this when diagnosing and treating suspected bites.
- Brown recluse spiders are notable for their characteristic violin pattern on the back of the cephalothorax. The violin pattern is seen with the base of the violin at the head of the spider and the neck of the violin pointing to the rear (Fig. 29.5). These small spiders are yellowish tan to dark brown in color with darker legs.
- They are not aggressive and bite only when threatened, usually when pressed up against the victim's skin. They seek out dark, warm, dry environments such as attics, closets, porches, barns, basements, woodpiles, and old tires.

CLINICAL MANIFESTATIONS

- The severity of symptoms can range from a minor reaction, a localized to slow-healing ulcerated lesion, to a systemic vascular reaction with renal damage that can be life-threatening with thrombocytopenia, disseminated intravascular coagulopathy, and renal failure.

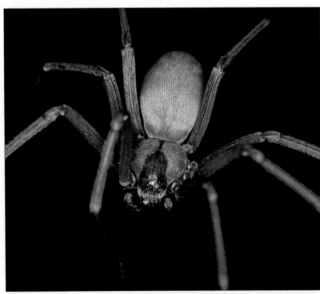

29.5 ***Brown recluse spider.*** 6 to 20 mm long, these spiders usually have markings with a black line that looks like a violin with the neck of the violin pointing to the rear of the spider, resulting in the nickname "fiddleback spider."

- The initial bite is typically painless, but symptoms develop about 2 to 8 hours later, area becomes painful and swollen.
- A "bull's eye" lesion may form.
- Over days the blister forms a crust, which hardens and falls off to leave behind an ulcerated depression.
- The ulcer heals over months and leaves behind a scar.

 MANAGEMENT

- An attempt should be made to identify the offending spider to ensure proper management.
- General measures that should occur after a spider bite include the following:
  - The bitten area should be washed with soap and water.
  - Application of an ice pack wrapped in cloth to the site.
  - Analgesics.
  - Seek immediate emergency care for further treatment.
- Treatment involves supportive care including the use of systemic antibiotics to prevent infections and antihistamines to reduce swelling.
- Antivenom for bites by *Loxosceles* genera is very effective if given soon after the bite.
- Systemic steroids may be of benefit.

 HELPFUL HINTS

- It is believed that the vast majority of reported brown recluse bites have been greatly overdiagnosed.
- Conditions that are far more common and more likely to be the source of necrotic wounds that have been initially misdiagnosed as recluse spider bites by medical professionals include: infection by *Staphylococcus, Streptococcus,* herpes simplex, diabetic ulcers, and pyoderma gangrenosum (Fig. 29.6).

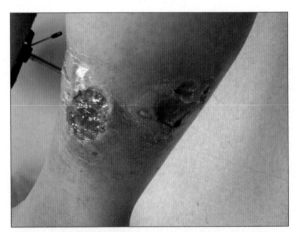

29.6 ***Pyoderma gangrenosum.*** This patient initially presented with an ulcer that was presumed to be a spider bite. Ultimately, it was discovered that she had Crohn disease which accounted for the undermined ulcers of pyoderma gangrenosum.

LYME DISEASE (LYME BORRELIOSIS)

BASICS

- Lyme disease, or Lyme borreliosis (LB), is a systemic infection caused by the spirochete *Borrelia burgdorferi,* which is transmitted by the bite of a tick.
- *B. burgdorferi* is the most common cause of LB in North America, and is most commonly associated with joint disease.
- In Europe, several *Borrelia* species are implicated in human disease; *Borrelia afzelii* is typically associated with skin disease and *Borrelia garinii* with neurologic symptoms.
- The tick has to be attached for 24 hours for the organism to be transmitted.
- Once in the skin, the spirochete may stay localized at the site of inoculation, or it may disseminate via the blood and lymphatics. Hematogenous dissemination can occur within days or weeks of the initial infection. The organism can travel to other parts of the skin, the heart, the joints, the central nervous system, and other parts of the body.
- The tick vector of Lyme disease, *Ixodes dammini,* is found in the northeastern and midwestern United States where most cases are reported. *Ixodes scapularis* in the southeastern United States, *Ixodes pacificus* on the Pacific coast, and *Ixodes ricinus,* the sheep tick, in Europe are also vectors. Because the disease depends on deer, mice, ticks, and bacteria, it is limited geographically to the areas where all these organisms are present.
- LB can occur in any season, although it is most prevalent during the warmer months from May through September during the nymphal stage of the tick. The ticks cling to vegetation (not trees) in grassland, marshland, and woodland habitats. They transfer to animals and humans via brushing up against the vegetation.

CLINICAL MANIFESTATIONS

Early Lyme Disease

- At the early stage of disease, flu-like symptoms, such as malaise, arthralgias, headaches, and a low-grade fever and chills, may occur. Other symptoms include stiffness of the neck and difficulty in concentrating.
- The EM rash itself is usually asymptomatic.

DESCRIPTION OF LESIONS

- Initially, the LB lesion is a red macule or papule at the site of a tick bite. The bite itself usually goes unnoticed (only 15% of patients report a tick bite). The rash appears approximately 2 to 30 days after infection.
- The lesion expands to form an annular erythematous lesion, erythema migrans (EM), which is the classic lesion of LB (Fig. 29.7). The lesion measures from 4 to 70 cm in diameter, generally with central clearing.
- The center of the lesion, which corresponds to the putative site of the tick bite, may become darker, vesicular, hemorrhagic, or necrotic (Fig. 29.8).

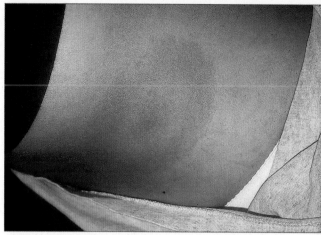

29.7 *Lyme disease, erythema migrans.* A solitary, annular, target-like, erythematous plaque of erythema migrans.

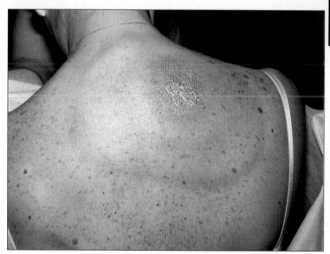

29.8 *Lyme disease.* In this patient, erythema migrans is manifested by concentric rings with resolving central vesicles.

- Lesions may be confluent (not annular), and concentric rings may form.
- Multiple lesions occur in approximately 20% of patients, likely a result of bacteremia (Figs. 29.9 and 29.10). The presence of multiple lesions of erythema migrans indicates early disseminated disease. These secondary lesions tend to be more uniform in morphology than the primary lesion.

DISTRIBUTION OF LESIONS

- Common sites are the thigh, groin, trunk, and axillae.
- Because secondary lesions spread hematogenously, they are less restricted than primary lesions in terms of location.

Intermediate, Chronic, and Late Lyme Disease

- Late Lyme disease refers to symptoms, primarily rheumatologic and neurologic in nature, that occur months to years after initial infection.

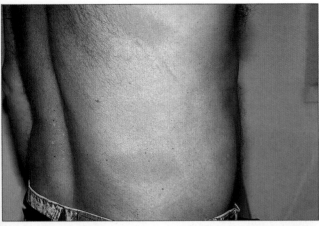

29.9 *Lyme disease.* Multiple confluent lesions of erythema migrans are noted.

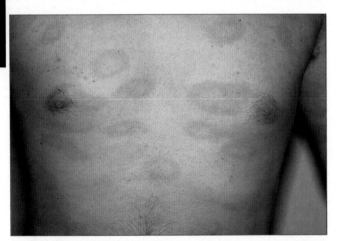

29.10 *Lyme disease.* Multiple annular lesions of erythema migrans are seen here.

- It is not unusual for patients to first present with late extracutaneous symptoms without ever having had an initial EM lesion or other overt symptoms of early Lyme disease. This may occur because the patient was asymptomatic or because early disease was not recognized by the patient or correctly diagnosed by the health care provider.
- The signs and symptoms of intermediate, chronic, and late Lyme disease include the following:
  - Arthritis in one or more large joints, nervous system problems that may include pain, paresthesias, Bell palsy, headaches, memory loss, and cardiac dysrhythmias.
  - Rarely, a lesion of lymphocytoma cutis may develop, usually occurring on the earlobe or nipple. These lesions are bluish-red nodules.
  - **Acrodermatitis chronica atrophicans** (ACA) is a manifestation of chronic LB that begins as an inflammatory eruption marked by edema and erythema, usually on the distal extremities. Later, atrophy occurs, and thin "cigarette-paper" skin is seen. Because of the loss of subcutaneous fat, underlying venous structures are more visible, and the skin becomes thin, atrophic, and xerotic.
  - Both lymphocytoma cutis and ACA are late cutaneous presentations of borreliosis and are very rare findings in the United States. They are seen primarily in Europe where the clinical differences probably result from the different antigenic strains of *Borrelia.*

DIAGNOSIS

- The diagnosis of LB is often difficult because the disease mimics many other conditions.

Early Diagnosis
To diagnose early LB, the following are important:

- There is a history of tick exposure or bite in an area endemic for LB.
- The specific tick is identified as a potential vector of LB.
- The various presentations of EM are recognized.

LABORATORY TESTING

- Serologic testing, using enzyme-linked immunosorbent assay (ELISA) and Western blot analyses for *B. burgdorferi,* is notoriously unreliable.
- At the early presenting stage of LB, serologic testing has been reported to be positive in only 25% of infected patients. After 4 to 6 weeks, approximately 75% of these patients test positive, even after antibiotic therapy.
- Patients with past LB and those who have been vaccinated may be persistently seropositive.
- The poor reputation of serologic testing is derived somewhat from the many false-negative test results of patients treated very early in the course of the disease and from the many misdiagnosed cases of supposed LB.
- In endemic areas, seropositivity may exist in as much as 50% of residents.
- The U.S. Centers for Disease Control and Prevention currently recommends a two-step testing procedure consisting of a screening ELISA or immunofluorescent assay followed by a confirmatory Western immunoblot test on any samples with positive or equivocal results on ELISA.
- Other diagnostic measures, such as polymerase chain reaction and cultures for *B. burgdorferi* have had some success; however, these techniques are time consuming and expensive. The *Borrelia* organism is fastidious, and culture of skin biopsy specimens is not readily available.

DIFFERENTIAL DIAGNOSIS—DIFFERENTIAL DIAGNOSIS

Tinea Corporis (see Discussion in Chapter 18)
- *There may be a history of exposure to fungus.*
- *Lesions are also annular (ring-like) and clear in the center; however, tinea corporis has an "active" scaly border that denotes epidermal involvement.*
- *Lesions are potassium hydroxide positive, or the fungal culture grows dermatophytes.*
- *Tinea corporis generally itches.*

Acute Urticaria (see Discussion in Chapter 27)
- *At times, this may be indistinguishable from erythema migrans.*
- *Lesions tend to be more eccentric in shape.*
- *Individual lesions disappear within 24 hours.*
- *Urticaria generally itches.*

Erythema Multiforme (see Discussion in Chapter 27)
- *Lesions evolve to form targetoid plaques (iris lesions) with a dark center that may become vesicobullous.*
- *Lesions persist (are "fixed") for at least 1 week.*

Other Considerations
- ***Viral infections,*** *such as* ***influenza*** *and* ***mononucleosis,*** *also may manifest with rash, aches, fever, and fatigue.*
- ***Drug eruptions*** *and* ***insect bite reactions*** *other than those caused by the Ixodes tick closely match the rash of early LB.*

 MANAGEMENT

Tick Recognition
- *Ixodes* ticks are much smaller than dog ticks. In their larval and nymphal stages, they are no bigger than a pinhead; unengaged adult ticks are the size of the head of a match (Fig. 29.11).

Tick Removal
- An attached tick should be removed carefully by using a pair of tweezers. The tick should be grasped by the head (not the body), as close as possible to the skin, to avoid force that may crush it. It is then gently pulled straight out of the patient's skin (Fig. 29.12).

Treatment of Erythema Migrans (Early Lyme Borreliosis)
- **Doxycycline** (100 mg twice per day for 21 days [do not use in children younger than 8 years or in pregnant women]) *or*
- **Amoxicillin** (500 mg three times per day for 14 to 21 days); this is the preferred medication in pregnancy *or*
- **Ceftriaxone** or **cefuroxime** (500 mg twice per day for 21 days); expensive; use only if patient is unable to tolerate the other antibiotics.
- Azithromycin (**Zithromax**) and erythromycin: second-line drugs that should also be considered in pregnant patients who are allergic to beta-lactam antibiotics.

Prevention
- Avoidance of tick bites. People who are outdoors in endemic areas in the summer should wear long pants and socks, use insect repellents, and frequently look for ticks on themselves, their children, and on their clothing.
- *B. burgdorferi* infection may be prevented through early removal of the tick, including the mouthparts (less than 36 hours after tick bite).
- No vaccines are currently available for humans.

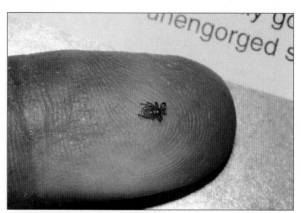

29.11 *Ixodes tick.* An adult tick is the size of the head of a match.

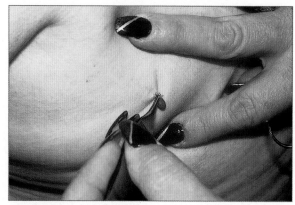

29.12 *Dog tick.* An intact engorged adult dog tick being removed by the head.

HELPFUL HINTS

- Patients can be reinfected. There is no lasting immunity to Lyme disease.
- An additional tick-borne coinfection by *Ehrlichia* species and *Babesia microti* has been reported with increasing frequency. Such coinfection is suggested by a very high fever or toxicity.
- Antibiotic prophylaxis after tick bites is controversial. Clearly, prevention of bites is a better means of avoiding disease.
- Wearing clothing with white colors improves the odds of seeing ticks on clothing before they attach.
- Regular tick inspections and removal of ticks before they have been attached for 24 hours is another important way to reduce the risk of contracting Lyme disease.

POINTS TO REMEMBER

- Most patients at the early EM stage are seronegative.
- Many late complications of Lyme disease may be prevented by systemic antibiotic therapy early in the course of infection.

 SEE PATIENT HANDOUT "Lyme Disease" AND "Lyme Disease: Prevention" IN THE COMPANION eBOOK EDITION.

SCABIES

BASICS

- Scabies is a skin infestation caused by the mite *Sarcoptes scabiei* var. *hominis.* It is usually spread by skin-to-skin contact, most frequently among family members and by sexual contact in young adults. Occasionally, epidemics occur in nursing homes and similar extended-care institutions, where scabies is spread by person-to-person contact and possibly by mite-infested clothing and bed linen.
- The diagnosis of scabies should be considered when an individual complains of intractable, persistent pruritus, especially when other family members, consorts, or fellow inhabitants of an institution such as a nursing home or school have similar symptoms.
- Although scabies is found more commonly in poor, crowded living conditions, it occurs worldwide and is not limited to the impoverished or those who practice poor personal hygiene. African-American and Afro-Caribbean individuals less frequently acquire scabies; the reason is unknown.

PATHOGENESIS

- A fertilized female mite (Fig. 29.13) excavates a burrow in the stratum corneum, lays her eggs, and deposits fecal pellets (scybala) behind her as she advances.
- The eggs, scybala (Fig. 29.14), and other secretions act as irritants or allergens, which may account for the itching and the subsequent delayed type IV hypersensitivity reaction that occurs approximately 30 days after infestation.

CLINICAL MANIFESTATIONS

- Because the incubation period from initial infestation to the onset of pruritus is approximately 1 month, it is not uncommon for contacts to be asymptomatic, especially if they have been recently infested.
- Itching, especially at night (nocturnal pruritus), has traditionally been considered a symptom that is characteristic of scabies; however, nocturnal pruritus commonly occurs in many other skin conditions because people are less distracted by their active daytime routines at night.

DESCRIPTION OF LESIONS

- The initial lesions of scabies include tiny pinpoint vesicles and erythematous papules, some of which evolve into burrows, the classic telltale lesions of scabies.
- The burrow is a linear or S-shaped excavation that is pinkish white and slightly scaly and ends in the pinpoint vesicle or papule. This is where the mites may be found. Burrows are easiest to find on the hands, particularly in the finger webs (Fig. 29.15) and flexor wrists (Fig. 29.16) in adults and on the palms and soles in infants.
- Sometimes burrows can be highlighted by applying black ink with a felt-tipped pen to the suspected areas.

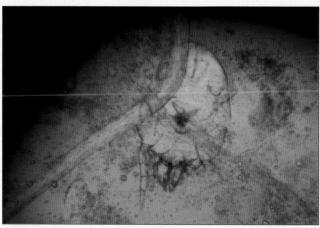

29.13 *Scabies.* A fertilized female mite. Note size relative to a human hair.

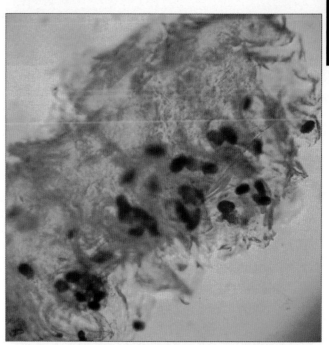

29.14 *Fecal pellets (scybala).* These are the hardened masses of the mite's feces.

DISTRIBUTION OF LESIONS

- Lesions are most often located on the interdigital finger webs, sides of the hands and feet, flexor wrists, umbilicus, waistband area, axillae, ankles, buttocks, groin, and penis (Figs. 29.17 and 29.18).
- Children and adults rarely have lesions above the neck; this is an important diagnostic sign.
- **Infants** tend to have more widespread involvement, including the face and scalp and especially the palms and soles.

Scabies in the Elderly

- Patients, particularly in an institutional setting, can have intense pruritus and few papular lesions, excoriations, or simply may be manifested by dry, scaly, itchy skin.

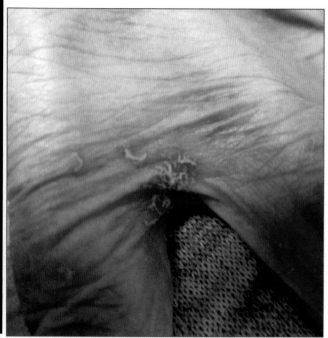

29.15 *Scabies.* Multiple burrows are evident in the web spaces of this patient's fingers.

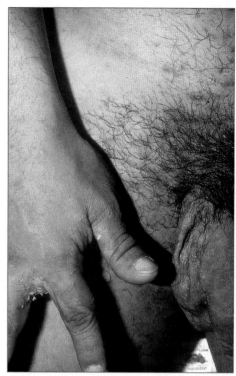

29.17 *Scabies.* Characteristic distribution of scabies infestation in finger webs and scrotum.

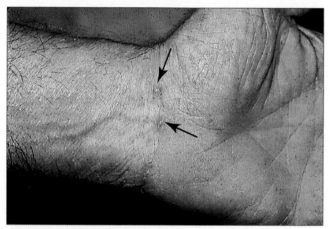

29.16 *Scabies.* Besides the web spaces of the fingers, the flexor wrists are a typical location to find lesions of scabies. Note burrows as indicated by arrows.

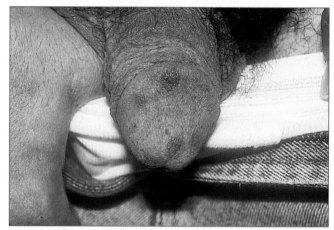

29.18 *Scabies.* Characteristic pruritic papules are present on this patient's penis.

Norwegian or Crusted Scabies

- Norwegian, or crusted, scabies occurs in people with varying degrees of immune deficiency such as that seen in Down syndrome (Fig. 29.19), leukemia, certain nutritional disorders, and acquired immunodeficiency syndrome (HIV/AIDS) (see also Chapter 33 and Figs. 33.13 and 33.14).
- The lesions tend to involve large areas of the body.
- The hands and feet may be scaly and crusted with a thick keratotic material that can also be seen under the nails.
- There may be wart-like vegetations on the skin; these are hosts to thousands of mites and their eggs.

Course and Secondary Lesions

- Initially, itching is rather mild and focal, but when lesions begin spreading rapidly, usually after 4 to 6 weeks, it can sometimes become intolerable.
- A generalized distribution of lesions is probably the result of a hypersensitivity reaction. In this case, a more pleomorphic array of lesions, such as "juicy" papules and nodules, may be seen.
- Hemorrhagic crusts and ulcerations may replace the primary lesions.
- In men, itchy papules and nodules, particularly on the penis and scrotum, are virtually pathognomonic for scabies.

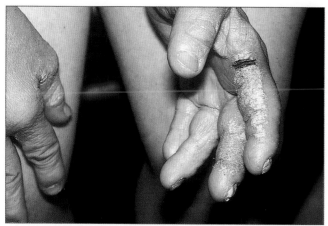

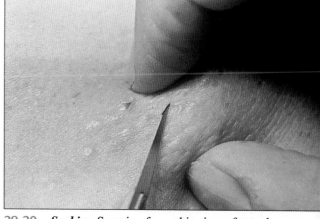

29.19 *Norwegian scabies.* This child with Down syndrome has verrucous plaques on his hands and thickened dystrophic nails. His lesions are teeming with scabies mites.

29.20 *Scabies.* Scraping for scabies is performed.

 DIFFERENTIAL DIAGNOSIS

Insect Bites
- *Generally spares areas that are covered (e.g., the groin and axillae).*

Atopic Dermatitis and Dyshidrotic Eczema
- *Often there is a personal or family history of atopy.*
- *Tends to be chronic.*

Pruritus Associated with Systemic Diseases
- *Renal disease, hepatic disease, lymphomas, HIV/AIDS, leukemias, and Hodgkin disease, should be excluded.*

Drug Eruptions and other Itchy Rashes
- *Urticaria, tinea infections, xerosis, and contact dermatitis, should also be kept in mind.*

DIAGNOSIS

- A conclusive diagnosis is made by finding scabies mites, eggs, or feces.
- A drop of mineral oil is applied to the most likely lesion (usually a vesicle on the finger web or wrist is chosen). The site is then scraped with a surgical blade (Fig. 29.20), the scrapings are placed on a slide, and a cover slip is then applied.
- Adults, who are more efficient scratchers than children, tend to remove the definitive evidence of scabies (i.e., mite) with their fingernails. Because mites are few and are particularly difficult to find in adults, the time and effort spent searching for the mite may be better used by taking a thorough history and counseling the patient and his or her contacts. Thus, if scabies is strongly suspected on clinical grounds, scabicidal treatment should be initiated.

MANAGEMENT

Treatment is directed at killing the mites with a scabicide as well as providing rapid symptomatic relief using appropriate oral antihistamines and topical corticosteroids, if necessary.

Management of Institutional Scabies
- Treatment must be conducted in an organized, cooperative fashion.
- A scabicide and/or oral ivermectin (see below) is administered to all patients, staff, family members, and frequent visitors.
- Laundering of all bed linen and clothes is necessary shortly after treatment.

Permethrin (Elimite and Acticin)
- The prescription drugs **Elimite** and **Acticin** both contain permethrin 5% cream. They are safe and effective scabicides that are currently considered the treatment of choice.
- Approved for use in infants 2 months or older and is pregnancy category B.
- The instructions for use are as follows:
  - After a warm bath, the cream is applied to all skin surfaces "from head to toe" (including the palms, soles, and scalp in small children) and is left on for 8 to 12 hours, usually overnight. It is washed off the next morning.
  - All household members should be treated simultaneously.
  - All bed linen and intimate undergarments should be washed in hot water after treatment is completed.
  - Treatment should be repeated in 7 days. The medication should not be applied repeatedly.
  - Patients should be advised that it is normal to continue itching for days or weeks after treatment, albeit less

continued on page 444

MANAGEMENT *Continued*

intensely. Systemic antihistamines and a potent class 3 or 4 topical corticosteroid can be used for these symptoms.

Precipitated Sulfur Ointment (5% to 10%)

- Applied topically to all skin overnight for three consecutive nights. This is often used in pregnant or lactating women and in infants younger than 2 months.
- Although it is messy and malodorous, it is effective and safe.

Ivermectin

- Ivermectin (**Stromectol**) is an anthelmintic that can be administered (off-label) in a single oral dose. This agent is not currently approved by the U.S. Food and Drug Administration for the treatment of scabies in humans, and no studies have been done to establish its safety for use in pregnancy or in children.
- It may be used when topical therapy is difficult or impractical (e.g., widespread infestations in nursing homes).
- It has been used safely and effectively in patients who are seropositive for human immunodeficiency virus and in some patients with Norwegian scabies.
- This agent may be administered adjunctively with a topical scabicide.
- It is available in 3- and 6-mg tablets.
- **Dosage:** 0.2 mg/kg in a single oral dose that is repeated on day 8 or 14. For 6-mg tablets, the dosages are given in Table 29.1.

Lindane

- **Lindane 1% cream (Kwell, Scabene)**, gamma benzene hydrochloride, was formally the mainstay of therapy for scabies; however, its potential neurotoxicity and reports of resistance have lead to its use only in selected cases.

Table 29.1	IVERMECTIN DOSAGE FOR TREATMENT OF SCABIES WITH 6-mg TABLETS	
WEIGHT (kg)	**NUMBER OF TABLETS**
15–24	0.5
25–35	1
36–50	1.5
51–65	2
66–79	2.5
>80	3–4

HELPFUL HINTS

Think scabies when you see:
- An infant with palmar or plantar vesicles or pustules.
- More than one family member, roommate, or sexual partner who is itching.
- Pruritic scrotal or penile papules or nodules.
- Small itchy vesicles or papules in the finger webs.

 SEE PATIENT HANDOUT "Scabies" IN THE COMPANION eBOOK EDITION.

POINTS TO REMEMBER

- Scabies mimics other skin diseases such as eczematous dermatitis.
- Scabies rarely occurs above the neck in immunocompetent children and adults.
- Contacts should be treated simultaneously to avoid "ping-ponging" (reinfection).
- Treatment failure may result from noncompliance (i.e., treating lesions only) or reinfection.
- Pruritic symptoms may persist after appropriate treatment.
- Because the scabies mite can survive away from the skin for 2 to 5 days on inanimate objects such as clothing of an affected person, it is believed that indirect contact with such personal items can transmit the organism.

BASICS

- Louse (plural: lice) is the common name for members of over 3,000 species wingless insects of the order Phthiraptera.
- **There are two species of sucking lice: *Pediculus humanus* and *Phthirus pubis* (pubic lice, sometimes called "crabs").**
- *P. humanus* is further divided into two subspecies: *P. humanus capitis* (the head louse) and *P. humanus corporis* (the body louse).

HEAD LICE (PEDICULOSIS CAPITIS)
(SEE DISCUSSION IN CHAPTER 9)

- Head lice spread from human to human; epidemics of head lice are most commonly seen in schoolchildren.
- The head louse is wingless insect (2.5 to 3 mm long). They spend their entire life on the human scalp and feed exclusively on human blood.
- They are grey in general, but their color varies. After feeding, consumed blood causes the louse body to take on a reddish color (Fig. 29.21).
- Head lice occur more often in girls and women than in boys and men; they are unusual in African-Americans, but not in African blacks.

BODY LICE (PEDICULOSIS CORPORIS)

- Body lice are most often found in situations of poor personal hygiene, such as in homeless people.
- They are historically prevalent in war conditions.

PUBIC LICE

- **Pediculosis pubis** (also known as "**crabs**" and "**pubic lice**") is a disease caused by the pubic louse, *P. pubis,* a parasitic organism notorious for infesting human pubic hair. The species may also live on other areas with hair, including the eyelashes, causing *pediculosis ciliaris.*
- Infestation usually leads to intense itching in the pubic area.
- Pubic lice are generally transmitted by sexual contact.

CLINICAL MANIFESTATIONS

Head, Pubic, and Body Lice
- Itching is the predominant symptom.
- Affected children with head lice may be asymptomatic.
- There is a possibility of secondary infection from scratching.
- With the exception of body lice, which have historically been known to carry epidemic typhus, trench fever, and relapsing fever, lice are not known to transmit any disease.

DESCRIPTION AND DISTRIBUTION OF LESIONS

Head Lice
- There are no primary lesions; however, secondary crusts and eczematous dermatitis resulting from scratching may be present.

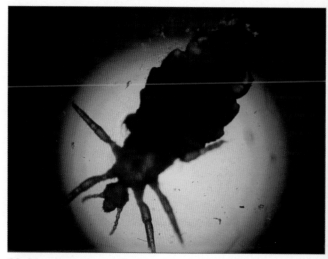

29.21   *Head louse.* The head louse is wingless insect (2.5 to 3 mm long). They are grey in general, but their color varies. After feeding, consumed blood causes the louse body to take on a reddish color.

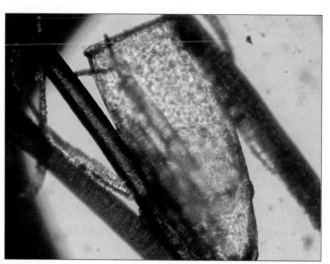

29.22   *Head louse nits.* The nits are attached to the hair shaft.

- Nits (louse eggs) are cemented to the hairs (Fig. 29.22).
- It is difficult to find living lice.
- Only the scalp is involved.

Body Lice
- Lesions begin as small papules.
- Later, secondary lesions develop from scratching and may produce crusted papules, infected papules, and ulcerations.
- Covered areas (under infested clothing) of the body may be affected.

Pubic Lice
- Small living brown lice may be seen at the base of hairs (Fig. 29.23).

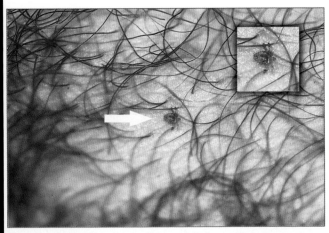

29.23 *Pubic lice.* A small brown living crab louse is seen at the base of hairs (*arrow*).

- Blue macules (*maculae ceruleae*), thought to result from enzymes present in louse saliva that breakdown bilirubin, may occur on nearby skin in chronic infestations.
- Pubic hair, eyebrows, eyelashes, and axillary hair may be infested.

DIAGNOSIS

Head Lice (see also Chapter 9)
- Knowledge of an epidemic at school generally alerts parents or school nurses to look for evidence of lice.
- A hair may be plucked and examined for nits using the low power of a microscope.
- A nit is attached to the base of a hair shaft when the egg is first laid and remains cemented to the growing hair.

Body Lice
- The diagnosis is made not from examining the patient but closely inspecting the seams of his or her clothing, where the lice are found.

Pubic Lice
- Lice may be present.
- Pruritus is noted.
- Blue macules may be seen.
- Often, a sexual partner has "crabs."

 DIFFERENTIAL DIAGNOSIS

Head Lice
Atopic Dermatitis of the Scalp
- *Should be considered if there is a positive atopic history.*

Body Lice and Pubic Lice
Atopic Dermatitis or Another Type of Eczematous Dermatitis
- *Should be considered as noted above.*

Scabies
- *Should be excluded (see above in this chapter).*

 MANAGEMENT

Head Lice
- Because head lice are predominantly an issue of school-aged children the management is presented in Chapter 9.
- Proper treatment of head lice involves the use of a pediculicide (two applications, 1 week apart) and manual nit removal.

Pubic Lice
- Topical agent such as **Elimite** (permethrin cream).
- **Kwell (Lindane) shampoo** USP 1%. Used in situations where treatment with other drugs have failed or cannot be tolerated.
- **RID** and **Nix** lotions are also effective.
- Treatment should include contacts of infested patients, especially sexual partners.

Body Lice
- A shower and clean clothing generally cure body lice.
- Clothing should be washed at hot temperatures to kill the lice.

 HELPFUL HINTS

- Shaving of pubic, scalp, or body hair is not necessary to treat lice.
- In resistant cases, particularly after repeated treatment failures, delusions of parasitosis should be considered in the differential diagnosis in adult patients.

Waterborne Stings and Seashore Infestations

JELLYFISH STINGS

BASICS

- Two types of stinging jellyfish are seen floating in the coastal waters of North America: the smaller sea nettle and the more rare, more dangerous, Portuguese man-of-war, whose poison can be fatal.
- The tentacles of jellyfish have many stinging nematocysts, which contain a hollow poisonous tip and hooks. The hooks hold the jellyfish onto the victim while the nematocysts discharge the toxic venom.

CLINICAL MANIFESTATIONS

- Victims of a common jellyfish sting usually describe a stinging or burning sensation.
- The sting of the Portuguese man-of-war is more painful than that of a jellyfish. It has been described as feeling like being struck by a lightning bolt, and some victims dread it more than a shark bite (Fig. 29.24).
- There have been reported cases of anaphylactic reactions and fatalities from both sea nettle and Portuguese man-of-war stings.

DESCRIPTION OF LESIONS

- The shape of the lesions, which resemble linear welts that develop at the site of contact, often give the victim the appearance of having been whipped (Fig. 29.25).
- Lesions may fade or may blister and become necrotic depending on the amount of injected venom and the victim's sensitivity.

DISTRIBUTION OF LESIONS

- The distribution is asymmetric and unilateral.

DIAGNOSIS

- The diagnosis is based on the reported sting occurring in an endemic area and its characteristic eruption.

 MANAGEMENT

- Mild stings may be treated symptomatically with cool soaks and topical steroids.
- For more severe reactions, the affected area should be washed with seawater, alcohol, or vinegar to remove nematocysts and to inactivate any toxins that remain.
- Topical lidocaine and hot water appear to be effective remedies against stings by jellyfish in North America and Hawaii.

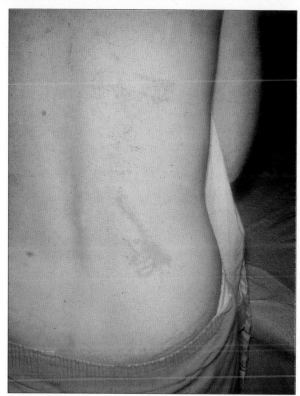

29.24 *Jellyfish sting.* Note the curvilinear, whip-like shape of the lesions.

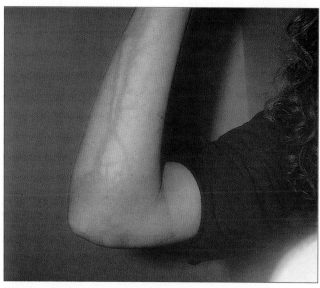

29.25 *Portuguese man-of-war sting.* Note the linear shape of the lesions. The sting of the Portuguese man-of-war is more painful than a common jellyfish sting.

 POINT TO REMEMBER

- Severe stings that result in systemic reactions may require life-support measures such as on-site resuscitation.

SEABATHER'S ERUPTION ("SEA LICE")

BASICS

- This intensely pruritic eruption develops *under* swimwear, presumably because the responsible larvae become trapped under the garments.
- The eruption occurs several minutes to 12 hours after exposure to the larvae of the thimble jellyfish (*Linuche unguiculata*) in the saltwater off the coast of Florida and in the Caribbean.
- This condition has also been noted off of coastal Long Island, New York, where it has been reputedly caused by the larvae of a sea anemone.

CLINICAL MANIFESTATIONS

- Erythematous macules and papules occur *under* swimwear (Fig. 29.26A,B). The eruption has a similar distribution as seen in hot tub folliculitis (see Fig. 16.12).
- The pruritus is worse at night and tends to prevent the patient from sleeping.
- Children may experience fever and malaise.
- Lesions last for 2 to 14 days and resolve spontaneously.

DIAGNOSIS

- The diagnosis can be made when the patient has bathed in an endemic area and displays inflammatory papules on the area covered by the bathing suit.

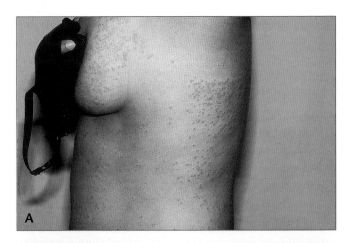

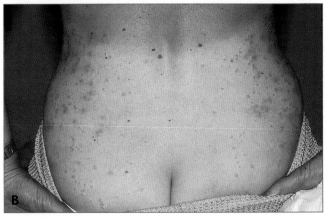

29.26 **A** and **B:** *Seabather's eruption.* This patient has just returned from bathing off the coast of Florida. The lesions are confined to the area covered by her bathing suit.

 DIFFERENTIAL DIAGNOSIS

Swimmer's Itch (Cercarial Dermatitis)
- *Occurs on **exposed sites** after freshwater swimming.*
- *Caused by Schistosoma organisms that invade the skin. These organisms are the microscopic larvae of the parasitic flatworm. After being released from host snails, the larvae swim in water until they penetrate the skin of a host such as a duck or a human.*

Other bites or stings should be considered.

 HELPFUL HINTS

- Treatment for both seabather's eruption and swimmer's itch is symptomatic.
- After bathing, immediate removal of the swimwear for washing, or rinsing of the swimwear while it is still being worn, may help prevent seabather's eruption.

CUTANEOUS LARVA MIGRANS ("CREEPING ERUPTION")

BASICS

- As the name suggests, cutaneous larva migrans is a cutaneous eruption that creeps or migrates in the skin. It results from the invasion and movement of various hookworm larvae that have penetrated the skin through the feet, hands, lower legs, or buttocks.
- *Ancylostoma braziliense, Ancylostoma caninum, Ancylostoma ceylanicum, Uncinaria stenocephala* (dog hookworm), *Bunostomum phlebotomum* (cattle hookworm), *Ancylostoma duodenale,* and *Necator americanus* are the primary hookworms that cause cutaneous larvae migrans in the United States.
- The adult hookworm (nematode) resides in the intestines of dogs, cats, cattle, and monkeys. The feces of these animals contain hookworm eggs that are deposited on sand or soil, hatch into larvae if conditions are favorable, and then penetrate human skin which serves as a "dead-end" host.
- At greatest risk are gardeners, farm workers, and people who sunbathe or walk on sandy beaches by the seashore.
- Larva currens, a distinct variant of cutaneous larva migrans, is caused by *Strongyloides stercoralis* and may produce visceral disease. Visceral larva migrans is caused by another species of hookworm.

CLINICAL MANIFESTATIONS

- This benign eruption is usually pruritic and self-limited because the larvae usually die within 4 to 6 weeks.
- Lesions have a characteristic curvilinear, serpentine shape (Fig. 29.27).
- Areas that come into contact with sand or contaminated soil, most commonly the feet (farmers) or buttocks (sunbathers on nude beaches) are affected.

DIAGNOSIS

- The diagnosis is based on the characteristic clinical appearance.
- If the patient has been vacationing on the beach in an area endemic for cutaneous larva migrans, consider the condition when diagnosing a local itchy eruption on one foot.

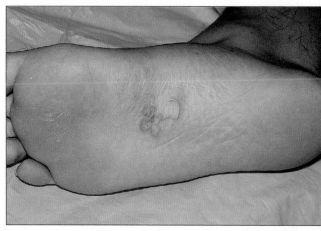

29.27 *Cutaneous larva migrans.* Note the serpiginous, erythematous, raised, tunnel-like lesions in typical locations.

 MANAGEMENT

- **Class 1 superpotent topical steroids** (e.g., clobetasol cream) for itching.
- **Topical thiabendazole** suspension (500 mg/5 mL under occlusion three times per day for 1 week).
- **Oral thiabendazole** (Mintezol; 50 mg/kg/day in two daily doses for 2 to 5 days) *or* Albendazole (400 mg daily for 3 days [this drug has fewer side effects than thiabendazole]).
- **Liquid nitrogen**, applied to the active, advancing end of the lesion.

 DIFFERENTIAL DIAGNOSIS

Granuloma Annulare
- *Lesions are annular.*
- *It lacks scale and vesicles and does not itch.*

Tinea Pedis
- *Potassium hydroxide examination is positive.*

Other Diagnoses
- *Other bites or stings (e.g., jellyfish) should be considered.*

30 Benign Cutaneous Neoplasms

OVERVIEW

Benign lesions such as melanocytic nevi (moles), skin tags, seborrheic keratoses, cherry angiomas, and epidermoid cysts are commonplace, and are consequences of the skin's normal hereditary, age-appropriate, maturation process.

Skin lesions—particularly pigmented skin lesions—often present a difficult and puzzling conundrum for the non-dermatologist health care provider. Questions such as "Am I missing a melanoma?" "Is this mole suspicious?" and "Is this a skin cancer?" may arise. In reality, the answer is not always apparent. In fact, the decision of whether a lesion is benign or malignant is often a challenge for many dermatologists as well. Distinguishing between a benign pigmented lesion such as a melanocytic nevus or a seborrheic keratosis and a potentially fatal skin cancer such as a melanoma creates the most concern among health care providers.

As with most skin lesions, familiarity breeds recognition. This chapter, along with Chapter 31, presents the various common benign and malignant neoplasms in their diverse clinical guises.

IN THIS CHAPTER...

➤ **MELANOCYTIC NEVI**

- Junctional melanocytic nevus
- Compound melanocytic nevus
- Dermal melanocytic nevus
- Blue nevus
- Halo nevus
- Spitz nevus
- Congenital melanocytic nevus (also see Chapter 1)
- Atypical melanocytic nevus (dysplastic nevus, Clark nevus)

➤ **SOLAR LENTIGO AND LENTIGO SIMPLEX**

➤ **SEBORRHEIC KERATOSIS**

- Stucco keratosis
- Dermatosis papulosa nigra
- Sign of Leser–Trélat

➤ **SKIN TAGS (ACROCHORDONS)**

➤ **SEBACEOUS HYPERPLASIA**

➤ **CYSTS**

➤ **LIPOMA**

➤ **CHONDRODERMATITIS NODULARIS HELICIS**

➤ **DERMATOFIBROMA**

➤ **FIBROUS PAPULE OF THE NOSE**

➤ **COMMON ANGIOMAS**

➤ **PYOGENIC GRANULOMA**

➤ **HYPERTROPHIC SCARS AND KELOIDS**

BASICS

- Melanocytic nevus (MN), commonly called moles or "beauty marks," are, most often, benign proliferations of normal skin components. They are composed of nevus cells that are derived from melanocytes, the pigment-producing cells that colonize the epidermis.
- The acquisition of MN is greatest in childhood and adolescence. In addition to a hereditary predisposition, there is also evidence that their onset is a response to sun exposure.
- During late adolescence and adulthood, the development of new lesions tapers off, and many existing lesions gradually lose their capacity to form melanin and become skin-colored or disappear completely.
- MN may be congenital or acquired, and they are more often noted in individuals with light or fair skin than in blacks or Asians.
- Acquired MN are sometimes associated with melanoma; however, the frequency of transformation into a melanoma is not known. Congenital nevi, on the other hand, especially when very large, hold the greater risk of malignant transformation (see discussion in Chapter 1).

JUNCTIONAL MELANOCYTIC NEVUS

- These small, macular (flat), frecklelike lesions are uniform in color. Individual lesions may be brown to dark brown to black (Fig. 30.1).
- Histologic examination reveals melanocytic nevus cells located at the dermoepidermal junction.
- Whether acquired or congenital, junctional MN are most prevalent on the face, arms, legs, trunk, genitalia, palms, and soles (Fig. 30.2).

COMPOUND MELANOCYTIC NEVUS

- Compound MN are elevated dome-shaped papules or nodules.
- Uniformly brown to dark brown, or black; they may contain hairs.

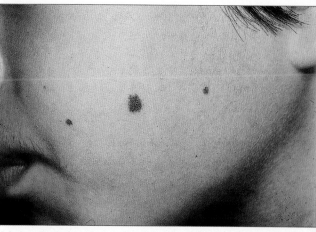

30.1 *Junctional melanocytic nevi.* These small, flat, lesions are uniform in color.

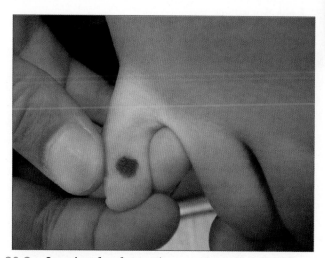

30.2 *Junctional melanocytic nevus (congenital).* This small lesion is unlikely to become malignant.

- Seen most often on the face (Figs. 30.3 and 30.4), arms, legs, and trunk.
- Their histologic findings combine features of junctional and dermal nevi.

 ### DIFFERENTIAL DIAGNOSIS

In Children
Freckles (Ephelides)
- *Small, tan macules appear on the sun-exposed skin of fair-skinned people.*
- *They darken after sun exposure and lighten when they are no longer exposed to the sun.*

In Adults
Dysplastic Nevus ([Atypical Nevus] see Discussion below)
- *Most often arise on the trunk, legs, and arms and spares the face.*

- *Usually larger than common nevi.*
- *Borders are generally irregular, notched, and ill-defined.*
- *The centers may be raised (sunny-side-up egg) appearance.*
- *Coloration (tan, brown, black, pink, or red) is irregular.*

In Adults and Elderly
Lentigo (Plural: Lentigines) or "Liver Spot" (see below)
- *Sun-exposed areas (face, flexor forearms).*

Lentigo Maligna and Melanoma (see Discussion in Chapter 31)

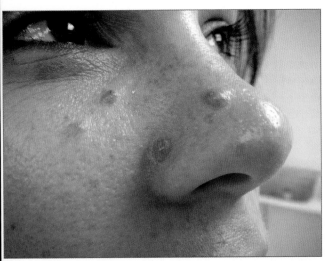

30.3 *Compound melanocytic nevi.* Elevated, dome-shaped, flesh-colored, papules.

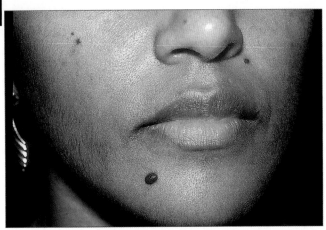

30.4 *Compound melanocytic nevi.* In individuals with dark skin, such lesions tend to be more intensely pigmented.

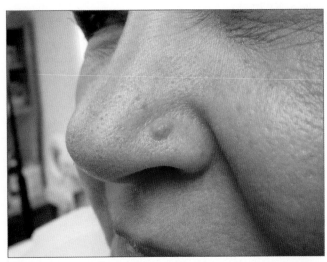

30.5 *Dermal melanocytic nevus.* Now skin-colored, old photographs demonstrate that this lesion was pigmented when the patient was in her teens and twenties.

DERMAL MELANOCYTIC NEVUS

- Dermal MN may be elevated and dome-shaped, wartlike, or pedunculated.
- Most often skin-colored, but they may also be tan or brown, or they may be dappled with pigmentation.
- Lesions tend to lose pigmentation with age and become skin-colored (Fig. 30.5).
- Most often noted on the face and neck.
- Microscopy reveals dermal MN cells located in the dermis.

CLINICAL MANIFESTATIONS OF DERMAL AND COMPOUND NEVI

- Both are asymptomatic unless irritated or inflamed.
- Very rarely do they transform into malignant melanoma.

DIAGNOSIS

- The diagnosis is based on clinical appearance or, if necessary, a histopathologic evaluation after removal.

 DIFFERENTIAL DIAGNOSIS OF DERMAL NEVUS AND COMPOUND NEVUS

Dermal nevi and compound nevi often are clinically indistinguishable from one another as well as the following:

Skin Tags (Acrochordons [see later in this chapter])
- *1- to 10-mm fleshy papules.*
- *Skin-toned, tan, or darker than the patient's skin.*
- *Most often arise on the neck, axillae, inframammary area, inguinal crease, and the eyelids.*

Seborrheic Keratosis (see later in this chapter)
- *Adults >50 years old.*
- *Warty, "stuck-on" appearance that ranges from tan to dark brown to black.*
- *Scaly, flat, or almost flat or small pigmented papules*
- *Most often are located on the back, chest, and face, the frontal hairline and scalp. They are also frequently found on the arms, legs, and abdomen.*

Basal Cell Carcinoma (see Discussion in Chapter 31)
- *Age generally >40 years old.*
- *Sun-exposed areas.*
- *Pearly papules with rolled (raised) border and telangiectases with or without ulceration.*

Angiofibroma (Fibrous Papule of the Nose [see later in this chapter])
- *Most are noted on the nose; less commonly, on the cheeks and chin.*

continued on page 453

DIFFERENTIAL DIAGNOSIS OF DERMAL NEVUS AND COMPOUND NEVUS *Continued*

- *May be difficult to distinguish from compound or dermal nevus or basal cell carcinoma.*
- *Generally dome-shaped, flesh-colored, pale, or pink firm papules with a shiny appearance.*

Neurofibroma/Neuroid Nevus
- *Very soft, flesh colored*

Nodular Melanoma (see Discussion in Chapter 31)

HELPFUL HINT

- With few exceptions such as blue nevi (discussed below), lesions that arise after the age of 30 are unlikely to be melanocytic nevi.

BLUE NEVUS

- Blue nevi are a benign variant of dermal melanocytic nevi (MN) that are heavily pigmented.
- They occur as blue-gray or blue-black macules, papules, or nodules (Fig. 30.6). They are rarely malignant.
- The dark brown pigment that creates a bluish color to these lesions is caused by the Tyndall phenomenon.
- Blue nevi usually begin to appear in adolescence, early adulthood, or middle age.

HALO NEVUS

- Halo nevi are MN that are encircled by a white halo of depigmentation. The halo represents a regression of a pre-existing nevus initiated by a lymphocytic infiltrate. Frequently, the entire nevus disappears, and the area regains normal pigmentation.
- Most often, halo nevi are initially seen on preadolescents; usually appearing on the trunk (Fig. 30.7).
- If a halo nevus is seen on an adult, two very rare possibilities should be considered: The lesion may be a melanoma or a melanoma may be present elsewhere on the body. Biopsy and removal are indicated in this situation.

SPITZ NEVUS

- These nevi are a distinctive variant of MN. In the past, they were referred to as "juvenile melanomas," but now they are mostly recognized as benign lesions in children.
- In children, the lesions may appear as pink papules or a heavily pigmented lesion that is jet black in color (see Chapter 1).
- A heavily pigmented, small, spindle-cell variant of Spitz nevus may be seen on the legs of women.

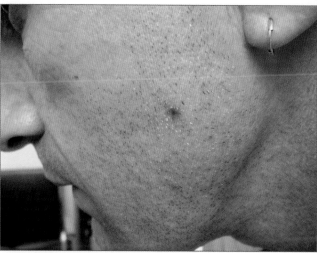

30.6 *Blue nevus.* This is a variant of melanocytic nevus. Note the characteristic blue-gray color.

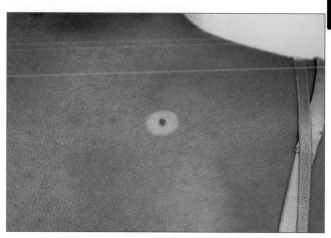

30.7 *Halo nevus.* An inflamed compound nevus has lost some of its original tan pigmentation. It is encircled by a white halo of depigmentation. Ultimately, the nevus often disappears, and the area will regain normal pigmentation.

- Treatment of Spitz nevi is controversial. Most pediatric dermatologists agree that most Spitz nevi are benign lesions; however, in adults, it is prudent to completely excise these lesions to minimize the risk of recurrence and possible confusion with a malignant lesion.

CONGENITAL MELANOCYTIC NEVUS (SEE CHAPTER 1)

- Often generating great concern in both patents and pediatricians, congenital melanocytic nevi (CMN) are MN that are present at birth or arise during the first year of life.
- By definition, CMN are present at birth or soon thereafter, although some small CMN are the so-called "tardive," and may appear as late as up to 2 years of age.
- CMN occur in about 1% of children.

MANAGEMENT OF MELANOCYTIC NEVI

- All MN should be carefully examined and biopsy should be considered, particularly if there is any suggestion of atypia clinically.
- However, for most MN, biopsy is not indicated. Persons with numerous MN, particularly atypical nevi (see later discussion), are at greater risk for developing malignant melanoma.

Indications for Removal
- Atypical appearance.
- Cosmetic reasons.
- Repeated irritation by clothing, such as a bra strap
- Persistent discomfort (e.g., a lesion that itches, hurts, or bleeds).

Methods of Removal
Lesions can be removed by shave excision (which is often followed by electrodesiccation) or by elliptic excision (see Chapter 35).

- **Shave (tangential) excision:** This method is fast and economical, and it generally provides satisfactory cosmetic results. Its disadvantage is that it often results in only partial removal of lesions, which infrequently necessitates a second excisional procedure.
- **Elliptical excision:** This technique is performed with the intent of removing lesions completely; thus surgical margins can be identified. However, an elliptical excision takes longer to do than a shave biopsy. It also requires suturing and suture removal, and it results in linear scars that may not be as cosmetically pleasing as scars that result from shave excisions.

POINTS TO REMEMBER

- Any pigmented lesion that changes rapidly in size or color or that has an atypical appearance should be removed for biopsy.
- A primary care physician should have a low threshold for referral to a dermatologist if there is any concern regarding the diagnosis and management of a pigmented lesion.
- All MN that are removed should be submitted for microscopic evaluation.
- Large CMN have a low but real risk of malignant transformation and the development of melanoma (see Chapter 1).

ATYPICAL MELANOCYTIC NEVUS (DYSPLASTIC NEVUS, CLARK NEVUS)

BASICS

- The atypical nevus, which is also called dysplastic nevus, an atypical mole, or Clark nevus, is a controversial and confusing lesion. Nevi that are clinically atypical are not always dysplastic under the microscope. Even among dermatopathologists, there is no consensus regarding the histopathologic criteria for a dysplastic nevus.
- Some individuals have only a few atypical nevi, and their risk of melanoma may not be much higher than those individuals without such nevi.
- This much is agreed: When a patient has numerous atypical nevi and there is a positive family history of melanoma, the potential for melanoma in that patient, as well as in his or her family is extremely high. Such atypical nevi may be inherited as an autosomal dominant trait (see discussion below of familial *atypical mole syndrome*).
- Atypical nevi are rarely seen in black, Asian, or Middle Eastern populations.

CLINICAL MANIFESTATIONS

Atypical nevi have some or all of the following features:

- Atypical nevi are most often found on the trunk (Fig. 30.8), legs, and arms; generally, the face is spared.
- They are usually larger than common moles and frequently measure 5 to 15 mm in diameter.
- Their borders are usually irregular, notched, and ill-defined.
- They have a macular appearance, but the centers may be raised (for this reason, they are sometimes called "sunny-side-up egg lesions") (Fig. 30.9).
- Their coloration (tan, brown, black, pink, or red) is irregular.
- The exact risk of an individual atypical nevus developing into a melanoma is uncertain.

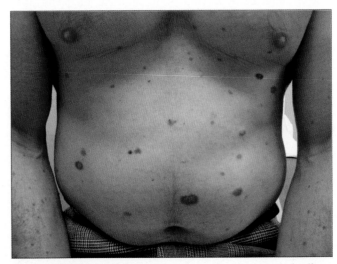

30.8 *Multiple dysplastic nevi.* Note the characteristic distribution on the trunk.

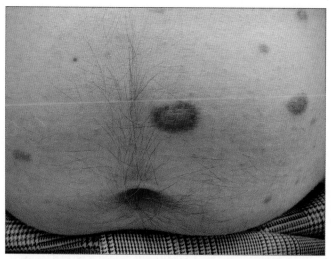

30.9 *Atypical nevus (dysplastic nevus).* **Close-up of** Figure 30.8. Note the raised center and indistinct border; such a nevus is sometimes called a "sunny-side-up egg lesion." It is generally larger than a common mole.

- Unlike dermal and compound nevi, these lesions often continue to appear into adulthood.
- Differentiating them clinically from melanoma is often difficult.

CLINICAL VARIANTS

SPORADIC ATYPICAL NEVI

- A patient with an isolated atypical nevus and no family history of multiple atypical nevi or melanoma probably carries little risk of developing melanoma and should not necessarily be identified as prone to melanoma.

MULTIPLE ATYPICAL NEVI

- The exact risk of an individual nevus developing into a melanoma is uncertain.
- In certain situations atypical nevi are considered possible precursors to, as well as potential markers for, the development of melanoma that may occur *de novo* without evolving from a precursor dysplastic nevus.

FAMILIAL ATYPICAL MOLE SYNDROME

- Those persons who meet the following criteria are considered to have an extremely high potential for developing malignant melanoma:
  1. Patients with a first-degree (e.g., parent, sibling, or child) or second-degree (e.g., grandparent, grandchild, aunt, uncle) relative who has a history of malignant melanoma have heightened risk.

2. Many nevi—often more than 50—are present, and some of them are atypical moles.
3. Having moles that show certain dysplastic features microscopically.

 DIFFERENTIAL DIAGNOSIS

Other Melanocytic Nevi (see earlier Discussion)
Malignant Melanoma
- Some or all of the A, B, C, D, E features of melanoma (see discussion in Chapter 31) may also be seen in atypical nevi.

Pigmented Basal Cell Carcinoma (see Chapter 31)
- Brownish to blue-black pigmentation are often seen in more darkly pigmented persons.

Seborrheic Keratosis (see below)
- May be indistinguishable from a nevus or a pigmented basal cell carcinoma.
- Dermoscopic evaluation of the lesion will help confirm the diagnosis.

 MANAGEMENT

- The method chosen for removing suspected atypical nevi depends on the purpose of treatment.
- If melanoma is suspected, complete excision should be performed.
- If melanoma is not suspected, the lesion can be removed and prepared for biopsy with a shave or punch biopsy technique.

Prevention
- Patients with many atypical nevi should avoid excessive sun exposure and should routinely use a broad spectrum sunscreen with a sun-protective factor of greater than 50.
- Patients who meet the criteria for familial atypical mole syndrome should examine their own skin every 2 to 3 months, in addition to having a full body examination and regular screening visits performed by a dermatologist.
- High-risk patients and their families should be taught self-examination to detect changes in existing moles and should be given printed material with photographs to help them recognize the features of malignant melanoma.

HELPFUL HINT

- Despite the fact that patients with many dysplastic nevi are at a higher risk of developing a melanoma, the notion of removing *all* of their dysplastic nevi to reduce their risk of melanoma is generally believed to be ill advised. To consider all of these nevi to be precursors of melanomas creates undo anxiety for patients but does not appear to decrease their potential for developing melanomas.

POINTS TO REMEMBER

- Once a diagnosis of multiple atypical nevi is established, other family members should be examined.
- Melanoma risk is greater in those persons who have one relative with melanoma than in those with no affected relative. The lifetime risk of melanoma may approach 100% in persons with atypical nevi who are from melanoma-prone families (i.e., individuals having two or more first-degree relatives with melanoma).
- Patients with the familial atypical mole syndrome (also known as the dysplastic nevus syndrome) should be monitored vigilantly.

 SEE PATIENT HANDOUT "Atypical Nevus (Mole)" IN THE COMPANION eBOOK EDITION.

Solar Lentigo and Lentigo Simplex

BASICS

SOLAR LENTIGO (PLURAL: LENTIGINES)

- These small, acquired tan macules, often referred to as "age" or "liver spots," occur on sun-exposed areas during middle and elderly years.
- They are uniform in color from light brown to black.
- Most often, they appear on the face (Fig. 30.10), dorsal hands (Fig. 30.11), extensor forearms, and anterior legs.
- Microscopically there is an increased number of normal melanocytes in the basal layer of the epidermis.

LENTIGO SIMPLEX

- This is the most common form of lentigo. A single lesion or multiple lesions may be present at birth or develop in early childhood.
- Darker in color than freckles, they do not further darken or increase in number on sun exposure, as do freckles.
- These lesions may occur anywhere on the skin or mucous membranes.
- Round- or oval-shaped macule(s) 3 to 15 mm in diameter.
- Multiple lentigines can occur with associated conditions such as Peutz–Jeghers syndrome.

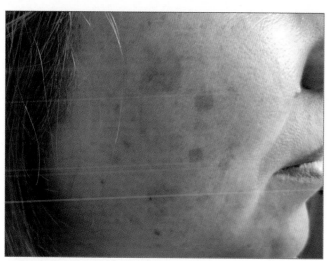

30.10 *Solar lentigines.* Note the uniformity in color of these lesions.

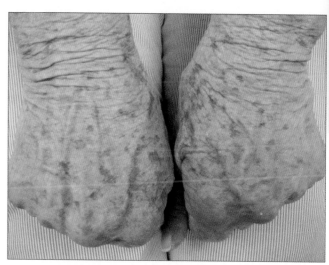

30.11 *Solar lentigines.* These extremely common tan macules arise on sun-exposed areas during middle age.

Seborrheic Keratosis

BASICS

- A seborrheic keratosis (SK) is an extremely common benign skin growth that becomes apparent in people older than 40 years of age. They are the most common neoplasm in the elderly and have virtually no malignant potential.
- The use of the word "seborrheic," a misnomer, stems from the occasional "greasy" or shiny appearance of the lesions; SKs are actually epidermal in origin, with no sebaceous derivation.
- Patients often report a positive family history of SKs; men and women are equally affected.
- SKs have been whimsically described as "barnacles in the sea of life" and "maturity spots"; these metaphors are intended to allay patients' anxieties.

CLINICAL MANIFESTATIONS

- SKs are generally asymptomatic; however, they may itch when irritated or inflamed.
- At times, they are cosmetically undesirable to the patient.
- The typical SK has a warty, "stuck-on" appearance that ranges from tan to dark brown to black.
- The appearance of individual lesions tends to vary considerably, even on the same patient.
- Lesions may be warty and tortoiseshell-like (Fig. 30.12); scaly, flat, or almost flat (Fig. 30.13); or small pigmented papules similar to skin tags (discussed below) (Fig. 30.14).
- Often the "dry," crumbly, keratotic surface of some lesions are sometimes rubbed or picked off, only to recur later.
- To the untrained eye, as well as to dermatologists, SKs can resemble melanomas since they may share similar features (i.e., they may be asymmetric, have irregular or notched borders, and vary in color [see Chapter 31]).

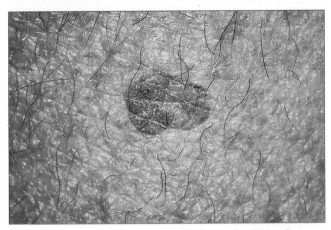

30.13 *Seborrheic keratoses.* This lesion is almost flat.

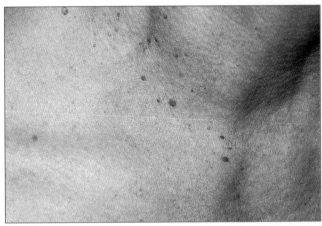

30.14 *Seborrheic keratoses.* Multiple pigmented papules, some of which are clinically indistinguishable from pigmented skin tags, are evident here.

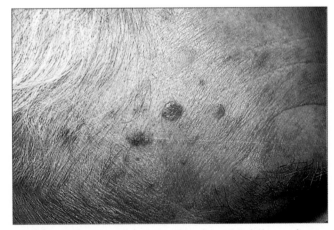

30.15 *Seborrheic keratoses.* The frontal hairline and temples are common locations.

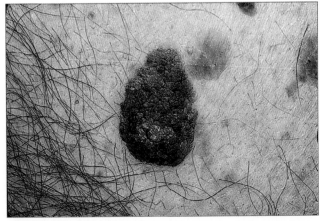

30.12 *Seborrheic keratoses.* The largest, darkest, lesion has a warty, rough-surfaced, tortoise shell–like appearance. The lesions in the background are also SKs; such lesions are unusual before 30 years of age.

DISTRIBUTION OF LESIONS

- SKs most often are located on the back, chest, and face, particularly along the frontal hairline (Fig. 30.15) and scalp.

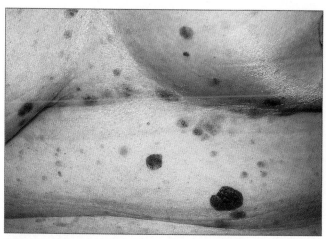

30.16 *Seborrheic keratoses.* These lesions are in a typical location. Note the different colors, sizes, and shapes of the various lesions in this patient.

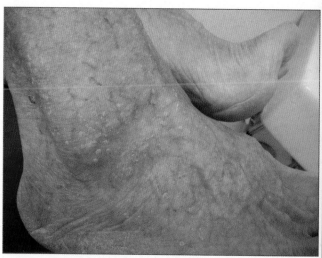

30.17 *Stucco keratoses.* These lesions have a whitish, "stuck-on" appearance. They occur especially on the dorsum of the foot and around the Achilles tendon area.

They are also frequently found on the arms, legs, and abdomen (Fig. 30.16).
- Smaller lesions similar to skin tags can be seen around the neck, under the breast, or in the axillae.
- In women, lesions are often seen under and between the breasts.
- When many lesions are present, the distribution is usually bilateral and symmetric.

CLINICAL VARIANTS

STUCCO KERATOSES

- Stucco keratoses are a nonpigmented variant of SK most often seen in the elderly.
- Stucco keratoses are skin-colored or whitish papules that become whiter and scalier when they are scratched. They typify the "dry, stuck-on" type of seborrheic keratosis.
- They are commonly found on the distal lower leg, particularly around the ankles (Fig. 30.17), less likely on the dorsal forearms.

DERMATOSIS PAPULOSA NIGRA

- This common manifestation is diagnosed primarily in African-American, Afro-Caribbean, and sub-Saharan African blacks; however, it is also seen in darker-skinned persons of other races. Lesions start appearing in adolescence and increase in number as persons age.
- Dermatosis papulosa nigra (DPN) lesions are histopathologically identical to SKs and are considered to be of autosomal dominant inheritance.
- Lesions are darkly pigmented and, in contrast to typical SKs, they have minimal, if any, scale.
- DPNs generally appear on the face, especially the upper cheeks and lateral orbital areas (Fig. 30.18).

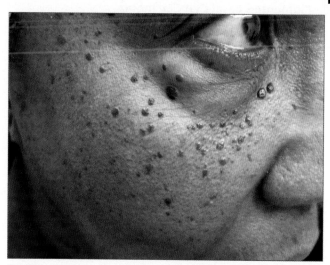

30.18 *Dermatosis papulosa nigra.* This common inherited condition appears as small, pigmented papules on the face that resemble SKs and are histologically indistinguishable from them.

SIGN OF LESER–TRÉLAT

- A condition that refers to the sudden appearance of multiple SKs in a short period or a rapid increase in their size.
- It is a rare phenomenon and is presumed by some observers to be a cutaneous sign of leukemia or internal malignant disease, especially of the gastrointestinal tract, prostate, breast, ovary, uterus, liver, or lung.
- However, in light of the frequency of malignant disease in the elderly, and the ubiquitous presence of SKs in this age group, the relationship is believed by some observers to be fortuitous.

DIAGNOSIS

- With experience, SKs are easily recognized.
- If necessary, a shave biopsy (using a no. 15 scalpel blade) or curettage may be performed for histologic confirmation (see Chapter 35).

DIFFERENTIAL DIAGNOSIS

Verruca Vulgaris (see Chapter 18)
- *An SK may be indistinguishable from a wart.*

Solar Lentigo (see above)
- *May be indistinguishable from a flat seborrheic keratosis.*

Melanocytic Nevus/Dysplastic Nevus (see earlier Discussion)

Malignant Melanoma (see Chapter 31)

Pigmented Basal Cell Carcinoma (see Chapter 31)

POINTS TO REMEMBER

- SKs are mainly a cosmetic concern, except when they are inflamed or irritated and can be an annoyance. The challenge for primary care clinicians is to distinguish these lesions from skin cancer, particularly malignant melanoma.
- Lesions may be quite numerous on some persons. Because SKs may, at times, be confused with melanoma, careful visual examination of all lesions should be performed.

MANAGEMENT

- Patients with SKs are often referred to dermatologists with a presumptive diagnosis of warts or moles or to have these lesions evaluated to rule out cancer, particularly melanoma.
- Learning to recognize SKs should obviate the need for many of these referrals. When a patient is referred, a biopsy (generally a shave biopsy) is performed if necessary to confirm the diagnosis or to distinguish SK from a pigmented basal cell carcinoma, melanocytic nevus, wart, or melanoma.
- Because some patients have numerous lesions, it is an impractical expenditure of time and money to perform multiple biopsies of lesions, as long as the clinical appearance is typical.
- An excisional biopsy should always be performed whenever malignant melanoma is suspected.

Treatment
- **Cryosurgery** is performed with liquid nitrogen spray, cotton swab application, or light electrocautery and curettage (treating the base of the lesion helps to prevent recurrence).
- **Excisional surgery**, which results in scar formation, is unnecessary, unless the clinical appearance is suggestive of a malignant disease such as melanoma.

HELPFUL HINT

- SKs present in many shapes, colors, and sizes. It is a good idea to become familiar with these lesions by consistently examining the skin of all adult patients.

BASICS

- These benign skin lesions are extremely common. They are sometimes referred to as *acrochordons, fibroepithelial polyps,* or, if large, *soft fibromas* or *pedunculated lipofibromas.* They are commonly seen in the body folds of many adults as well as obese individuals.
- Skin tags were formerly suspected by several investigators to be markers for intestinal polyps or, possibly, internal malignant diseases, but current evidence suggests that this association is not justifiable.

CLINICAL MANIFESTATIONS

- Skin tags are generally 1- to 10-mm fleshy papules.
- They may be skin-toned, tan, or darker than the patient's skin. They are sessile or pedunculated in shape.
- Skin tags are primarily of cosmetic concern; however, they may become a nuisance from the irritation of necklaces and underarm shaving, for example.
- In women, they tend to grow larger and more numerous over the course of a pregnancy.
- They are often seen in association with acanthosis nigricans (see Chapter 23).

DISTRIBUTION OF LESIONS

- They are most often found on the neck (Fig. 30.19), the axillae, the inframammary area, the groin (especially the inguinal creases), the upper thighs, and the eyelids (Fig. 30.20).

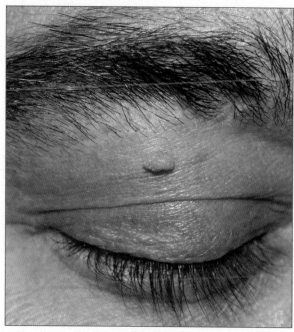

30.20 *Skin tag (acrochordon).* A solitary, skin-colored skin tag is present on the eyelid.

DIAGNOSIS

- Skin tags are easy to recognize; a skin biopsy is rarely necessary.

DIFFERENTIAL DIAGNOSIS

Small Pedunculated SKs (see Fig. 30.14)

Compound or Dermal Nevus (see earlier in this chapter)

Neurofibroma
- *Very soft upon palpation.*

MANAGEMENT

- Small skin tags are easily removed by snipping them off at their base using iris scissors, with or without prior local anesthesia (see Chapter 35). The crushing action of the scissors results in little bleeding or pain.
- Skin tags, if disregarded, occasionally may spontaneously self-destruct. After torsion, they become necrotic and autoamputate.

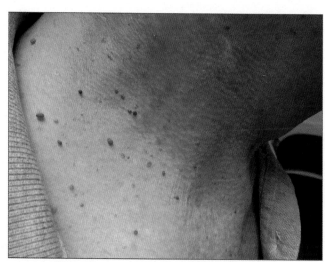

30.19 *Skin tags (acrochordons).* Pigmented papules are present around this patient's neck.

HELPFUL HINT

- A rapid and painless treatment for small skin tags is to dip a needle holder or nontoothed forceps into liquid nitrogen for 5 to 10 seconds and then gently grasp each skin tag for about 5 to 10 seconds. There is little or no collateral damage, just a narrow rim of erythema.

Multiple lesions can be treated using this method. The frozen skin tag will be shed in approximately 10 days. This is a good approach for skin tags hanging on the eyelids (Figs. 30.21A,B and 30.22).

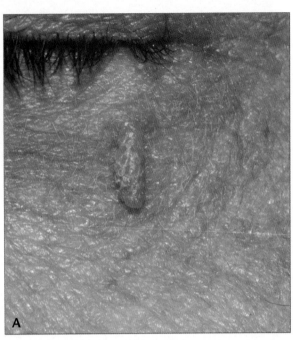

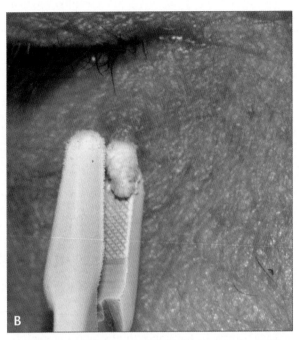

30.21   **A** and **B:** *Pedunculated fibroepithelioma (skin tag).* **A:** Skin tag on lower eyelid. **B:** Treatment is performed with liquid nitrogen. Frost appears at the tip of the needle holder and on the skin tag. The frozen skin tag will be shed in 7 to 10 days.

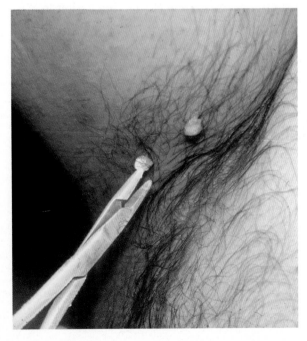

30.22   *Skin tags (acrochordons).* Axillary lesions treated with liquid nitrogen.

BASICS

- Sebaceous hyperplasia refers to small, benign papules on the face of adults representing hypertrophy of the sebaceous glands.
- These fairly common lesions are often confused with basal cell carcinomas.

CLINICAL MANIFESTATIONS

- Lesions are asymptomatic but are of cosmetic concern to some patients.
- Lesions typically occur on the forehead and cheeks.
- Lesions are yellow or cream-colored papules are often doughnut-shaped with a dell (umbilication) in the center (Fig. 30.23) and are generally small ~1 to 3 mm in diameter.
- Telangiectasias radiate in a spoke-like fashion (Fig. 30.24).

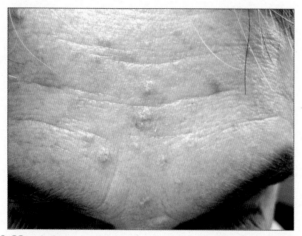

30.23 Sebaceous hyperplasia. Multiple yellowish papules are present. Note the central dell and telangiectasias.

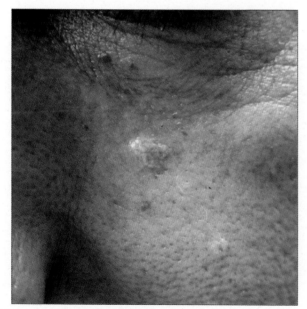

30.24 Sebaceous hyperplasia. Compare vessels to those of basal cell carcinoma (see Fig. 31.23).

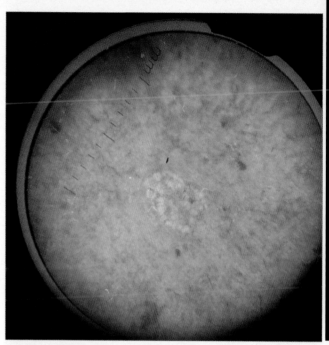

30.25 Sebaceous hyperplasia. This is a 10× magnification of Figure 30.24 above visualized with a dermoscope. This demonstrates the "popcorn-like" appearance. The dermoscope allows inspection of skin lesions unobstructed by skin surface reflections.

DIAGNOSIS

- The diagnosis is made by the lesion's typical clinical appearance (little bagels).
- "Popcorn" appearance on dermoscopy (Fig. 30.25).
- Biopsy is indicated if basal cell carcinoma is suspected.

👤 DIFFERENTIAL DIAGNOSIS

Basal Cell Carcinoma (see Chapter 31)
- *Telangiectasias are more tortuous, "hairpin" shaped.*

🛠 MANAGEMENT

- The patient should be reassured about the benign nature of this condition.
- If desired, light electrocautery, shave biopsy, or laser ablation may be performed to remove lesions, although, these lesions tend to recur.

Cysts

BASICS

- A cyst is a sac containing semisolid or liquid material. The sac contains keratin and lipid-rich debris and has an epithelial lining that produces keratin.
- Cysts tend to be hereditary, arise in adulthood, and may occur as multiple lesions.
- **Epidermoid cysts** (Fig. 30.26), are commonly, but erroneously, termed "sebaceous cysts" are the most common type. They are derived from the epithelium of the hair follicle and connect to the surface of the skin with a keratin-filled central pore that looks like a blackhead.
- **Pilar cysts** (Fig. 30.27), the second most common type, have a thicker wall that develops from a stratified epithelium. Pilar cysts lack a central pore.
- **Scrotal** (Fig. 30.28) and **vulvar cysts** are also commonly seen.

CLINICAL MANIFESTATIONS

- Cysts are usually asymptomatic, unless inflamed or infected; consequently, they may become tender and painful (Fig. 30.29).
- More often, they are of cosmetic concern to the patient.
- Lesions appear as smooth, discrete, freely movable, dome-shaped nodules.
- Cysts that have previously been infected, ruptured, drained, or scarred may be firmer to palpation and less freely movable.
- Lesions range from 0.5 to 5.0 cm in diameter.
- A cheesy-white, malodorous keratin material can be expressed from the central pore.
- Pilar cysts are generally devoid of overlying scalp hair.
- Scrotal and pilar cysts may calcify.

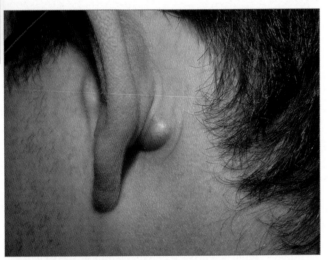

30.26 *Epidermoid cyst.* The retroauricular area is a common site for cysts to appear.

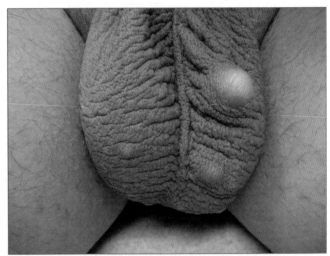

30.28 *Scrotal cysts.* Epidermoid cysts can be white, skin-colored or yellow, as seen on the scrotum.

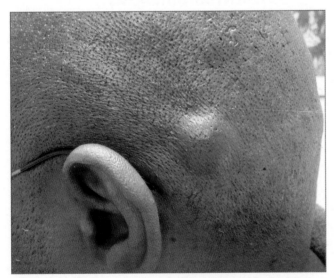

30.27 *Pilar cyst.* Note the absence of hair. The pressure from the enlarging cyst has destroyed the hair follicles. These lesions are freely movable.

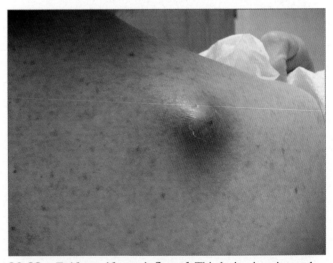

30.29 *Epidermoid cyst, inflamed.* This lesion is quite tender.

DISTRIBUTION OF LESIONS

- Epidermoid cysts occur most often on the face, behind the ears, and on the neck, trunk, scrotum, and labia.
- Pilar cysts are most often located on the scalp.

DIAGNOSIS

- On palpation, an intact epidermoid or pilar cyst feels smooth; when compressed, it feels like one's eyeball or a fully expanded balloon (Fig. 30.30A,B).
- If necessary, a biopsy or an incision and drainage can be performed to confirm the diagnosis.

CLINICAL VARIANTS

MILIA (SEE ALSO IN CHAPTER 2)

- Milia (singular, milium) are extremely common epidermal cysts that contain keratin.
- They can occur in people of any age. They may arise in traumatic scars or in association with certain scarring skin conditions, such as porphyria cutanea tarda.
- Benign, asymptomatic.
- 1 to 2 mm in diameter and are white to yellow (Figs. 30.31 and 30.32).
- Milia are most often noted on the face, especially around the eyes and on the cheeks and forehead.

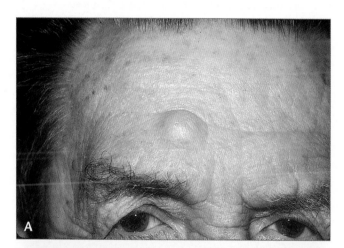

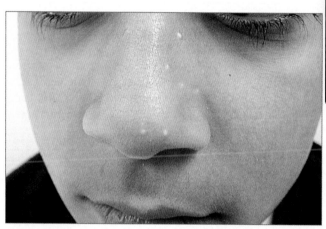

30.31 *Milia.* These epidermal cysts contain keratin. They are 1 to 2 mm in diameter and are white to yellow.

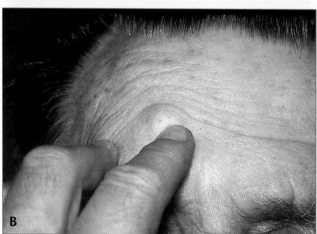

30.30 A and B: *Clinical diagnosis of an epidermoid cyst.* They appear as smooth, discrete, freely movable, dome-shaped ballotable masses. A: Cyst. B: Compression of the lesion, which has the same consistency as an eyeball or a fully inflated balloon.

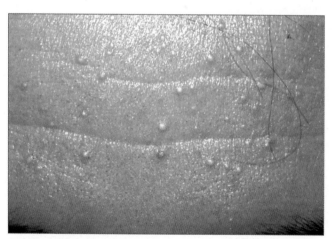

30.32 *Milia.* These lesions are often mistaken for the closed comedones of acne ("whiteheads").

DIFFERENTIAL DIAGNOSIS CYSTS AND MILIA

Lipoma (see below)

- *Should be considered when cyst-like lesions are found on the trunk, the back of the neck, and extremities. However, the consistency of a lipoma is rubbery and somewhat softer when palpated than that of a cyst. Lipomas are also irregular in shape.*

Closed Comedones

- *Milia are often mistaken for closed comedones of acne ("whiteheads").*

POINT TO REMEMBER

- Erythematous, tender, or draining epidermal and pilar cysts are often misdiagnosed as being infected rather than inflamed, and patients are often treated unnecessarily with oral antibiotics.

MANAGEMENT

Epidermoid and Pilar Cysts
Options

- **No treatment** and reassure the patient of the benign nature of these lesions.
- **Total surgical excision** that includes the cyst wall and its contents.
- **Incision and drainage:** An alternative approach is to create a small aperture in the cyst by a punch biopsy tool or no. 11 blade followed by extrusion of the cyst contents, and, if possible, much or all of the cyst wall (see Chapter 35). The entire cyst wall does not have to be completely removed to prevent recurrence.
- Incision and drainage of an inflamed tender or infected cyst may be performed with a no. 11 blade, followed by drainage and packing with iodoform gauze.
- The contents of inflamed or so-called "infected" cysts are most often sterile or contain normal skin flora; thus pre- or postoperative antibiotics are probably unnecessary.

Milia

- In contrast to closed comedones (which they resemble), milia must first be incised (usually with a no. 11 blade) before their contents can be expressed.
- Alternatively, they can be destroyed with light electrodesiccation.

BASICS

- A lipoma is a benign, slowly growing subcutaneous tumor composed of fat cells. They generally arise in young adults and are uncommon in children.

CLINICAL MANIFESTATIONS

- With the exception of **Dercum disease** and **angiolipomas** (see below), lipomas are asymptomatic.
- Rubbery, lobulated subcutaneous nodules of 2 to 10 cm in diameter (Fig. 30.33).
- Solitary lipomas are more common in females.
- Multiple lipomas are most common in males.
- Overlying skin is normal and not connected to lipoma.
- **Dercum disease** is a syndrome of multiple tender lipomas that develop in middle-aged women.
- **Angiolipomas** may be tender or painful (Fig. 30.34).
- Lipomas occur most commonly on the trunk, the back of the neck, the upper arms, and the forearms.

DIAGNOSIS

- The diagnosis is made on clinical grounds.
- A biopsy should be performed if the diagnosis is uncertain. Pathology appears as normal fat.

DIFFERENTIAL DIAGNOSIS

Cysts

- *As noted earlier, a lipoma may be confused with an epidermoid cyst; however, the latter has semi-solid contents and "feels like an eyeball."*

MANAGEMENT

- Lesions may be ignored, excised, or evacuated using liposuction

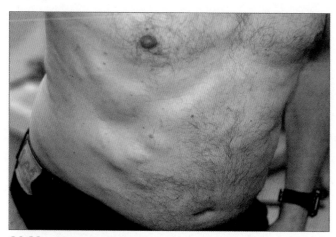

30.33 *Lipomas.* Multiple, rubbery, flesh-colored nodules are palpable on this patient.

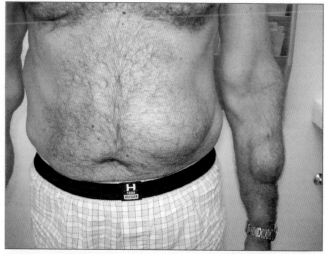

30.34 *Angiolipomas.* This patient has tender, tumor-sized, fatty subcutaneous lesions.

Chondrodermatitis Nodularis Helicis

BASICS

- Chondrodermatitis nodularis helicis (CNH) is a relatively common, benign, tender inflammatory condition of the apex of the helix or on the antihelix (inner cartilage) of the ear.
- Lesions typically arise on the lateral rim of the helix.
- CNH is characterized by one or more spontaneously appearing tender papules.
- Occurs most commonly in fair-skinned individuals who have severely sun-damaged skin.
- CNH can occur in patients at any age but mostly affects middle-aged to older individuals. It more often occurs in men; 10% to 35% of cases involve women. Age at onset is similar in men and women.
- Spontaneous resolution is unusual; the condition often continues unless treated.
- The cause of CNH is unknown.
- Neural hyperplasia and a secondary perichondritis probably account for the tenderness associated with this condition.

CLINICAL MANIFESTATIONS

- The onset of CNH may be precipitated by pressure, trauma, or cold. Sleeping on the affected side or holding a telephone instrument to the involved ear can be quite painful.
- The nodule—actually papular in size—usually enlarges rapidly to a maximum size, approximately 4 to 8 mm, and remains stable.
- Firm, often quite tender, well demarcated, and round to oval with a raised, rolled edge, and central ulcer or crust (Fig. 30.35).
- Most often seen as a tender papule(s) on the apex of the helix of the ear.
- Lesions on the antihelix (Fig. 30.36) are more commonly seen in women.

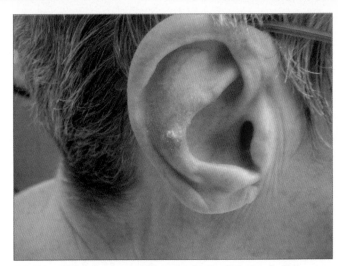

30.36 *Chondrodermatitis nodularis chronica helicis.* This tender papule with surrounding erythema is located on the antihelix.

 DIFFERENTIAL DIAGNOSIS (SEE ALSO CHAPTER 31)

Actinic Keratosis
- *Nontender papule on top rim of helix.*
- *Rough textured.*

Keratoacanthoma
- *Nontender nodule with central hyperkeratosis (volcano-like).*

Squamous Cell Carcinoma
- *May be indistinguishable from an actinic keratosis (AK).*

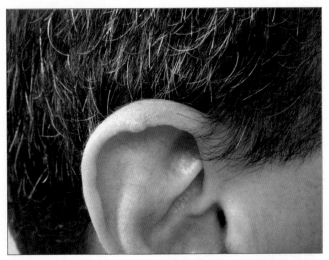

30.35 *Chondrodermatitis nodularis chronica helicis.* This tender papule is located on the lateral margin of the helix.

MANAGEMENT

- Intralesional injections of steroids such as triamcinolone (**Kenalog**; 20 to 40 mg/mL) (Fig. 30.37) may relieve discomfort and result in resolution. Several visits for these injections may be necessary.
- If the patient sleeps on the affected side, changing sides or using pressure-relieving pillows or pads may be helpful.
- Biopsy is indicated if the diagnosis is in doubt.
- If conservative methods to relieve symptoms are unsuccessful, surgical approaches are almost always needed.
- Wedge excision, curettage, electrocauterization, carbon dioxide laser ablation, and excision of the involved skin and cartilage are often curative.

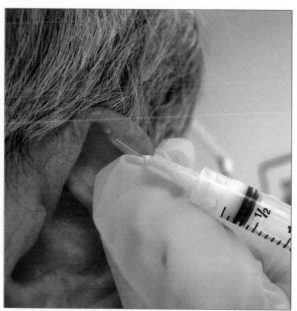

30.37 *Chondrodermatitis nodularis chronica helicis.* Treatment with intralesional triamcinolone is sometimes effective in relieving tenderness and may result in resolution of this lesion.

 HELPFUL HINTS

- Most often the patient with CNH seeks medical attention because of the pain associated with the skin lesion(s). In contrast, the cutaneous tumors listed in the differential diagnosis of CNH are usually painless and nontender.
- Actinic keratoses, basal cell carcinomas, squamous cell carcinomas, and keratoacanthomas typically arise on the sun-exposed *top rim* of the helix, whereas CNH lesions are generally found on the *lateral* rim of the helix (see Fig. 30.35).

BENIGN CUTANEOUS NEOPLASMS

Dermatofibroma

BASICS

- Also known *as fibrous histiocytoma* and *sclerosing hemangioma,* a dermatofibroma (DF) is a common dermal fibrous tumor of unknown cause.
- DFs occur most commonly on the legs, trunk, and arms, especially in women older than 20 years of age. The lesions are benign growths that are usually brought to medical attention either to rule out skin cancer or because of cosmetic concerns.

CLINICAL MANIFESTATIONS

- Generally asymptomatic.
- A lesion may be a papule or a nodule. It may be elevated with a dome shape, flat, or depressed below the plane of the surrounding skin (Fig. 30.38).
- The color can vary, even in a single lesion, and can appear as skin-colored, chocolate brown, red, or even purple.
- The surface may be smooth or scaly, depending on whether the lesion has been traumatized (e.g., by shaving).

DIAGNOSIS

- Typically, a dermatofibroma feels like a firm, pea-sized, buttonlike papule that is fixed to the surrounding dermis (accounting for the "dimple" or "collar button" sign) (Fig. 30.39A,B).
- It is freely movable over deeper adipose tissue.

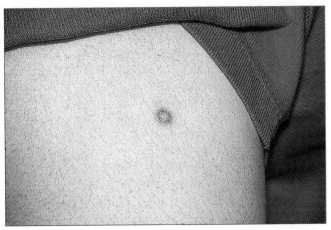

30.38 *Dermatofibroma.* This pigmented, firm papule is a very common finding on the extremities in many patients.

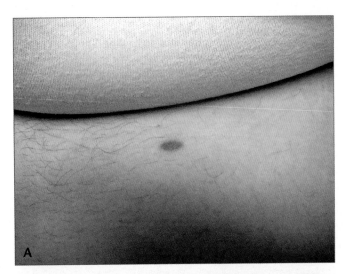

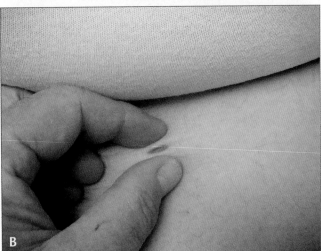

30.39 **A** and **B:** *Dermatofibroma.* **A:** This papule is in a typical location. **B:** Note the "dimple" or "collar button" (retraction) sign that is elicited on compression of the lesion.

 DIFFERENTIAL DIAGNOSIS

Cysts and Lipomas
- *Compressible or feel rubbery on palpation*

Melanocytic Nevus
- *Not firm as dermatofibromas*

Melanoma (Nodular Type)
- *Is more variable in shape and size than a dermatofibroma*

Dermatofibrosarcoma Protuberans
- *This is a locally aggressive tumor with a high recurrence rate. Dermatofibrosarcoma Protuberans (DFSP) is an uncommon soft tissue neoplasm with intermediate- to low-grade malignancy; metastases rarely occur.*

MANAGEMENT

- No treatment is necessary; however, local excision can be performed for biopsy confirmation or cosmetic concerns, or if the lesion is symptomatic.
- Deep shave excision is another alternative; however, the lesion may recur.

 HELPFUL HINTS

- If there is any doubt about the diagnosis, a biopsy should be performed.
- The patient should be informed that if the lesion is removed, the scar may be more cosmetically objectionable than the original lesion.

Fibrous Papule of the Nose

BASICS

- A fibrous papule of the nose is a relatively common benign lesion that may be difficult to distinguish from a compound or dermal nevus; furthermore, it may resemble a basal cell carcinoma.

CLINICAL MANIFESTATIONS

- Asymptomatic.
- Generally they are dome-shaped, pale or pink firm papules with a shiny appearance. They usually range from 1 to 5 mm in diameter (Fig. 30.40).
- Lesions appear in late adolescence or adulthood most often as a single lesion, but, occasionally, several lesions may be present.
- Most are noted on the nose; less commonly, they are found on the cheeks and chin.

DIAGNOSIS

- Histopathology reveals a combined vascular and fibrous proliferation.

 DIFFERENTIAL DIAGNOSIS

Melanocytic Nevus (see earlier in this chapter)
- *Compound or dermal nevi are typically "old" lesions that have been present since adolescence.*

Basal Cell Carcinoma (see Chapter 31)
- *Typically have "pearly", shiny, semi-translucent, color; a rolled (raised) border, telangiectasias, a possible history of bleeding, and ulceration.*

 MANAGEMENT

- No treatment is necessary.
- A shave biopsy if the diagnosis is in doubt or to rule out a basal cell carcinoma.
- They may also be removed for cosmetic reasons.

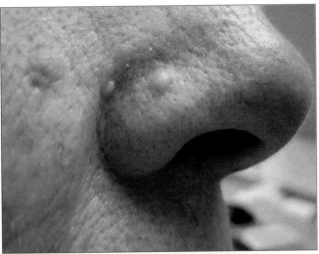

30.40 *Fibrous papules (angiofibromas, fibrous papules of the nose).* These are dome-shaped, pale or pink, firm papules with a shiny appearance and may be difficult to distinguish from compound or dermal nevi. They often may resemble a basal cell carcinoma.

Common Angiomas

BASICS

- There are various kinds of benign vascular growths that consist of small blood vessels. These neoplasms can be located anywhere on the body. Some of the different types include spider angiomas, cherry angiomas, and angiokeratomas.

CLINICAL VARIANTS

CHERRY ANGIOMAS

- Also known as Campbell De Morgan spots, ruby spots, and senile angiomas; cherry angiomas are extremely common benign vascular neoplasms.
- They are asymptomatic, easily diagnosed, cherry- to plum-colored papules that develop primarily on the trunk (Fig. 30.41).
- The angiomas are found in fair-skinned adults older than 40 years of age.

VENOUS LAKES

- Venous lakes (venous varices) are another common benign vascular neoplasm. They are generally macules or papules that are dark blue to purple and may be seen on the lower lip (Fig. 30.42), face, ears (Fig. 30.43), and eyelids.
- The lesions usually occur in patients older than 60 years of age.

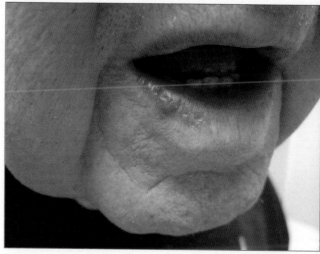

30.42 *Venous lake.* This is a common lesion among seniors. If a patient is concerned about its appearance, the lesion can be removed with electrocautery or laser destruction. They appear on the lower lip and on the external ears.

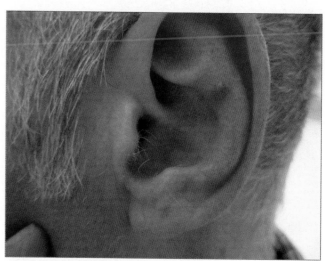

30.43 *Venous lake.* This lesion is located on the antihelix of this patient.

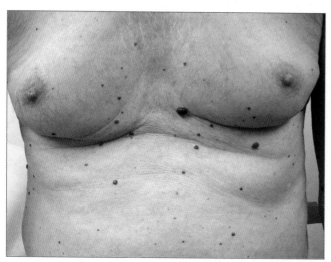

30.41 *Multiple cherry angiomas.* These cherry- and plum-colored papules are common in fair-skinned persons older than 40 years of age.

ANGIOKERATOMA (FORDYCE ANGIOKERATOMA)

- Angiokeratomas are most often found on the scrotum (Fig. 30.44) or vulva (Fig. 30.45), and they consist of multiple red-purple asymptomatic papules ("caviar spots").
- They are usually first noticed in young adulthood.

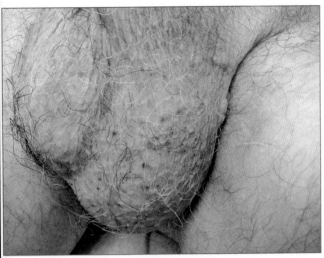

30.44 *Angiokeratomas.* These red-purple papules are most often found on the scrotum; they are usually first noticed when the patient is a young adult.

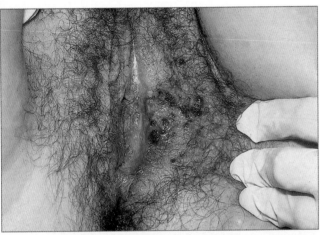

30.45 *Angiokeratomas.* Lesions are seen here on the vulva.

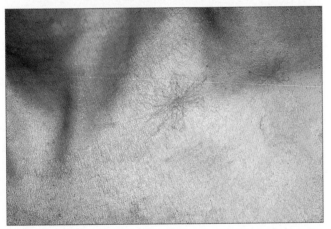

30.46 *Spider angioma.* This lesion is actually a cluster of telangiectasias radiating from a central arteriole. Compression of the central arteriole completely blanches the lesion.

SPIDER ANGIOMA (SPIDER TELANGIECTASIA)

- A spider angioma is a cluster of telangiectasias, or dilated capillaries, that radiate from a central arteriole (Fig. 30.46).
- More commonly seen in women and may be associated with pregnancy or oral contraceptive use, spider angiomas are also seen in patients with hyperestrogenic conditions, such as chronic liver disease. They may also arise in healthy children.
- Lesions appear as spoke-like capillaries radiating from a slightly raised central arteriole. Compression of the central arteriole completely blanches the lesions.
- Spider angiomas most often occur on the face and trunk. Lesions are asymptomatic and are primarily of cosmetic concern.

DIAGNOSIS

- The diagnosis of all these lesions is usually made clinical grounds.

 MANAGEMENT

- Reassure the patient that the lesions are benign.
- If the lesions are a cosmetic concern, they may be treated with electrocautery, cryosurgery with liquid nitrogen, or laser therapy.
- Spider angiomas often regress spontaneously, especially in children.
- Other types of telangiectasias may serve as a clue to an underlying collagen vascular disease, such as the periungual telangiectasias of systemic lupus erythematosus and dermatomyositis or the telangiectasias seen in scleroderma and the CREST syndrome (*C*alcinosis, *R*aynaud's phenomenon, *E*sophageal motility disorders, *S*clerodactyly, and *T*elangiectasia) (see Chapter 33).

Pyogenic Granuloma

BASICS

- A pyogenic granuloma (PG) is a common vascular hyperplasia that arises on the skin and mucous membranes. PGs are most often in children and young adults.
- Lesions may also arise during pregnancy (such a lesion is known as a *granuloma gravidarum*). PGs are also associated with oral contraceptive use.
- The cause of PGs is unknown, but minor trauma and hormonal factors appear to be factors in their development.

CLINICAL MANIFESTATIONS

- PG lesions are benign, rapidly developing, red, purple, or red-brown, dome-shaped papules or nodules. They resemble hemangiomas or granulation tissue ("proud flesh").
- Lesions are asymptomatic but tend to readily bleed after minor trauma.
- PGs are generally solitary and range in size from a few millimeters to 3 to 4 cm in diameter (Fig. 30.47).
- The bases of lesions are often surrounded by a collarette of skin.
- PG papules or nodules may be crusted.
- PGs most frequently occur at sites of minor trauma, such as the fingers (Fig. 30.48) and toes, but they also may be seen on the trunk.
- During pregnancy, lesions tend to occur on the lips (Fig. 30.49), gums, and buccal mucosa. Spontaneous resolution often occurs after childbirth.

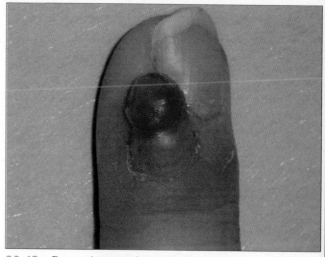

30.48 *Pyogenic granuloma.* The fingers and toes are common sites where PGs tend to arise.

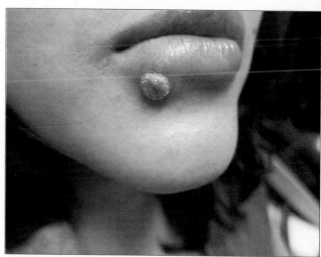

30.49 *Pyogenic granuloma.* This patient is pregnant (see also Fig. 32.5).

DIAGNOSIS

- The diagnosis is usually based on the typical clinical appearance or a shave biopsy, if necessary.

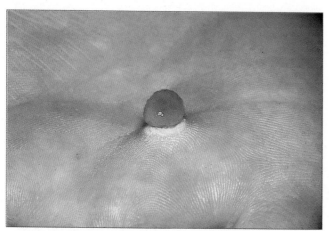

30.47 *Pyogenic granuloma.* This patient has a typical dusky red nodule with a collarette of skin. These lesions tend to bleed when traumatized.

DIFFERENTIAL DIAGNOSIS

In Children and Adults
Hemangioma (see Chapter 1)

In Adults
Nodular (Amelanotic) Melanoma
- *Blue, blue–black, or nonpigmented.*
- *May ulcerate and bleed with minor trauma.*
- *May be indistinguishable from a PG.*

Kaposi Sarcoma (see Chapter 33)
- *Lesions most commonly asymptomatic violaceous macules, papules, or nodules.*
- *Most arise acrally: on the nose, penis, and extremities.*
- *May be disseminated in advanced HIV infection; localized to lower legs in classic Kaposi sarcoma.*

 MANAGEMENT

- If there is any doubt about the diagnosis, a biopsy should be performed.
- The lesion is generally destroyed by electrocautery, curettage, laser therapy, cryosurgery, or excisional surgery. Recurrences may occur if the lesion is not completely removed.

 POINT TO REMEMBER

- The clinical presentation of a rapidly developing, friable, vascular lesion in a child or pregnant woman suggests a PG.

Hypertrophic Scars and Keloids

BASICS

- A hypertrophic scar is defined as a widened or unsightly scar that does not extend beyond the original boundaries of the original injury. Hypertrophic scars appear within weeks of skin injury.
- A keloid is an overgrowth of dense fibrous tissue, a scar whose size far exceeds that which would be expected from the extent and margins of an injury to the skin. Keloid, derived from the Greek *chele* (crab's claw), describes the lateral growth of tissue into unaffected skin.
- Hypertrophic scars and keloids represent an exaggerated formation of scar tissue in response to skin injuries such as lacerations, insect bites, ear piercing, and surgical wounds.
- Such scars may also result from healed inflammatory lesions (e.g., acne, chickenpox) (Fig. 30.50).
- In recent years, the popularity of skin piercing procedures and tattooing has increased the frequency of these undesirable scars and has expanded the sites on the body where they may occur.
- Exaggerated scars occur less frequently at the extremes of age—the very young and elderly—however, increasing numbers of presternal keloids, as well as hypertrophic scars may be seen in older age groups and result from coronary artery bypass surgery or intravenous Port-A-Caths (peripherally inserted central venous catheters) used to deliver fluids and medications.
- Keloids are more likely to occur in Hispanics, Asians, and particularly individuals of African descent than in Caucasians. There is no racial preponderance noted with hypertrophic scarring.

PATHOGENESIS

- In susceptible individuals an overproduction of collagen becomes piled up in fibrous masses resulting in an exaggerated formation of scar tissue.

- **Hypertrophic scars:** Scanning electron microscopy reveals flattened collagen bundles that are parallel in orientation.
- **Keloid:** Unlike hypertrophic scar formation, the electron microscope reveals a number of distinguishing features, including randomly organized collagen fibers in a dense connective tissue matrix.

CLINICAL MANIFESTATIONS

- Hypertrophic scars and keloids are firm, flesh-colored, tan, shiny, hairless papules, nodules, or tumors.
- If lesions are inflamed or are of recent onset, they may be red (erythematous) or purple (violaceous).
- Both hypertrophic scars and keloids may be tender, painful, or pruritic; however, keloids, by virtue of their excessive size, are generally more problematic and are of much greater cosmetic concern to patients.
- Unlike keloids, the hypertrophic scar reaches a certain size and subsequently stabilizes or regresses, whereas keloids do not regress without treatment and tend to recur after excision.
- Both hypertrophic scars and keloids tend to arise in the same anatomic locations: the sternum (Fig. 30.51), the shoulders, the deltoid region of the upper arm, and the upper back.
- The most common sites on the head and neck are the earlobes, mandibular border, and posterior neck. The earlobe is typically affected secondary to earring posts (Figs. 30.52 and 30.53).

DIAGNOSIS

- The diagnosis of hypertrophic scars and keloids is made on the basis of clinical appearance.

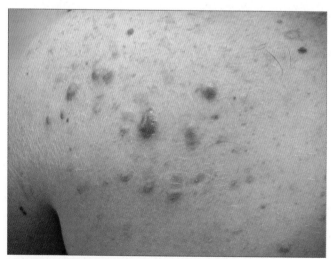

30.50 *Hypertrophic scars.* The scars on this boy's shoulders resulted from scarring acne lesions.

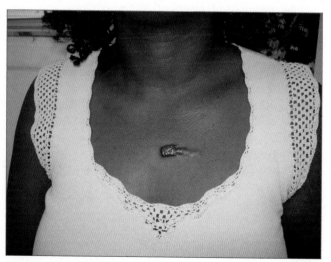

30.51 *Keloid.* This presternal lesion is a very common site for keloids to emerge.

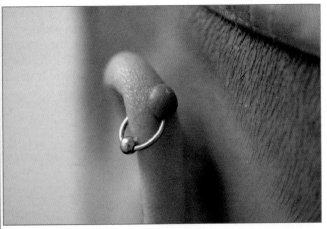

30.52 *Keloid.* Sites of ear piercing is a common location. This violaceous lesion is inflamed.

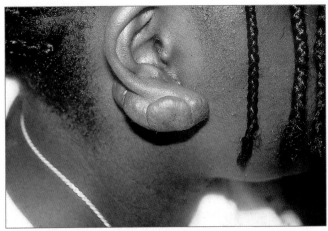

30.53 *Keloid.* This lesion was also caused by earlobe piercing. Large lesions such as this are more likely to occur in African Americans.

 MANAGEMENT

Prevention

- Prevention is essential. Patients who tend to develop hypertrophic scars or keloids should be advised to discontinue or avoid repetitive skin trauma such as tattooing and skin piercing, particularly in areas that are prone to abnormal scarring such as the presternal areas and earlobes.
- Conditions such as inflammatory acne and cutaneous infections should be treated promptly to prevent scarring. Despite preventive measures, keloids may form in simple clean wounds or may occur in the absence of trauma.

Treatment

Hypertrophic Scars

- **Intralesional corticosteroids** with triamcinolone acetate (ILTAC) in varying concentrations (5 to 40 mg/mL) are injected directly into the scar (Fig. 30.54); this has been the mainstay of treatment for hypertrophic scars and keloids. Use of a 25- to 27-gauge needle at 4- to 6-week intervals often helps flatten the lesions. Additionally, these injections are also useful for diminishing itching and tenderness. Side effects from these injections include hypopigmentation, atrophy, and telangiectasias (Fig. 30.55).
- **Topical corticosteroids:** A clear surgical tape (Cordran Tape) that is uniformly impregnated with flurandrenolide, a corticosteroid, has been shown to soften and flatten keloids over time.
- **Pulsed-dye lasers** have been used successfully and safely on some persistent hypertrophic scars.
- If they are in amenable locations, hypertrophic scars can sometimes be removed by **simple excision**, provided that wound closure can occur without undue tension on the surgical site.

Keloids

- As described above, intralesional corticosteroid injections directly into keloids are utilized; however, there is a high recurrence rate after treatment. As with hypertrophic scars, intralesional triamcinolone, often in concentrations as high as 40 mg/mL, can help flatten keloids and diminish itching and erythema.

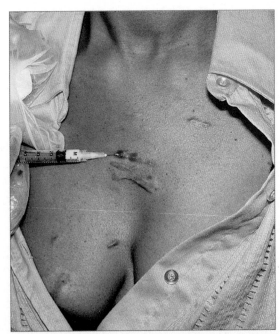

30.54 *Treatment of keloids with intralesional cortisone.* Triamcinolone (Kenalog) is being injected into this patient's presternal lesions.

continued on page 479

MANAGEMENT *Continued*

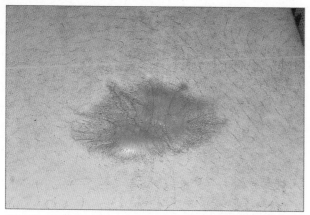

30.55 *Keloid after intralesional cortisone injection.*
This shiny scar shows the possible untoward after effects of intralesional steroid injections: atrophy, telangiectasias, and perilesional hypopigmentation.

- Such high concentrations are generally necessary for denser, more recalcitrant lesions. Similarly, complications of repeated corticosteroid injections include atrophy, telangiectasias, and pigmentary alteration.
- Excision, in combination with other postoperative modalities, such as ILTAC injections, compression dressings, radiotherapy, or injected interferon, is sometimes effective.
- Careful operative technique that closes surgical wounds with minimal tension is important. This is followed by postoperative injection of ILTAC 2 to 3 weeks postoperatively, followed by repeat injection in 3 to 4 weeks.
- After excisional treatment alone, keloids frequently recur (more than 50% of the time); however, when excision is combined with injected steroids or other modalities, the recurrence rate may be diminished.
- **Laser therapy.** Lasers have been used as alternatives to cold excision for keloids. As with excisional therapy, results are best when laser therapy is combined with postoperative injected steroids.
- Combined modality treatment of keloids. Effective treatment may involve excision followed by pressure dressings (compression therapy) during the postoperative period.
- **Compression therapy** is based on the finding that pressure has long been known to have thinning effects on skin. Occlusive dressings such as silicone gel sheeting may also be helpful.
- Topical imiquimod (**Aldara**) cream: Postoperative application of imiquimod 5% cream induces local production of interferon alpha, which, in turn, is known to enhance keloidal collagenase activity and reduce the synthesis of collagen.
- **Other medications:** In addition to topical imiquimod, other methods that are sometimes used to treat keloids and hypertrophic scars include intralesional interferon, oral verapamil, intralesional bleomycin, 5-fluorouracil, and botulinum toxin.

 HELPFUL HINT

- Intralesional corticosteroid injections must be administered cautiously to avoid overtreatment, which may result in skin atrophy, telangiectasias, and over-depressed scars.

CHAPTER 31
Premalignant and Malignant Cutaneous Neoplasms

OVERVIEW

This chapter is intended to help healthcare providers distinguish skin cancers from precancers and benign growths. The ability to make clinical diagnoses, to identify benign versus malignant lesions, especially in less classic presentations, is an important skill that comes with focused, repetitive visual scrutiny. By far, the most important skin lesion for the healthcare provider to recognize is melanoma.

BASICS

- An aging population that is living longer in an atmosphere with a declining ozone layer, coupled with more outdoor and leisure time to bask in the sun, has led to a dramatic increase in sun-related skin damage (*dermatoheliosis*), skin cancers, as well as precursors to skin cancer such as actinic keratoses.
- Actinic keratosis (AK), also known as *solar keratosis,* is the most common sun-related skin growth. Whether this lesion is benign (premalignant) or malignant (squamous cell carcinoma *in situ*) from its onset is a controversial issue. What is accepted, however, is that AKs have the potential to develop into invasive squamous cell carcinomas.
- The development of AKs, is directly related to cumulative sun exposure, and is estimated that 60% of predisposed people older than 40 have at least one AK.
- AKs are most common in persons who are fair-skinned, burn easily, and tan poorly particularly those who work, or have worked, in outdoor occupations, such as farmers, sailors, and gardeners, and those who participate in outdoor sports.
- The incidence of AKs, as with all of the skin cancers described in this chapter, is highest in Australia and in the Sun Belt area of the United States.
- It is estimated that 1 in 20 AKs eventually becomes a squamous cell carcinoma, the vast majority of which, are very slow-growing, indolent, unaggressive, and have an excellent prognosis. Distant metastases are rare. Consequently, among dermatologists, there is an ongoing debate regarding the need to be aggressive or to be somewhat *laissez-faire* in the approach to treatment of these lesions.

HISTOPATHOLOGY

- Cellular atypia is present, and the keratinocytes vary in size and shape. Mitotic figures are common.
- The histologic changes of individual cells are indistinguishable from those seen in squamous cell carcinomas.

CLINICAL MANIFESTATIONS

- AKs are usually asymptomatic, but they may itch and become tender or irritated.
- They are of cosmetic concern to some patients.
- Lesions usually appear singly or as multiple discrete, flat or elevated, verrucous, scaly papules. Their texture typically feels gritty or rough to the touch (Fig. 31.1).
- AKs often have an erythematous base covered by a white, skin-toned, yellowish, or brown hyperkeratotic scale.
- Found chiefly on sun-exposed areas: the face, especially on the nose, temples, and forehead. They are also commonly noted on the bald areas of the scalp (Figs. 31.2 and 31.3), helix of the ears in men (Fig. 31.4), pretibial legs in women (Fig. 31.5), dorsal forearms (Fig. 31.6), dorsal hands (Fig. 31.7), and the sun-exposed areas of the neck.

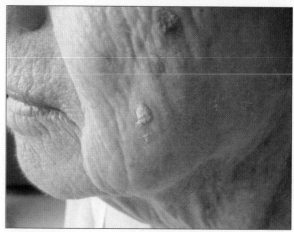

31.1 *Actinic keratosis.* This rough-textured papule on an erythematous base occurs in an area of sun-exposed skin. Note two seborrheic keratoses are located superior to this lesion.

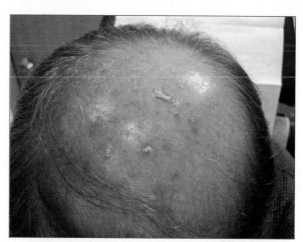

31.2 *Actinic keratoses.* Rough, scaly papules are present on the scalp. This is a typical finding in bald, elderly men with fair complexions who have spent much of their lives working outdoors.

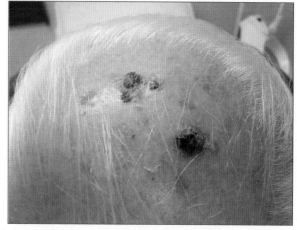

31.3 *Actinic keratoses.* Thicker, crusted, hyperkeratotic lesions are more obvious in this patient's scalp. The largest lesion proved to be a squamous cell carcinoma.

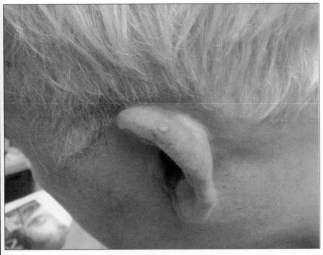

31.4 *Actinic keratosis.* The pinna of the ear is a very common site for these lesions in men. (Note the similarity to Fig. 30.35, an illustration of chondrodermatitis nodularis chronica helicis.)

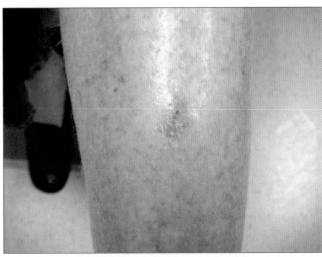

31.5 *Actinic keratosis.* A pretibial lesion in this woman who played tennis frequently.

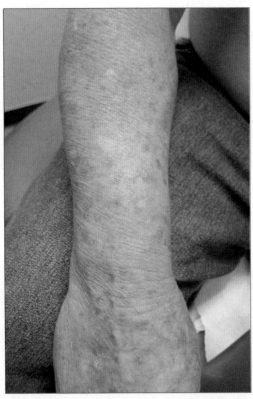

31.6 *Actinic keratoses.* Numerous small, gritty feeling, AKs on the sun-exposed dorsal forearms of this man with fair skin.

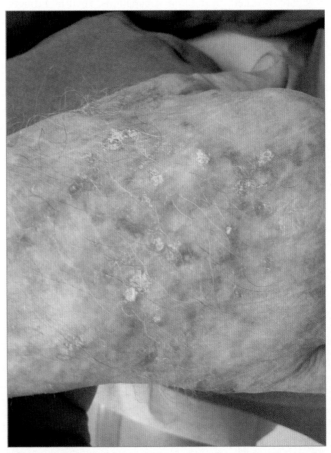

31.7 *Actinic keratoses.* AKs on dorsal hands in this elderly man.

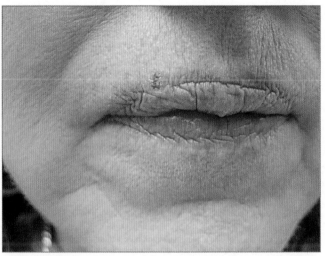

31.8 *Actinic keratosis.* The vermilion border of the upper lip is a common site of sun damage and AKs. These lesions are often better palpated than visualized.

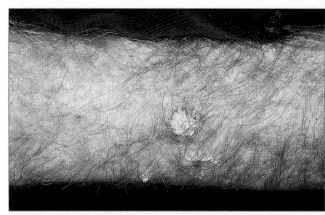

31.10 *Actinic keratoses, hypertrophic.* These thick, hyperkeratotic papules arose on areas of sun-exposed skin in this elderly individual.

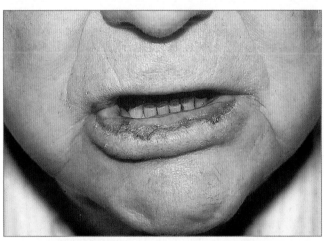

31.9 *Actinic cheilitis.* This patient is undergoing treatment with topical 5-fluorouracil for multiple actinic keratoses of his lower lip.

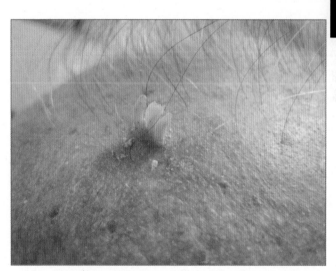

31.11 *Actinic keratosis/cutaneous horn.* This cutaneous horn was produced by an underlying actinic keratosis.

- The vermilion border of the upper lip is another very common site for actinic keratoses (Fig. 31.8).
- Extensive involvement of the mucosal lower lip is referred to as *actinic cheilitis* (Fig. 31.9).
- AKs are usually 3 to 10 mm in size and can gradually enlarge, thicken, and become more elevated and thus develop into **hypertrophic actinic keratoses** (Fig. 31.10) or a **cutaneous horn** (Fig. 31.11).

DIAGNOSIS

- Clinically, very small lesions are often better felt than seen. Palpation of these scaly growths reveals a gritty, sandpaper-like texture.
- A shave biopsy is performed if the diagnosis is in doubt.

DIFFERENTIAL DIAGNOSIS

Cutaneous Squamous Cell Carcinoma (see later Discussion)

- *An AK may be indistinguishable from a squamous cell carcinoma.*
- *Untreated, squamous cell carcinoma becomes indurated, with a tendency to ooze, ulcerate, or bleed.*

Basal Cell Carcinoma (see later Discussion)

- *Classically, this lesion is a pearly, shiny papule with telangiectasias.*
- *It may be indistinguishable from actinic keratosis, particularly when it is small, ulcerated, manipulated, or pigmented.*

Verruca Vulgaris (Wart)

- *May be indistinguishable from an AK.*

Seborrheic Keratosis (see Chapter 30)

- *Has a "stuck-on" appearance and may occur in areas not exposed to the sun.*
- *Most often more darkly pigmented than AKs.*
- *May be indistinguishable from an AK.*

Chondrodermatitis Nodularis Helicis (see Chapter 30)

- *Often confused with AKs on the helix of the ears.*
- *Always tender.*
- *Arise on less sun-exposed sides of helices (lateral rim of helix).*

MANAGEMENT

- Prevention begins with educating the patient to limit sun exposure by using sunscreens and wearing protective clothing.

Destructive Methods

- **Liquid nitrogen** (LN₂) is the traditional mainstay of treatment for AKs. LN₂ is most useful when lesions are few in number. It is applied to individual lesions for 3 to 5 seconds.
- For thick, hyperkeratotic lesions, a **shave biopsy** followed by **electrocautery** or **electrocautery** alone may be performed.

Patient Applied

Immunotherapy

- Imiquimod (**Aldara**) 5% cream is a local inducer of interferon. It is applied twice weekly to involved skin for 16 weeks until a response similar to that described with 5-FU agents is elicited.
- Imiquimod activates immune cells through a toll-like receptor. Activated cells secrete cytokines (primarily interferon-α [INF-α], interleukin-6 [IL-6], and tumor necrosis factor-α [TNF-α]) that leads to activation of the adaptive immune system. Other cell types activated by imiquimod include natural killer cells, macrophages, and B-lymphocytes.
- Besides actinic keratoses, imiquimod has been approved for the treatment of superficial basal cell carcinomas (see below), Bowen disease (squamous cell carcinoma *in situ*), as well as genital warts (see Chapter 28).
- **Zyclara** (imiquimod) cream, 2.5% and 3.75%, available in pump dispensers, are less concentrated imiquimod cream preparations that only need to be applied over the course of a shorter period of 2 weeks on and 2 weeks off for 2 months.

Chemotherapy

- Topical application of **Efudex**, a 5-fluorouracil (5-FU) 5% cream, is used when lesions are too numerous to treat individually.
- 5-FU interferes with the synthesis of DNA; it destroys dysplastic cells and spares normal cells. Enough medication is applied to cover the entire area with a thin film. This is done twice daily for 2 to 4 weeks for facial lesions. Other body sites require longer treatment (e.g., 6 to 8 weeks for the arms).
- Alternatively, a 0.5% 5-FU cream (**Carac**) may be applied only once daily. This preparation is less irritating than the 5-FU 5% agents.
- During treatment with 5-FU, lesions become increasingly red and crusted, and subclinical lesions become visible. This situation can result in a very red, disfiguring complexion; however, if the patient completes the treatment, lesions usually heal within 2 weeks of stopping treatment, the skin becomes smooth, and the majority of the actinic keratoses are gone (Fig. 31.12A,B).

Other Treatments

- **Photodynamic therapy** can be used to treat multiple actinic keratoses. In this treatment, topical 5-aminolevulinic acid accumulates preferentially in the dysplastic cells. On exposure to irradiation with light of the appropriate wavelength, oxygen-derived free radicals are generated, and cell death results.

continued on page 485

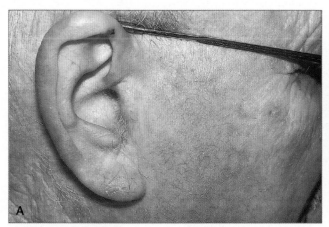
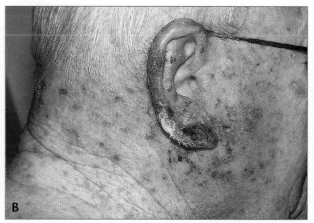

31.12 *Actinic keratoses.* **A:** Before treatment, few lesions are clinically visible. **B:** Two weeks after treatment with topical 5-FU, crusting and erythema are evident in areas that had lesions that were not initially apparent.

- **Chemical peels** and **dermabrasion** are also used in patients with numerous facial actinic keratoses.
- Diclofenac sodium 3% **(Solaraze)** gel is a nonsteroidal anti-inflammatory preparation that has been introduced as a topical treatment for actinic keratoses. These agents appear to be less irritating than the standard 5-FU products and **Aldara**, however, they are less effective.
- Ingenol mebutate 0.015% and 0.05% gel **(Picato)**, derived from the sap of the plant *Euphorbia peplus,* is

an inducer of cell death via mitochondrial swelling and a secondary immune response via activation of protein kinase C delta.

- For the face and scalp the 0.015% gel is used for 3 consecutive days.
- For the trunk and extremities the 0.05% gel is used for 2 days.
- The most common side effects are skin redness, flaking/scaling, crusting and swelling.

 HELPFUL HINTS

- Because actinic keratoses are more often easily felt than seen, the clinician should run ungloved fingers over the patient's skin to detect all lesions.
- Sunscreens should also be applied to the lower lip to prevent actinic cheilitis.
- Topical 5-FU treatment can be likened to using a "smart bomb" in which the "bomb" (in this case 5-FU) targets only the "enemy" (the rapidly growing dysplastic cells).

- Imiquimod **(Aldara, Zyclara)** cream may "immunize" patients against their own dysplastic keratinocytes.
- When treating with multiple AK lesions over large areas of skin, field-directed treatment with a topical agent is most effective.

 SEE PATIENT HANDOUTS "Actinic Keratosis" and "Sun Protection Advice" IN THE COMPANION eBOOK EDITION.

Cutaneous Squamous Cell Carcinoma

BASICS

- Squamous cell carcinoma (SCC) is a malignant epithelial tumor arising from keratinocytes. Cutaneous (nonmucous membrane) SCC is the second most common form of skin cancer, occurring much less frequently than basal cell carcinoma (BCC) and in an older age group than does BCC.
- Lesions most frequently occur on sun-exposed sites of elderly, fair-skinned individuals.
- Most SCCs arise in actinic keratoses (*solar keratoses*) and these are slow-growing, minimally invasive, unaggressive, and have an excellent prognosis because distant metastases are extremely rare.
- An SCC may also appear *de novo* without a preceding actinic keratosis or emerge from a pre-existing human papilloma virus infection (*verrucous carcinoma*).
- SCCs may develop from causes other than sun exposure such as within an old burn scar or on sites previously exposed to ionizing radiation.
- Metastases are more likely to occur in thicker tumors >6 mm deep. Other risk factors for metastases include lesions that arise on the ears, the vermilion border of the lips, or on mucous membranes.
- Although SCC is very rare in people of African and Asian descent, an SCC tends to be more aggressive in these populations.
- Also apt to be more aggressive are the non–sun-related SCCs such as an SCC in long-standing scars or in sites previously exposed to ionizing radiation or long-term psoralen and ultraviolet A (PUVA) light, on chronic inflammatory lesions (e.g., discoid lupus erythematosus), cutaneous ulcers (e.g., venous stasis ulcers), or other nonhealing wounds.
- As with AKs and BCCs (see later discussion), SCC is related to sun exposure and is noted more frequently in those with a greater degree of outdoor activity.

HISTOPATHOLOGY

- In the *in situ* type of SCC (**Bowen disease**), the full thickness of the epidermis is involved. The basement membrane remains intact. Atypical keratinocytes (squamous cells) show a loss of polarity and an increased mitotic rate.
- An invasive SCC penetrates into the dermis. It has various levels of anaplasia and may manifest relatively few to multiple mitoses and may display varying degrees of differentiation such as keratinization.

RISK OF METASTASIS

- The risk of metastasis of SCC depends on its degree of differentiation, depth of penetration, and location.
- *In situ* SCC (Bowen disease) has a low incidence of metastasis.
- An SCC arising in an actinic keratosis also has a low incidence of metastasis.
- Lesions that appear on mucous membranes and transplant recipients have the highest risk of metastasis.

- Tumors that are induced by ionizing radiation or those that arise in old burn scars or in inflammatory lesions are also more likely to metastasize.

CLINICAL MANIFESTATIONS

- Most SCCs are asymptomatic, although bleeding, pain, and tenderness may be noted.
- Slow-growing, firm papules with the ability to produce scale (keratinization) tend to be more clearly differentiated and are less likely to metastasize (Fig. 31.13).
- Softer, nonkeratinizing lesions are less well differentiated and are more likely to metastasize (Fig. 31.14).

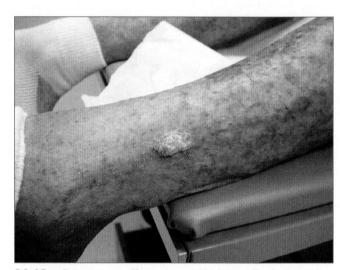

31.13 *Squamous cell carcinoma.* This nodular lesion arose from an actinic keratosis. The thick scale (keratinization) suggests greater cellular differentiation. This lesion is less likely to metastasize.

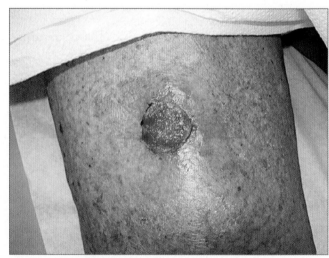

31.14 *Squamous cell carcinoma.* This poorly differentiated nodule arose in an immunocompromised patient in a site previously exposed to ionizing radiation. It has a greater potential to metastasize.

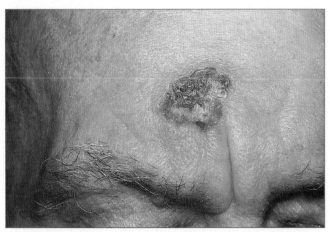

31.15 *Squamous cell carcinoma.* This neglected tumor has ulcerated.

- SCCs typically present as papules, plaques, or nodules that grow slowly.
- Lesions may be scaly or ulcerated (Fig. 31.15) or have a smooth or thick hyperkeratotic surface.
- As with actinic keratoses, an SCC may also produce a cutaneous horn on its surface.
- An SCC may appear as a reddish brown nodule. It may, at times, be indistinguishable from a hypertrophic actinic keratosis or a BCC.
- With the exception of mucous membrane SCCs, lesions of cutaneous SCC occur in exactly the same locations as do actinic keratoses: sun-exposed areas such as the face, the dorsa of the forearms and hands, and the "V" of the neck.
- In men, SCCs tend to arise on the bald areas of the scalp and on the tops of the ears as well as the posterior neck below the occipital hairline.
- In women, lesions tend to occur on the legs as well as other relatively sun-exposed locations.
- In individuals of African origin there is an equal frequency of skin cancers in sun-exposed and unexposed areas.

CLINICAL VARIANTS

INTRAEPITHELIAL SQUAMOUS CELL CARCINOMA

- **Bowen disease** (Fig. 31.16) is one of the few skin cancers that should be considered as a diagnosis in African-American, Afro-Caribbean, and African blacks. This non–sun-related skin cancer may arise on the extremities *de novo* (Fig. 31.17), in an old scar or in a lesion of discoid lupus erythematosus.
- **Bowen disease** (SCC *in situ*) and **erythroplasia of Queyrat** are intraepithelial SCCs that often arise in sites that are not exposed to the sun. When an SCC *in situ* lesion occurs on the penis, it is referred to as erythroplasia of Queyrat (Fig. 31.18).

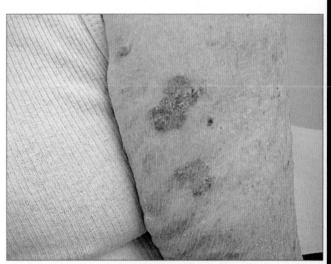

31.16 *Bowen disease (squamous cell carcinoma in situ).* These well-circumscribed lesions closely resemble psoriatic plaques.

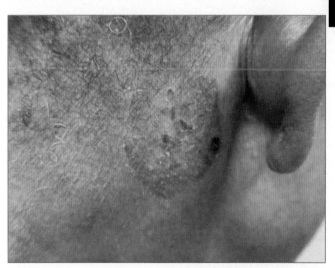

31.17 *Bowen disease in an African-American woman.* This plaque arose *de novo* in a non–sun-exposed location.

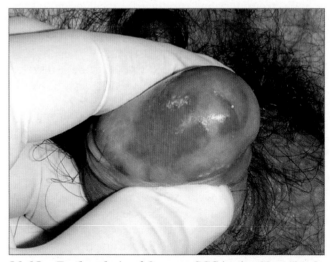

31.18 *Erythroplasia of Queyrat. SCC in situ.* Note "beefy red," nonhealing erosions on the glans penis.

SQUAMOUS CELL CARCINOMA OF MUCOUS MEMBRANES

- This condition (Fig. 31.19) may initially present as leukoplakia, nonhealing fissures, or ulcerations. Such lesions have significant metastatic potential.
- Treatment is beyond the scope of this publication.

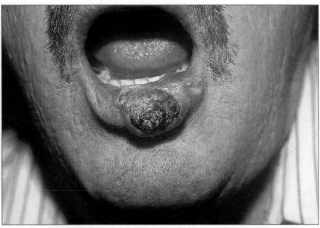

31.19 *Squamous cell carcinoma of the lip.* This lesion also has a significant metastatic potential.

 ## DIFFERENTIAL DIAGNOSIS

Actinic Keratosis (see above)
- *Early SCC lesions may be clinically difficult, if not impossible, to distinguish from a precursor AK.*

Basal Cell Carcinoma (see below)
- *Typically pearly and telangiectatic.*
- *Appear at a younger age than do SCCs.*
- *May be indistinguishable from SCC, particularly if the lesion is ulcerated.*

Keratoacanthoma (see below)
- *This lesion also may be clinically and, at times, histopathologically, indistinguishable from a SCC; considered by some to be a low-grade variant of an SCC.*
- *It is fast growing and less aggressive.*
- *Has a central hyperkeratotic crater.*

Melanoma (see below)
- *An amelanotic melanoma (lacking typical pigmentation) or an ulcerated melanoma may also be impossible to distinguish from an SCC.*

Psoriasis/Eczema
- *Bowen disease resembles a scaly solitary psoriatic or eczematous plaque (see Chapters 13 and 14).*

Seborrheic Keratosis (see Chapter 30)
- *"Stuck on" appearing.*

Verruca Vulgaris
- *The appearance of common warts is often similar to that of SCC lesions.*

 ## MANAGEMENT

Treatment
- **Electrocautery and curettage** for small lesions (generally less than 1 cm in diameter). This is done in a fashion similar to that performed for BCC treatment (see subsequent discussion). It is particularly useful on flat surfaces (e.g., forehead, cheek) and SCC *in situ* (Bowen disease).
- As with superficial BCCs, selected SCCs may be treated using **cryosurgery** with LN₂.
- **Total excision**, the preferred method of therapy for SCC, permits histologic diagnosis of the tumor margins.

Immunotherapy
- Imiquimod **(Aldara)** 5% cream is approved for the treatment of actinic keratoses (see previous discussion), for superficial BCCs (see later discussion), and is used "off-label" for SCC *in situ* (Bowen disease).

- **Aldara** may also have some utility in treating selected patients who have highly differentiated SCCs and in some renal transplant patients who tend to develop numerous SCCs.
- **Micrographic (Mohs) surgery** (see Fig. 35.25A–D) is useful for excessively large or invasive carcinomas, for recurrent lesions, for lesions with poorly delineated clinical borders, for SCCs within an orifice (e.g., ear canals or nostrils), and for carcinomas in locations where preservation of normal tissue is extremely important (e.g., tip of the nose, eyelids, nasal alae, ears, lips, and glans penis). It is also a treatment of choice for a lesion in an area of late radiation change.
- **Radiation therapy** is used for those patients who are physically debilitated or who are unable to, or refuse to, undergo, excisional surgery. It is also suitable for larger, advanced lesions.

continued on page 489

MANAGEMENT *Continued*

- For metastatic squamous cell carcinoma, oral **5-FU** has been used alone or in combination with SC interferon. More recently, epidermal growth factor receptor (EGFR) inhibitors, such as cetuximab, are used in combination with systemic chemotherapy for metastatic disease.

Surgery/Other Procedures
- Complete lymphadenectomy of the draining nodal basin for high-risk tumors.
- Metastatic disease requires aggressive management by a multidisciplinary team, involving plastic, ENT/ maxillofacial, and general surgeons, or a surgical oncologist.

Prevention
- Sun avoidance measures
- Sunscreens, sun-protective garments, and hats
- Sunglasses with ultraviolet protection
- Tinted windshields and side windows in cars
- Avoidance of contact with known carcinogenic compounds

 HELPFUL HINTS

- A subungual SCC can easily be mistaken for a verruca.
- High-risk SCCs may require imaging studies.
- Lymph node biopsy is indicated for suspected nodal involvement.

 SEE PATIENT HANDOUT "Sun Protection Advice" IN THE COMPANION eBOOK EDITION.

SEE PATIENT HANDOUT "Squamous Cell Carcinoma" IN THE COMPANION eBOOK EDITION.

 POINTS TO REMEMBER

- Bowen disease (SCC *in situ*) and frank SCC are two of the few skin cancers that should be considered in African-Americans. Such non–sun-related SCCs tend to arise on the extremities *de novo,* in an old scar, or in a lesion of discoid lupus erythematosus.
- An early lesion of SCC is difficult to distinguish from a precursor actinic keratosis.
- SCCs that develop from AKs are generally unaggressive.
- An SCC that is histopathologically "poorly differentiated" should be treated more aggressively.
- SCCs arising on a mucous membrane, in a chronic ulcer, or in an immunocompromised are at higher risk of metastasis.

Keratoacanthoma

BASICS

- A keratoacanthoma (KA) is a unique lesion with a characteristic clinical appearance. There is controversy about the benign versus malignant nature of this lesion. A KA resembles an SCC histologically; consequently some dermatologists and dermatopathologists consider it to be a low-grade variant of an SCC and believe that it should be treated as such. Lesions may be clinically impossible to differentiate from SCCs.
- KAs generally occur in persons older than 65 years of age.
- If ignored, some KAs have been reported to regress spontaneously. This fact lends support to the theory that this lesion is benign in nature.

CLINICAL MANIFESTATIONS

- Lesions arise quickly, usually developing in 3 to 4 weeks.
- Spontaneous regression may result in a small depressed scar.
- A KA usually occurs as a single, dome-shaped, erythematous or skin-colored nodule with a central keratin core (central crater) with an overlying crust (Figs. 31.20 and 31.21). It resembles the appearance of a volcano.
- It generally attains a diameter of 1.0 to 2.5 cm.

DISTRIBUTION OF LESIONS

- As with the nonmelanoma skin cancers such as BCC and SCC, lesions tend to appear on the sun-exposed areas of the face, ears, neck, dorsa of hands, and forearms.

DIAGNOSIS

- An excisional or incisional biopsy is often recommended so that the complete architecture of the lesion can be evaluated histologically. An insufficient biopsy, such as a shave biopsy, may result in a histology that is indistinguishable from an SCC.
- When KAs appear on areas where it is difficult to perform an excisional biopsy, such as the nose and external ears, a deep shave biopsy is often adequate to obtain sufficient tissue.

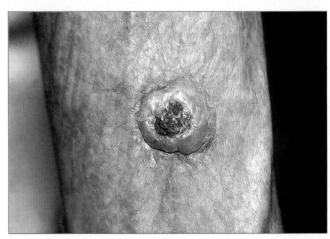

31.20 *Keratoacanthoma.* This "volcano-like" nodule arose over a period of 2 weeks. Note the characteristic crusting in the center.

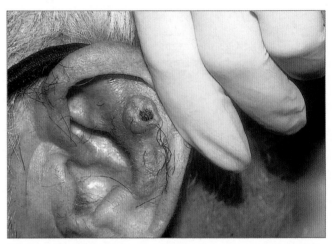

31.21 *Keratoacanthoma.* This nodule arose over a period of 4 weeks in a characteristic location.

⚒ MANAGEMENT

- A deep shave biopsy with or without electrodesiccation in selected cases often results in a permanent cure.
- Intralesional 5-FU has been used.
- Micrographic (Mohs) surgery may be necessary for recurrences.

😊 DIFFERENTIAL DIAGNOSIS

Squamous Cell Carcinoma
- *Lacks central crater.*
- *Arises over a longer period of time.*

Verruca Vulgaris
- *Lacks central crater.*
- *Appears in younger age group.*

BASICS

- The basal cell carcinoma (BCC) is the most common skin cancer and the most common cancer overall.
- Although this lesion qualifies as a cancer, its morbidity, if recognized and treated early, is frequently inconsequential. A BCC is usually slow growing and very rarely metastasizes, but it can result in significant local invasion and considerable destruction if it is neglected or treated inadequately.

HISTOPATHOLOGY

- Cells of nodular BCC typically have large, hyperchromatic, oval nuclei and very little cytoplasm. The cells appear rather uniform, and, if present, mitotic figures are usually scant.
- Nodular tumor aggregates may be of varying sizes, but tumor cells tend to align more densely in a *palisade pattern* at the periphery of these nests. Cleft formation, known as "retraction artifact," commonly occurs between BCC nests and stroma because of shrinkage of mucin during tissue fixation and staining.

RISK FACTORS

- Many of the same risk factors that predispose to actinic keratoses and SCCs are responsible for the development of BCCs, although BCCs tend to occur at a younger age than actinic keratosis, SCC, and KA.
- Risk factors for BCC include the following:
  - Age older than 40 years.
  - Male sex.
  - Positive family history of BCC.
  - Light complexion (as in SCCs and actinic keratoses, BCCs are rare in blacks and Asians) with poor tanning ability.
  - A history of long-term sun exposure.

CLINICAL MANIFESTATIONS

- Lesions are often ignored, asymptomatic, and slow growing.
- Very mild trauma, such as face washing or drying with a towel, may cause bleeding.
- In time, lesions may ulcerate (e.g., "the sore that will not heal").
- The classic lesion, the nodular BCC, is also the most common type. Occur most commonly on the head, neck, and upper back and may have some of the following features:
  - A pearly, shiny, semi translucent, papule or nodule.
  - A rolled (raised) border (Figs. 31.22 and 31.23).
- Telangiectases over the surface account for a history of bleeding with minor trauma.
- Erosion or ulceration ("rodent ulcer") caused by a gnawed appearance (Fig. 31.24).

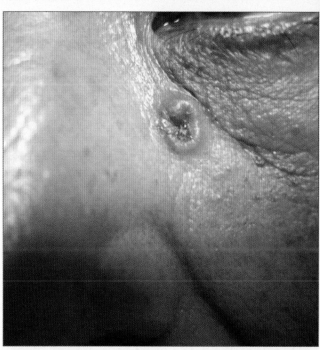

31.22 *Basal cell carcinoma.* A pearly papule with ulceration ("rodent ulcer") and telangiectasias is the "classic" presentation of a nodular BCC.

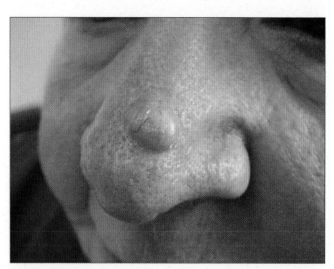

31.23 *Basal cell carcinoma.* Here the lesion is a shiny, pearly, translucent papule with telangiectasias.

- A lesion can sometimes present as a small, nonhealing erosion.
- Brownish to blue-black pigmentation (pigmented BCC) is seen in more darkly pigmented persons (Figs. 31.25 and 31.26).

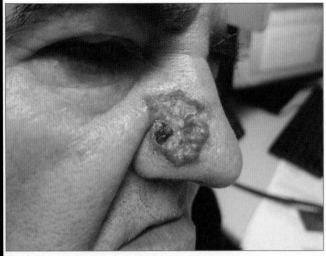

31.24 *Basal cell carcinoma.* This lesion shown had been ignored for several years.

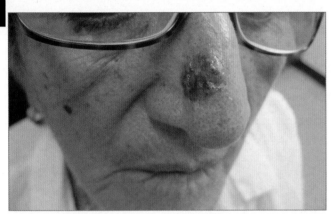

31.25 *Basal cell carcinoma, pigmented.* Note the pearly surface and telangiectasias.

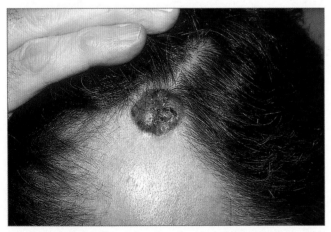

31.26 *Basal cell carcinoma, pigmented.* This lesion could easily be mistaken for a melanoma.

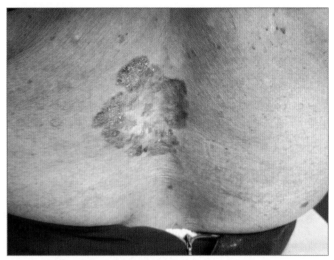

31.27 *Superficial basal cell carcinoma.* The back is a common place to find a superficial BCC. Note the distinct thread-like border. Often patients are not aware of these lesions, which resemble psoriatic plaques as well as Bowen disease.

DISTRIBUTION OF LESIONS

- Lesions occur on the head and neck in 85% of all affected persons.
- Occur on sun-exposed areas, for example, the face, especially on the nose, cheeks, forehead, periorbital area, lower face, and the back of the neck.

CLINICAL VARIANTS

SUPERFICIAL BASAL CELL CARCINOMA

- A superficial BCC occurs as a scaly pink to red-brown patch with a thread-like border (Fig. 31.27).
- The lesions tend to be indolent, asymptomatic, and the least aggressive of BCCs.
- Lesions are sometimes multiple, occurring primarily on the trunk and proximal extremities.
- When solitary, a lesion of superficial BCC may resemble psoriasis, eczema, a seborrheic keratosis, or Bowen disease (SCC *in situ*).
- There is no clear association between superficial BCC and sun exposure.

MORPHEAFORM BASAL CELL CARCINOMA

- This is the least common and most aggressive form of BCC.
- Lesions appear as whitish, scarred atrophic plaques with surrounding telangiectasia (Fig. 31.28).
- The margins of these lesions are often difficult to evaluate clinically; as with icebergs, what is seen on the surface is not always what lies under the surface.
- Consequently, morpheaform BCCs are generally more difficult to treat than other BCCs.
- A morpheaform BCC may be mistaken for scar tissue.

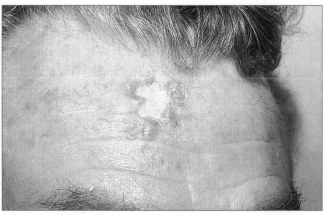

31.28 *Morpheaform basal cell carcinoma.* A whitish, atrophic, scar-like plaque is present, with surrounding telangiectasias and pearly papules surrounding it.

DIAGNOSIS

- The diagnosis is generally made by shave or excisional biopsy.
- A shave biopsy suffices for the diagnosis of most BCCs (see Chapter 35).

SCC (see earlier discussion)

Actinic keratosis (see earlier discussion)

Intradermal nevus (see Chapter 30)

Melanoma pigmented (see later discussion)

Angiofibroma (fibrous papule of the nose [see Fig. 30.45]), easily confused with BCC

Sebaceous Hyperplasia
- *Yellow or cream-colored papules are often dough-nut-shaped with a dell (umbilication) (see Fig. 30.28).*
- *Telangiectasias radiate in a spoke-like fashion (see Fig. 30.29).*
- *Generally dome-shaped, flesh-colored, pale or pink firm papules with a shiny appearance.*

Seborrheic Keratosis
- *May be indistinguishable from a pigmented BCC.*

Trichoepithelioma
- *Individual lesions may be confused clinically and pathologically with BCC, which is more common but usually arises as a solitary lesion.*

 MANAGEMENT

Prevention
- Techniques involve sun avoidance, use of sunscreens with a sun protection factor (SPF) of at least 15, and wearing protective clothing.
- People with a history of skin cancer should learn skin self-examination and should have annual skin examinations.

Treatment
- **Electrodesiccation and curettage** (see Chapter 35). The overall cure rate exceeds 90% for low-risk BCCs. This method is quick, simple, and less expensive than most other procedures.
- **Excision** allows for histologic diagnosis of margins. Cosmetic results compare favorably with those of curettage; however, surgical excision is more time-consuming and costly than curettage.
- **Immunotherapy** with 5% imiquimod cream (**Aldara**), a topical immunomodulator, is approved for the treatment of superficial BCCs. It is applied five times per week for a full 6 weeks.
- **Micrographic (Mohs) surgery** (see Chapter 35 [Figs. 35.25A–D]) for morpheaform, recurrent, or large lesions, as well as for lesions in "danger zones" (e.g., the nasolabial area, around the eyes, behind the ears, in the ear canal, and on the scalp).
  - Mohs micrographic surgery is a microscopically controlled method of removing skin cancers that allows for controlled excision and maximum preservation of normal tissue. Excisions are repeated in the areas proven to be cancerous until a completely cancer-free plane is reached.
  - Mohs surgery is time-consuming and expensive, and it may require extensive reconstruction of surgical wounds. However, it provides the most reliable method of determining adequate margins, it has a very high cure rate of 98% to 99% for BCCs, and it preserves the maximum amount of normal tissue around the cancer.
- **Radiation therapy** for elderly debilitated patients or for those who are physically unable to undergo excisional surgery. The disadvantages include the potential for late radiation changes in the skin, as well as the inability to examine skin margins because tissue is not obtained. It is less often used today.
- **Cryosurgery** with LN_2. Superficial BCCs may be treated rapidly using this method. However, nodular basal cell carcinomas, particularly selected lesions on the eyelid and ear, are ideally treated with a temperature probe before cryosurgery is performed. Successful treatment is highly dependent on the experience of the operator. This technique is also less often used today.
- **Vismodegib (Erivedge)** is an oral inhibitor of the Hedgehog pathway approved by the FDA as a targeted treatment for locally advanced or metastatic basal cell carcinoma that is not amenable to surgery and radiation.

HELPFUL HINTS

- Avoidance of exposure to ultraviolet radiation is encouraged. Preventive measures include carefully planning outdoor activities before 10 AM and after 4 PM, wearing a broad-brimmed hat during outdoor activities, and using sunscreens with an SPF of 15 or greater.
- In the rare instances of an advanced or metastatic BCC or one that is inoperable, treatment with an oral anti-cancer medication vismodegib (**Erivedge**), a selective hedgehog pathway inhibitor, given as a 150-mg tablet daily, has shown an overall response rate of 43% and 30% in patients who are not candidates for surgery, and those with advanced and metastatic BCC.

POINTS TO REMEMBER

- BCC is, by far, the most common type of skin cancer.
- As with SCC and AKs, BCCs are induced by ultraviolet radiation in susceptible persons.
- Almost 50% of patients with BCC will have another one within 5 years.
- Recurrent BCCs are generally more aggressive than primary lesions.
- Patients with BCC have an increased risk of melanoma.

 SEE PATIENT HANDOUT "Sun Protection Advice" IN THE COMPANION eBOOK EDITION.

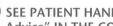 SEE PATIENT HANDOUT "Basal Cell Carcinoma" IN THE COMPANION eBOOK EDITION.

BASICS

- Malignant melanoma, more appropriately referred to (non-redundantly) as melanoma, is a cancer of melanocytes, the cells that produce pigment. Melanoma generally occurs in the skin and, much less commonly, in the eyes, ears, gastrointestinal tract, leptomeninges of the central nervous system, as well as oral and genital mucous membranes.
- It is the most common cancer in women aged 25 to 29 years and is second only to breast cancer in women aged 30 to 34 years.
- Melanoma is also commonly seen in patients with defects of DNA repair such as *xeroderma pigmentosum* and in patients with *familial atypical mole syndrome* (see Chapter 30).
- It is also more often seen in patients who have an abundance of melanocytic nevi.
- Although BCC and SCC (nonmelanoma skin cancers) are associated with long-term exposure to sunlight, melanoma is more likely to occur with infrequent but strong exposures that result in sunburns. Nonmelanoma skin cancers are more likely to be found on chronically sun-exposed areas such as the face; in contrast, melanomas are more likely to occur on areas that are less often exposed and more frequently burned, specifically the backs of men and the legs of women.
- By far, the most important skin lesion for the healthcare provider to recognize is melanoma. It is one of the only skin diseases that can be fatal if neglected; consequently, early recognition and prompt removal of a melanoma can save a life.

RISK FACTORS

- Persons at greatest risk for melanoma have the following characteristics:
  - Age generally older than 20 years, particularly older than 60 years.
  - A light complexion, an inability to tan, and a history of sunburns.
  - Moles that are numerous, changing, or atypical (dysplastic nevi).
  - A personal or family history of melanoma (first-degree relatives).
  - A personal or family history of BCCs or SCCs.

HISTOPATHOLOGY

- Superficial spreading melanoma (SSM), lentigo maligna melanoma (LMM), and acral lentiginous melanoma (ALM) have an early *in situ* (radial growth) phase characterized by increased numbers of intraepithelial melanocytes, which are large and atypical as well as being arranged haphazardly at the dermal–epidermal junction. They show upward (pagetoid) migration and lack the biologic potential to metastasize.
- Invasion into the dermis may confer metastatic potential and is characterized by a distinct population of melanoma cells with mitoses and nuclear pleomorphism within the dermis (papillary, reticular) and, possibly, the subcutaneous fat.

CLINICAL MANIFESTATIONS

WARNING SIGNS

- New, changing (evolving), or unusual nevi; the most common sign of melanoma.
- Symptomatic nevi (e.g., those that itch, burn, or are painful).
- An initial slow horizontal growth phase, if left untreated, is followed in months or years by a vertical growth phase (lesions that extend vertically in the skin), which indicates invasive disease and potential metastasis.
- White coloration may indicate regression or scarring.

DISTRIBUTION OF LESIONS

- In white women, the most common lesion sites for SSM are the upper back, the lower leg between the knees and ankle, and the arms and is less common on covered areas such as under bras and swimsuits.
- In white men, the most common lesion sites for SSM are the upper back, anterior torso, and the upper extremities.
- In both white women and white men, other types of melanoma such as lentigo malignant melanoma may occur on the head, neck, and sun-exposed arms. Nodular melanomas tend to arise on the legs and trunk.
- Melanoma is very rare in dark-skinned persons and Asians. However, when it does occur, it tends to present on acral, non–sun-exposed areas such as the palms of the hands, soles of the feet, or in the nail bed. In such cases, it is referred to as acral lentiginous melanoma (ALM).

SUPERFICIAL SPREADING MELANOMA

- Of the four major clinicopathologic types of melanoma, SSM is by far the most common.
- SSM may arise *de novo* or in a pre-existing nevus.
- The lesions of SSM may conform to some, or all, of the "ABCDE" criteria for melanoma, in which the primary lesion is a macular (flat) lesion or an elevated plaque that displays the following (Figs. 31.29–31.34):
  - **A: Asymmetry.** If you draw an X and a Y axis through the middle of a lesion and "fold" the lesion on itself, the halves will not match.
  - **B: Border** that is irregular or notched (like a jigsaw puzzle).
  - **C: Color** that is varied or has different shades (may have brown, black, pink, blue gray, white, or admixtures of these colors). A blue color results from the Tyndall effect, an optical illusion that occurs when light reflects off brown or black pigment in the deeper layers of the skin. The red color results from an inflammatory response that the immune system is mounting against the tumor. An ivory-white color suggests regression.
  - **D: Diameter** greater than 6 mm (the size of a pencil eraser), but a lesion may be smaller when first detected.

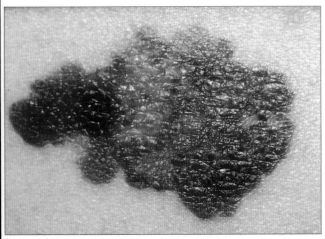

31.29 *Superficial spreading melanoma.* Note the "ABCD" features: asymmetry, notched border, varied colors, and diameter of more than 6 mm.

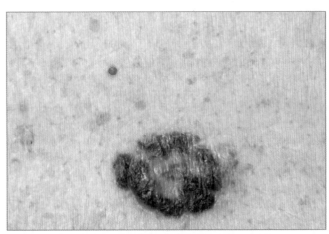

31.31 *Superficial spreading melanoma/evolving.* Note the central area (whitish gray) that represents regression.

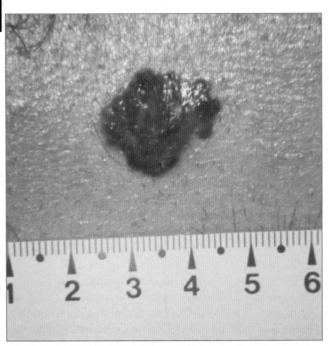

31.30 *Superficial spreading melanoma.* Asymmetry, notched border, varied colors, and diameter of more than 6 mm is evident in this lesion.

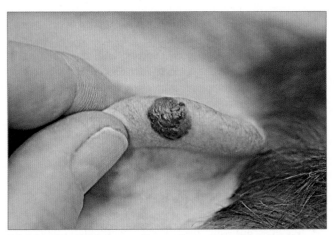

31.32 *Superficial spreading melanoma/evolving.* Melanoma of the helix of the ear. Note the subtle superficial spreading component (brown color) at the base and the darker nodule arising from it.

- **E: Evolution**, or change in a pre-existing lesion, that is, any change in size, color, elevation, or any new symptom such as bleeding, itching, or crusting should prompt suspicion.

DIAGNOSIS

- Clinical diagnosis is based on ABCDE criteria.
- Elliptic excisional biopsy should include the entire visible lesion.

DIFFERENTIAL DIAGNOSIS

Seborrheic Keratosis (see also Chapter 30)
- *Particularly if the lesion is variegated in color or jet black.*

Pigmented Basal Cell Carcinoma
- *May be clinically indistinguishable from SSM or other types of malignant melanoma (see Fig. 30.27).*

Dysplastic or Atypical Nevus (see Chapter 30)
- *A dysplastic nevus or a melanocytic nevus with an atypical appearance may also be clinically indistinguishable from melanoma.*

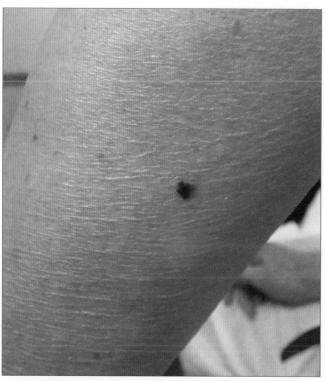

31.33 *Superficial spreading melanoma.* A very small early melanoma was present on this patient's leg. This lesion illustrates two colors. The presence of dark pigmentation and irregular shape prompted biopsy of the lesion.

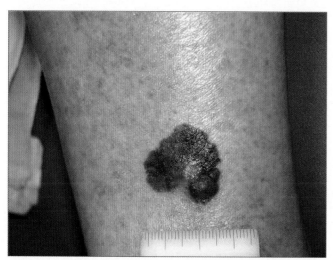

31.34 *Superficial spreading melanoma.* The scale in this lesion represents ulceration and is a poor prognostic sign.

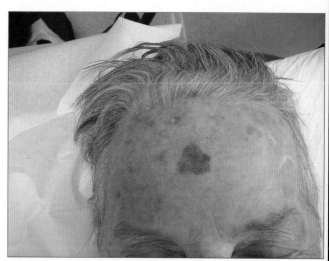

31.35 *Lentigo maligna.* Note in the darker parts of this lesion the irregular border of this malignant melanoma *in situ*. Note similarity to actinic lentigo (see Fig. 30.15).

CLINICAL VARIANTS

LENTIGO MALIGNA AND LENTIGO MALIGNA MELANOMA

- Lentigo maligna (LM) is a type of lentigo that is found on the face of elderly patients with chronically sun-damaged skin. LM is considered to be a potential precursor to melanoma (Fig. 31.35).
- LM lesions are characterized by:
  - a gradually enlarging tan to brown macule with irregular borders.
  - slow growth over 5 to 20 years.
  - an irregular color and border.
  - when an LM invades the dermis, it is then referred to as a lentigo maligna melanoma (LMM). The prognosis of LMM is similar to that of other subtypes of melanoma and is dependent on the thickness of the tumor (Fig. 31.36A,B).

NODULAR MELANOMA

- The lesion of a nodular melanoma may arise from a pre-existing melanocytic nevus or it may appear *de novo* as a nodule or plaque (Figs. 31.37 and 31.38). It occurs in 10% to 15% of patients. Because of a rapid vertical growth phase, lesions become invasive at an early stage.

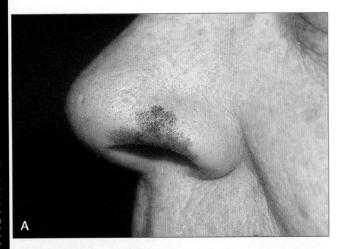

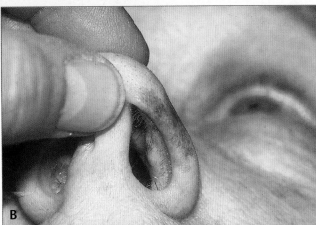

31.36 *Lentigo maligna melanoma.* **A:** Biopsy of this pigmented lesion demonstrated invasion into the dermis. **B:** The same patient; note involvement of the nasal mucosa.

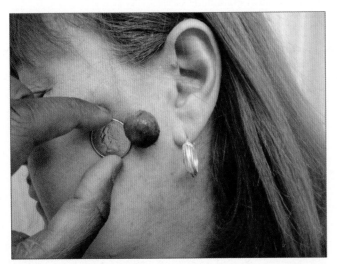

31.37 *Nodular amelanotic melanoma.* This rapidly growing nodule was initially considered to be a pyogenic granuloma.

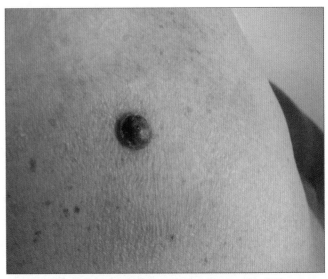

31.38 *Nodular melanoma.* Prior to biopsy this lesion was initially considered to be a seborrheic keratosis.

- Nodular melanoma lesions have the following characteristics:
  - They are blue, blue-black, or nonpigmented (as in amelanotic melanoma); their color is more uniform than that of SSM.
  - May ulcerate and bleed with minor trauma.
  - Occur most commonly on the legs and trunk.
  - May be indistinguishable from a pyogenic granuloma (see Fig. 30.52).

ACRAL LENTIGINOUS MELANOMA

- ALM is the least common subtype of melanoma.
- Although relatively rare compared to other types of melanoma, especially in Caucasians, ALM most often appears in blacks and Asians. It is the most common subtype in people with darker skins. It is not related to sun exposure.
- Lesions of ALM tend to occur on areas that do not bear hair, such as the palms, soles, and periungual skin (Figs. 31.39 and 31.40).
- ALM has a tendency toward early metastasis.
- A subungual ALM presenting as diffuse nail discoloration or a longitudinal pigmented band within the nail plate is potentially confused with subungual hematoma (see Fig. 22.5) or junctional nevus (Fig. 31.41). Pigment spread to the proximal or lateral nail folds **(Hutchinson sign)** is a hallmark of ALM (Fig. 31.42).

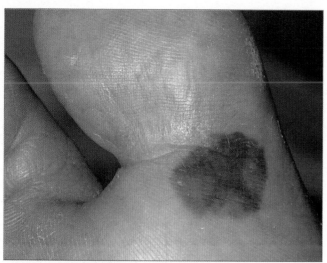

31.39 *Acral lentiginous melanoma.* Note the size and variegated pigmentation of this lesion. (Courtesy of Charles Miller, MD, San Diego Naval Hospital.)

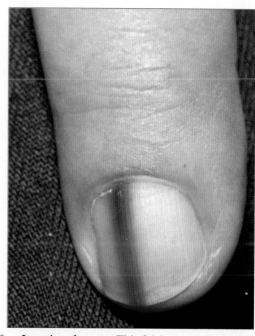

31.41 *Junctional nevus.* This fairly common lesion may present a worrisome quandary (to biopsy or not to biopsy). Note the even, linear bands of pigmentation in this patient's nail bed.

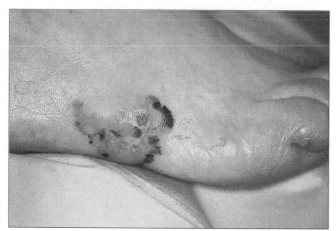

31.40 *Acral lentiginous melanoma.* A podiatrist who was treating the lesion as a wart referred this patient; the lesion did not resolve with destructive therapy. It was, in fact, a level V melanoma (melanoma cells were located in the subcutaneous tissue). (Courtesy of Art Huntley, MD, University of California at Davis.)

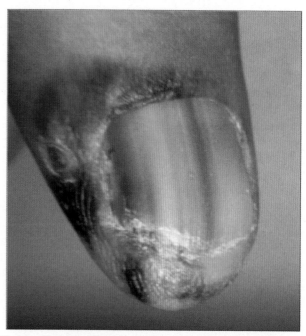

31.42 *Acral lentiginous melanoma.* Hutchinson sign shows uneven pigmentation spreading beyond the nail into surrounding skin.

MANAGEMENT

Workup for Patients with Melanoma

- The most important aspects of the initial workup for patients with cutaneous melanoma are a careful history, review of systems, and physical examination.
- Recently published data have shown that baseline and surveillance laboratory studies (e.g., lactate dehydrogenase level, liver function tests); chest radiography; and other imaging studies (e.g., computed tomography, positron emission tomography, bone scanning, magnetic resonance imaging) are not typically beneficial for patients without signs or symptoms of metastasis.
- A metastatic workup should be initiated if physical findings or symptoms suggest disease recurrence or if the patient has documented nodal metastasis based on results from a Sentinel Lymph Node Biopsy (SLNB).

Sentinel Lymph Node Biopsy

- SLNB is a method used to detect the first lymph node draining from the site of a melanoma.
- It is generally indicated for pathologic staging of the regional nodal basin(s) for primary tumors of at least 1 mm depth and when certain high-risk histologic features (e.g., ulceration, extensive regression) are present in thinner melanomas.
- The probability of sentinel node positivity increases with increasing tumor thickness.
- This minimally invasive procedure allows the pathologist to detect micrometastases.
- A negative sentinel node obviates the need for further lymph node dissection.
- Sentinel node status (positive or negative) is the most important prognostic factor for recurrence and is the most powerful predictor of survival in melanoma patients.

Surgical Treatment

- **Elliptic excision** should include the entire visible lesion down to the subcutaneous fat.
- Surgical margins of 5 mm are currently recommended for melanoma *in situ*.
- For lesions with a thickness of less than 1 mm, a 1-cm margin of normal skin is usually adequate.
- **Amputation, regional lymph node dissection**, and **regional chemotherapy perfusion** are sometimes necessary for ALMs.

Long-Term Management

- Patients who have had melanoma should be followed every 3 months for the first 2 years and annually thereafter.
- At each visit, the patient's entire cutaneous surface and lymph nodes should be examined.
- Patients with invasive disease require an annual chest radiograph, complete blood count, and liver function studies.

Metastatic Melanoma

- It is beyond the scope of this discussion to describe the emerging novel therapies for metastatic melanoma; however, there are several targeted therapies with BRAF and MEK inhibitors that are now available have been shown to incrementally increase long-term survival for those with metastatic disease (Figs. 31.43 and 31.44).

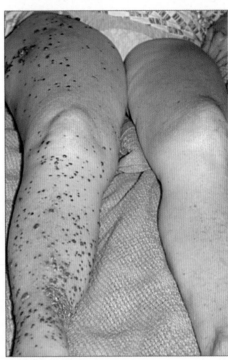

31.43 *Metastatic melanoma.* Note the lymphedema and multiple metastatic nodules on this patient's leg. The skin is the most common organ to which melanoma metastasizes.

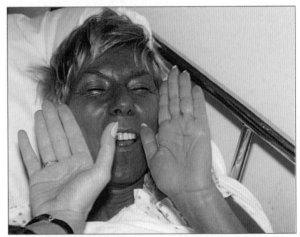

31.44 *Metastatic melanoma.* The unusual brown-blue coloration in this patient is the result of widespread melanin pigmentation in the tissues.

PROGNOSIS OF MELANOMA

- Five-year survival is based on the thickness of the tumor on a scale known as the Breslow measurement (Table 31.1). The thickness of the lesion is measured from the top of the granular layer of the skin to the deepest tumor cell. Melanomas that are thicker than 4 mm are associated with a high rate of distant and nodal metastasis.
- Prognosis may also be determined by the grade of the melanoma, as determined by its location in the dermis using Clark levels (Table 31.2).
- Sentinel lymph node status is also used for prognostication (see above).
- Other important prognostic factors include the sex of the patient (women have a better prognosis than men), age (the prognosis worsens with increasing age), and the presence of ulceration or regional or distant spread.

Table 31.1 BRESLOW MEASUREMENT

TUMOR THICKNESS (mm)	5-YR SURVIVAL (%)
<0.75	98–99
0.76–1.50	94
1.51–2.25	83
2.26–3.00	72–77
>3	<50

Table 31.2 CLARK'S LEVELS

GRADE	LOCATION IN DERMIS
I	*In situ* disease confined to the epidermis
II	Melanoma cells in papillary dermis
III	Melanoma cells filling papillary dermis
IV	Melanoma cells in reticular dermis
V	Melanoma cells in subcutaneous fat

HELPFUL HINTS

- Trauma from rubbing or irritation does not cause malignant degeneration of moles.
- Total skin examination that includes the legs should be performed when evaluating a female patient for possible skin cancer.
- To identify growing lesions, total body photographs allow for the assessment of existing and new lesions anywhere on the body.
- The use of the "ugly duckling" sign, wherein skin examination is focused on recognition of a lesion that simply looks different from the rest, may assist with detection of lesions that lack the classic ABCDE criteria for melanoma (Figs. 31.45 and 31.46).
- African-Americans are more likely than whites to be initially seen with advanced disease and have a worse prognosis.

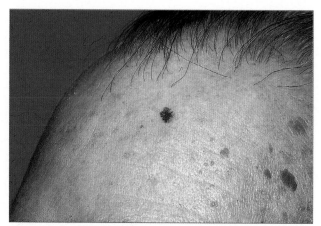

31.45 *In situ melanoma/"ugly duckling" lesion.* Note jet-black coloration of the lesion on this man's forehead in comparison to the surrounding brown seborrheic keratoses. This patient's wife noticed the "ugly duckling" lesion, which was out of character with his usual seborrheic keratoses.

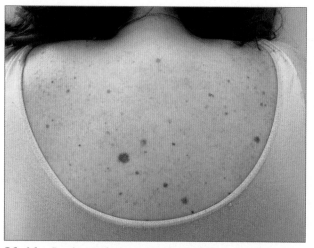

31.46 *In situ melanoma/"ugly duckling" lesion.* The lesion on this patient's midback appeared to be different from the rest of her nevi.

POINTS TO REMEMBER

- Sun protection should be stressed in those with a personal or family history of melanoma.
- Anyone who has a history of melanoma needs lifelong skin surveillance, because 3% of these patients will develop a second melanoma within 3 years.
- Patients should be taught self-examination.
- Patients should be advised to have all first-degree relatives undergo a dermatologic examination to check for dysplastic nevi or melanoma.
- Any lesion that looks suspicious must be examined by biopsy.
- An amelanotic melanoma is easily overlooked because of its lack of pigmentation.

- Removal of thin lesions (less than 0.76 mm) is curative in almost all patients.
- Early detection is the key to saving lives, because the treatments for metastatic melanoma are limited. Once a melanoma is metastatic, there is no uniformly effective adjuvant chemotherapy.
- No definite proof of survival benefit has been found for performing SLNB versus a group of people who had similar melanomas but no SLNB.

 SEE PATIENT HANDOUT "Sun Protection Advice" IN THE COMPANION eBOOK EDITION.

BASICS

- Paget disease of the breast (PDB) and extramammary Paget disease (EMPD) are intraepidermal skin cancers that are often indicative of more severe underlying malignancies.
- Both diseases—particularly EMPD—can have a subtle, insidious course and tend to be ignored, misdiagnosed, or unrecognized. A high index of suspicion and prompt identification and treatment of these conditions can be lifesaving.

PAGET DISEASE OF THE BREAST

- PDB is a relatively uncommon clinical presentation of intraductal carcinoma of the breast. It occurs almost exclusively in postmenopausal women; men are rarely affected.
- PDB accounts for 1% to 4% of breast cancers.
- In more than half of the cases, there is no associated palpable breast mass, and mammography results are often normal.
- PDB is often mistakenly diagnosed as a chronic eczematous condition.
- Not infrequently, an elderly patient may be too embarrassed to mention the lesion to her family or clinician, thereby further delaying diagnosis and treatment.

PATHOPHYSIOLOGY

- PDB is an underlying intraductal carcinoma of the breast, with retrograde extension into the overlying epidermis through mammary duct epithelium.
- The epidermis becomes infiltrated with characteristic Paget cells that cause thickening of the nipple and the areolar skin.

CLINICAL MANIFESTATIONS

- The PDB lesion is usually insidious and slow growing, and it is often asymptomatic.
- Patients with PDB often present with a chronic *unilateral* eruption on the nipple, areola, or surrounding skin; less commonly, the lesion originates and remains on the nipple.
- Typically, the lesion appears as a sharply marginated red plaque with an irregular border and eczema-like appearance (Fig. 31.47).
- When the nipple is involved, it may become scaly, crusted, have a bloody nipple discharge, become deformed, or retracted.

DIAGNOSIS

- Punch, wedge, or excisional biopsy of the lesional skin of the nipple–areola complex, including the dermal and subcutaneous tissue for microscopic examination.

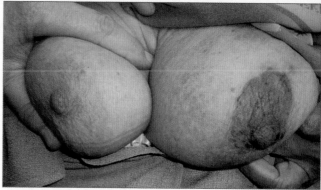

31.47 *Paget disease of the breast.* This patient had an eczema-like lesion of the nipple, areola, and surrounding skin for several years. On biopsy, the patient was found to have an infiltrating ductal carcinoma of the underlying breast tissue.

👤 DIFFERENTIAL DIAGNOSIS

Atopic Dermatitis

- *In addition to various unusual neoplasms, atopic dermatitis of the nipples and areolae should be included in the differential diagnosis.*
- *Atopic dermatitis often presents bilaterally (Fig. 31.48), but may present unilaterally.*
- *Atopic dermatitis occurs in association with a personal or family history of atopy (see Chapter 13) and it should respond rapidly to topical corticosteroid therapy.*

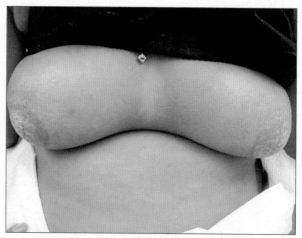

31.48 *Atopic dermatitis on the nipples and areolae (bilateral).* Note the obliteration of the margins of the nipples and areolae, as well as the oozing and fissuring of the left breast. These lesions responded readily to topical corticosteroids.

Extramammary Paget Disease

BASICS

- EMPD is a rare condition that is similar to PDB; the primary difference is the anatomic location. EMPD targets the genital skin, perianal skin, and other cutaneous sites rich in apocrine glands.
- EMPD is four to five times more likely to occur in women than in men. The condition most commonly appears in patients of ages 50 to 60.

PATHOPHYSIOLOGY

- EMPD arises as a primary cutaneous adenocarcinoma in most cases. The epidermis becomes infiltrated with characteristic Paget cells—neoplastic cells that show glandular differentiation.

CLINICAL MANIFESTATIONS

- The initial lesion may present as a unilateral, erythematous, sharply marginated, eczema-simulating, slow-growing plaque that may be indistinguishable from PDB (Fig. 31.49).
- Not infrequently, lesions may be ill-defined and resemble eczema, intertrigo, tinea cruris, candidiasis, as well as other neoplastic and inflammatory conditions before the diagnosis is made.
- EMPD has usually been present for a long time before biopsy is performed to confirm the diagnosis.

DIAGNOSIS

- The diagnosis of EMPD requires a high degree of clinical suspicion, followed by skin biopsy with pathologic correlation.
- Histologic features of PDB and EMPD disease are similar.

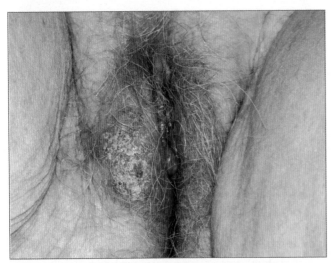

31.49 *Extramammary Paget disease.* This persistent vulvar plaque is suggestive of Paget disease and requires a biopsy. (From Craft N, Fox LP. *Visual Dx: Essential Adult Dermatology.* Philadelphia, PA: Lippincott Williams & Wilkins, 2010.)

DIFFERENTIAL DIAGNOSIS

The differential diagnosis of EMPD is more extensive than that of PDB, and **EMPD may simulate various neoplastic and inflammatory conditions.**

Atopic Dermatitis
- *Responds to topical steroids.*

MANAGEMENT

- As in other types of confirmed breast carcinoma, treatment of PDB can include surgery, radiation therapy, chemotherapy, and hormonal treatment as indicated.
- Mastectomy (radical or modified) and lymph node clearance are appropriate for patients with PDB who have a palpable mass and underlying invasive breast carcinoma.
- Because EMPD often extends beyond the visibly involved clinical margins, a wide, controlled surgical excision of all the involved epidermis is the most effective treatment.

POINTS TO REMEMBER

- PDB is uncommon and unilateral, whereas eczematous dermatitis of the nipples is common and tends to present bilaterally.
- Any unilateral, chronic eczematous lesion of the breast or nipple ("nipple eczema") that is unresponsive to topical corticosteroid therapy should be biopsied.
- EMPD is a rare disorder that is easily overlooked, but it must be considered in the differential diagnosis of patients with chronic genital or perianal dermatitis.
- Both PDB and EMPD closely resemble eczema; therefore, it is important to consider PDB or EMPD among patients in whom supposed eczema of the breast or perineum does not clear with appropriate therapy.

BASICS

- Merkel cell carcinoma (MCC), traditionally considered to be a rare form of skin cancer, has become more commonly reported in recent years. MCC may be very aggressive and often metastasizes.
- Believed to arise from Merkel cells, which are pressure receptors in the skin, this skin cancer is more common in the elderly >50 years of age. It occurs on areas commonly exposed to sunlight, most often the head and neck.
- Ultraviolet radiation has been implicated as a factor in developing MCC, due to the frequent occurrence of the tumor on sun-exposed skin. Immunosuppression following organ transplantation and other immune-deficiency states are also associated with its development.
- Polyomavirus has been detected in about 80% of MCCs tested.

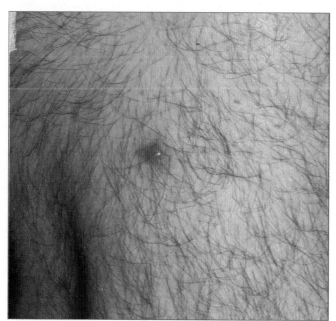

31.50 *Merkel cell carcinoma.* Shiny, slightly tender pink papule on the thigh of a 55-year-old male.

CLINICAL MANIFESTATIONS

- MCC usually presents as a solitary reddish pink, shiny papule or nodule (Fig. 31.50).
- May be tender.
- MCCs spread through the lymphatic system and multiple smaller seedlings can develop around the main tumor. With a nearly 40% recurrence rate, MCC may spread to lymph nodes in the neck, axillae, and groin.

DIAGNOSIS

- Excisional biopsy.
- Unless there is a high degree of suspicion, the diagnosis of MCC is usually made *after* a biopsy is performed.
- After general examination, including evaluation of local lymph nodes, staging imaging investigations may be arranged to determine whether the tumor has spread to other sites.

 MANAGEMENT

- For early stage disease that is localized to the skin, a wide surgical excision followed by radiotherapy is often used as primary treatment.
- The relevant lymph nodes may also be surgically removed or irradiated as a prophylactic measure. In some cases the lymph nodes may be sampled using a sentinel lymph node biopsy (see earlier in this chapter). This helps in staging the tumor but may not influence outcome.

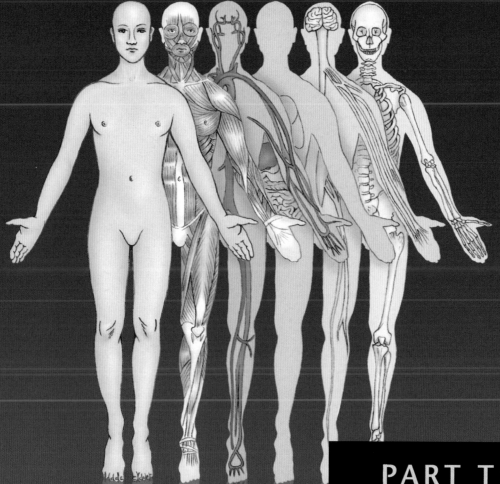

PART THREE

Systemic Conditions
and the Skin

Cutaneous Manifestations of Pregnancy

OVERVIEW

During pregnancy, hormonal shifts may result in physiologic alterations in the skin, hair, and nails. Many of these changes are seen so frequently, that they are considered to be normal. Pregnancy can also alter the course of certain pre-existing skin conditions and systemic diseases that have cutaneous involvement, for example:

- Systemic lupus erythematosus and scleroderma may flare.
- Acne may improve, or it may worsen.
- Dyshidrotic eczema may appear *de novo,* or a flare-up of pre-existing lesions may occur.
- Condylomata acuminata may enlarge considerably and may proliferate.

   It should always be kept in mind that common skin diseases unrelated to pregnancy should also be considered when evaluating a pregnant patient with a skin disorder.

IN THIS CHAPTER...

➤ **PHYSIOLOGIC CHANGES DURING PREGNANCY**

- Hyperpigmentation
- Connective tissue changes
- Vascular phenomena
- Hair changes
- Other findings

➤ **DERMATOSES OF PREGNANCY**

- Pruritic urticarial papules and plaques of pregnancy (PUPPP)
- Pruritus gravidarum
- Recurrent cholestasis of pregnancy
- Pemphigoid gestationis

HYPERPIGMENTATION

- Hyperpigmentation is presumed to be secondary to increased levels of estrogens and melanocyte-stimulating hormone.
- It frequently manifests as follows:
  - Darkening of the linea alba which becomes the linea nigra (Fig. 32.1).
  - Darkening of the nipples and surrounding areolae, as well as darkening of the axillae, thighs, umbilicus, perineum, and external genitalia, may occur.
  - Melasma (see Chapter 23). The "mask of pregnancy" (formerly known as chloasma) occurs in more than 50% of women during pregnancy. It is worsened by exposure to the sun. Melasma is also seen in women taking oral contraceptives and, on occasion, it appears *de novo* in women in whom there is no obvious explanation.
  - Darkening of pre-existing freckles and nevi.

 MANAGEMENT

- For patients with melasma caused by pregnancy, it is usually best to keep sun exposure to a minimum and to wait for fading, which often takes place spontaneously. Treatment of persistent nongestational melasma consists of diligent sun avoidance and, frequently, the use of skin bleaching hydroquinone creams (see Chapter 23).
- Darkened freckles, nevi, and linea nigra usually regress after termination of pregnancy.

CONNECTIVE TISSUE CHANGES

- **Striae gravidarum** (striae cutis distensae related to pregnancy) or "stretch marks" are caused by the combination of increased adrenocortical activity and rapid tissue growth and distention, which results in the tearing of the dermal collagen matrix and a weakening of elastic fibers.
- Typically, striae are reddish pink to violaceous linear atrophic bands that are located on the abdomen, hips, buttocks, and breasts. The striae are permanent, but the purplish color fades with time.
- **Proliferation and enlargement of skin tags**, with some persisting after pregnancy.
- **Growth of pre-existing keloids.** For example, this may occur in the scars of an abdominal hysterectomy or a cesarean section (Fig. 32.2). A problem more often noted in women of African descent.

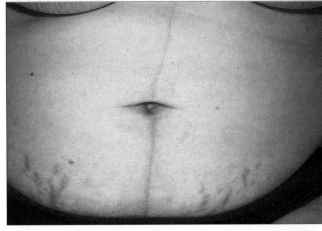

32.1 *Linea nigra and striae gravidarum.* The linea alba darkens during pregnancy, but the normal color usually returns after delivery. In contrast, although the purplish color of striae gravidarum fades over time, the striae themselves are permanent.

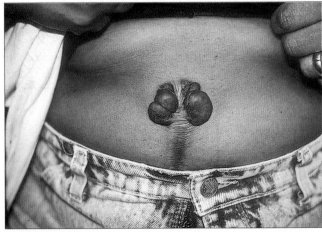

32.2 *Keloids.* These lesions are growing well beyond the border of cesarean section scar.

 MANAGEMENT

- There is no proven effective treatment or preventative strategy for striae.
- **Cocoa butter, Mederma stretch mark cream**, and **Bio-Oil** are over-the-counter emollients that have been used during pregnancy for both prevention and treatment of stretch marks with varying degrees of success.
- If desired, skin tags may be easily removed (see Chapter 30).
- Keloids may diminish in size postpartum; if they do not, treatment with intralesional steroids may be helpful (see Chapter 30).

VASCULAR PHENOMENA

- **Spider telangiectasias and angiomas** presumably are a consequence of the high levels of estrogens in pregnancy (Fig. 32.3).
- **Scattered petechiae** in the lower extremities are the result of increased capillary fragility and increased hydrostatic pressure in this region.
- **Palmar erythema**, flushing, and increased sweating (Fig. 32.4).
- **Venous varicosities** of the legs and feet.
- **Hemorrhoids.**
- **Edema** of the leg, face, or eyelids.

MANAGEMENT

- Most vascular phenomena resolve postpartum. However, varicosities may persist and may worsen with future pregnancies.

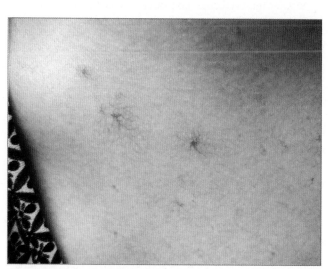

32.3 *Spider telangiectasias.* These can result from the high levels of estrogens in pregnancy.

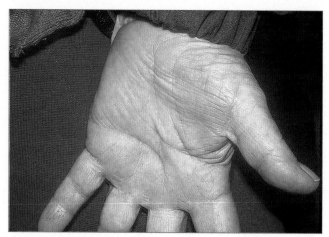

32.4 *Palmar erythema.* Flushing and increased sweating may also occur during pregnancy.

HAIR CHANGES

- **Hirsutism:** Mild degrees of hirsutism are common during pregnancy. The face is frequently affected, although hair growth may be pronounced on the extremities as well. Hirsutism normally regresses after delivery, but it may recur in subsequent pregnancies.
- **Telogen effluvium:** Increased hair shedding that occurs anywhere from 1 to 5 months postpartum and is generally followed by total regrowth. Rarely, the regrowth may not be as thick as prepregnancy hair growth (see Chapter 19).

MANAGEMENT

- Because both telogen effluvium and hirsutism usually resolve spontaneously, no specific management is needed. Excessive hirsutism, however, warrants investigation for an endocrinologic abnormality.

OTHER FINDINGS

Other skin changes during pregnancy:

- Increased nail fragility, brittleness, and distal separation of the nail plate (onycholysis).
- Edema and hyperemia of the gums ("pregnancy gingivitis").
- Pyogenic granulomas often develop on the lips and gums and usually regress shortly postpartum (Fig. 32.5).
- Erythema nodosum, an apparently autoimmune skin condition, is usually associated with infections, sarcoidosis, malignant diseases, and drugs, but it can also be precipitated by pregnancy alone (Fig. 32.6).
- Erythema multiforme has a variety of causes, including pregnancy.

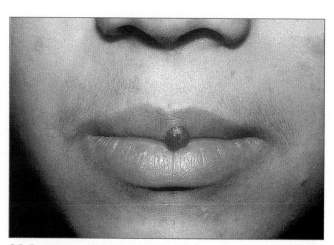

32.5 *Pyogenic granuloma.* Lesions tend to occur on the lips and gums.

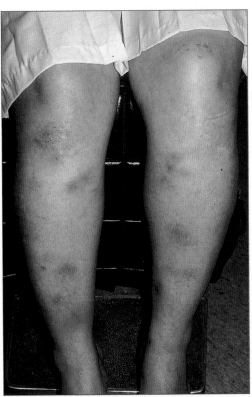

32.6 *Erythema nodosum.* These tender nodules occurred during pregnancy and resolved postpartum.

 MANAGEMENT

Pregnancy Gingivitis

- Good dental hygiene (adequate brushing and flossing) is essential, because the problem is exacerbated by plaque and calculus.

Pyogenic Granulomas

- Treatment may be deferred until after delivery or performed during pregnancy. Options include **cryodestruction, electrodesiccation**, and **excisional surgery** (see Chapter 30).

Erythema Nodosum

- Erythema nodosum tends to clear postpartum and to recur in subsequent pregnancies. Treatment consists of bed rest and mild analgesics.

Erythema Multiforme

- As with erythema nodosum, erythema multiforme resulting from pregnancy tends to clear spontaneously and is managed symptomatically. Underlying causes other than pregnancy (e.g., infection) should be sought and treated (see Chapters 27 and 34).

BASICS

- The specific dermatoses of pregnancy are a group of cutaneous eruptions that are unique to pregnancy. Historically, these eruptions have been variously classified, resulting in overlapping and confusing terminology. The following discussion should help to simplify the approach to these entities.

PRURITIC URTICARIAL PAPULES AND PLAQUES OF PREGNANCY

- A common dermatosis of late pregnancy, pruritic urticarial papules and plaques of pregnancy (PUPPP) is, as its name suggests, a pruritic eruption consisting of urticarial papules that coalesce into plaques (Figs. 32.7 and 32.8).

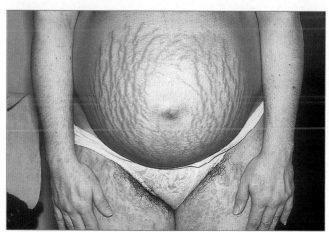

32.7 *Pruritic urticarial papules and plaques of pregnancy.* Lesions are located in the stretch marks. Note the periumbilical sparing.

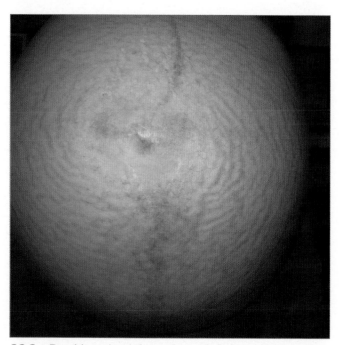

32.8 *Pruritic urticarial papules and plaques of pregnancy.* A closer view.

- PUPPP more frequently arises in primigravidae and multiple pregnancies.

CLINICAL MANIFESTATIONS

- The itching, which can become quite intense, generally begins in the last few weeks of the third trimester of pregnancy.
- Initially, the papules are found in the striae cutis distensae (i.e., stretch marks) of the abdomen, that typically spares the area surrounding the umbilicus. Later, lesions can be found on the thighs, proximal limbs, and buttocks, where they coalesce to form urticarial plaques. PUPPP tends to spare the face, palms, soles, and mucous membranes.
- The onset of PUPPP is in the third trimester and remission occurs within a few days of delivery.
- PUPPP can be sufficiently discomforting to require potent topical—and sometimes oral—corticosteroids.
- The natural history of PUPPP is spontaneous resolution within a few days of delivery in most cases. It does not appear to increase infant morbidity. Recurrences in subsequent pregnancies are unlikely, and if they do appear, they tend to be less severe.
- A broader clinical description of PUPPP has been described to include the following:
  - A rash resembling that of a drug eruption
  - A target-like rash that resembles erythema multiforme
  - A vesicular eruption

Consequently, some dermatologists suggest that PUPPP be renamed "polymorphic eruption of pregnancy."

DIAGNOSIS

- Diagnosis is usually made clinically.
- Direct immunofluorescence is negative, unlike pemphigoid gestationis (see below).

 MANAGEMENT

- Medium- to high-potency topical steroids and sedative oral antihistamines provide relief of symptoms.
- In severe cases, systemic steroids may be necessary.

PRURITUS GRAVIDARUM

CLINICAL MANIFESTATIONS

- Characterized by generalized itching that begins in the later stages of pregnancy.
- The patient's complaints often seem to be out of proportion to the visible changes on the skin. There are no primary skin lesions, and the condition clears after delivery.
- Pruritus gravidarum is considered by some investigators to be possibly a variation of PUPPP without lesions.

- Management of pruritus gravidarum is aimed at symptomatic control of pruritus with the use of bland emollients and topical antipruritic agents. Oral antihistamines are sometimes effective.

RECURRENT CHOLESTASIS OF PREGNANCY

CLINICAL MANIFESTATIONS

- Also known as *intrahepatic cholestasis of pregnancy,* recurrent cholestasis of pregnancy is a rare form of reversible cholestasis that appears in the second half of pregnancy. It generally occurs during the second or third trimester.
- This condition is caused by hyperbilirubinemia and bile acid accumulation in the skin.
- It initially manifests as severe, generalized pruritus followed by the clinical appearance of jaundice. The degree of itching correlates with levels of serum and skin bile acid. There are no primary skin lesions; however, excoriations may result from the patient's scratching.
- The condition clears after delivery but may recur in future pregnancies. The incidence of premature birth, intrapartal fetal distress, stillbirth, and low birth weight appear to be increased in the children of affected women.
- Ideally, treatment should be directed to decrease maternal bile acid levels; however, symptomatic therapy that includes bland emollients, cholestyramine resins, topical antipruritic agents, and, sometimes, oral antihistamines, have been used effectively.

PEMPHIGOID GESTATIONIS

- Pemphigoid gestationis, previously known as *herpes gestationis,* is a rare, intensely pruritic vesicobullous autoimmune dermatitis that may be clinically confused with PUPPP. The term "herpes" derives from the grouped herpetiform clustering of blisters that sometimes occurs; however, there is no relation to herpesvirus infection.

CLINICAL MANIFESTATIONS

- The skin lesions are polymorphic, ranging from urticarial papules or plaques to bullae that are small and vesicular or large and tense (Fig. 32.9).
- The onset of pemphigoid gestationis is most often in the second trimester (weeks 13 to 26), but it may arise at any stage and may even occur postpartum.

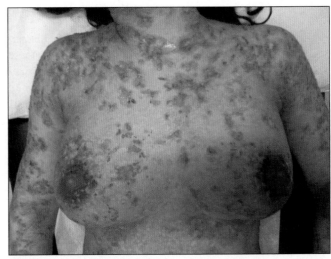

32.9 *Pemphigoid gestationis.* This pregnant woman has multiple erosions that represent evolving vesicles and bullae.

- Some reports have suggested that women with pemphigoid gestationis may have an increased risk of fetal morbidity and mortality, as well as an increased chance of giving birth prematurely and of having an infant with a lower birth weight, however, the extent, if any, of this increased risk remains controversial. Postpartum flares and symptoms may recur with menses or with administration of oral contraceptives, findings suggesting that hormonal factors play a strong role.
- Pemphigoid gestationis often recurs in subsequent pregnancies, with earlier and more florid consequences; however, it has been known to skip an ensuing pregnancy.

DIAGNOSIS

- The diagnosis can be confirmed by skin biopsy with direct immunofluorescent testing that shows deposition of C3, IgG and/or other antibodies.

 MANAGEMENT

- Treatment generally requires systemic corticosteroids in gradually tapered doses.
- In mild cases, topical corticosteroids and oral antihistamines may be sufficient.

CHAPTER 33

Cutaneous Manifestations of HIV Infection

OVERVIEW

The first organ that may be affected in human immunodeficiency virus (HIV) infection is the skin. Before the advent of highly active antiretroviral therapy (HAART), the inevitable decrease in CD4 cells with disease progression was accompanied by a variety of HIV-associated skin diseases. HIV infection was often suspected initially based on the occurrence of cutaneous diseases, such as Kaposi sarcoma (KS) or extensive molluscum contagiosum, or in a patient with particularly severe or recalcitrant manifestations of a common skin disease, such as psoriasis.

With the use of HAART, the number and frequency of cutaneous manifestations have plummeted in the United States and other countries. Furthermore, in patients with advanced HIV infection, the cutaneous manifestations often remit spontaneously when HAART is started. Nonetheless, some patients have viral resistance to these drugs or personal or economic reasons for not taking HIV medications, and in this group, the severe cutaneous manifestations of advanced HIV infection may still be seen.

Acute HIV infection is characterized by a morbilliform rash resembling measles, fever, lymphadenopathy, sore throat, and malaise may accompany the eruption.

As the number of CD4 cells decreases to fewer than 200 during the course of infection, signaling the onset of acquired immunodeficiency syndrome (AIDS), skin manifestations become more severe and increase in number.

IN THIS CHAPTER...

- ➤ HIV-ASSOCIATED HERPES SIMPLEX
- ➤ HIV-ASSOCIATED HERPES ZOSTER
- ➤ HIV-ASSOCIATED MOLLUSCUM CONTAGIOSUM
- ➤ HIV-ASSOCIATED (EPIDEMIC) KAPOSI SARCOMA
- ➤ HIV-ASSOCIATED BACILLARY ANGIOMATOSIS
- ➤ HIV-ASSOCIATED CONDYLOMA ACUMINATUM
- ➤ HIV-ASSOCIATED SYPHILIS
- ➤ HIV-ASSOCIATED NORWEGIAN SCABIES
- ➤ HIV-ASSOCIATED EOSINOPHILIC FOLLICULITIS
- ➤ HIV-ASSOCIATED ORAL HAIRY LEUKOPLAKIA
- ➤ HIV-ASSOCIATED ORAL CANDIDIASIS
- ➤ HIV-ASSOCIATED APHTHOUS ULCERS
- ➤ HIV-ASSOCIATED DRUG ERUPTIONS
- ➤ HIV-ASSOCIATED PRURITUS
- ➤ HIV-ASSOCIATED SEBORRHEIC DERMATITIS
- ➤ HIV-ASSOCIATED PSORIASIS
- ➤ HIV-ASSOCIATED LIPOATROPHY

HIV-Associated Herpes Simplex

BASICS

- In the immunocompromised host, the clinical manifestations and course of herpes simplex virus (HSV) infection differ in patients with defective cell-mediated immunity, as seen in HIV infection (see Chapters 6, 17, and 28 for a full discussion of HSV infections in immunocompetent hosts).
- Recurrent lesions may affect mucous membranes and possibly become chronic, centrifugally expanding ulcerations. These ulcerations may persist for 1 month or more in an HIV-positive patient and are an AIDS-defining diagnosis.
- Lesions may become resistant to acyclovir, or they may develop into chronic keratotic papules. Because acyclovir resistance is associated with prior treatment of suboptimal doses, it is important not to undertreat HIV-positive patients who also have HSV infections.

CLINICAL MANIFESTATIONS

- Initially, there are the typical grouped vesicles on an erythematous base, which evolve into pustules, erosions, and crusts.

Ultimately, the following lesions may occur:

- Severe or chronic erosions, ulcerations, or keratotic lesions should alert the clinician to the presence of advanced immunosuppression (Figs. 33.1 and 33.2).
- Mucosal erosions or papules.

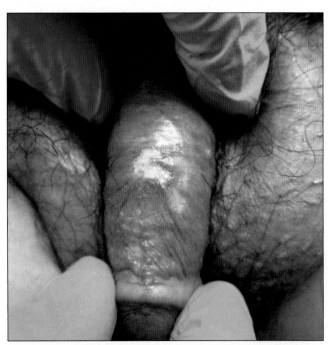

33.1   Herpes simplex. Chronic ulcerated lesions. Shown here is human immunodeficiency virus–associated chronic ulcerated genital herpes simplex that is resistant to acyclovir. This patient is receiving intravenous foscarnet.

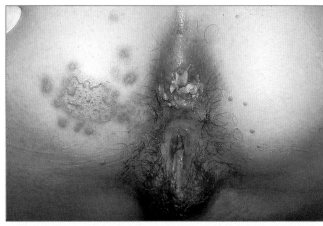

33.2   Herpes simplex. Chronic ulcerated lesions and scattered intact vesicles are present with involvement of the gluteal cleft.

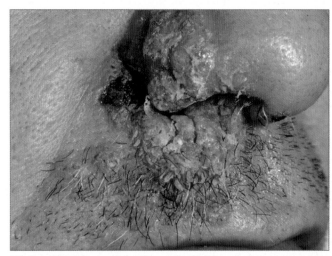

33.3   Herpes simplex. Crusted wartlike plaques are noted.

- Centrifugally expanding ulcerations with scalloped borders.
- Keratotic or wartlike papules or plaques (Fig. 33.3).
- Lesions may be more severe and more extensive than in immunocompetent hosts.

DISTRIBUTION OF LESIONS

- Intraoral areas, including the tongue, buccal mucosa, palate, and gingivae may be involved.
- Chronic ulcerative lesions in perianal areas may occur. These lesions can extend into the intergluteal cleft (see Fig. 33.2).
- Keratotic lesions may occur in any location.

DIAGNOSIS

- See Chapters 6, 17, and 28 for detailed discussion.

DIFFERENTIAL DIAGNOSIS

Herpes Zoster

- *Lesions of herpes zoster may involve only part of a dermatome and may be clinically indistinguishable from HSV lesions.*

Decubitus Ulcer

- *These lesions affect bony prominences in debilitated patients and do not extend to the intergluteal cleft.*

Cutaneous Cytomegalovirus Infection

- *In cytomegalovirus infection, perianal ulcers develop as an extension of gastrointestinal involvement. Skin biopsy shows characteristic viral inclusion bodies.*
- *In the keratotic type of cytomegalovirus infection, disseminated infection is associated with retinal findings, so an ophthalmologic examination is essential.*

Disseminated *Mycobacterium Avium-Intracellulare* Complex

- *Patients may have oral ulcerations.*
- *This infection is associated with severe systemic disease and fever in HIV-infected patients.*

Disseminated Histoplasmosis

- *Patients may have oral and cutaneous ulcerations.*
- *Disseminated histoplasmosis is associated with systemic disease.*

 ## MANAGEMENT

Recalcitrant Herpes Simplex

- If the patient has malabsorption or if lesions do not respond to other treatment, **acyclovir** (5–10 mg/kg every 8 hours) is infused over 1 hour. The dosage interval should be increased in patients with renal failure.

Acyclovir Resistance

- Failure to respond to intravenous acyclovir indicates acyclovir resistance.
- Acyclovir resistance can be prevented by avoiding undertreatment and intermittent treatment.
- **Foscarnet** (40 mg/kg intravenously every 8 hours) is used in acyclovir-resistant patients.
- Strains that recur after treatment with foscarnet are usually acyclovir sensitive.

 ## POINTS TO REMEMBER

- Long-term suppressive therapy with acyclovir has been associated with acyclovir resistance.
- Treatment should continue until clinical lesions resolve completely.
- Clinicians should be careful not to underdose with antiviral agents.

BASICS (SEE CHAPTER 17)

- Herpes zoster is most common in elderly patients and in immunocompromised persons, although it may occur in anyone who has a history of chickenpox.

CLINICAL MANIFESTATIONS

- Prodromal symptoms of pain and itching may be severe enough to lead to a suspicion of serious illness. For example, the prodromal pain of thoracic zoster has led to critical care unit admission to rule out myocardial infarction.
- Regional adenopathy may occur.
- Varicella pneumonia may develop.
- Cutaneous lesions may become chronic in patients with AIDS.
- Grouped vesicles or bullae on an erythematous base affect all or part of a dermatome.
- Lesions evolve into pustules and crusts and may erode. Chronic ulcerations and crusted or verrucous lesions may occur.
- Severe scarring may result (Fig. 33.4).

DISTRIBUTION OF LESIONS

- Any dermatome can be affected.
- Disseminated herpes zoster virus may occur. Occasional dissemination may lead to 25 or more lesions outside of the primary and two contiguous dermatomes (Fig. 33.5A,B). The disease usually begins with typical dermatomal herpes zoster virus that becomes widespread and chronic. The eruption may be indistinguishable from varicella.

🔧 MANAGEMENT

Recalcitrant Herpes Zoster

- **Intravenous acyclovir** (10 mg/kg every 8 hours) is given for 10 to 14 days.
- Dosage intervals are increased in patients with renal failure.
- If lesions improve but persist beyond 10 to 14 days, treatment is continued until all lesions resolve.

Acyclovir Resistance

- If lesions fail to resolve, the virus may be resistant to acyclovir.
- Acyclovir-resistant varicella-zoster virus infection responds to **foscarnet** (40 mg/kg every 8 hours until lesions resolve).

🎯 POINTS TO REMEMBER

- Undertreatment may lead to viral resistance.
- Patients with herpes zoster can transmit the virus as chickenpox to nonimmune persons.

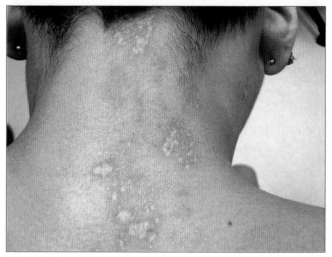

33.4 *Herpes zoster.* This patient developed scarring from HZV infection.

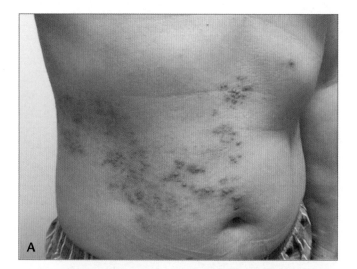

A

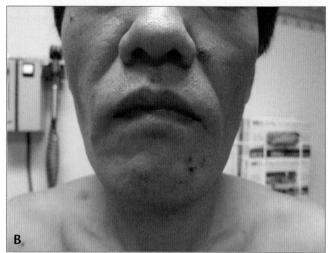

B

33.5 *Disseminated herpes zoster.* Note the initial dermatomal involvement on the abdomen in this patient (**A**), who also has scattered vesicles on the face (**B**).

BASICS (SEE CHAPTER 17)

- Molluscum contagiosum is caused by a poxvirus; the condition is most commonly seen in immunocompetent children and less commonly in healthy adults.
- Multiple and extensive facial lesions, as well as lesions with atypical morphology, should alert the practitioner to the possibility of HIV infection.

CLINICAL MANIFESTATIONS

- There is occasional tenderness or inflammation.
- Lesions are often a great cosmetic concern to patients.
- Papules may be dome-shaped or, more commonly, are atypical in appearance.
- Size may be up to, or greater than, 1 cm (*giant molluscum contagiosum*) (Fig. 33.6).
- Lesions may lack central umbilication or may have several umbilications.
- Lesions on hairy areas tend to penetrate hair follicles.
- Lesions may be extensive (hundreds to thousands in number) in patients with advanced AIDS.
- Patients receiving HAART tend to have rare molluscum, with the more typical morphology seen in immunocompetent hosts.
- The appearance of new lesions may follow a downward fluctuation in immunity caused by a concurrent infection, such as influenza.

DISTRIBUTION OF LESIONS

- All areas of the body may be affected, but lesions are most common on the face and genitals (Fig. 33.7).
- In men, possible extensive involvement of the beard area may result from shaving.

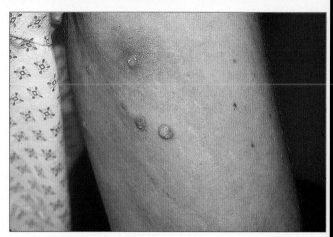

33.6 *Molluscum contagiosum.* This patient has "giant" molluscum lesions on his arm.

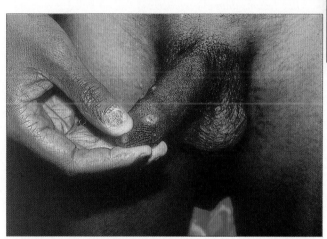

33.7 *Molluscum contagiosum.* This HIV-positive patient has a large molluscum contagiosum lesion on the shaft of his penis as well as other scattered smaller lesions. Also note onychomycosis of his thumbnail which is another sign of immunodeficiency.

DIFFERENTIAL DIAGNOSIS

Disseminated Cryptococcosis

- *Cutaneous lesions may be clinically identical to those of molluscum contagiosum (Fig. 33.8).*
- *Affected patients are usually systemically ill, although cutaneous involvement may be the first sign of illness.*
- *Crush preparation with India ink shows encapsulated yeast.*
- *When in doubt, lesions can be identified by biopsy.*
- *Patients with cutaneous dissemination have neurologic involvement, and a faster diagnosis can be made by cerebrospinal fluid examination.*

Disseminated Histoplasmosis

- *This is a less common cause of molluscum contagiosum–like lesions than cryptococcosis.*
- *Cutaneous histoplasmosis is always indicative of systemic infection.*

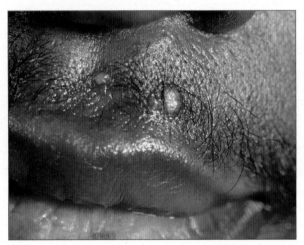

33.8 *Disseminated cryptococcosis.* Note the resemblance of these papules to those of molluscum contagiosum.

 MANAGEMENT

- Treatment is individualized for each patient. No specific treatment is universally more effective than any other.
- **Topical tretinoin** is a useful adjunctive treatment in cases of molluscum contagiosum of the beard.
- Surgical treatment is with **curettage** or **liquid nitrogen cryosurgery**.
- **Trichloroacetic acid** 25% to 75% may be applied to individual lesions.
- **Podofilox** (Condylox) 5% may be applied to lesions twice per day, 3 days per week.
- Imiquimod 5% (**Aldara**) cream may be effective and should be used daily if possible.
- Treatment is long term and is unlikely to eradicate all lesions unless the patient's immunity improves. Lesions may remit spontaneously after the patient is started on HAART, and knowing this will sometimes influence a reluctant patient to start and adhere to treatment for HIV infection.

POINT TO REMEMBER

- Cutaneous lesions of disseminated cryptococcosis and histoplasmosis may look identical to lesions of molluscum contagiosum.

HIV-Associated (Epidemic) Kaposi Sarcoma

BASICS

- Epidemic KS is an AIDS-defining diagnosis.
- Because it is found almost exclusively in men who have had homosexual contact, KS is thought to be sexually transmitted.
- KS is exceedingly rare in women, and women with KS are presumed to have had sexual contact with bisexual men.
- KS is associated with infection of human herpesvirus 8 (HHV-8), which has been detected in saliva and in semen of affected patients.
- Lesions may resolve spontaneously as immunity improves. A similar phenomenon has been observed in immunocompromised renal transplant recipients.

CLINICAL MANIFESTATIONS

- Violaceous macules, papules, or nodules occur (Figs. 33.9 and 33.10).
- Limb edema with subtle violaceous discoloration of the skin may be present.

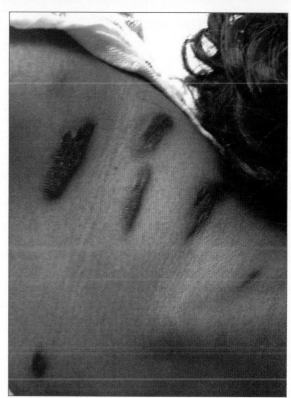

33.10 *Epidemic Kaposi sarcoma.* Multiple darkly pigmented linear nodules are present on this patient's neck and shoulder.

- Lesions are most commonly asymptomatic.
- Edema occurs with lymphatic involvement, usually in the extremities, but sometimes it affects the face.
- Oral lesions can cause pain, difficulty with eating, and loss of teeth.

DISTRIBUTION OF LESIONS

- Lesions are most common acrally, on the nose, penis, and extremities.
- Mucous membranes may be affected.
- Lesions may be disseminated in advanced HIV infection.

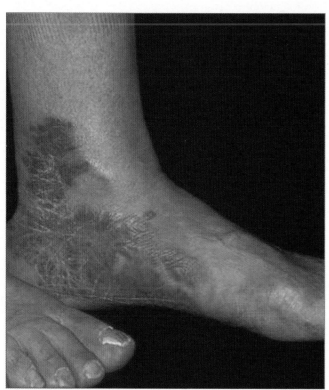

33.9 *Epidemic Kaposi sarcoma.* Note the characteristic violaceous plaques.

DIFFERENTIAL DIAGNOSIS

Pyogenic Granuloma
- *May be clinically identical to lesions of bacillary angiomatosis.*

Bacillary angiomatosis (see below)

 POINTS TO REMEMBER

- KS in an HIV-infected patient is an AIDS-defining diagnosis.
- Treatment of individual lesions does not prevent the occurrence of new lesions.
- Lesions may resolve spontaneously in patients receiving effective antiretroviral therapy, so it is beneficial to delay surgical treatment until the patient has been receiving HAART for several months.

 MANAGEMENT

- All forms of KS regress spontaneously with successful treatment of immunodeficiency with **HAART**.

Disseminated Cutaneous Kaposi Sarcoma
- Disseminated involvement that does not regress with HAART requires systemic chemotherapy.

Lymphangitic Kaposi Sarcoma
- Lymphatic involvement that does not respond to HAART requires systemic chemotherapy.
- Intermittent sequential compression boots can be used to decrease edema and to increase the comfort level of the patient.

Localized Cutaneous or Mucosal Kaposi Sarcoma
- **Radiation therapy** is used, particularly for facial lesions.
- **Intralesional vinblastine** is given at doses of 0.1 to 0.6 mg/mL.
- **Liquid nitrogen cryosurgery** is used for macular lesions.
- A retinoid gel, alitretinoin (**Panretin**), applied three to four times daily as tolerated, is useful for macular lesions.

HIV-Associated Bacillary Angiomatosis

BASICS

- Bacillary angiomatosis, which was first reported in 1983, is seen almost exclusively in HIV-positive patients with advanced disease. Cases have been extremely rare in recent years.
- Bacillary angiomatosis is caused by the bacilli *Bartonella henselae* and *B. quintana.*
- Bacillary angiomatosis is a systemic infection, and lesions have been described in nearly every organ of the body.
- Untreated bacillary angiomatosis can be fatal.

CLINICAL MANIFESTATIONS

- Lesions may occur as erythematous dome-shaped papules and nodules (Fig. 33.11); they can also be flatter, violaceous lesions, subcutaneous nodules, or rarely, necrotic tumors.

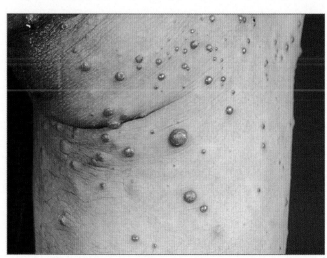

33.11 *Bacillary angiomatosis.* Dome-shaped papules and nodules are present.

- There may be associated fever.
- Bacillary angiomatosis can occur on any location of the skin or internally.
- Untreated lesions can lead to respiratory obstruction, gastrointestinal bleeding, and local or systemic infection.
- Deaths have been reported from laryngeal obstruction and disseminated intravascular coagulopathy.

DIAGNOSIS

- Skin biopsy shows a lesion resembling pyogenic granuloma, with characteristic clusters of bacilli.
- Culture is available only in research centers.

 DIFFERENTIAL DIAGNOSIS

Pyogenic Granuloma
- *May be clinically identical to lesions of bacillary angiomatosis (see Figs. 30.52 and 30.53).*

Epidemic KS (HIV-Associated)
- *May also be clinically identical to lesions of bacillary angiomatosis (see above).*

 MANAGEMENT

- **Doxycycline** (100 mg twice per day) *or*
- **Erythromycin** (250 to 500 mg four times per day)
- Treatment until lesions have resolved (usually 3 to 4 weeks)

BASICS

- Of HIV-infected men, 90% have anal human papilloma virus (HPV) infection.
- Of HIV-infected men, 73% with HPV have multiple subtypes.
- The most common subtype is the oncogenic subtype HPV 16.
- The increasing rate of anal cancer that has been seen in the United States over the last three decades is due to the increasing rate of HIV infection with HPV coinfection.
- More than half of HIV-infected men with anal condyloma will develop anal intraepithelial neoplasia (AIN). HIV-infected patients with AIN are more likely to develop invasive cancer than nonimmunocompromised persons.
- There have been fewer studies on HIV-infected women, but it is known that 49% of HIV-infected women have latent cervical HPV infection, with high oncogenic risk types, persistent infection, and an increased risk of cervical dysplasia and cancer.

CLINICAL MANIFESTATATIONS

- Four morphologic types of anogenital condyloma acuminata have been described.
- The verrucous type (Fig. 33.12) is associated with coinfection with at least four subtypes, including HPV 16. These patients are at high risk for the development of high-grade AIN.
- In the leukoplakic type, a majority of patients have HPV 16, but with fewer numbers of coinfecting subtypes, and a lower risk of high-grade AIN.
- The other types are erythroplakic and bowenoid.
- Lesions may occur anywhere on the anogenital skin.
- Lesions may also occur on skin at the angles of the mouth, or on the intraoral, vaginal, or rectal mucous membranes. Rectal condylomata may be a cause of recurrent anal condyloma, and such patients should be referred for evaluation by a rectal surgeon.

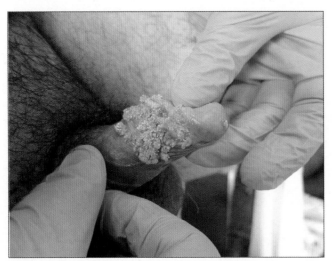

33.12 *Condyloma acuminata.* Exuberant warts in this HIV-positive patient.

DIAGNOSIS

- Diagnosis is made on clinical grounds.
- Lesions that appear to be atypical (e.g., with ulcerations) that fail to respond to several treatments, or that grow in spite of treatment should be biopsied to evaluate for malignant degeneration.

DIFFERENTIAL DIAGNOSIS

Squamous Cell Carcinoma
- *This is the most important diagnosis to exclude. This can only be done by skin biopsy of atypical lesions, or of an atypical area within a lesion.*

Inflammatory Conditions
- *Atypical, nonverrucous lesions may be confused with an inflammatory dermatosis such as perianal psoriasis, lichen planus, or lichen simplex chronicus. For a detailed discussion of the differential diagnosis of condyloma acuminatum, please refer to Chapter 28.*

MANAGEMENT

- The treatment of condyloma acuminata in HIV-infected patients is the same as that in HIV-negative patients, although it is more difficult to eradicate because intact cellular immunity is necessary to clear the skin of viral lesions.
- Some experts advocate anal cytology smears in HIV-infected patients with anogenital HPV. This is not currently recommended by the Centers for Disease Control (CDC) because rate of progression of AIN to invasive cancer, the reliability of the screening method, and the safety and the effectiveness of treatment for AIN are all unknown.

POINTS TO REMEMBER

- HIV-infected patients appear to have an increased susceptibility to malignant degeneration when they are infected with oncogenic subtypes of human papillomavirus, with the development of anal cancers in homosexual men and cervical cancer in women.
- Condylomata that appear to be clinically atypical, do not respond to treatment, or enlarge in spite of treatment should be biopsied to evaluate for malignant degeneration.

BASICS (SEE ALSO CHAPTER 28)

- Unusual manifestations of syphilis have been reported in patients with coinfection with HIV.

CLINICAL MANIFESTATIONS

- Unusual manifestations include negative serologic examination for syphilis in the presence of active secondary syphilis.
- Relapse after treatment that should have been adequate.
- Fulminant cutaneous lesions with induration.
- Necrosis and fulminant neurosyphilis resulting in permanent neurologic deficits.

 POINTS TO REMEMBER

- If syphilis is suspected in an HIV-infected patient and the serologic test is negative, then a skin biopsy should be performed.
- The only medication for the treatment of syphilis that adequately penetrates the blood–brain barrier is intravenous **aqueous penicillin**, which should be given at a dosage of 2 to 4 million units every 4 hours for 10 to 14 days in cases of suspected or proven neurosyphilis. Patients allergic to penicillin should undergo desensitization.

BASICS (ALSO SEE CHAPTER 29)

- "Norwegian" scabies is an infestation with *Sarcoptes scabiei* var. *hominis* in an immunocompromised host.
- Immunocompetent hosts are able to limit the number of mites (10 to 12) that remain in the epidermis.
- The rash and itching are the result of a delayed hypersensitivity response to the mite, its eggs, and its fecal products.
- Immunocompromised hosts are not able to contain the population of mites and may be infested with millions of mites. These patients may not itch because of their defective cell-mediated immunity.
- HIV-infected patients with Norwegian scabies infestation pose a significant risk for transmission of scabies to household contacts and medical personnel.

CLINICAL MANIFESTATIONS

- Fine white linear lesions from female mites may be visualized burrowing into the skin (Fig. 33.13).
- Crusted, keratotic plaques are characteristic of Norwegian scabies (Fig. 33.14).
- Atypical acral lesions may be seen in HIV-infected patients.

DIAGNOSIS

- Mineral oil preparation is done by scraping the epidermal surface of a burrow with a scalpel that has been dipped in mineral oil. The scraping is examined with a low-power microscope. Mites, ova, or fecal pellets are seen (Fig. 33.15).

DIFFERENTIAL DIAGNOSIS

Psoriasis
- *Psoriatic lesions tend to be located on extensor aspects of the extremities.*
- *Predominance of scale in the finger webs should lead to suspicion of Norwegian scabies.*

Solar Keratoses
- *Norwegian scabies on sun-exposed areas in elderly patients can mimic solar keratoses (see Fig. 33.14).*

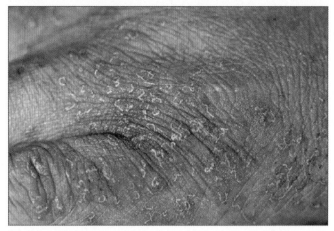

33.13 *Norwegian scabies in a patient with AIDS.* Note the white curvilinear burrows.

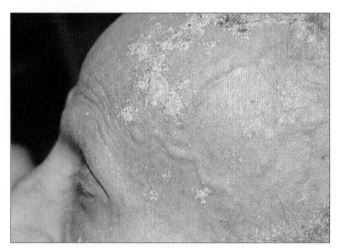

33.14 *Norwegian scabies in a patient with AIDS.* The lesions resemble solar keratoses (see also Figs. 29.13 to 29.20 and 31.1 to 31.6).

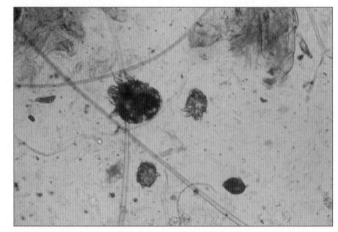

33.15 *Scabies.* Mites, ova, and fecal pellets are shown.

MANAGEMENT

Scabicides

- Permethrin 5% (**Elimite**) cream is applied, after a warm bath, to all skin surfaces from head to toe, including the palms and soles and scalp in small children; it is left on for 8 to 12 hours, usually overnight, and is washed off the next morning, *or*
- Lindane 1% (**kwell**) lotion is applied from head to toe after bathing. Treatment should be continued once weekly until there is no evidence of residual lesions. Lindane is not as effective as permethrin and may cause neurologic toxicity, particularly in children and in elderly patients.
- **Ivermectin**, 0.2 mg/kg by mouth, has been shown to be effective in eradicating infection. It is not approved by the United States Food and Drug Administration for this use.

Keratolytic Agents

- Keratolytic agents, such as 10% to 40% **salicylic acid**, remove crusts and allow penetration of the scabicides.

 POINTS TO REMEMBER

- Norwegian scabies is an infestation with millions of scabies mites and is highly contagious. Failure to treat patients promptly has led to epidemics affecting dozens of people.
- Because of the immunodeficiency in patients with Norwegian scabies, prolonged treatment may be necessary.
- Household contacts and medical staff who come into contact with the patient or the patient's bedclothes should undergo treatment as for scabies in an immunocompetent host, regardless of symptoms.

HIV-Associated Eosinophilic Folliculitis

BASICS

- HIV-associated eosinophilic folliculitis, also known as eosinophilic pustular folliculitis, is an extremely pruritic rash that is seen in the later stages of HIV infection.
- Eosinophilic folliculitis appears to be a hypersensitivity reaction because of the large numbers of eosinophils that are seen in the skin, but no consistent association with specific allergens has been reported.
- Very few patients with eosinophilic folliculitis respond to antihistamines.
- HIV-infected patients have high circulating levels of interleukin 4 and 5, the cytokines that are chemotactic for eosinophils, so a seemingly allergic manifestation such as eosinophilic folliculitis may be a result of the general immunologic derangement in these patients.
- Eosinophilic folliculitis has become rare since the use of HAART has decreased the number of cases of advanced HIV infection.

CLINICAL MANIFESTATIONS

- Severe pruritus may interfere with the patient's ability to function.
- Primary lesions are urticarial papules measuring 3 to 5 mm that look like insect bites (Fig. 33.16).
- Pustules may be present, but they are not the predominant lesions.
- In many cases, only excoriations are present because of the intense pruritus.
- Patients with long-standing eosinophilic folliculitis may develop lichenification secondary to repeated scratching.

DISTRIBUTION OF LESIONS

- Lesions may occur anywhere, but they are prominent on the "seborrheic areas" of the skin (e.g., scalp, face, chest, and upper back).

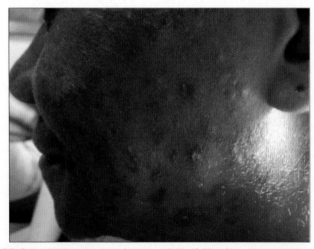

33.16 *HIV-associated eosinophilic folliculitis.* These lesions are urticarial papules measuring 3 to 5 mm that resemble insect bites.

DIAGNOSIS

- Skin biopsy shows perifollicular and follicular infiltration by eosinophils.
- Occasional peripheral eosinophilia may be present.

 DIFFERENTIAL DIAGNOSIS

Bacterial Folliculitis (see also Chapter 16 for a more Complete Discussion)
- *May be clinically indistinguishable from eosinophilic folliculitis.*
- *Gram's stain, bacterial culture, and skin biopsy help to make the distinction.*

Pityrosporum Folliculitis
- *May be clinically indistinguishable from eosinophilic folliculitis.*
- *Potassium hydroxide preparation of pus shows yeast and hyphae.*
- *Periodic acid–Schiff stain of skin biopsy specimen shows yeast and hyphae.*

Arthropod Bite Reaction
- *Also may be clinically and histologically indistinguishable from eosinophilic folliculitis.*
- *Lesions are less likely to be folliculocentric.*
- *The patient's history should include possible exposure to arthropods (e.g., fleas, lice, scabies, bed bugs, and mosquitoes).*

 MANAGEMENT

- **Topical steroids, antihistamines**, and **antibiotics** are usually ineffective.
- **Ultraviolet B phototherapy** is effective. Patients should be referred to a qualified phototherapy center. In the summer, sunlight is effective.
- **Isotretinoin** (40 mg per day) is usually effective. Treatment must be continued for at least 3 months and may need to be continued on a long-term basis. Once the lesions have resolved, an attempt to taper the dosage to the lowest effective dose should be made. Cholesterol and triglyceride levels require monitoring on a monthly basis because of the side effect of hyperlipidemia. Because the protease inhibitors also cause hyperlipidemia, patients may need to be started on a cholesterol-lowering medication concomitantly.
- **Itraconazole** (200 mg twice daily) may be effective.

POINT TO REMEMBER

- Eosinophilic folliculitis, as described herein, is almost always associated with HIV infection.

BASICS

• Oral hairy leukoplakia is a marker of HIV infection that is thought to be caused by Epstein–Barr virus infection of the oral mucosa. It is rarely seen in patients receiving HAART (see Chapter 21 for a detailed discussion).

CLINICAL MANIFESTATIONS

• Lesions are usually asymptomatic.
• Patients occasionally complain of a burning sensation of the tongue.
• White plaques resembling "corrugated cardboard" (Fig. 33.17; see also Fig. 21.14) are fixed to the mucosa; they are not friable, as in candidiasis (see below).

DISTRIBUTION OF LESIONS

• Lesions most often appear on the lateral aspects of the tongue.

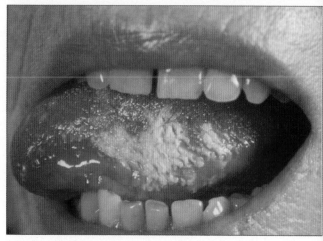

33.17 *Oral hairy leukoplakia.* White plaques resembling "corrugated cardboard" are fixed to the mucosa.

MANAGEMENT

• Treatment is necessary only in symptomatic cases.
• **Surgical excision** can be performed, but lesions recur at the margins.
• **Acyclovir** (3.2 g per day) is given with recurrence of lesions on cessation of treatment. The use of acyclovir for oral hairy leukoplakia may result in the development of acyclovir-resistance of concurrent HSV infection.
• **Topical tretinoin** 0.05% solution may be applied for 15 minutes once daily using a gauze sponge.
• **Podophyllin 25% solution** is applied sparingly to one side of the tongue at a time and is allowed to air dry. This is repeated once weekly.

HIV-ASSOCIATED ORAL CANDIDIASIS

BASICS

- Candidiasis ("thrush") is also seen in immunocompromised patients and in neonates.
- Curdlike or erosive lesions can easily be removed with gauze or a tongue blade (Fig. 33.18).
- Lesions are more common on the dorsal aspect of the tongue, oropharynx, angles of mouth, and buccal mucosa.
- The potassium hydroxide preparation shows yeast.

 MANAGEMENT

- In patients with severe immunosuppression, intermittent or prolonged topical or oral antifungal treatment is usually necessary.
- Meticulous dental hygiene and an oral rinse containing 0.12% **chlorhexidine gluconate** may be effective.
- Oral therapy with fluconazole (**Diflucan**) produces remission within approximately 1 week. Fluconazole 100 mg qd is more effective than **nystatin** 500,000 U qid or **clotrimazole** troche 10 mg 5 times per day.
- Maintenance therapy or intermittent therapy with fluconazole is essential to prevent relapse.

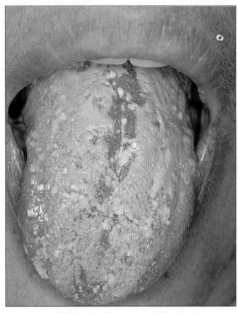

33.18 *Oral candidiasis.* These curdlike lesions can easily be removed with gauze.

HIV-ASSOCIATED APHTHOUS ULCERS

BASICS

- Aphthous ulcers may be severe in HIV-infected patients (Fig. 33.19).
- The pain may interfere with the patient's ability to eat.
- Mucosal pain leads to difficulties with eating and drinking, with resultant weight loss and dehydration (see the discussion of mucous membranes in Chapter 21; see Figs. 21.1 to 21.4).

 MANAGEMENT

- **Topical steroids** may be applied directly to the ulcerations.
- **Stomatitis elixir**, consisting of equal parts of magnesium carbonate or magnesium hydroxide suspension, viscous lidocaine, diphenhydramine elixir 12.5 mg/5 mL, and 1 g tetracycline powder, to be swished and spat out of the mouth as needed, is useful for pain.
- **Thalidomide** (100 mg by mouth twice per day) is effective with notable toxic effects of sedation, neutropenia, peripheral neuropathy, and teratogenicity.

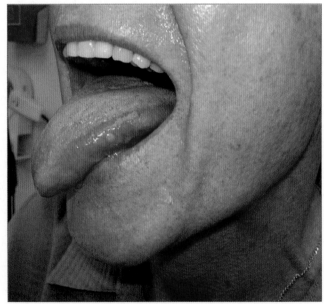

33.19 *Aphthous ulcer in a patient with AIDS.* These lesions can be quite painful.

HIV-ASSOCIATED DRUG ERUPTIONS

BASICS

- Drug eruptions are common in the HIV-infected population because of the large number of medications taken by these patients. The most commonly implicated medications are sulfamethoxazole-trimethoprim, to which at least 60% of patients with AIDS develop an allergy, followed by the aminopenicillins.
- When the drug allergy causes a typical morbilliform eruption, it is possible to continue the offending medication and treat the patient's symptoms with antihistamines and topical steroids. More serious drug eruptions are characterized by urticaria, mucosal involvement, target lesions, erythroderma, and tenderness of the skin. Any of these signs or symptoms requires prompt discontinuation of the offending medication.
- Mucosal involvement and target lesions are indicative of erythema multiforme or Stevens–Johnson syndrome, whereas erythroderma and skin tenderness are seen in toxic epidermal necrolysis. The non-nucleoside reverse transcriptase inhibitor nevirapine has been associated with severe cases of Stevens–Johnson syndrome. For a complete discussion of drug eruptions, see Chapter 26.

HIV-ASSOCIATED PRURITUS

BASICS

- Pruritus is a common and troubling symptom in HIV-infected patients. It often has a multifactorial origin.
- Many patients use antibacterial or deodorant soaps with the mistaken belief that these will decrease the risk for infection. In fact, these soaps dry the skin and make the patients itchy and more susceptible to cutaneous infection because of the excoriations that results.
- Patients may become itchy because of subclinical drug eruptions or as a medication-related side effect.
- Patients may be colonized with *Staphylococcus aureus,* which is known to be a cause of pruritus in HIV-infected patients.

 MANAGEMENT

- Careful history taking and a physical examination rule out dermatologic disease as the cause.
- Patients should discontinue use of deodorant and antibacterial soaps; superfatted soaps are the least drying.
- Patients should be instructed to limit bathing to once per day.
- **Emollients** should be applied after the patient has bathed and pats dry; ointments are more emollient than creams, which are more emollient than lotions.
- Patients need to try different preparations to find which is most cosmetically acceptable and effective.
- Patients who do not obtain relief with over-the-counter moisturizers often do well with ammonium lactate 12% lotion or cream (**Lac-Hydrin**).
- Anti-itch preparations containing calamine, pramoxine, menthol, camphor, and oatmeal may be soothing.
- Sedating **antihistamines** are useful, especially before bedtime.
- **Topical steroids** should be prescribed for dermatitis, which may result from dry skin.
- **Ultraviolet B phototherapy** is palliative.
- For further discussion of pruritus, see Chapter 24.

HIV-ASSOCIATED SEBORRHEIC DERMATITIS

BASICS

- Seborrheic dermatitis is a scaly skin condition that affects up to 5% of the human population.
- In immunocompetent patients, it may be associated with an overgrowth of saprophytic *Pityrosporum* yeast on the scalp and face; it is not known whether the same is true in HIV-infected patients.
- The frequency and severity of seborrheic dermatitis are increased in HIV-infected patients, for unknown reasons.
- Seborrheic dermatitis appears commonly in hospitalized patients, probably because of the changes in hygiene (e.g., inability to shampoo the hair) experienced during illness.

For description and distribution of lesions, as well as management, see Chapter 15.

POINT TO REMEMBER

- Seborrheic dermatitis is common in HIV-infected patients, and the sudden onset of severe, recalcitrant, seborrheic dermatitis should lead to an enquiry regarding risk factors and HIV testing.

HIV-ASSOCIATED PSORIASIS

BASICS

- Psoriasis is a scaly skin disease that affects 1% to 2% of the general population.
- Psoriasis is not more common in HIV-infected patients, but it may present in a more severe or unusual form and may be recalcitrant to the usual treatments.

- Reactive arthritis that often mimics psoriasis is the most severe manifestation (see Chapter 34) symptoms may include psoriatic lesions, arthritis, urethritis, and conjunctivitis. A new onset of severe psoriasis in a patient at risk for HIV should lead to HIV testing.
- The combination of treatment with methotrexate and sulfonamides can lead to fatal bone marrow suppression.
- The use of systemic steroids for treatment of psoriasis may result in life-threatening pustular psoriasis (see Chapter 14 for a more complete discussion).

HIV-Associated Lipoatrophy

BASICS

- The complete syndrome of HIV-associated lipodystrophy consists of lipoatrophy of the face and extremities, truncal obesity with the development of a buffalo hump, triglyceridemia, and insulin resistance.
- The cause is multifactorial. It is associated with treatment with nucleoside reverse transcriptase inhibitors (NRTIs), notably stavudine (**Zerit**®) and with protease inhibitors. In addition, host factors play a role, in that white patients with CD4 counts less than 100 cells/mm^3 and body mass index less than 24 kg/m^2 have a significant risk of developing lipoatrophy independently of HIV medications.
- Facial lipoatrophy is a marker of a person who is infected with HIV, and causes severe psychological problems and depression in many of them, even when the treatment has lowered the viral load to undetectable levels.

CLINICAL MANIFESTATIONS

- Lesions are usually asymptomatic.
- There is loss of facial fat to varying degrees.
- In severe cases, there is hollowing of the cheeks and development of a "nasolabial band" between the nasolabial lines and the cheeks (Fig. 33.20). Loss of the temporal, periorbital, and the fat of the cheeks gives prominence to the underlying bony structure, giving a skeletal look.

DISTRIBUTION OF LESIONS

- Initially the cheeks are affected.
- Later the temporal and the periorbital fat disappears.

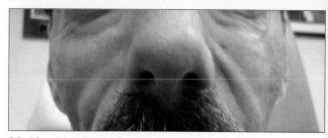

33.20 *Lipodystrophy.* Note the linear subcutaneous atrophy in this patient who has AIDS.

MANAGEMENT

- Avoidance of NRTIs, especially stavudine.
- Careful selection of protease inhibitors. Atazanavir (**Reyataz**®) does not cause the same lipid abnormalities or body fat changes that some of the other protease inhibitors do.
- Switching therapy may stop the progression of lipoatrophy.
- Filler substances have been used successfully to treat facial lipoatrophy and to reduce the stigma that is felt by patients with HIV infection. In the United States, poly-L-lactic acid (**Sculptra**®) and calcium hydroxylapatite microspheres (Radiesse®) are currently approved for the treatment of HIV-associated lipoatrophy. There are many more filler substances being used in other countries for this indication.
- Treatment of patients with severe lipoatrophy with Sculptra® requires an average of 6 treatments over 6 months by a skilled injector to achieve good results, which last for an average of 2 years. Results are not immediate, but develop 4 to 6 weeks after injection as the skin begins to form new collagen on the poly-L-lactic acid matrix.
- Treatment with **Radiesse**® does result in immediate correction, and may require only a single treatment. The microspheres which contain the calcium provide a matrix on which new collagen is formed by the skin. Because the reabsorption of the microspheres may occur more rapidly than new collagen formation, a touch-up treatment may be required approximately 3 months after the initial treatment. Results last for a year or more.
- When lipoatrophy is treated by a skilled injector, side effects are rare.

POINTS TO REMEMBER

- NRTIs and protease inhibitors are the main causes of facial lipoatrophy.
- Patients with HIV are extremely stressed by facial lipoatropy.
- Facial lipoatrophy can be treated with injections of poly-L-lactic acid or calcium hydroxylapatite microspheres.

Cutaneous Manifestations of Systemic Disease

OVERVIEW

The cutaneous surface, nails, hair, and oral cavity often afford clues to many underlying disorders. The skin is sometimes referred to as a "window to disease." For example, the presence of jaundice, palmar erythema, pruritus, and spider telangiectasias point to liver disease. The appearance of pyoderma gangrenosum, erythema nodosum, or severe aphthous stomatitis may indicate inflammatory bowel disease. By appreciating skin signs of systemic diseases, the healthcare provider can often lead his or her patient to an early diagnosis and appropriate treatment. This chapter reviews some of the cutaneous manifestations of systemic diseases and highlights some of the recent developments in their management.

IN THIS CHAPTER...

➤ **CUTANEOUS MANIFESTATIONS OF DIABETES MELLITUS**

- Necrobiosis Lipoidica Diabeticorum
- Diabetic Bullous Disease
- Diabetic Neuropathic Ulcers

➤ **CUTANEOUS MANIFESTATIONS OF THYROID DISEASE**

➤ **CUTANEOUS MANIFESTATIONS OF LIPID ABNORMALITIES**

- Xanthomas

➤ **CONNECTIVE TISSUE DISEASES**

- Systemic Lupus Erythematosus
- Drug-induced Lupus Erythematosus
- Subacute Cutaneous Lupus Erythematosus
- Chronic Cutaneous Lupus Erythematosus
- Dermatomyositis
- Morphea (aka Localized Scleroderma)
- Limited and Diffuse Systemic Sclerosis

➤ **ERYTHEMA NODOSUM**

➤ **CUTANEOUS SARCOIDOSIS**

➤ **CUTANEOUS MANIFESTATIONS OF REACTIVE ARTHRITIS**

➤ **PYODERMA GANGRENOSUM**

➤ **EXFOLIATIVE DERMATITIS**

Cutaneous Manifestations of Diabetes Mellitus

BASICS

- Many different skin manifestations are seen in conjunction with endocrine disorders. Some cutaneous lesions are directly related to the degree of endocrine dysfunction and may be caused by an excess or deficiency of a hormone acting on a specific tissue, such as warm and moist skin associated with hyperthyroidism or dry and cool skin associated with hypothyroidism.
- In diabetes, it may be difficult to link the skin findings to the degree of hyperglycemia (e.g., necrobiosis lipoidica diabeticorum).

DIABETES MELLITUS–ASSOCIATED LESIONS

- Diabetes mellitus is a disease characterized by a disturbance in the production of insulin or a resistance to insulin activity, which results in abnormal glucose metabolism.
- Diabetes causes cellular changes, such as microangiopathy of small blood vessels, which can result in organ damage, retinal disease, renal dysfunction, and cutaneous lesions.
- Diabetes can also affect immune function and can lead to an increase in bacterial, fungal, and yeast infections.

Necrobiosis Lipoidica Diabeticorum

BASICS

- Necrobiosis lipoidica diabeticorum (NLD) is an idiopathic chronic granulomatous disease characterized by collagen degeneration, granuloma formation, fat deposition, and vascular endothelial wall thickening.
- NLD is seen more frequently in type 1 than in type 2 diabetes and may occur before the onset of clinical diabetes.
- A minority of patients have no clinical evidence or family history of diabetes; in these patients, the term *necrobiosis lipoidica* is used.
- Currently, the term *necrobiosis lipoidica* is used to encompass all patients with the same clinical lesions regardless of whether diabetes is present or not, since these lesions have also been described in patients with sarcoidosis, inflammatory bowel disease, and in otherwise healthy patients.

CLINICAL MANIFESTATIONS

- NLD is more commonly seen in women than in men.
- Lesions appear most commonly on the pretibial areas; rarely they may arise on other sites such as the scalp, face, groin, and upper extremities.
- Lesions typically arise as one to three asymptomatic papules and nodules with erythematous borders that coalesce into atrophic plaques.
- The plaques are characteristically translucent yellow-red to brown in color as epidermal atrophy and telangiectasias become evident (Fig. 34.1). As lesions progress, the center becomes depressed and yellowish in color (Fig. 34.2).
- Ulceration resulting in pain may occur.
- The condition is typically chronic with variable progression and scarring.

DIAGNOSIS

- Usually made on clinical appearance.
- A skin biopsy is performed if the diagnosis is in doubt.

DIFFERENTIAL DIAGNOSIS

- The lesions of NLD can be similar to those of **morphea** (see later discussion) and **other localized sclerosing lesions**.

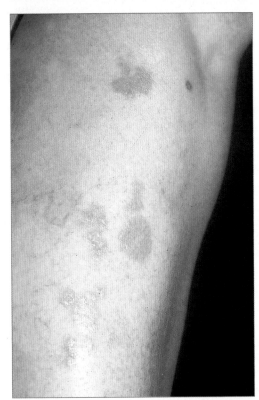

34.1 *Necrobiosis lipoidica diabeticorum.* This diabetic patient has early lesions that consist of yellow-red plaques. Epidermal atrophy and telangiectasias tend to occur later.

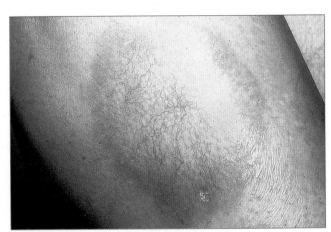

34.2 *Necrobiosis lipoidica diabeticorum.* This diabetic patient has more advanced lesions than those seen in Figure 34.1. Epidermal atrophy and telangiectasias are seen here.

MANAGEMENT

- High-potency **topical steroids** or **intralesional steroid injections** are used to lessen the inflammation of early active lesions and the active borders of enlarging lesions, but these have little beneficial effect on atrophic plaques. In fact, steroid use may cause further atrophy.
- Because localized trauma can cause NLD to ulcerate, protection of the legs with **support stockings** is helpful.
- Antiplatelet aggregation therapy with **aspirin** and **dipyridamole** has produced varied results.
- Pentoxifylline (**Trental**) may be prescribed because of its inhibition of platelet aggregation, and its fibrinolytic activity.

- Topical application of **bovine collagen** is believed to improve granulation tissue by supporting fibroblast activity and promote wound debridement by increasing the number of macrophages and neutrophils at the wound site.
- **Ticlopidine, nicotinamide, clofazimine**, and **perilesional heparin** injections have been used in uncontrolled studies and appeared to benefit some patients with NLD.
- Immunosuppressants, intralesional infliximab, colchicine, photodynamic therapy, and topical calcineurin inhibitors (**Protopic ointment** [tacrolimus] 0.1% or **Elidel cream** 1% [pimecrolimus]) have been used with reported efficacy.

Diabetic Bullous Disease

BASICS

- Lesions tend to arise in patients with long-standing diabetes mellitus who have multiple complications of the disease.

CLINICAL MANIFESTATIONS

- Diabetic bullous disease (bullosis diabeticorum) manifests as large, tense, subepidermal, noninflammatory blisters (Fig. 34.3).

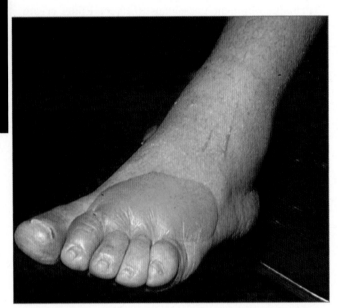

34.3 *Diabetic bullous disease.* This large, tense blister arose spontaneously in a characteristic location.

- Lesions most often arise spontaneously on the lower extremities, especially the ankles and feet. Multiple lesions may develop.
- Bullae are asymptomatic unless secondarily infected.

DIAGNOSIS

- Usually made on clinical appearance and by the exclusion of other diagnostic possibilities.

 DIFFERENTIAL DIAGNOSIS

Bullous Pemphigoid
- *Biopsy demonstrates subepidermal bullae.*
- *Positive direct and/or indirect immunofluorescence of skin biopsy.*

Edema Bullae (also Known as "Hydrostatic Bulla" and "Stasis Blister")
- *Develop in patients with an acute exacerbation of chronic edema, particularly of the lower extremities, and in the setting of anasarca.*

 MANAGEMENT

- Blisters generally heal spontaneously within 2 to 6 weeks of onset.
- Topical antibiotics are recommended until the lesions heal.

BASICS

- Diabetic neuropathic ulcers (*mal perforans*) are a major complication of diabetes mellitus. Other factors, such as mechanical changes in conformation of the bony architecture of the foot and atherosclerotic peripheral arterial disease, may be contributing causes.

CLINICAL MANIFESTATIONS

Lesions most often occur at sites of pressure (e.g., the heel), particularly in areas of poor sensory function and poor circulation (Fig. 34.4).

- Ulcers are usually painless as a result of peripheral neuropathy.

DIAGNOSIS

- Diabetic neuropathic ulcers should be distinguished from infections and other ulcerations and cutaneous neoplasms that may present as ulcers.

DIFFERENTIAL DIAGNOSIS

Venous Stasis Dermatitis Ulceration
- *Most cases are located on the medial malleolus.*
- *Large venous varicosities may be evident proximal to the eruption.*

Arterial Ulceration
- *Painful, located acrally on digits.*

MANAGEMENT

- It is beyond the scope of this discussion to describe all therapies for diabetic foot ulcers; however, management may include glycemic control, special footwear, topical wound management, daily saline soaks, surgical debridement, and skin grafting when necessary.
- Becaplermin (**Regranex**), a recombinant human platelet-derived growth factor, is available in gel form for topical therapy and (in conjunction with good ulcer care) is reported to promote healing of diabetic neuropathic foot ulcers.
- Hyperbaric oxygen therapy may be useful.

OTHER FINDINGS IN DIABETIC PATIENTS

- **Acanthosis nigricans** (Fig. 34.5) sometimes occurs in insulin-resistant diabetes (also see Figs. 23.19 and 23.20).
- **Cutaneous candidiasis** may also occur (see Figs. 18.17–18.22)
- **Eruptive xanthomas** are seen as skin markers for various primary genetic disorders such as certain types of hyperlipidemias or secondary to diabetes (see discussion later in this chapter).
- **Diabetic dermopathy** is characterized by small brownish, atrophic, scarred, hyperpigmented plaques (Fig. 34.6).
  - Lesions occur primarily on the anterior lower legs in patients with type 1 and type 2 diabetes.
  - It is typically a late manifestation of diabetes and is usually asymptomatic.
  - Diabetic dermopathy must be differentiated from lesions caused by trauma.

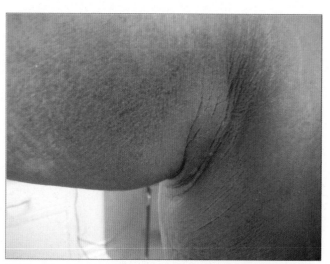

34.4 *Diabetic ulcer of the heel (mal perforans).* These lesions are noted at sites of pressure, such as the heel in this patient.

34.5 *Acanthosis nigricans.* Note the characteristic hyperpigmentation in a typical location. This patient has insulin-resistant diabetes.

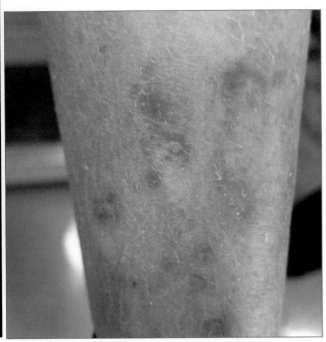

34.6 *Diabetic dermopathy.* Small, asymptomatic, brownish, atrophic, scarred, hyperpigmented plaques are seen on the shins of this diabetic patient.

- **Perforating folliculitis** (Kyrle disease) consists of firm, rough, hyperkeratotic papules, which are often hyperpigmented in dark-skinned people.
  - There is a high incidence of perforating folliculitis in patients with long-standing diabetes who are undergoing long-term hemodialysis.

- Lesions are found most commonly on the extensor surfaces of the extremities. Itching can be intense.
- **Disseminated granuloma annulare** consists of annular dermal papules (see Chapter 15) that occur both in patients with clinical diabetes and sometimes in individuals with only abnormal glucose levels.
- **Scleredema of Buschke–Löwenstein** is a rare manifestation of diabetes mellitus. The lesion is a sclerotic, thickened plaque characteristically seen on the upper back.

DIAGNOSIS

- The diagnosis of many of these entities is generally based upon clinical findings.
- A skin biopsy may be necessary to confirm the diagnosis.

LABORATORY EVALUATION

- Serum glucose levels and glycosylated hemoglobin A1C are determined to confirm the diagnosis of diabetes mellitus.
- Skin biopsies of lesions of necrobiosis lipoidica and granuloma annulare demonstrate palisading granulomas with degeneration of collagen.
- Skin biopsy of perforating folliculitis demonstrates basophilic material in the dermis, with transepidermal elimination.
- Skin biopsies of diabetic dermopathy show thickening of blood vessels and mild perivascular infiltrate.
- Diabetic bullous lesions have subepidermal blistering on hematoxylin and eosin staining of skin biopsy tissue; direct immunofluorescence of skin biopsies in these lesions is negative for immunoglobulins.

Cutaneous manifestations of Thyroid Disease

BASICS

- Thyroid hormones profoundly influence the growth and differentiation of epidermal and dermal tissues.
- Abnormal levels of thyroid hormone produce striking changes in the texture of the skin, hair, and nails.
- Some of the associated skin alterations in thyroid disease are the result of a deficiency or a high toxic level of tissue thyroid hormone.
- Other skin disorders that are considered to be autoimmune in etiology may coexist with thyroid disease such as vitiligo and alopecia areata, but are not directly related to thyroid hormone function.
- Findings such as pretibial myxedema are caused by circulating autoimmune γ-globulin, which acts as a thyroid-stimulating hormone.
- Hyperthyroidism may be caused by Graves disease, subacute thyroiditis, toxic goiter, and thyroid carcinoma.
- Hypothyroidism may be caused by iodine deficiency (cretinism), Hashimoto thyroiditis, pituitary dysfunction with thyroid-stimulating hormone deficiency, and surgical or radiation ablation of the thyroid.
- Patients with thyroid disease may be hyperthyroid at one point in their clinical course and hypothyroid at another time.

CLINICAL MANIFESTATIONS

- Hyperthyroid skin changes result from a hypermetabolic state (e.g., warm, moist, flushed skin) during the active thyrotoxic stage of thyroiditis, active Graves disease, or in patients with toxic goiters. These skin changes may gradually resolve when the patient returns to a euthyroid state.

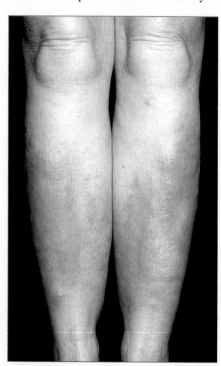

34.7   *Pretibial myxedema, Graves disease.* Erythematous plaques with early involvement.

- Hyperthyroid skin lesions may include the following:
  - Warm, moist, and velvety skin.
  - Alopecia with diffuse hair loss.
  - Nail changes with onycholysis (Plummer nails).
  - Hyperpigmentation.
  - Pretibial myxedema lesions—flesh-colored or erythematous waxy, infiltrated, translucent plaques (Figs. 34.7 and 34.8).
- Graves disease lesions (pretibial myxedema) occur in up to 4% of patients with this disease. The skin lesions and eye lesions (exophthalmos, Fig. 34.9) usually do not resolve, even after treatment of the thyroid disease brings a return to a euthyroid state.

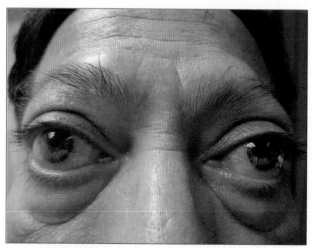

34.8   *Pretibial myxedema, Graves disease.* Note the progressive exuberant hypertrophy with folding of the skin on the shins and tops of this patient's feet.

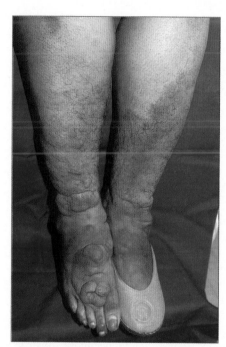

34.9   *Exophthalmos.* Eye proptosis and lid retraction is characteristic of Graves disease.

- Hypothyroid skin changes (e.g., cool, dry skin) are related to the length and severity of the clinical hypothyroid state. These skin lesions gradually improve some months after the patient returns to a euthyroid state.
- Hypothyroid skin lesions may include the following:
  - Myxedema of the skin with generalized thickening and a dry, coarse feel, yellow skin secondary to carotenemia.
  - Hair changes—coarse, sparse hair; lateral third of eyebrows lost.

DIAGNOSIS

- Diagnosis of both hyperthyroid and hypothyroid disease is made by specific thyroid function tests.
- Pretibial myxedema is often diagnosed in the clinical context of Graves disease; a skin biopsy should be performed if there is any doubt.

LABORATORY EVALUATION

- Elevated thyroid-stimulating hormone levels are the most sensitive screening test for hypothyroidism.

- Serum thyroid hormone levels can be most accurately measured by obtaining free thyroxine and free triiodothyronine levels.
- Antithyroglobulin antibodies and antithyroid microsomal antibodies are often positive in Graves disease and Hashimoto thyroiditis.
- Long-acting thyroid stimulator is elevated in 50% of patients with Graves disease.
- Skin biopsies in Graves disease show increased staining of hyaluronic acid with mucin stains in the reticular and papillary dermis.

MANAGEMENT

- Functional symptoms (e.g., increase or decrease in sweating, dry skin, hair and nail changes) of hyperthyroidism and hypothyroidism may improve after appropriate treatment of thyroid disease and return to a euthyroid state.
- Treatment of pretibial myxedema lesions can be attempted with **high-potency topical steroids** and **intralesional steroids,** although the response is generally poor.

DIFFERENTIAL DIAGNOSIS

Pretibial myxedema should be differentiated from other skin diseases such as:

Elephantiasis nostras verrucosa
- *Nonpitting edema, skin fibrosis, cobblestone-like plaques, and massive enlargement of the lower legs*
- *A progressive cutaneous hypertrophy due to chronic lymphedema, characterized by repeated inflammatory episodes, long-standing lymphatic obstruction, stasis dermatitis, or low-grade recurrent cellulitis* (Fig. 34.10)

Stasis Dermatitis (see Chapter 13)
- *Medial malleolar eczematous dermatitis.*

Lichen Simplex Chronicus (see Chapter 13)
- *Pruritus and lichenification.*

Lichen Amyloidosis
- *Pruritus and positive Congo Red stain for amyloid.*

Lichen Planus (see Chapter 15)
- *Pruritus and possible lichen planus elsewhere on the body.*

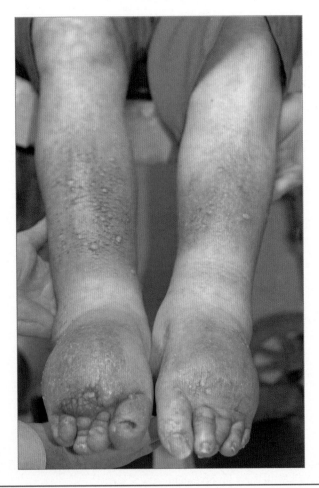

34.10 *Elephantiasis nostras verrucosa.* Nonpitting edema, hyperkeratotic papules, cobblestone-like plaques, and massive enlargement of the lower legs are evident. (From Goodheart HP. *Goodheart's Same-Site Differential Diagnosis.* Philadelphia, PA: Lippincott Williams & Wilkins, 2011.)

Cutaneous Manifestations of Lipid Abnormalities

XANTHOMAS

BASICS

- Abnormalities of lipid metabolism, with high circulating levels of various lipoproteins can result in deposition of cholesterol and other lipids in the skin, tendons, and other organs.
- Xanthomas consist of the lipids found in tissue macrophages in the skin and tendons. Lipoprotein abnormalities have been classified into primary (genetic) lipoproteinemia and secondary lipoproteinemia resulting from underlying diseases.
- There is also a high correlation between abnormal lipoproteinemia and the development of atherosclerosis.
- Primary lipoproteinemias are phenotypic expressions of various genetic disorders of lipid metabolism with the following characteristics:
  - Type I, familial lipoprotein lipase deficiency: elevated chylomicrons
  - Type IIA, familial hypercholesterolemia: elevated low-density lipoproteins
  - Type IIB, familial hyperlipidemia: elevated low-density lipoproteins and very-low-density lipoproteins
  - Type III, familial dysbetalipoproteinemia: elevated intermediate-density lipoproteins
  - Type IV, endogenous familial hypertriglyceridemia: elevated triglycerides
  - Type V, familial combined hyperlipidemia: elevated chylomicrons and elevated very-low-density lipoproteins
  - Secondary hyperlipoproteinemias result from disturbances in cholesterol and triglyceride metabolism caused by cholestatic liver disease, diabetes mellitus, pancreatitis, multiple myeloma, and nephrotic syndrome. These disorders may mimic any of the genetic lipoprotein abnormalities and may produce similar xanthomatous deposits in tissues.

CLINICAL VARIANTS

Eruptive Xanthomas

- Smooth, yellow, papular lesions (2 to 5 mm) (Fig. 34.11A,B). Sometimes a red halo appears around the lesions.
- Appear suddenly over the extensor surfaces and pressure points (Fig. 34.12).
- These lesions are usually seen in association with very high levels of triglycerides (2,000 to 4,000 mg/dL). Uncontrolled diabetes mellitus and acute pancreatitis are both common underlying causes of their surfacing on the skin.

Planar Xanthomas

- Flat to slightly palpable yellowish lesions are usually asymptomatic.
- Palmar xanthomas are seen with type III lipoproteinemia. Diffuse planar xanthomas are found in patients with multiple myeloma.

Xanthelasma

- Also known as xanthoma palpebrarum, xanthelasma is a form of planar xanthoma (Fig. 34.13).

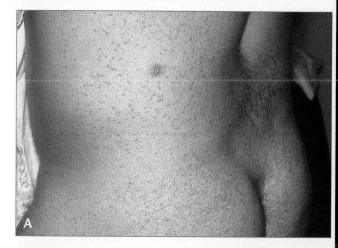

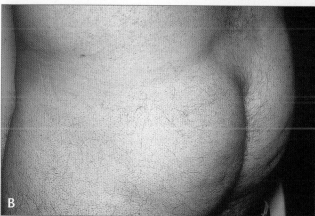

34.11 *Eruptive xanthomas.* **A:** This 28-year-old male patient has a triglyceride level of 31,000 and a cholesterol level of 580 mg/dL. **B:** This is the same patient after 2 months of a low-fat diet and a cholesterol-lowering drug.

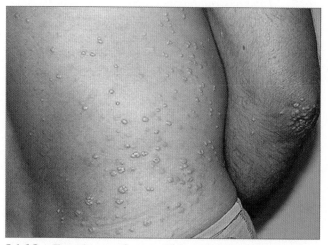

34.12 *Eruptive xanthomas.* This patient has widespread yellow-orange papules.

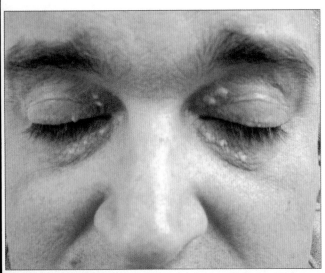

34.13 **Xanthelasma.** Periorbital yellow-orange papules are present on the upper inner eyelids. This patient was nor-molipemic when this photograph was taken.

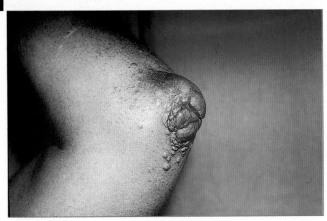

34.14 **Tuberous xanthomas.** These are firm papules and nodules in a patient with hyperlipidemia type II.

- Lesions grow slowly over years. More than 50% of patients with xanthelasma have normal lipoprotein levels.

Tuberous Xanthomas
- Small (0.5 cm) to large (3 to 5 cm), firm, yellow papules and nodules (Fig. 34.14).
- Lesions are also slow growing. They are associated with familial hypercholesterolemia but can also occur in patients with high triglyceride levels.

Tendinous Xanthomas
- Subcutaneous thickenings around tendons and ligaments.
- Occur in patients with hypercholesterolemias.

DISTRIBUTION OF LESIONS
- Eruptive xanthomas appear most frequently over the knees, elbows, and buttocks.
- Planar xanthomas are found in the palmar creases but may also be generalized.

- Xanthelasma lesions are usually found on the eyelids and medial canthus.
- Tuberous xanthomas are found on the elbows, knees, and buttocks.
- Tendinous xanthomas affect the Achilles tendon, extensor tendons of the wrists, elbows, and knees.

DIAGNOSIS
- The diagnosis is made by clinical evaluation of skin and subcutaneous lesions.
- Skin biopsy is confirmatory for xanthomas.

LABORATORY EVALUATION
- Fasting blood levels of triglycerides and cholesterol should be determined.
- Lipoprotein electrophoresis demonstrates specific lipoprotein abnormalities.
- Skin biopsy of xanthomas demonstrates collections of lipids in foamy macrophages in the dermis.
- Serum glucose levels and glycosylated hemoglobin A1C are determined to rule out diabetes mellitus.
- Serum amylase levels should be examined to rule out pancreatitis.
- Serum protein electrophoresis should be performed to rule out multiple myeloma.

 DIFFERENTIAL DIAGNOSIS

A skin biopsy may be necessary to distinguish cutaneous xanthomas from the following:
- **Cutaneous sarcoid** (see later in this chapter)

Rarely:
- **Cutaneous histiocytosis**
- **Rheumatoid nodules**
- **Subcutaneous granuloma annulare**

 MANAGEMENT

- Patients with lipid disorders and xanthomas must be appropriately evaluated for primary and secondary lipoprotein abnormalities. Treatment of the underlying cause may reverse both eruptive and tuberous xanthomas over time.
- **Dietary restrictions** and **cholesterol-lowering drugs** may reverse some changes associated with hypercholesterolemia.
- Xanthelasmas of the eyelids can be removed by application of 25% to 80% **trichloroacetic acid**, by local **electrodesiccation, laser therapy**, and **excision**; however, lesions may recur.

BASICS

- Systemic lupus erythematosus (SLE) is a chronic, idiopathic, multisystemic, autoimmune disease associated with polyclonal B-cell activation.
- Fibrinoid degeneration of connective tissue and the walls of blood vessels associated with an inflammatory infiltrate involving various organs may result in arthralgia or arthritis, kidney disease, liver disease, central nervous system disease, gastrointestinal disease, pericarditis, pneumonitis, myopathy, splenomegaly, as well as skin disease.
- The cutaneous manifestations of SLE result from the production of multiple autoantibodies that deposit immune complexes at the dermal–epidermal junction.
- Lupus skin lesions may be classified into three distinct groups:
  - **Acute cutaneous lupus erythematosus (ACLE)** lesions are strongly associated with active SLE; however, ACLE lesions may occasionally be seen in **subacute cutaneous lupus erythematosus** (SCLE).
  - **SCLE** comprises the second category.
  - **Chronic cutaneous lupus erythematosus (CCLE)** traditionally referred to as discoid lupus erythematosus (DLE). DLE lesions may be seen in both SLE and CCLE.
- SLE is seen in a 9:1 female-to-male ratio; it is more common in blacks and Hispanics.
- Approximately 10% of patients with SLE have a first-degree relative with the disease. An association of lupus and human leukocyte antigens (HLA) -DR2 and -DR4 has been seen.

CLINICAL MANIFESTATIONS

The following are considered to be **SLE-specific skin lesions:**

- The classic malar or **"butterfly" rash** (Fig. 34.15) is a persistent erythema over the cheeks that tends to spare the nasolabial creases. Sometimes, this is the initial symptom of lupus, and it often occurs after sun exposure.
- **Photosensitivity** occurs as an exaggerated or unusual reaction to sunlight. Lesions tend to occur in sun-exposed areas such as the face, dorsa of the forearms, the hands, and the sun exposed "V" of the neck.
- **Discoid lesions (discoid lupus erythematosus)** are erythematous lesions that evolve into scaly, atrophic scarring plaques (Fig. 34.16). Such discoid lesions affect 10% to 15% of patients with SLE.
- **Oral ulcerations** may develop, more often on the hard palate or nasopharynx.
- **Nonspecific lesions** of lupus that may be seen in SLE and other connective tissue diseases include the following:
  - The **"spider" type of telangiectasia** is usually seen in SLE, scleroderma, as well as dermatomyositis.
  - On dorsal hands, violaceous plaques that *spare the skin overlying the joints* are characteristic of SLE. Conversely,

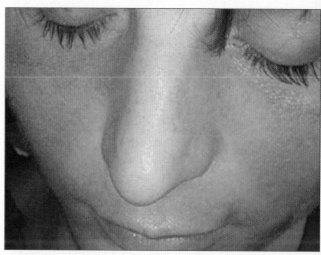

34.15 Systemic lupus erythematosus. A "butterfly rash" is evident. Note the sparing of the nasolabial areas that are often involved with seborrheic dermatitis.

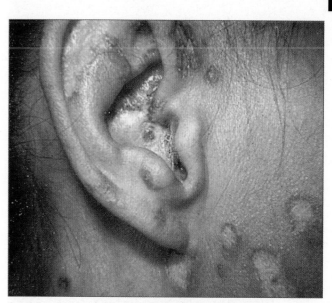

34.16 Systemic lupus erythematosus (discoid lupus erythematosus). Characteristic atrophic, disc-shaped scarring plaques.

in dermatomyositis, the *skin over joints* are affected (*Gottron papules [see 34.26 below]*).
  - **Periungual telangiectasias** are seen in SLE (Fig. 34.17), as well as in dermatomyositis and scleroderma.
  - **Palmar telangiectasias, palmar erythema.**
  - **Livedo reticulitis** (Fig. 34.18), panniculitis, thrombophlebitis, urticaria, urticarial vasculitis, frontal alopecia ("lupus hair") and diffuse nonscarring alopecia, and bullae are associated primarily with SLE.
  - **Vasculitis,** palpable purpura, and vasculitic ulcers (Figs. 34.19 and 34.20).
  - **Raynaud phenomenon** is associated with SLE and scleroderma.

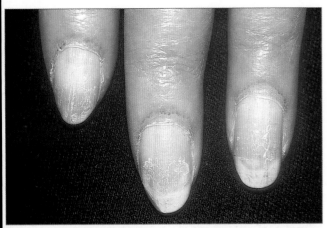

34.17 *Systemic lupus erythematosus.* Periungual telangiectasias are present. There is also thickening of the cuticles and nail dystrophy.

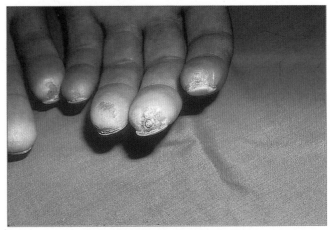

34.20 *Systemic lupus erythematosus.* Necrotic, painful, vasculitic ulcers are present on the fingertips.

SYSTEMIC SIGNS OF SLE

- Fatigue, fever, and malaise may be the presenting nonspecific symptoms.
- Signs or symptoms related to the specific organ or area involved (e.g., arthralgia).
- Associated hematologic abnormalities: idiopathic thrombocytopenic purpura, hemolytic anemia, leukopenia, and clotting abnormalities, which may be related to the anticardiolipin syndrome.
- Other associated conditions and symptoms that may be noted include rheumatoid arthritis, Sjögren syndrome, seizures, and the occurrence of multiple spontaneous abortions.

DIAGNOSIS

According to the American Rheumatologic Association, a person is considered to have SLE if four or more of the following criteria are present:

- "Butterfly" rash
- Lesions of CCLE or DLE
- Photosensitivity
- Oral ulcers
- Arthritis in two or more joints
- Serositis
- Renal disorder
- Neurologic disorder
- Hematologic disorder
- Immunologic disorder: anti-DNA, anti-Smith (anti-Sm) antibody, or a false-biologic–positive syphilis serologic result
- Antinuclear antibodies (ANAs)

LABORATORY EVALUATION

- Antinuclear antibody (ANA) titers are positive in 95% of patients with SLE. The peripheral rim pattern is associated most strongly with lupus erythematosus, although other patterns commonly are present.

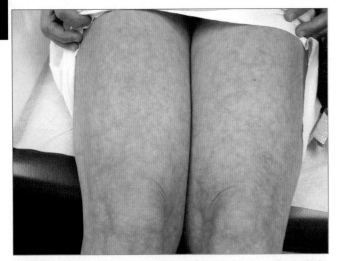

34.18 *Systemic lupus erythematosus.* Livedo reticularis is present here.

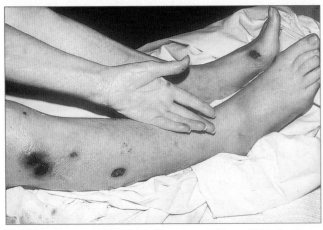

34.19 *Systemic lupus erythematosus.* Vasculitic ulcers are seen on this patient's legs.

- Anti-dsDNA (antibody to native double-stranded DNA) is present in 60% to 80% of patients and is more specific for SLE.
- Anti-Sm antibody has a strong specificity for SLE. This is particularly relevant in patients in whom anti-dsDNA results are negative and may help exclude underlying systemic involvement.
- Antiphospholipid antibodies are present in 25% of patients.
- The erythrocyte sedimentation rate is usually elevated.
- Hypocomplementemia occurs in 70% of patients and is noted especially when there is renal involvement in active SLE.
- The lupus band test involves the direct immunofluorescence of uninvolved, non–sun-exposed skin. When positive, it is suggestive of the presence of renal disease. This test has been largely supplanted by the aforementioned serologic tests.

 DIFFERENTIAL DIAGNOSIS

Rosacea (also see Chapter 12)
- *Presence of acne-like papules and pustules in addition to malar erythema.*
- *Absence of systemic complaints.*
- *Negative ANA titers.*

Seborrheic Dermatitis (see Chapter 13)
- *Involvement of nasolabial creases.*
- *Patients respond readily to topical steroids.*
- *Lack of systemic complaints.*
- *Negative ANA titers.*

Other Conditions
- Other connective tissue diseases, such as **scleroderma** and **dermatomyositis** (see discussion below).
- Other **photosensitivity conditions**, such as polymorphous light eruption.
- **Other causes of vasculitis:** renal, hematologic, and central nervous system (CNS) disease.

Drug-Induced Lupus Erythematosus

BASICS

- The clinical and serologic picture of drug-induced lupus erythematosus is often indistinguishable from that of SLE.
- A syndrome resembling SLE can be induced by certain drugs: hydralazine, procainamide, phenytoin, isoniazid, quinidine, beta-blockers, sulfasalazine, minocycline, and lithium; however, patients with drug-induced lupus syndromes develop cutaneous lesions much less commonly than is typically seen in SLE.
- Arthralgia or arthritis, generally affecting the small joints, is often the only clinical symptom. Myalgia, pleuritis, pericarditis, fever, and hepatosplenomegaly may occur.
- The classic SLE-type skin lesions such as the butterfly rash and mucosal ulcerations are usually absent in drug-induced lupus erythematosus. CNS manifestations and renal involvement are also rare.
- In 90% of patients, ANAs are present in a homogenous or speckled pattern.
- Withdrawal of the offending drug, followed by a regression of symptoms, helps confirm the diagnosis.

MANAGEMENT

Sun-related Symptoms

- Excessive sun exposure should be avoided and the patient should be counseled in the use of broad-spectrum sunscreens.

Severely Ill Patients

- The mainstays of therapy for systemic disease are systemic steroids (prednisone), given in a dosage of 0.5 to 1 mg/kg/day.
- Administration of oral antimalarials such as hydroxychloroquine (**Plaquenil**) and chloroquine (**Aralen**) are sometimes used as first-line therapy. They both may be very effective in the treatment of skin lesions and as steroid-sparing agents.

Other therapeutic agents include the following:

- **Dapsone, gold, oral retinoids** such as isotretinoin (**Accutane**), and immunosuppressive drugs such as azathioprine (**Imuran**) and cyclophosphamide (**Cytoxan**) and **methotrexate** may be helpful.
- Mycophenolate (**CellCept**) as well as interferon alpha-2a and alpha-2b (**Roferon and Intron** A) may also be administered.
- Immunosuppressive agents are used as adjuvant therapy to treat systemic disease due to their steroid-sparing effects.
- **Thalidomide** and **intravenous γ-globulin** are used to control recalcitrant cases.

Subacute Cutaneous Lupus Erythematosus

BASICS

- Subacute Cutaneous Lupus Erythematosus (SCLE) tends to be less severe than SLE and rarely progresses to renal or CNS involvement.
- SCLE is characterized by photodistributed erythematous lesions that are nonscarring.
- SCLE occurs most commonly in young and middle-aged white women.
- Patients may have some of the American Rheumatologic Association criteria for SLE, but serious disease with renal involvement is uncommon.

CLINICAL MANIFESTATIONS

- The eruption is typically papulosquamous and often closely resembles psoriasis or pityriasis rosea.
- Lesions are often annular and heal without scarring (Fig. 34.21).
- Fatigue, malaise, and arthralgias may be noted.

34.21 *Subacute cutaneous lupus erythematosus.* This patient has multiple scaly, annular, papulosquamous lesions.

- Sjögren syndrome, idiopathic thrombocytopenic purpura, urticarial vasculitis, and morphea have been reported in association with SCLE.
- Lesions most often occur on the upper trunk, the "V" of the neck, and the extensor surfaces of the arms and hands.
- The face is often spared.

DIAGNOSIS

- Sjögren anti–SS-A (anti-Ro) and anti–SS-B (anti-La) antibodies are often found, although the absence of these antibodies does not exclude the diagnosis.
- Low titers of ANA may be present.

DIFFERENTIAL DIAGNOSIS

Psoriasis
- *Papulosquamous lesions of SCLE are often confused with psoriasis.*

Pityriasis Rosea (see Chapter 15)
- *Self-limiting.*

MANAGEMENT

- Treatment of SCLE is much like that of CCLE and SLE.
- Management focuses mainly on the avoidance of excessive sun exposure and the use of **broad-spectrum sunscreens, topical steroids, oral antimalarials, dapsone, gold, oral retinoids, thalidomide**, and **immunosuppressive drugs**.
- Because patients with SCLE have a better prognosis than patients with SLE, the clinician must weigh the potential toxicities of these agents against their benefits before initiating therapy.

BASICS

- CCLE consists of scarring plaques.
- DLE is, by far, the most common form of CCLE.
- Other CCLE variants include hypertrophic lupus erythematosus, lupus erythematosus panniculitis, and lupus profundus.
- DLE is a chronic, scarring, photosensitive dermatosis that may occur in approximately 25% of patients with SLE.
- If the initial workup of patients who present solely with localized lesions of DLE shows no evidence of SLE, then those patients are considered to be at low risk (less than 5%) for SLE to ultimately develop.

CLINICAL MANIFESTATIONS

- Lesions begin as well-defined, erythematous plaques that evolve into atrophic, disc-shaped plaques, characterized by scale, accentuated hair follicles, follicular plugging, and a combination of hypopigmentation and hyperpigmentation.
- DLE often involves the scalp and produces scarring alopecia (Fig. 34.22), which can be quite extensive.
- Lesions of DLE are relatively asymptomatic, but they may itch or be tender.
- Rarely, squamous cell carcinoma develops into hypertrophic chronic lesions.

CCLE VARIANTS

- **Hypertrophic lupus erythematosus** is a warty-appearing form of CCLE.
- **Lupus erythematosus panniculitis** is an inflammation of subcutaneous tissue.
- When lupus panniculitis occurs with an overlying lesion of CCLE, it is then referred to as **lupus profundus**.

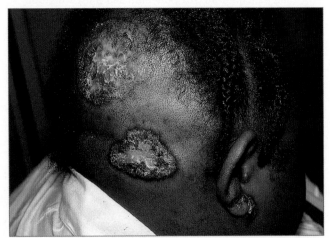

34.22   Chronic cutaneous lupus erythematosus. Lesions of DLE have caused scarring alopecia in this patient who has no evidence of SLE.

DISTRIBUTION OF LESIONS

- Patients with DLE are often divided into two groups: those with localized disease and those with widespread disease. Localized DLE occurs when only the head, neck, and external ears (Fig. 34.23) are affected, whereas widespread DLE occurs when other areas are involved (Fig. 34.24).

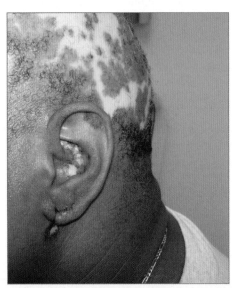

34.23   Chronic cutaneous lupus erythematosus. Extensive, progressive scarring alopecia and external ear involvement are evident in this patient, who has neither serologic nor clinical evidence of systemic disease.

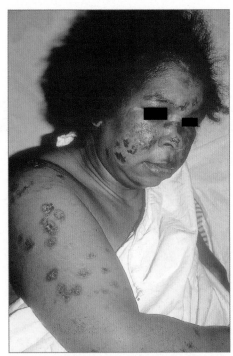

34.24   Chronic cutaneous lupus erythematosus in patient with SLE. Widespread lesions of DLE are noted. SLE is more likely to develop in patients with such extensive involvement of DLE.

DIAGNOSIS

- The clinical appearance is confirmed by a punch biopsy.

DIFFERENTIAL DIAGNOSIS

Cutaneous Sarcoidosis (see below)
- *Atrophic lesions of sarcoidosis may resemble DLE.*

Lichen Planus
- *Atrophic lesions may also closely resemble those of DLE (see image on page 4 Introduction).*

HELPFUL HINTS

- **Sun protection** whenever possible between 10 AM and 2 PM.
- Encourage smoking cessation.
- Most patients with CCLE do not have, and will not develop, SLE. Even so, many patients who are given the diagnosis of CCLE describe themselves as having "lupus" or systemic lupus erythematosus, and are mistakenly convinced that they have the more serious systemic disease.

POINT TO REMEMBER

- Patients with widespread DLE involvement are more likely to develop SLE.

MANAGEMENT

- **Broad-spectrum sunscreens** that block both ultraviolet A (UVA) and ultraviolet B (UVB) are recommended.
- **Potent topical steroids** are generally effective for treating isolated lesions. Facial lesions should be treated with low- to medium-potency agents. If necessary, high-potency or superpotent agents may be used for short periods.
- **Intralesional steroid injections** are helpful in CCLE lesions that are refractory to topical therapy.
- Systemic agents may be indicated when lesions are widespread or unresponsive to topical or intralesional therapy. Agents such as the antimalarials hydroxychloroquine (**Plaquenil**) and chloroquine (**Aralen**) comprise the first line of systemic therapy.
- **Systemic steroids, dapsone, oral retinoids, gold, intravenous immunoglobulin, clofazimine, cyclosporine, cyclophosphamide, low-dose methotrexate, thalidomide, tetracycline** or **erythromycin combined with niacinamide**, and **mycophenolate mofetil (CellCept)**, have proved to be helpful in selective cases.
- **Biological response modifiers** with anti–tumor necrosis factor-alpha therapy, particularly **adalimumab** and **infliximab**, are promising options for patients with recalcitrant disease.

Dermatomyositis

BASICS

- Dermatomyositis is an inflammatory skin and muscle disease that is related to polymyositis; in fact, both conditions are considered to be the same disease except for the presence or absence of any skin findings. Cutaneous manifestations without detectable muscle disease are known as *amyopathic dermatomyositis.*
- The female-to-male ratio is 2:1.
- An autoimmune origin, which may be initiated by a virus in genetically susceptible people, has been proposed as a possible cause of dermatomyositis. As a result, antibodies that attack the skin and muscle are produced.
- An overlap syndrome with scleroderma or lupus (**mixed connective tissue disease**) is characterized by the presence of antiribonucleoprotein (anti-RNP) antibodies.
- Adults with dermatomyositis appear to have an increased risk of certain malignant diseases and the skin disease often follows the clinical course of exacerbations and remissions of the cancer. Most malignant diseases are the common cancers (e.g., colon, ovarian, and breast cancer). Usually dermatomyositis antedates tumor by 1 to 2 years.

CLINICAL MANIFESTATIONS

- The **heliotrope rash** consists of red or violaceous coloration around the eyes and is associated with periorbital edema (Fig. 34.25). The change in color may be a subtle clinical finding, particularly in dark-skinned patients.
- **Gottron papules** consist of erythematous or violaceous, flat-topped papules on the dorsa of the hands (Fig. 34.26). Lesions are located on the joints of the fingers; they begin as papules and subsequently become atrophic and hypopigmented.
- **Poikiloderma** is a characteristic eruption of dermatomyositis, consisting of telangiectasia, atrophy, hyperpigmentation, and hypopigmentation. Poikiloderma occurs on the extensor aspects of the body, upper back (*shawl sign*), forearms, and "V" of the neck (Figs. 34.27 and 34.28). Atrophic lesions may occur particularly on the knees and elbows.

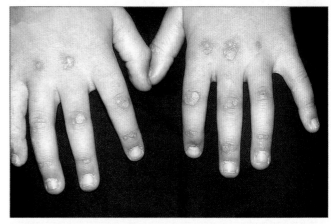

34.26 *Dermatomyositis.* Gottron papules are violaceous, flat-topped papules located *on the knuckles* of the fingers in this patient who has dermatomyositis.

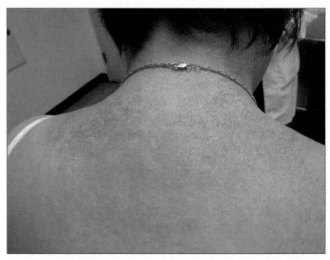

34.27 *Dermatomyositis or "shawl sign."* Poikiloderma consisting here of telangiectasia, atrophy, and hypopigmentation on the upper back.

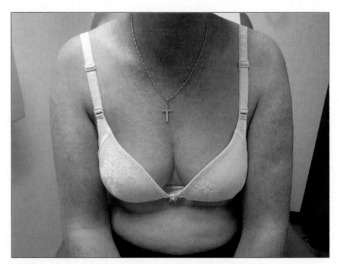

34.28 *Dermatomyositis or "shawl sign."* This is the same patient as in Fig. 34.27. Note the involvement of sun-exposed areas of the forearms and "V" of the neck.

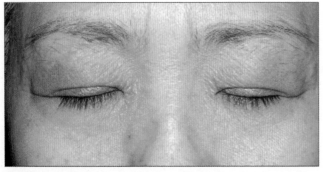

34.25 *Dermatomyositis.* Note the characteristic heliotrope (pink-purple) erythema of the upper eyelids.

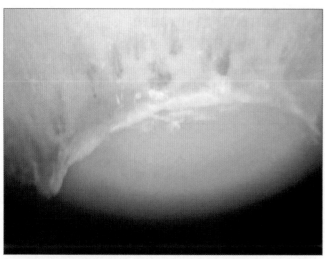

34.29 *Dermatomyositis.* Dermatoscopic view showing dilated capillaries.

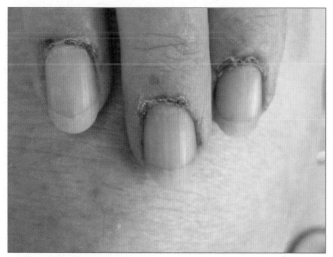

34.30 *Dermatomyositis or "ragged cuticles."* Thickened hypertrophic cuticles in a patient with dermatomyositis.

- Progressive, bilateral, symmetric, proximal muscle weakness develops, as suggested by difficulty with brushing or combing hair and standing from a seated position.
- Muscle tenderness or pain is usually not a complaint.
- Photosensitivity is evidenced in areas of poikiloderma.
- Arthralgias occur in one third of patients.
- Pulmonary fibrosis affects 10% of patients, particularly in the presence of anti-Jo 1 (histidine) or anti-PL 12 (alanine) antibodies.
- Evidence of vasculitis (e.g., palpable purpura or ulcers) may be present.
- Calcinosis cutis is seen in the juvenile form of dermatomyositis (see Chapter 10).
- Myocardial disease may be an associated finding.
- Dysphagia may occur.
- There may be features of an overlap syndrome or a mixed connective tissue disease.

DIAGNOSIS

- The diagnosis is usually made on clinical grounds
- A magnetic resonance imaging (MRI) is the most useful study for the assessment of a myositis.
- Elevation of creatine phosphokinase levels is often a reliable indicator of muscle involvement.
- Aldolase levels may be increased.
- Electromyography (abnormal in about 90% of active cases).
- A muscle biopsy may aid in the diagnosis.
- Findings on skin biopsy are often nonspecific but are generally suggestive of a connective tissue disease resembling systemic lupus erythematosus.
- The presence of autoantibodies, such as anti-DNA, anti-RNP, and anti-Ro, may be found. Anti–M-1 antibody is highly specific for dermatomyositis, but it is present in only 25% of patients.

- **Periungual telangiectasias** (Fig. 34.29) and nail dystrophy occur (see Fig. 34.17). Nail fold changes also may display a characteristic hypertrophy of the cuticles (*ragged cuticles* [Fig. 34.30]).
- **"Mechanics hands"** describe a roughening and fissuring of the tips and sides of the fingers, resulting in irregular, dirty-appearing lines that resemble those of a manual laborer.
- Scalp involvement in dermatomyositis is relatively common and manifests as an erythematous to violaceous, psoriasiform dermatitis that can be very itchy. Clinical distinction from seborrheic dermatitis or psoriasis is occasionally difficult.

 DIFFERENTIAL DIAGNOSIS

SLE should be considered (see above):

- *On dorsal hands, violaceous plaques that spare the skin overlying the joints.*

Mixed connective tissue disease or overlap syndrome is another possibility.

When only the muscle is involved, **other myopathies** should be considered.

MANAGEMENT

Skin

- Minimize sun exposure.
- Use of broad-spectrum sunscreens.
- Antimalarial drugs: hydroxychloroquine (**Plaquenil**). 5 mg/kg/day for 4 to 6 weeks; then titrate according to clinical response.
- Low-dose methotrexate using a weekly pulse.
- Azathioprine (**Imuran**) 2 to 3 mg/kg/day.

For Systemic Symptoms

- **Systemic steroids, physical therapy,** immunosuppressive therapy, including **low-dose oral methotrexate, cyclosporine, cyclophosphamide,** azathioprine (**Imuran**), **plasmapheresis, intravenous high-dose γ-globulin, interferons.**
- Results with rituximab (**Rituxan**) have been mixed.

 POINT TO REMEMBER

- The adult form of dermatomyositis may be associated with internal malignant diseases; patients older than age 50 years should be evaluated with this possibility in mind.

Morphea (aka Localized Scleroderma)

BASICS

- Morphea, also known as localized scleroderma, is an inflammatory skin disease that affects the dermis and subcutaneous fat and leads to a scar-like sclerosis.
- Morphea can present in a patchy distribution or as a linear plaque.
- Morphea can occasionally extend deep to the underlying fascia, muscle, or bone.
- Unlike systemic sclerosis, patients with morphea do not have involvement of internal organs or Raynaud phenomenon.
- The female-to-male ratio is 3:1.

CLINICAL MANIFESTATIONS

- Morphea can be seen as a single plaque, multiple plaques in a widespread distribution (generalized morphea), or a single linear plaque.
- An individual lesion initially appears as a localized, pink-red to violaceous slightly raised plaque. Subsequently, the plaque becomes an indurated, hairless lesion with a characteristic "active" "lilac" border that represents disease expansion (Fig. 34.31).
- As plaques expand the central part becomes white and scar-like and progressively indurated.
- Lesions are commonly found on the trunk or extremities or they may become widespread (generalized morphea).
- Linear morphea usually begins as a single plaque that then expands longitudinally most often on an extremity.
- Occasionally, linear morphea can severely affect the mobility of the affected extremity, especially if the condition crosses a joint.
- Morphea is generally asymptomatic, but itching may occur in the initial stages

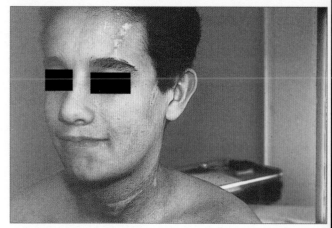

34.32   Linear morphea. A linear *en coup de sabre* lesion is present on this boy's forehead and neck.

- Morphea usually "burns out" spontaneously, and leaves post-inflammatory hyperpigmentation or a scar.

CLINICAL VARIANTS

- Linear morphea of the head is referred to as "morphea *en coup de sabre*" and is usually located on the lateral forehead and extends into the frontal scalp.
- The affected area is likened to a cut from a saber (Fig. 34.32).
- *En coup de sabre* morphea can involve the underlying muscles and bones or rarely, the meninges and even the brain.
- *Parry–Romberg syndrome,* also called hemifacial atrophy, is considered a very severe variant of linear morphea seen on the face in the distribution of the trigeminal nerve.
- Deep, guttate, or nodular forms are less common variants.

DIAGNOSIS

- The diagnosis is generally made on clinical grounds and skin biopsy.
- The serologic examination is generally negative.

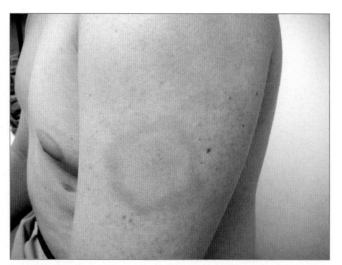

34.31   Morphea. This ivory-colored plaque has the characteristic "lilac" border.

👤 DIFFERENTIAL DIAGNOSIS

Lichen Sclerosis (also Known as Lichen Sclerosis et Atrophicus [LSA])
- *Atrophic isolated plaque(s) that resembles morphea.*
- *May coexist with morphea.*
- *Lesions consist of white plaques with epidermal atrophy and "cigarette paper" wrinkling.*
- *May involve genitals.*

MANAGEMENT

- **Topical, intralesional**, and **systemic steroids** may be helpful in the early inflammatory stage.
- Topical vitamin D analogs (**calcitriol, calcipotriene**) are sometimes effective.
- Treatment with **UVB, UVA,** and **methotrexate** may also be of some benefit.
- For more extensive cases and linear morphea that crosses a joint systemic corticosteroids and methotrexate are often used to halt progression of the disease.

HELPFUL HINTS

- Some evidence suggests that some European cases of morphea (Lyme disease) may result from *Borrelia burgdorferi* infection. This connection has not been demonstrated in the United States.
- Resolution of the advancing lilac border is a clinical indication that the morphea is no longer active.

Limited and Diffuse Systemic Sclerosis

BASICS

- Systemic sclerosis, also called systemic scleroderma, is a systemic autoimmune connective tissue disease that is categorized according to degree of skin involvement into the following:
  - **Limited systemic sclerosis**, includes **CREST syndrome** (defined below) and is associated with delayed appearance of visceral involvement.
  - **Diffuse systemic sclerosis (DSS)** (formerly referred to as progressive systemic sclerosis) which has more extensive skin involvement and often affects the internal organs and has a very poor prognosis.
- Limited systemic sclerosis accounts for 90% of the cases of systemic sclerosis.
- In DSS the female-to-male ratio is 4:1.

PATHOGENESIS

- The exact etiology of scleroderma is unknown.
- Vascular inflammation and infiltration of activated T4 cells results in an increase in number and activity of fibroblasts and excess collagen. Induration, thickening and sclerosis of the skin, and subcutaneous tissues result.

CLINICAL MANIFESTATIONS

- Thickening and fibrotic skin changes present symmetrically on the hands and fingers. These changes are termed *acrosclerosis.*
- Initially patients may report a tightening sensation of the fingers.
- In limited systemic sclerosis the sclerosis is restricted to the fingers, hands, and face.
- In diffuse systemic sclerosis the fibrotic skin changes start on the fingers but then become generalized to involve the arms, trunk, face, and legs.
- **Raynaud phenomenon**, often an early symptom, occurs in both limited and diffuse systemic sclerosis.
- Raynaud phenomenon consists of pain and a characteristic sequence of color changes of the distal fingers from white to purple to red in response to cold exposure (Fig. 34.33).
- **Sclerodactyly**, the result of long-standing disease, appears as thickened, sausage-shaped digits with a shiny, waxy atrophic look to the skin (Figs. 34.34 and 34.35).
- Other skin findings include the following:
  - Dyspigmentation characterized by either diffuse hyperpigmentation or depigmentation with perifollicular sparing ("leukoderma of scleroderma").
  - Dystrophic calcinosis cutis.
  - Matted telangiectasias of face, lips, or palms.
  - Capillary abnormalities of the proximal nail fold.

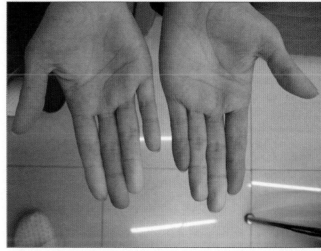

34.33 *Raynaud phenomenon in patient with CREST syndrome.* Note the blanching of this patient's distal fingers.

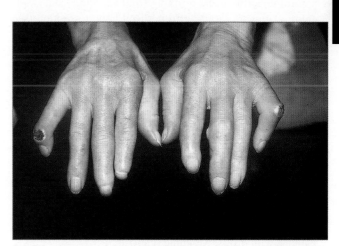

34.34 *Progressive systemic sclerosis with acrosclerosis and sclerodactyly.* The patient has tapered, shiny, stiff, waxy fingers. Note the painful vasculitic lesions on the distal fingers.

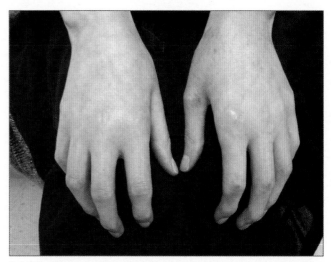

34.35 *Progressive systemic sclerosis or sclerodactyly.* The same patient as in Figure 34.36 has tapered fingers and shiny, stiff, waxy bound down skin.

CREST syndrome is considered a clinical subset of limited systemic sclerosis and consists of the following:

- *C*alcinosis cutis, most commonly occurring on the palms, fingertips, and bony prominences.
- *R*aynaud phenomenon.
- *E*sophageal dysfunction.
- *S*clerodactyly ("claw deformity").
- *T*elangiectasia (macular lesions) on the face, lips, palms, back of hands, and trunk.

DIFFUSE SYSTEMIC SCLEROSIS

- Diffuse involvement and symptoms secondary to the tightening of the skin, with difficulty in opening the mouth, masklike facies, "pinched" nose, numerous telangiectasias, and retraction of the lips (Fig. 34.36).
- Loss of manual dexterity; later, contractures of the hands, painful fingertip ulcers resulting from vasculitis, and shortening of fingers resulting from distal bone resorption (see Fig. 34.34 above).
- Esophageal dysfunction, dysphagia, bloating, and diarrhea.
- Systemic symptoms may include shortness of breath, difficulty in swallowing, and arthralgia.
- Possibly, rapid progression of kidney disease, reduced breathing capacity, cardiac disease, and renal failure.

DIAGNOSIS

- Based on clinical findings and laboratory abnormalities.
- Positive anticentromere antibody is seen in 70% of patients with CREST syndrome.
- The Scl-70 antibody is present in approximately 30% of patients with diffuse systemic sclerosis.
- Antihistone antibodies can be observed in the course of systemic sclerosis.

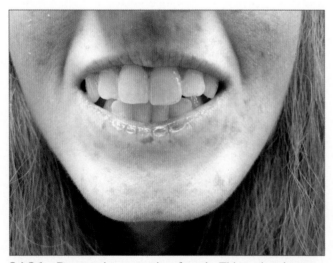

34.36 ***Progressive systemic sclerosis.*** This patient is unable to expand her smile any further. Note numerous telangiectasias, and retraction of her lips.

 DIFFERENTIAL DIAGNOSIS

Scleredema
- *Rare connective tissue disease.*
- *Excess mucin deposition leads to woody induration and hardening of the skin.*

Generalized Morphea
- *Plaques of morphea may coalesce resulting in a diffuse appearance of skin hardening.*
- *Rarely systemic associations.*

Mixed Connective Tissue Disease
- *Has signs and symptoms that tend to occur in sequence over a number of years and consist of a combination of disorders—primarily of lupus, scleroderma, and polymyositis; sometimes referred to as an* **overlap syndrome***.*

 MANAGEMENT

- Treatment regimens are diverse, difficult to treat, and remain a great challenge. Currently, no standard therapy is available for skin sclerosis. Raynaud phenomenon often responds to calcium channel blockers such as **nifedipine** and scleroderma kidney disease often responds to angiotensin-converting enzyme and angiotensin II inhibitors.
- The following are just some of the drugs and measures that have been tried or are currently under investigation: **systemic steroids, minocycline, prostaglandins, aspirin, immunosuppressive agents, tacrolimus, thalidomide, D-penicillamine, colchicine, alpha** and **gamma interferon,** and **relaxin.**
- Psoralen and UVA light, photopheresis, **lung transplantation, autologous stem cell transplantation, and etanercept.**

 HELPFUL HINTS

- Therapy of systemic scleroderma should include full range-of-motion exercises.
- When Raynaud phenomenon is present, the most effective nonpharmacologic method of preventing episodes is avoiding exposure to cold temperature and wearing layers of warm, loose-fitting clothing, including socks and gloves. Also, smoking cessation is advised.

 POINT TO REMEMBER

- CREST syndrome has a more favorable prognosis than progressive systemic sclerosis, although visceral involvement may occur late in the course of the disease.

BASICS

- Erythema nodosum (EN) is an acute inflammatory reaction of the subcutaneous fat. It is considered a delayed hypersensitivity reaction to various antigenic stimuli.
- EN is three times more common in females than in males and has a peak incidence between 20 and 30 years of age.
- Sarcoidosis (see below), streptococcal infections, pregnancy, and the use of oral contraceptives are the most common causes of EN in the United States.
- In children, streptococcal pharyngitis is the most likely underlying cause.
- Approximately 40% of cases are idiopathic.
- In addition to sarcoidosis and pregnancy, EN is associated with a variety of conditions: deep fungal infections (in endemic areas), including coccidioidomycosis, histoplasmosis, and blastomycosis; tuberculosis; *Yersinia enterocolitica* infection; inflammatory bowel disease, including ulcerative colitis and Crohn disease; malignant disease, including lymphoma and leukemia; radiation therapy; and Behçet syndrome. Drugs such as sulfonamides, penicillin, gold, amiodarone, and opiates also have been implicated as causes of EN.

CLINICAL MANIFESTATIONS

- Lesions begin as bright red, deep, extremely tender nodules (Fig. 34.37).
- During resolution, lesions become dark brown, violaceous, or bruiselike macules ("contusiform") (Fig. 34.38).
- EN tends to occur in a bilateral distribution on the anterior shins, thighs, knees, and arms.
- Malaise, fever, arthralgias, and periarticular swelling of the knees and ankles may accompany the panniculitis.
- Other symptoms may also be present, depending on the cause of EN.
- Spontaneous resolution of lesions occurs in 3 to 6 weeks, regardless of the underlying cause.
- Generally, EN indicates a better prognosis in patients who have sarcoidosis.

DIAGNOSIS

- The diagnosis of EN is usually made on clinical grounds, but a biopsy may be helpful for confirmation.

LABORATORY EVALUATION

- Usually, a complete blood count, erythrocyte sedimentation rate, throat culture, antistreptolysin titer, purified protein derivative skin test (PPD), and chest film are all that are necessary.
- If indicated, an excisional skin biopsy will show panniculitis with infiltration of lymphocytes in the septa of the fat.

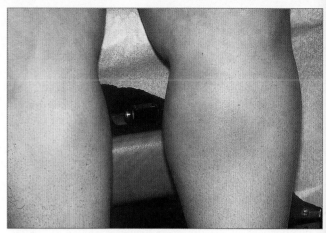

34.37 *Erythema nodosum.* Acute red, tender nodules appeared in this patient after she began taking oral contraceptives.

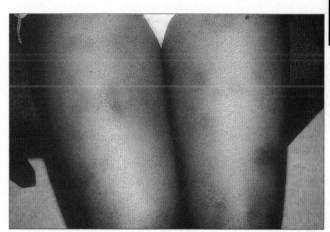

34.38 *Erythema nodosum.* These are healing "contusiform" lesions.

- Additional tests, such as gastrointestinal tract evaluation and serum angiotensin-converting enzyme determination, can be performed if suggested by the review of systems and physical examination.

 MANAGEMENT

- Treatment is symptomatic, consisting of **bed rest, leg elevation, nonsteroidal anti-inflammatory drugs** (NSAIDs), or **iodides**.
- **Systemic corticosteroids**, which often bring dramatic improvement, can be used if an infectious cause is excluded.
- Treatment or avoidance of the underlying cause, if discovered, should be attempted.

Cutaneous Sarcoidosis

BASICS

- Sarcoidosis is an example of a systemic disease in which cellular granulomatous infiltrates produce dermal skin lesions.
- Sarcoidosis is a chronic multisystemic disease of unknown origin. Most often, it presents with bilateral hilar adenopathy, pulmonary infiltration, eye lesions, and arthralgias; less commonly, there is involvement of the spleen and salivary and lacrimal glands, as well as gastrointestinal and cardiac manifestations.
- Sarcoidosis is seen most commonly in young adults, particularly in blacks in the United States and South Africa. It is also more common in Scandinavians.
- Of patients with sarcoidosis, 20% to 35% have cutaneous involvement. It usually accompanies systemic symptoms but may be the only site of involvement.
- African Americans have a greater risk of developing more serious problems such as cystic bone lesions, chronic uveitis, and chronic progressive disease.

CLINICAL MANIFESTATIONS

- Skin lesions are generally asymptomatic; however, they are often of great cosmetic concern because they occur commonly on the face.
- Specific lesions of cutaneous sarcoid include the following:
  - Dermal papules, nodules, or plaques that are brown or violaceous (Fig. 34.39).
  - Lesions may be annular, serpiginous, or atrophic.
  - Lesions may also appear on dorsa of hands, fingers, toes, and forehead.
  - **Lupus pernio**, a distinct variant, consists of reddish purple plaques around and on the nose, ears, lips, and face (Fig. 34.40). Lupus pernio also occurs with a higher frequency in African Americans and Puerto Ricans.
  - Subcutaneous nodules (**Darier–Roussy nodules**). These usually nontender, firm, oval, flesh-colored, or violaceous 0.5- to 2-cm nodules are found on the extremities or trunk.
  - **Löfgren syndrome** (erythema nodosum and arthritis) is a clinical variant of sarcoidosis.

Nonspecific cutaneous lesions associated with sarcoid include the following:

- Erythema nodosum (see above in this chapter), which more commonly affects Scandinavian populations. When associated with sarcoidosis, EN generally resolves spontaneously and suggests a better prognosis.
- Acquired ichthyosis may also be noted.

DISTRIBUTION OF LESIONS

- Lesions tend to be located periorificially (e.g., around the eyelids, nasal ala, tip of nose, earlobes, and lips).
- Lesions may occur in old scars anywhere on the body (Fig. 34.41). Scars from previous traumas, surgery, venipuncture, or tattoos may become infiltrated and may be red or purple.

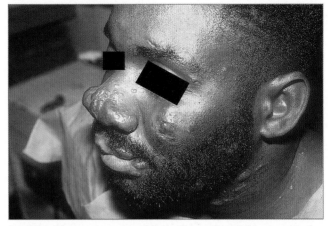

34.39 *Cutaneous sarcoidosis.* Dermal nodules are seen in a periorificial distribution (i.e., around the mouth, eyes, and nares).

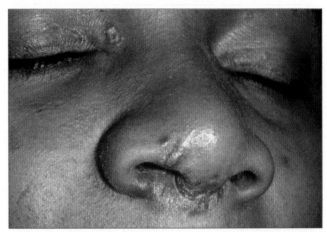

34.40 *Cutaneous sarcoidosis.* These flesh-colored papules are located perinasally.

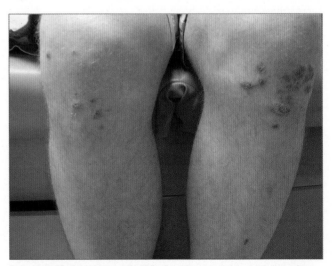

34.41 *Cutaneous sarcoidosis.* These violaceous papules are located on the knees.

- Scalp lesions may produce scarring alopecia.
- Ichthyosiform and lesions of EN tend to occur on the pretibial area.

DIAGNOSIS

- "Apple jelly" nodules are seen on blanching lesions with a glass slide (diascopy). These nodules represent the gross appearance of granulomas.
- Skin biopsy demonstrates noncaseating granulomas (sarcoidal granulomas).
- A chest radiograph may demonstrate bilateral hilar adenopathy and other characteristic changes.

Abnormal laboratory evaluations may include the following:

- Elevated angiotensin-converting enzyme levels.
- Hypergammaglobulinemia.
- Hypercalcemia.

 DIFFERENTIAL DIAGNOSIS

Granuloma Annulare (Discussed in Chapter 15)
- *Lesions most often arise symmetrically on the dorsal surfaces of hands, fingers, and feet (acral areas).*
- *Annular GA may be indistinguishable from cutaneous sarcoidosis.*

The following should also be considered in the differential diagnosis:

Lichen planus
Cutaneous tuberculosis (lupus vulgaris)
Discoid lupus erythematosus
Lymphocytoma cutis
B-cell lymphoma
Foreign body reaction
Cutaneous leprosy

 MANAGEMENT

- **Potent topical steroids** are applied under occlusion, if necessary.
- **Intralesional steroid injections** can help flatten lesions.
- **Minocycline** may help to arrest lesion progression.
- Oral **antimalarial agents** such as hydroxychloroquine (**Plaquenil**) and chloroquine (**Aralen**) are administered for therapeutically unresponsive or widespread disease.
- **Oral corticosteroids** should be used only on a short-term basis.
- If corticosteroids are not effective, **low-dose methotrexate, azathioprine, cyclosporine, oral isotretinoin, allopurinol, thalidomide,** anti–tumor necrosis factor-alpha therapy, particularly adalimumab (**Humira**) and infliximab (**Remicade**), are promising options for patients with recalcitrant or disfiguring disease.

 HELPFUL HINTS

- Systemic steroids should not be used routinely to treat cutaneous lesions; rather, potent topical steroids, intralesional steroids, or oral antimalarials should be tried first. If possible, systemic steroids are best reserved for more serious systemic involvement.
- Oral antimalarials can lead to irreversible retinopathy and blindness. Eye examination is necessary before and during antimalarial therapy.

Cutaneous Manifestations of Reactive Arthritis

BASICS

- Reactive arthritis, formerly referred to as Reiter syndrome, is an idiopathic inflammatory process affecting the skin, joints, and mucous membranes. The classic triad of **urethritis, conjunctivitis**, and **arthritis** is found in only 40% of cases at the time of the initial clinical presentation.
- Lesions and symptoms do not usually appear at the same time. Lesions may come on quickly and severely or more slowly, with sudden remissions or recurrences.
- Reactive arthritis primarily affects sexually active males between the ages of 20 and 40. Those with human immunodeficiency virus (HIV) are at a particularly high risk (see Chapter 33).
- HLA-B27 is frequently positive in patients with reactive arthritis, which generally portends a poorer prognosis.

CLINICAL MANIFESTATIONS

- Skin lesions are often indistinguishable from psoriasis; however, reactive arthritis often manifests certain characteristic findings such as the following:
  - **Keratoderma blennorrhagicum** (Fig. 34.42) consists of scaly, red, inflammatory, psoriasislike lesions on the palms and soles. The lesions may have a thick scale and may be pustular.
  - Scaling red plaques or erosions may be found on the glans penis (**circinate balanitis**) (Fig. 34.43). Lesions may also be seen on the scalp, elbows, knees, and buttocks, shaft of the penis, and scrotum.

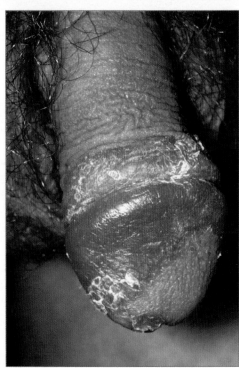

34.43   *Reactive arthritis/circinate balanitis.* Here lesions similar to psoriasis occur on the glans penis and the scrotum.

- Nail changes may include onycholysis and subungual hyperkeratosis (similar to psoriasis); furthermore, subungual pustules with resultant shedding of nails may occur.
- Oral lesions are usually painless, irregularly shaped, white plaques on the tongue that resemble geographic tongue.
- Initial symptoms often occur after nongonococcal urethritis (e.g., chlamydial infection) or infection with an enteric pathogen (e.g., *Shigella* and *Yersinia*).
- Reactive arthritis is a multisystemic disease that may present with fever, malaise, dysuria, arthralgias as well as red irritated eyes with accompanying cutaneous lesions.
- Frequently, it has a self-limited course, but it may become a chronic, relapsing condition.
- The arthritis of reactive arthritis is an asymmetric oligoarthritis that commonly involves large joints (elbows, knees); although it may also involve smaller joints. Sacroiliitis and ankylosing spondylitis may occur.
- Ocular disease may include conjunctivitis with intense red conjunctival injection and, less commonly, iritis and keratitis.
- Urethritis is a nonspecific urethral inflammation with a purulent exudate and dysuria.

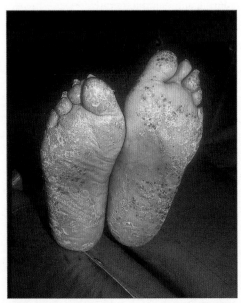

34.42   *Reactive arthritis/keratoderma blennorrhagicum.* Scaly, red-brown, inflammatory, pustular, psoriasis-like lesions are present on the soles of this patient.

DIAGNOSIS

- The diagnosis is generally made on clinical grounds.

LABORATORY EVALUATION

- HLA-B27 is positive in 75% of patients.
- ANA and rheumatoid factor are usually negative.
- The histopathologic features of skin lesions are indistinguishable from those of psoriasis.
- HIV testing should be performed.

 DIFFERENTIAL DIAGNOSIS

Psoriasis with Arthritis (see Chapter 14)
- *Psoriasiform skin lesions.*
- *Arthritis similar to that seen in reactive arthritis.*
- *No ocular symptoms.*
- *No urethritis.*

Behçet Syndrome
- *Painful oral ulcers.*
- *Arthritis.*
- *Iritis.*
- *Vasculitic skin lesions.*

Candidal Balanitis
- *Positive potassium hydroxide examination or fungal culture.*

 MANAGEMENT

Mild Cases
- May be treated with **topical steroids** for the skin lesions.
- **NSAIDs** for pain.

Severe Cases
- Oral **methotrexate** is sometimes used on a weekly basis for severe cases.
- **Oral steroids** may be necessary; however, tapering of steroids can produce an extreme flare of the pustular lesions.
- Oral retinoids such as 13-*cis*-retinoic acid (**Accutane**) and acitretin (**Soriatane**) have also been used to treat skin lesions.
- **Methotrexate, cyclosporine, UVB/UVA**, and infliximab (**Remicade**) have also been used to treat the cutaneous manifestations.

 POINT TO REMEMBER

- During initial or recurrent episodes, most patients with reactive arthritis do not manifest the complete triad of urethritis, conjunctivitis, and arthritis.

Pyoderma Gangrenosum

BASICS

- Pyoderma gangrenosum (PG) is an uncommon condition of uncertain origin.
- It is a unique, painful, inflammatory, ulcerative process of the skin.
- PG is often seen in association with certain systemic diseases including ulcerative colitis, regional enteritis, rheumatoid arthritis, symmetrical polyarthritis that may be either seronegative or seropositive, or monoclonal gammopathies, and leukemia.
- Patients often describe the initial lesion as a "pimple" or bite reaction, with a small, red papule or pustule rapidly changing into a larger, ulcerative lesion. Often, they give a history of a spider bite, but generally they have not seen or documented the presence of a spider, nor do they have any evidence that a spider actually caused the initial lesion.

CLINICAL MANIFESTATIONS

- Lesions are characterized by a rapidly expanding, painful, deep skin ulcer with a violaceous border that overhangs the ulcer bed.
- Skin ulcers are 2 to 10 cm in diameter.
- An undermined border can be demonstrated by a probe that can be placed under the overhanging edge of the lesion.
- Lesions may be multiple.
- Lesions typically heal with so-called cribiform scarring (Fig. 34.44).
- PG is usually self-limited and spontaneous healing may occur.
- Patients may have an associated oligoarticular arthritis.
- Ulcerations of PG occur after trauma or injury to the skin in some patients; this process is termed *pathergy.*
- PG is most commonly found on the lower extremities (shins and ankles), around stoma site (peristomal pyoderma gangrenosum), but lesions may occur anywhere on the body (Fig. 34.45).

DIAGNOSIS

- Generally made on a clinical basis, after exclusion of other causes of similar-appearing cutaneous ulcerations including infection, stasis ulcers, malignant disease, vasculitis, collagen vascular diseases, diabetes, and trauma.

LABORATORY EVALUATION

- Skin biopsy of the edge of the ulcer may be performed to rule out other causes of skin ulcers, however, the pathologic findings for PG are nonspecific.

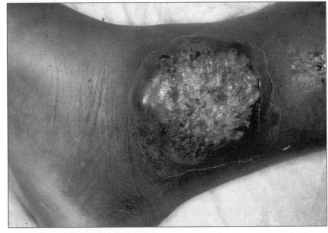

34.44 *Pyoderma gangrenosum.* This large ulceration is beginning to heal with a craterlike (cribriform) scar.

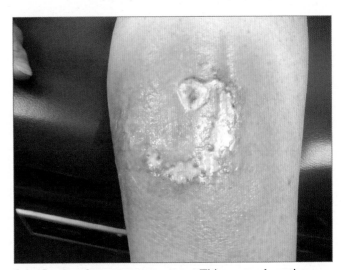

34.45 *Pyoderma gangrenosum.* This acute ulceration was initially considered to be a necrotic reaction to a spider bite. The patient was found to have regional enteritis (Crohn disease).

- Bacterial, fungal, and viral cultures of the ulcer are performed if clinically indicated.
- Workup for systemic disease should include complete blood count with differential, erythrocyte sedimentation rate, ANA, Venereal Disease Research Laboratory test, rheumatoid factor, and a chest radiograph.
- Serum or urine protein electrophoresis, peripheral smear, and bone marrow aspirate are performed, if indicated, to evaluate for hematologic malignant diseases.
- A gastrointestinal series for inflammatory bowel disease should be done if clinically indicated.

DIFFERENTIAL DIAGNOSIS

Cutaneous Malignant Diseases
Basal cell carcinoma.
Squamous cell carcinoma.

Infectious Processes
Bacterial infections
Deep fungal infections
Herpes simplex virus infections

Inflammatory Processes and Vasculitis
Collagen vascular diseases
Polyarteritis nodosa
Behçet disease
Wegener granulomatosis
Antiphospholipid antibody syndrome
Leukocytoclastic vasculitis

Also consider:
Factitial disease
Traumatic ulceration
Hidradenitis suppurativa
Insect bites
Atypical mycobacterial infections
Acute febrile neutrophilic dermatosis (Sweet syndrome)
Behçet disease
Ecthyma
Ecthyma gangrenosum

POINT TO REMEMBER

- Surgical debridement of the lesions of PG should be avoided, if possible, because of the pathergy that may occur with surgical manipulation or grafting. This can result in further wound enlargement.

MANAGEMENT

- The treatment of underlying associated diseases does not necessarily promote the healing of PG.

Topical and Intralesional Therapy
- Local compresses, antiseptic washes, and topical antibiotics may be useful.
- **Superpotent topical corticosteroids, cromolyn sodium 2% solution, nitrogen mustard**, and **5-aminosalicyclic acid** may be tried.
- **Intralesional steroid injections** (triamcinolone acetonide, 10 mg/mL) are administered into the edge of the ulcer.

Systemic Therapy
- **Oral steroids** for several weeks to months (starting at 60 to 80 mg prednisone daily and tapering the steroid slowly). Systemic steroids may be given alone or in combination with **dapsone, azathioprine**, or **chlorambucil.** In patients with steroid-resistant PG, **oral cyclosporine** has been shown to be effective.
- The following drugs have also met with some success: **mycophenolate mofetil** (*CellCept*), **tacrolimus, cyclophosphamide, thalidomide**, and **nicotine** chewing gum.
- Intravenous therapy can be administered using **pulsed methylprednisolone, pulsed cyclophosphamide**, or **human immunoglobulin.**
- **Surgical grafting** and **microvascular free flaps** are best reserved for after the disease has become inactive.

Other Therapies
- Hyperbaric oxygen.
- Biologics such as etanercept (**Enbrel**), adalimumab (**Humira),** and infliximab (**Remicade**) may prove useful.

Exfoliative Dermatitis

BASICS

- Exfoliative dermatitis (ED), known as *erythroderma* in the United Kingdom and *l'homme rouge* in France, refers to a total, or almost total, redness or scaling of the skin.
- It is an uncommon disorder seen more often in male patients; 50 years is the average age of occurrence.
- In children, ED most often is secondary to severe atopic dermatitis.
- In adults, psoriasis is the most frequently associated skin disease (see Chapter 14).
- ED may appear suddenly or gradually, occasionally accompanied by fever, chills, and lymphadenopathy.
- Less commonly, ED has been reported as a finding in the following skin disorders:
  - Allergic contact dermatitis.
  - Stasis dermatitis with secondary autoeczematization.
  - Papulosquamous dermatitis of acquired immunodeficiency syndrome.
  - Graft-versus-host disease.
  - Seborrheic dermatitis (Leiner disease) in infants.
  - Pemphigus foliaceus.
  - Pityriasis rubra pilaris (a rare disorder of keratinization).
- ED may occur as a reaction to the following drugs: sulfonamides; penicillins; antimalarials; lithium; phenothiazines; ED may be a stage in the natural history of severe eczematous dermatitis or psoriasis. Barbiturates; gold; allopurinol; NSAIDs, including aspirin; captopril; codeine; and phenytoin.
- It also may be a complication or presenting symptom of the following malignant diseases:
  - Mycosis fungoides (cutaneous T-cell lymphoma).
  - Sézary syndrome (leukemic variant of mycosis fungoides).
  - Hodgkin disease.
  - Non-Hodgkin lymphoma and leukemia.
- It is an idiopathic phenomenon in 20% to 30% of cases without any preceding dermatosis or systemic disease.

CLINICAL MANIFESTATIONS

- Unless patients have a known preexisting skin condition or concurrent physical evidence of a skin disease such as psoriasis, the clinical appearance and symptoms of most cases of ED tend to be similar, consisting of the following:
  - ED usually begins in a limited area; however, it may rapidly become generalized.
  - Pruritus may develop and may be severe.
  - Marked **generalized erythema** is followed by scaling (Figs. 34.46 and 34.47).
  - There is edema and increased warmth of the skin.
  - Lymphadenopathy, usually a reactive type (**dermatopathic lymphadenopathy**), is often present.
  - Unlike toxic epidermal necrolysis, ED spares the mucous membranes.
  - Thermoregulatory disturbances are manifested by fever or, more frequently, by hypothermia. If widespread inflammation occurs, the barrier efficiency of the skin may be impaired secondary to extensive vasodilatation.

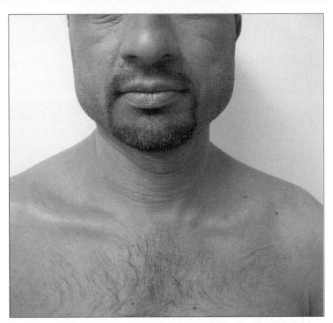

34.46 *Exfoliative erythroderma (exfoliative dermatitis).* This patient has generalized erythema (l'homnie rouge, "red man syndrome"). The etiology of his erythroderma was never determined. (From Goodheart HP. *Goodheart's Same-Site Differential Diagnosis*. Philadelphia, PA: Lippincott Williams & Wilkins, 2011.)

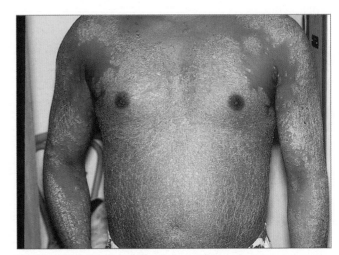

34.47 *Exfoliative erythroderma.* This patient has severe, widespread psoriasis. Note the marked scaling. (From Goodheart HP. *Goodheart's Same-Site Differential Diagnosis*. Philadelphia, PA: Lippincott Williams & Wilkins, 2011.)

- Protein loss secondary to a massive shedding of scale may occur, with resultant hypoalbuminemia.
- Rarely, high-output cardiac failure may develop, particularly in patients with a history of cardiac disease.
- The following chronic changes may also be seen:
  - Scaling of palms and soles (keratoderma).
  - Thickening and lichenification of the skin.
  - Scalp involvement, occasionally producing nonscarring alopecia.

- Nail dystrophy, onycholysis (separation of the nail plate from the nail bed), or nail shedding.
- Pigmentary changes (postinflammatory hypopigmentation or hyperpigmentation).
- Persistent generalized erythema.
- Conjunctivitis, keratitis, or ectropion.

DIAGNOSIS

- The diagnosis of ED is made on a clinical basis and the underlying cause is often elusive.
- Clinical findings, such as the characteristic lichenification and crusting of atopic dermatitis or nail pitting that suggests psoriasis, may be found.
- Eliciting a history of drug ingestion or a preexisting dermatosis may be valuable.
- Laboratory testing can provide serologic evidence of Sézary syndrome or leukemia.
- Patch testing during a period of remission may uncover a contact allergen.

LABORATORY EVALUATION

The following are possible positive laboratory findings:

- Anemia (usually the anemia of chronic disease).
- Decreased serum levels of protein and albumin.
- Leukocytosis.
- Eosinophilia.
- Elevated sedimentation rate.
- Elevated immunoglobulin E level (possibly supporting the diagnosis of atopic dermatitis).
- Leukemia (noted on peripheral blood smear).
- Imaging studies with computed tomography or magnetic resonance imaging if lymphoma or Hodgkin disease is suspected.

 DIFFERENTIAL DIAGNOSIS

Toxic Epidermal Necrolysis (see Chapter 26)

- *A potentially fatal condition that involves the skin and mucous membranes.*
- *Marked erythema is quickly followed by sloughing of the skin.*
- *Often the result of a severe drug reaction.*

 POINTS TO REMEMBER

- In its more severe manifestations, ED is a medical and dermatologic emergency. Consultation and ongoing management, using the expertise of both disciplines, are often necessary.
- In many cases, the underlying cause is never established.

 MANAGEMENT

- Treatment is directed toward the underlying cause, if it is known. For example, suspected etiologic drugs or contactants should be eliminated.
- **Bed rest, cool compresses, lubrication** with emollients, antipruritic therapy with **oral antihistamines,** and **low- to intermediate-strength topical steroids** are used.
- Systemic antibiotics can be administered if signs of secondary infection are observed
- In severe cases, patients frequently require hospitalization, where measures such as fluid replacement, temperature control, expert topical skin care, and systemic corticosteroids may be used.
- Isotretinoin (**Accutane**) has been used when pityriasis rubra pilaris is the underlying cause

Exfoliative Dermatitis Secondary to Psoriasis

- Possible precipitating factors (e.g., ultraviolet exposure) or drugs that are suspected to provoke ED (e.g., antimalarials) should be avoided.
- **Systemic and topical steroids** are helpful, except that they may worsen psoriasis and have been known to precipitate ED or an acute fulminant form of pustular psoriasis, known as pustular psoriasis of Von Zumbusch. This worsening of psoriasis tends to occur after steroid withdrawal.
- If conservative therapy fails, **methotrexate, cyclosporine**, and **retinoids** (e.g., acitretin) are additional therapeutic options.
- Phototherapy, photopheresis, and photochemotherapy, as well as monoclonal antibodies such as infliximab (**Remicade**) and Adalimumab (**Humira**), may be effective.
- For a further discussion of psoriasis (see Chapter 14).

Prognosis

- The course of ED depends on its underlying origin.
- ED resulting from a drug eruption may clear in days to weeks, after the drug is stopped.
- In some cases, ED may persist for many years, with exacerbations and remissions with no apparent diagnosis.
- In patients with an identified underlying cause, the course and prognosis generally parallel the primary disease.
- Acute, severe episodes, particularly in elderly persons or in persons with preexisting heart disease, have a more guarded prognosis.
- In patients with idiopathic ED, the prognosis is poor, and recurrences are not uncommon.

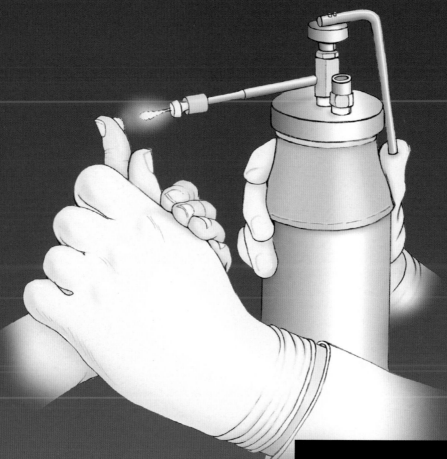

PART FOUR

Dermatologic Procedures

35 Diagnostic and Therapeutic Techniques

OVERVIEW

Because evaluation of the skin is so readily available, a number of diagnostic measures—many of which are noninvasive—can lead to a specific diagnosis. Examples include: KOH examination and fungal culture, Tzanck preparation, scabies preparation, Wood light examination, and patch testing. Skin biopsies using a punch, shave, snip, or excisional methods are relatively free of complications. Cryosurgery (see below), phototherapy (discussed in Chapter 14), and advanced surgical procedures such as Mohs micrographic surgery (see below) are but a few of the many available therapeutic modalities available for skin disorders.

Potassium Hydroxide Test and Fungal Culture*

BASICS

- The potassium hydroxide (KOH) examination provides an immediate diagnosis of a superficial fungal infection, whereas the results of a fungal culture may take weeks. It is a simple, rapid method to detect fungal elements in skin, nails, and hair.

TECHNIQUE

COLLECTION OF SPECIMEN

- Collection is optimal when no surface artifacts (e.g., topical medications) are present.

Skin

- Gently scrape scale from the "active border" with a no. 15 scalpel blade (Fig. 35.1).

Nails

- Trim the nail.
- Use a no. 15 scalpel blade or a 1- to 2-mm curette (Fig. 35.2) under the nail surface to obtain fine scale (thick specimens do not allow for cover slip application).

Hair

- Pluck broken hairs with forceps or use a toothbrush to obtain scale and hairs (Fig. 35.3).

PREPARATION

- Use a KOH solution such as Swartz–Lamkins Fungal Stain or a KOH solution with dimethyl sulfoxide.
- Gather a thin layer of scale, or scale plus hair on a slide and cover it with a coverslip.

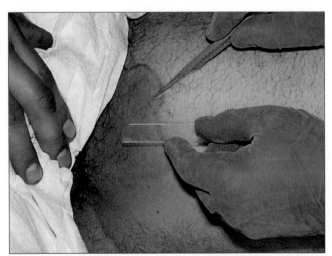

35.1 *Potassium hydroxide examination*. Collection of scale from the "active border" of a lesion.

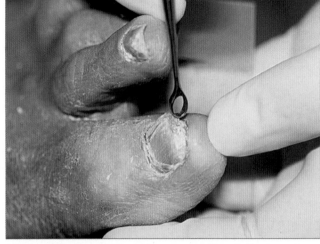

35.2 *Potassium hydroxide examination*. Collection of scale from under the nail after trimming.

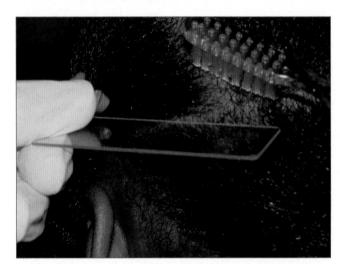

35.3 *Potassium hydroxide examination*. Collection of scale from the scalp of a child using a toothbrush.

- With an eyedropper, place a single drop of a KOH solution at the edge of the coverslip and allow it to spread under the coverslip by capillary action (Fig. 35.4).
- Heat the undersurface of the slide gently with a lighter or a match until bubbling begins. Wipe undersurface of slide to remove black residue of heating (KOH solution with dimethyl sulfoxide does not require heating).

OBSERVATION

- Begin with a low-power scan to identify scale and possibly hyphae.
- Become aware of artifacts that are easily confused with hyphae and spores, such as hairs, clothing fibers, keratinocyte cell borders, and air bubbles.
- Use higher power (40×) to confirm the presence of hyphae or spores (Figs. 35.5 to 35.11).

---

*N.B. Clinical Laboratory Improvement Act guidelines may require the practitioner to use outside laboratory facilities for conducting KOH examinations and fungal cultures.

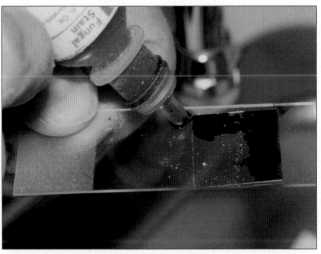

35.4 *Potassium hydroxide examination*. A single drop of a KOH solution is placed at the edge of the coverslip.

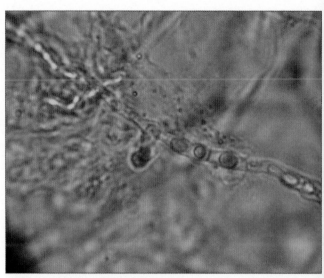

35.6 *Potassium hydroxide examination (40×). Dermatophyte.* Note septate hyphae and spores.

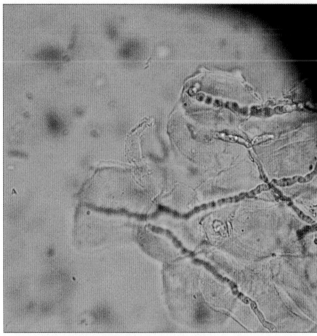

35.5 *Potassium hydroxide examination*. *Dermatophyte.* Note the wavy-branched hyphae with uniform widths coursing over anucleated cell borders.

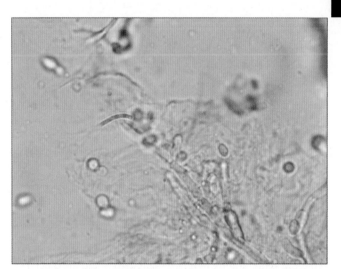

35.7 *Potassium hydroxide examination*. *Candida.* Spores and pseudohyphae (hyphae lack septae).

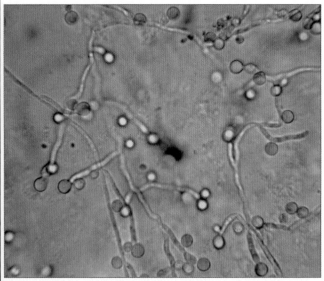

35.8 *Potassium hydroxide examination (40×). Candida.* Pseudohyphae with budding spores.

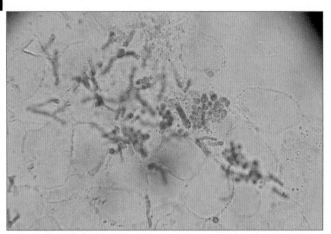

35.9 *Potassium hydroxide examination. Tinea versicolor.* Note the short, stubby hyphae ("spaghetti") and the clusters of spores ("meatballs").

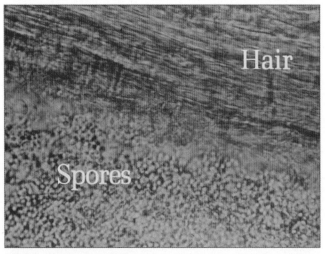

Hair

Spores

35.10 *Potassium hydroxide examination. Ectothrix.* Note the spores *outside* the hair shaft.

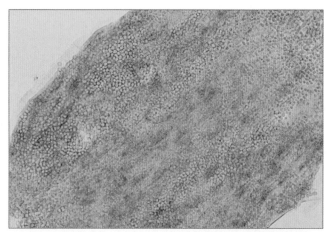

35.11 *Potassium hydroxide examination. Endothrix.* Note spores inside the hair shaft ("sack of marbles").

FUNGAL CULTURE

• Place scales and/or hair collected as described above on Sabouraud agar or on Dermatophyte Test Medium and incubate for 1 to 4 weeks (Fig. 35.12).

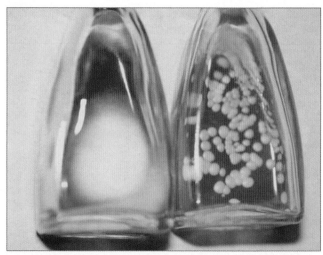

35.12 *Fungal culture using the Dermatophyte Test Medium.* Note the positive result on the *left* as indicated by the color change from yellow to red and the monomorphic colony growth. On the *right* are discrete mucoid growths of a yeast contaminant, despite the false-positive color change to red.

Skin Biopsy

BASICS

- Various skin biopsy techniques are available to the practitioner including shave biopsy, scissor or snip biopsy, punch biopsy, and excisional biopsy. The surgical tools and approaches vary according to size, shape, depth, and site of a lesion.
- When deciding on which biopsy technique to use, it is most important factor to use the technique that will provide the appropriate amount of tissue for a pathologic diagnosis, for example, a shave biopsy on the scalp would not provide enough tissue to make a diagnosis of alopecia areata, a condition of inflammation around the deeper hair bulb.

CHOOSING SITE TO BIOPSY

- Do not choose the biopsy specimen site indiscriminately.
- Evaluate the site according to the clinical impression, the lesion's location, the estimated depth of the pathologic process, the planned tissue studies, and the ensuing cosmetic result. When possible, it is best to biopsy the newest or "freshest" lesion.
- The choice of biopsy technique requires some knowledge of where in the skin (epidermis, dermis, or fat) the pathologic process is likely to be located.

LOCAL ANESTHESIA

- For skin biopsies (and most skin surgery procedures), local anesthesia with 1% **lidocaine with epinephrine** (1:1000,000 or 1:2000,000 dilution) is recommended.
- The epinephrine decreases bleeding and keeps the anesthetic in the area it was injected.
- Draw up 1 to 2 mL for shave or punch biopsies and 3 mL for larger biopsies.
- Methods to decrease pain caused by injections include the following:
  - Add a buffer (sodium bicarbonate) which may be added to the lidocaine.
  - Use a small, 30-gauge needle.
  - Inject very slowly.
  - Help distract the patient by talking continuously.
  - Inject down a hair follicle.
  - Minimize the number of injection sites by reinjecting into areas that are already numb.

SHAVE BIOPSY AND SHAVE REMOVAL

- This is used for the diagnosis and therapeutic removal of superficial (epidermal and upper dermal) skin lesions, such as melanocytic nevi, warts, seborrheic and solar keratoses, pyogenic granulomas, and skin tags, as well as other benign and certain malignant skin tumors.
- It is used to obtain biopsy specimens to confirm skin disease before a more definitive surgical procedure that may be required (e.g., basal or squamous cell carcinoma).

- It is very useful for flattening and diagnosing nevi, particularly in the facial area.

ADVANTAGES

- It is fast and economical.
- The technique is easy to learn.
- Wound care is simple.
- Cosmetic results are generally excellent.
- It does not require sutures.
- It is useful for difficult-to-reach sites (e.g., ear canal, periocular skin).
- It is also advantageous in areas of poor healing (e.g., the lower leg in elderly or diabetic patients).

DISADVANTAGES

- It is not indicated for lesions or diseases that extend into the subcutaneous layer.
- It is not indicated when a full-thickness biopsy is necessary (e.g., deep inflammatory dermatoses).
- It should not be performed on lesions suspected of being melanoma because of the difficulty in clinically determining the maximum thickness or extent of a lesion.

TECHNIQUE

- Anesthetize the area adjacent to the lesion with an injection of 1% plain lidocaine with or without epinephrine into the superficial dermis using a 30-gauge needle. Use lidocaine without epinephrine in finger and toe areas to avoid vascular compromise (Fig. 35.13A,B).
- Inject so that the lidocaine creates a wheal and elevates the lesion above the surrounding skin.
- Applying traction with the thumb and index finger of the free hand on either side of the lesion stabilizes it.
- Place a no. 15 scalpel blade flat on the skin; use in a slight sawing motion with smooth strokes parallel to the skin surface and draw the middle of the blade through the lesion.
- Release traction when the lesion becomes sufficiently free; use small forceps with teeth to hold and elevate the lesion to complete the "shave" and then to deliver it to a bottle of formalin.
- Use low-intensity electrocautery or further shaving to "feather" jagged edges.
- Apply **Monsel solution** (ferric subsulfate) or aluminum chloride 35% with a cotton pledget (**Q-Tip**) to rapidly achieve hemostasis. Hemostasis is possible only if the field is wiped dry of blood.
- Send all pigmented lesions to a pathologist; obvious nonpigmented skin tags do not need to be sent for pathologic evaluation.

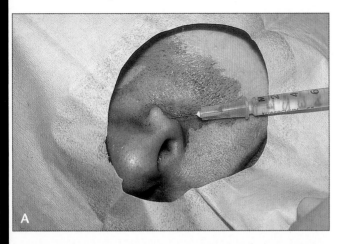

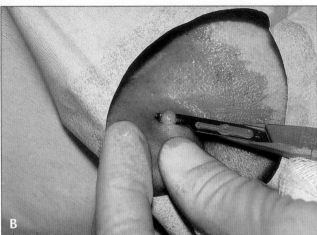

35.13   **A:** *Shave biopsy*. Local anesthesia creates a wheal that elevates the lesion above the surrounding skin. **B:** The lesion is stabilized with the free hand; the blade, which is parallel to the skin surface, is drawn through the lesion.

SCISSOR (SNIP) BIOPSY AND SNIP EXCISION

- Certain elevated or pedunculated lesions, such as warts, nevi, seborrheic keratoses, and skin tags, are ideally suited for removal with a shave or snip (with a scalpel or scissors).
- Many can be precisely removed level to the skin very quickly.

ADVANTAGES

- It is fast; many lesions can be removed in one visit.
- It is economical.
- It frequently can be performed without anesthesia.

DISADVANTAGES

- None exist, except for the possibility of obtaining an inadequate amount of tissue if a specimen is to be sent for histopathologic examination.

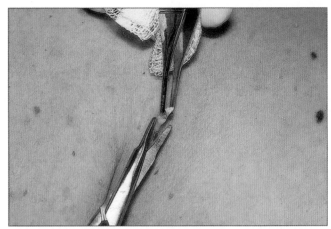

35.14   *Snip excision*. This filiform wart is snipped off after having been anesthetized with lidocaine.

TECHNIQUE

- It may be possible to snip off thin, small lesions without any anesthesia; larger lesions require the administration of local anesthesia. Anesthetize the area of larger lesions in the same manner as for scalpel shave excisions (see above) (Fig. 35.14).
- Gently hold the lesion with small forceps and pull it to cause slight tenting of the epidermis and upper dermis.
- Use straight or curved sharp iris scissors with fine points to snip off the lesion.
- Use light electrodesiccation at the base of the lesion, or apply a styptic (e.g., **Monsel solution**) or aluminum chloride 35% to cause hemostasis (stinging or burning may result if lesion has not been anesthetized). Local pressure is also effective in preventing blood flow.
- Trim away any slight elevation or irregularity of the margin with scissors.

PUNCH BIOPSY

- A punch biopsy involves the use of a 3- to 5-mm cylindric cutting instrument ("punch") to remove all or part of a lesion.
- This method is most useful for biopsy of relatively flat, inflammatory lesions such as seen in psoriasis, lichen planus, and vasculitis.

ADVANTAGES

- The specimen obtained is uniform.
- This is an effective method to evaluate inflammatory skin diseases.
- It is an efficient biopsy method for full-thickness skin.
- The operative site heals rapidly. Skin closure establishes a barrier to infection almost immediately after the procedure.

DISADVANTAGES

- The sample may not adequately show the entire lesion; a second technique (i.e., an elliptical biopsy) may be necessary for adequate demonstration of complete tumor architecture.
- It is not suited for lesions primarily located in the subcutaneous tissue.
- Areas to be avoided are the digits, around the facial nerve, or in any region where the operator is unfamiliar with the underlying anatomy.

TECHNIQUE

- In contrast to shave biopsy, a more thorough approach to sterile technique is necessary (Fig. 35.15).
- Cleanse the lesion and surrounding skin with 70% isopropyl alcohol, povidone-iodine (**Betadine**), or chlorhexidine (**Hibiclens**).
- Anesthetize the area with an injection into the deep dermis with **1% lidocaine** with or without epinephrine, using a 30-gauge needle.
- With the fingers of the nondominant hand, stretch the skin at a 90-degree angle to the natural wrinkle lines.
- Hold the punch between the thumb and forefinger.
- Gently push the punch downward into the dermis while advancing it slowly and twirling it back and forth until it "gives." Caution should be used over thin tissue or over vital structures.
- It is important to push the punch deep enough to obtain underlying fat tissue for an adequate sample.

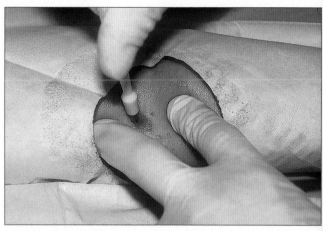

35.15 *Punch biopsy*. Traction of surrounding skin is performed with fingers while the punch is rotated.

- Withdraw the punch along with the tissue sample. If the sample does not come out with the punch, cut it at the base while depressing the surrounding skin.
- Remove the tissue specimen using forceps with teeth and then, if necessary, cut the specimen with iris scissors. Take care to avoid crushing the specimen and distorting the tissue sample.
- Place firm pressure on the circular skin wound to curtail bleeding.
- A one or two sutures for closure is all that is usually necessary.

Simple Elliptical Excision

BASICS

- Excisions are useful for obtaining tissue samples for biopsy and for the removal of many benign and cancerous lesions.
- Excisional biopsies may be performed on discrete lesions, such as cysts, basal or squamous cell carcinoma, malignant melanoma, or other solitary tumors and nevi.
- An incisional biopsy is the incomplete or partial removal of a lesion that may be too big or poorly located to perform a complete excision (e.g., a suspected melanoma that is too large to remove).

ADVANTAGES

- An excision provides a more extensive sample of a lesion that is too large for a shave or a punch biopsy.
- The margins of submitted tissue can be examined for possible involvement (e.g., basal cell carcinoma, squamous cell carcinoma, and melanoma).
- It often affords a definitive cure for many benign and malignant lesions.

DISADVANTAGES

- It is time-consuming.
- It is less economical than shaves or snips.
- It usually requires a return visit for suture removal.

TECHNIQUE

- The operator should be familiar with the underlying and surrounding anatomy.
- A thorough approach to sterile technique is necessary: sterile gloves and sterile drapes should be used.
- To achieve the best cosmetic results, place the lines of incision in or parallel to the relaxed skin. This placement is demonstrated by observing wrinkle lines and the effect of pinching the skin.
- Once a direction for the long axis of the ellipse has been chosen, draw an ellipse using gentian violet or a surgical skin marker around the lesion before administering a local anesthetic. This approach minimizes tissue distortion.
- Make sure that the excision has a length-to-width ratio of at least 3:1 and that the apices are at a 30-degree angle.
- Anesthetize the area by local infiltration with lidocaine and epinephrine 1:100,000.

- Use a no. 15 scalpel blade to make the incision. Use the dominant hand with the index finger and thumb of the other hand placed on either side of the incision. This pushes the skin under tension downward and away from the scalpel (Fig. 35.16A).
- Start the incision using the point of the scalpel held in a vertical position at the apex of the ellipse. Use the belly of the scalpel along the side of the ellipse to elongate the incision (Fig. 35.16B).
- Obtain an optimal tissue sample for histologic examination. The scalpel should cut through the upper subcutaneous fat so that the specimen includes the full thickness of the skin.
- Dissect the tissue free of the underlying fat after making incisions on both sides of the ellipse. Use forceps with teeth to hold the apex of the skin being removed.
- If the defect is large, dissect (undermine) the ellipse by using curved, blunt-tipped scissors (e.g., Steven tenectomy or Gradle scissors), making certain that the plane of the dissection is at the same level throughout. Undermining allows for the mobilization of tissue so that it can be advanced to close the defect; it also allows skin edges to come together with less tension and allows eversion of the wound edges with suturing (Fig. 35.16C).

UNDERMINING TECHNIQUE

- To perform undermining, use blunt-tipped scissors while elevating the skin edge by forceps with teeth or a skin hook.
- Advance scissors to the desired degree and open them to stretch the underlying skin. If necessary, repeat this procedure several times to achieve the desired skin mobility for wound closure.
- Remove any remaining tissue septa using the open blades of the scissors.
- Undermining is most effective when performed at the level of superficial fat tissue. This reduces the possibility of injury to nerves and blood vessels in the facial and neck areas.
- Wound repair is facilitated if an adequate ellipse has formed, the edges are perpendicular to the skin, and skin lines are followed.
- Meticulous hemostasis must occur after undermining. Apply direct pressure or perform electrocoagulation (Fig. 35.16D).
- Place subcutaneous sutures after undermining, to allow approximation of the edges of the wound to close the wound (Fig. 35.16E).

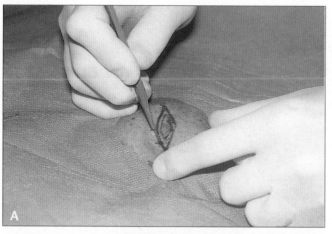

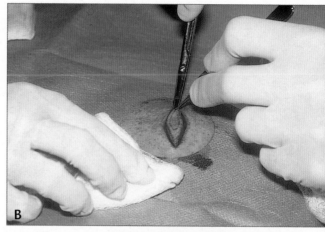

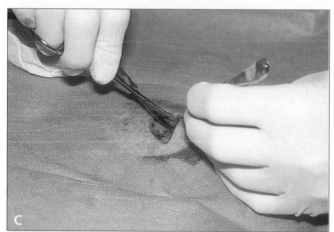

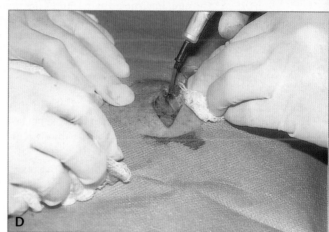

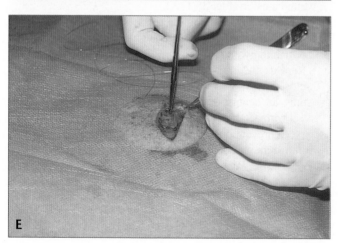

35.16 *Excision.* **A:** The incision is started using the point of the scalpel, held in a vertical position, at the apex of the lesion. Traction is accomplished with the nondominant hand. **B:** The tissue is dissected free of the underlying fat. Forceps are used to hold the apex of the skin being removed. **C:** Undermining is performed using blunt-tipped scissors while the skin edge is elevated by forceps. **D:** Hemostasis is achieved with an electrocautery device. **E:** Deeper, nonabsorbable sutures are used to approximate the wound edges.

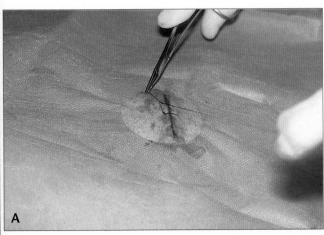

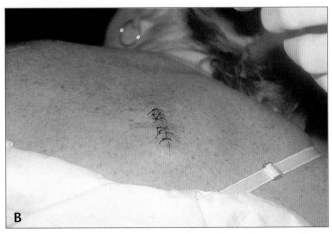

35.17 *Suturing.* **A:** Closure. Interrupted skin sutures are placed using the method of "halving." The first suture was placed in the center of the ellipse. **B:** Dressing. A transparent dressing overlying Steri-Strips allows for visualization of the wound as it heals.

WOUND CLOSURE

- Wounds should be closed in layers (Fig. 35.17A–B).
- The closure of dead space is necessary when large, subcutaneous vacuities have been created, such as after removal of subcutaneous cysts.
- Dermal, buried sutures are important on areas of the body that overlie large muscle groups, such as the upper trunk.

SUTURE MATERIAL

- Obtain hemostasis (a "dry field") before initiating wound closure.
- Choice of suture material depends on the size and degree of tension on the wound and the location on the body.
- For closure of the dermis and deeper subcutaneous layers, absorbable sutures such as polyglactin 910 (**Vicryl**) or polyglycolic acid (**Dexon**) are used. Absorbable sutures are fully absorbed and do not require removal.
- For surface closure of the skin, nonabsorbable sutures such as nylon (**Ethilon**) or polypropylene (**Prolene**) are used.
- For the face and cosmetically sensitive areas, smaller diameters such as 5-0 or 6-0 sutures are recommended. For the limbs or trunk, and areas with greater tension, larger 3-0 or 4-0 sutures are required.

- **Monocryl** is an absorbable suture that is very easy to handle and has excellent tensile strength. It causes little tissue reaction and thus is most often used when minimal tissue reactivity is essential.

SUTURING

- Simple, interrupted skin sutures are most commonly used.
- The method of "halving" is the most effective technique for wound closure. "Halving" allows for equal distribution of wound tension (Fig. 35.17A).
  - Place the first suture in the center of the ellipse.
  - Place the second and third sutures in the centers of the remaining wound lengths.
  - Repeat this procedure until the wound is completely closed.
- Apply an occlusive dressing (a perforated plastic film or sheet with an absorbable pad) or pressure dressing, if necessary, to prevent postoperative bleeding (Fig. 35.17B).
- Suture removal depends on wound tension, location, and depth of placement.
- Generally, removal of facial sutures should occur in 5 to 7 days and removal of sutures on the trunk should be in 1 to 2 weeks.

BASICS

- Electrodesiccation and curettage (ED and C) is a method to remove or destroy many types of benign superficial skin lesions such as warts, seborrheic keratoses, solar keratoses, pyogenic granulomas, and skin tags.
- In experienced hands, it is often used as a method to treat skin cancers such as small basal cell and squamous cell carcinomas.
- Electrodesiccation uses monopolar high-frequency electric currents to destroy lesions; curettage is a scraping or scooping technique performed with a dermal curette, which has a round or oval sharp ring.
- Electrodesiccation without curettage (as an alternative to shave procedures) is often used to eliminate warts, skin tags, and spider angiomas and to flatten lesions (e.g., melanocytic nevi). Conversely, curettage without electrodesiccation may also be used to remove many of these epidermal lesions.
- Curettage is a blind technique in which the specimen cannot always be examined for margin control.

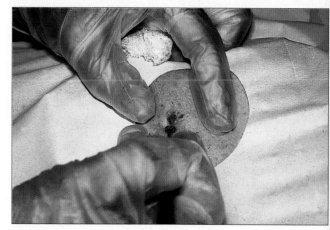

35.18 *Curettage.* Note the traction exerted by the operator's fingers.

ADVANTAGES

- It is fast and economical.
- It is useful for difficult-to-reach sites—ear canal, orbit of the eye.
- It is useful in areas of poor healing—the lower leg in elderly or diabetic patients.
- Secondary infection is uncommon.

DISADVANTAGES

- The procedure is "blind"; margins of lesions can only be guessed.
- Cosmetic results are unpredictable; hypopigmentation and scarring may result.
- Healing is by secondary intention and takes 2 to 3 weeks, which is longer than healing after an excisional procedure.
- Obtaining biopsy specimens from curettage is discouraged.

CURETTAGE

TECHNIQUE

- Anesthetize the area to be biopsied in a similar manner to that described for a skin biopsy (see above). The local anesthetic creates a wheal and elevates the lesion above the surrounding skin.
- Applying traction with the thumb and index finger of the free hand on either side of the lesion stabilizes it and keeps it taut.
- Hold a sharp curette like a pencil and draw it through the tissue with strokes pushed away with the thumb until an adequate amount of tissue is removed (usually when the dermis is reached) (Fig. 35.18).
- Obtain hemostasis by using **Monsel solution** (ferric subsulfate) or aluminum chloride 35% after wiping the field dry of blood.

ELECTRODESICCATION

- Electrodesiccation may be used before or after curettage or used alone.
- It causes superficial destruction with a charring of the skin.

TECHNIQUE

- Perform this procedure after administering local anesthesia.
- Use the lowest possible setting to prevent unnecessary tissue destruction.

Cryosurgery

BASICS

- Cryosurgery entails the destruction of tissue by freezing in a controlled manner, to produce sharply circumscribed necrosis. Tissue destruction results from intercellular and extracellular ice formation, denaturing liquid protein complexes, and cell dehydration.
- A repeat freeze–thaw cycle results in more cellular damage than a single cycle.
- Liquid nitrogen (LN_2) at $-195.8°C$ is the standard agent used. It is applied with a cotton swab, a cryospray gun, or a cryoprobe, and it is stored in a special vacuum container.
- Cryosurgery should be used only when a confident, clinical diagnosis is made.
- It is most commonly used on warts and solar keratoses.

ADVANTAGES

- Cryosurgery is an inexpensive, rapid, and simple technique that does not require complicated apparatus.
- Anesthesia is usually not necessary.
- Postoperative pain is minimal.
- Bleeding is not a problem during or after treatment.
- Sutures are not necessary, and scarring is generally minimal or absent.
- It is a relatively risk-free treatment for the cryosurgeon who treats some skin conditions in patients who are infected with human immunodeficiency virus. These include patients with molluscum contagiosum, condylomata acuminatum, Kaposi sarcoma, and warts.

DISADVANTAGES

- Young children do not tolerate cryosurgery well.
- Scarring may occur, particularly if lesions are overzealously frozen or if the patient tends to heal with hypertrophic scars or keloids.
- Postinflammatory pigmentary alterations may occur; more often, hypopigmentation results because of the destruction of melanocytes.

TECHNIQUE

COTTON TIP APPLICATOR TECHNIQUE

- Place LN_2 in a **Styrofoam** cup.
- Dip a cotton swab into the cup.
- Touch the lesion with the saturated cotton-tipped applicator, with a minimal amount of pressure, and create a 2- to 3-mm zone of freeze around the lesion for a total of 4 to 5 seconds (Fig. 35.19).
- The skin turns white. Care must be taken to avoid dripping onto surrounding, normal skin.

CRYOSPRAY TECHNIQUE

- The standard instrument used is a handheld **Cryogun,** which operates under a working pressure of approximately 6 psi (Figs. 35.20 to 35.23).
- Nozzle attachments with apertures of varying diameter for spray application are available (the "A" nozzle applies the greatest amount of spray; the "D" has the least amount for delicate work).
- Generally, no local anesthesia is necessary.
- For smaller lesions, this procedure involves treating the center of the lesion and allowing the freeze to spread laterally.

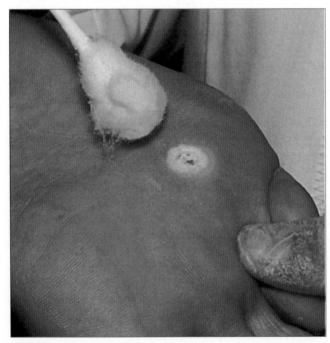

35.19 *Cryosurgery.* Liquid nitrogen is applied with a cotton pledget.

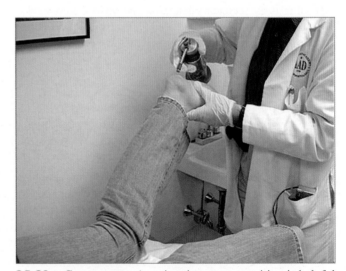

35.20 *Cryosurgery.* A patient in a prone position is helpful in examining and treating plantar lesions.

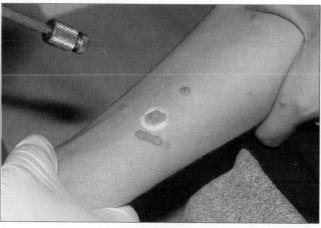

35.21 *Cryosurgery.* Here liquid nitrogen is delivered with a cryospray gun. Note the 2- to 3-mm zone of freeze around the lesion.

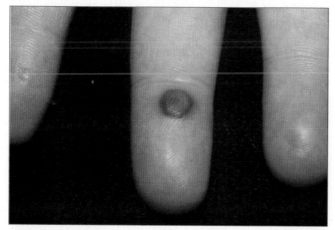

35.22 *Cryosurgery.* Note the wart on the surface of a hemorrhagic blister that appeared 24 hours after treatment with liquid nitrogen.

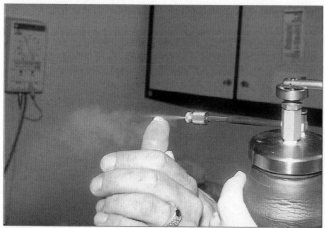

35.23 *Cryosurgery.* Application with a Cryogun apparatus (freezing the lesion at a right angle may lessen the pain).

- The time of application varies, depending on the thickness of the lesion.
- Standardization of freeze times is difficult to categorize for the treatment of benign and premalignant lesions. The goal is to produce, with either the swab or spray technique, a solid ice ball that extends 2 mm onto the surrounding normal skin.

POSTOPERATIVE COURSE AND WOUND CARE

- Mild to moderate swelling may occur at the lesion site.
- A blister or blood blister may form within 24 hours and resolves in 2 to 7 days.
- The lesion site may be cleansed with soap and water during the exudative stage.
- The lesion site starts to dry at the end of the exudative stage and then sloughs.
- A crust, which loosens spontaneously, commonly occurs.

HELPFUL HINTS

- It is best to underfreeze lesions; they can be retreated at a later date.
- For anxious children, a topical anesthetic such as **EMLA cream** (eutectic mixture of local anesthetics) can be applied under occlusion 1 hour before cryosurgery to decrease the discomfort associated with the procedure.
- Alternative delivery methods that can help minimize pain are shown in Figs. 35.23 and 35.24.

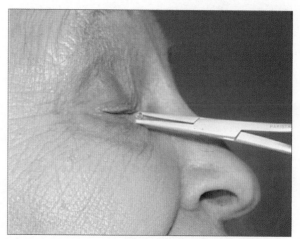

35.24 *Cryosurgery.* Treatment of a cutaneous horn with a hemostat that has been immersed for 10 seconds in liquid nitrogen. This simple, relatively painless procedure causes very little collateral damage to the surrounding skin.

Mohs Micrographic Surgery

BASICS

- Mohs micrographic surgery is a microscopically controlled method of removing skin cancers that allows for controlled excision and maximum preservation of normal tissue.

ADVANTAGES

- Most reliable method in determining adequate margins
- Cure rate between 98% and 99% for basal cell carcinomas
- Preserves the maximum amount of normal tissue around the cancer

DISADVANTAGES

- Time-consuming
- Expensive
- May require extensive reconstruction of surgical wounds

INDICATIONS

Mohs surgery is mostly suited for:

- Recurrent basal and squamous cell carcinomas, particularly those on the face

- Excessively large (>2 cm) or invasive carcinomas
- Carcinomas within an orifice (e.g., ear canals or nostrils)
- Carcinomas in locations where preservation of normal tissue is extremely important (e.g., tip of the nose, ala nasi, eyelids, ears, lips, glans penis)
- Carcinomas in locations known to have a high rate of recurrence (e.g., ala nasi, nasal labial folds, medial canthi, pinnae of the ears, postaurical sulcus)
- Morpheaform or sclerotic (desmoplastic) basal cell carcinoma
- Lesions of the finger or penis

TECHNIQUE

- Excise the tissue in a circular pie-shaped fashion; then systematically map it and examine it by means of frozen sections (Fig. 35.25A–D).
- While the patient waits in the examining room, submit the tissue to a histotechnician for the surgeon to review.
- Repeat excisions in the areas proven to be cancerous until a complete cancer-free plane is reached. Several stages may be necessary.
- Surgical wounds may be left to heal by secondary intention or corrected by plastic reconstructive procedures.

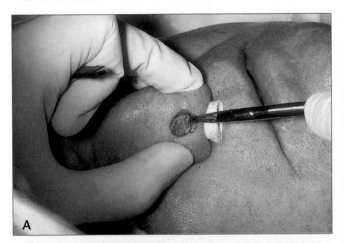

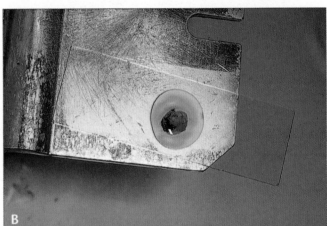

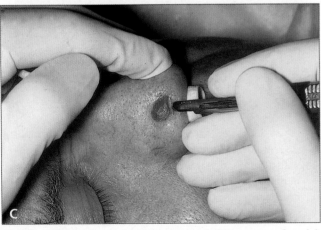

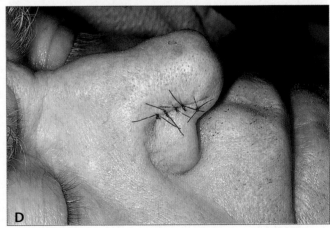

35.25 *Mohs micrographic surgery.* **A:** First stage of excision of lesion. **B:** Excised tissue color-coded, then evacuated by frozen section. **C:** Second stage of excision because the first had positive margins. **D:** Primary closure after the second stage was free of malignancy. (Images courtesy of Michael J. Mulvaney, MD.)

WOUND CARE AND HEALING

- Infections after simple skin surgery are unusual.
- Administration of systemic antibiotics is generally unnecessary.
- Meticulous hemostasis during surgery is essential.
- Small amounts of necrosis normally occur in wound healing.
- Hemostasis induced by electrosurgery, suture ligature, or cautery always produces tissue necrosis.
- Wound healing is delayed when necrosis is extensive.
- Hemostasis can be achieved with a pressure dressing, which is applied for 24 hours.
- When wounds are closed with a considerable amount of tension or if the patient has been taking steroids, the wound should be closed with sutures that are nonabsorbable and buried (nylon or polypropylene) or have prolonged tensile strength (**PDS, Dexon, or Vicryl**). Under the former conditions, skin sutures may be left in place for longer periods of time.
- External splinting using tape provides additional support until the tensile strength of the wound increases after suture removal.
- Exercise that stretches the skin should be avoided to minimize spreading of the scar.

DRESSINGS AND WOUND MANAGEMENT

- For small ellipses, dry, sterile gauze covered with paper tape may be all that is necessary.
- An occlusive dressing or pressure dressing should be applied, if necessary, to prevent postoperative bleeding.
- After 24 hours, the patient can remove the dressing and compress the wound with tap water or hydrogen peroxide. The hydrogen peroxide mechanically softens the wound and removes any debris.
- A topical antibiotic such as bacitracin or plain petroleum jelly (**Vaseline**) is applied to the surface of the wound before applying a clean, occlusive dressing.
- Patients repeat this procedure daily at home until the wound is covered with fresh epidermis.
- Patients are advised to return for follow-up if there is any pain, swelling, tenderness, purulent drainage, discharge, or bleeding of the wound.
- Postoperative pain usually is negligible, and patients are advised to call the surgeon should any pain occur.

Other Procedures

COMEDO EXTRACTION

- Removal of comedones involves a comedo extractor, an instrument that minimizes skin injury. A round loop extractor is used to apply uniform pressure sufficient to dislodge comedonal contents (Fig. 35.26A,B).
- To loosen lesions that offer resistance, insert a pointed instrument such as a lancet or a needle, or a no. 11 blade to carefully incise and expose the contents.
- Extraction can be a useful adjunct to topical therapy when blackheads and whiteheads are somewhat resistant to topical retinoids.

- Pretreatment with a topical retinoid for 4 to 6 weeks often facilitates the procedure.

SIMPLE PUNCH BIOPSY METHOD TO REMOVE CYSTS

- A large lesion such as an epidermoid or pilar cyst can be removed through a small hole and heals with excellent aesthetic results.
- If the results of this procedure are not completely satisfactory, a standard excision can be performed at a future date.

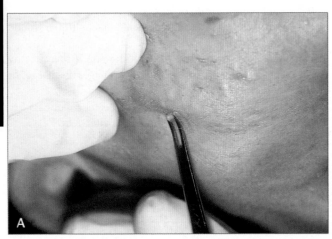
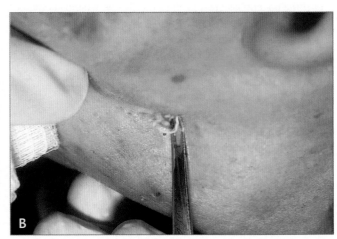

35.26 *Comedo extraction.* **A:** Gentle pressure is exerted along the rim of this closed comedo. **B:** The contents are extruded.

TECHNIQUE

- Superficially administer local anesthesia over the cyst (Fig. 35.27A–D).
- Punch the center of the cyst (the "pore") with a 4-, 6-, or 8-mm disposable punch.

- Dissect the cyst wall using forceps, iris scissors, and manual pressure around the cyst. A chalazion curette can be useful to scrape out any residual cyst wall.
- Close the defect with a 4-0 nylon stitch.

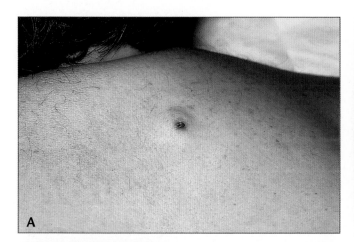

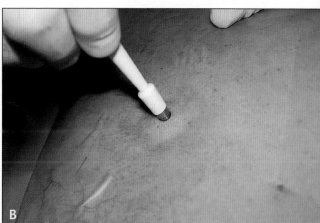

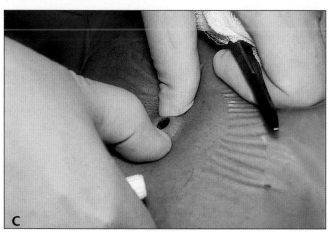

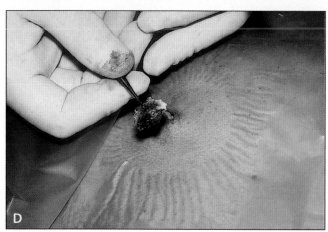

35.27 *Punch biopsy removal of a cyst.* **A:** This epidermoid cyst has a central "pore." **B:** A 6-mm disposable punch creates an opening. **C:** After dissection with iris scissors, pressure is exerted with the operator's thumbs. **D:** The cyst wall is extracted.

Index

Note: Page numbers followed by "f" indicate figure, and "t" indicate table.

hypopigmentation, 371–375 (*See also* Hypopigmentation)
idiopathic guttate hypomelanosis, 375, 375f
melanogenesis and, 370
other hypomelanosis, 375
overview of, 370
Pigmentary mosaicism, 44f, 45f
Pilomatricomas, 144, 144f
Pimecrolimus (Elidel), 18–19
for aphthous stomatitis, 343
for atopic dermatitis, 83
for inverse psoriasis, 251
for necrobiosis lipoidica diabeticorum, 536
for periorificial dermatitis, 74
for perlèche, 348
for pityriasis alba, 89
for seborrheic dermatitis, 92
for vitiligo vulgaris, 373
Pimozide, for delusions of parasitosis, 386
Pincer nails, 365, 365f
Pinworm infestation, 103
Pioglitazone, for lichen planopilaris, alopecia from, 328
Pitted keratolysis, 104, 104f
Pityriasis alba, 45, 89, 89f, 374, 374f
Pityriasis amiantacea, 91
Pityriasis rosea (PR), 9, 9f, 260–262, 260f–261f
basics of, 260
clinical manifestations of, 260, 260f
clinical variants of, 261
diagnosis of, 261
differential diagnosis of, 262
lesion distribution in, 260–261, 261f
lines of cleavage, 14, 14f
management of, 262
pathogenesis of, 260
points to remember on, 262
Pityriasis versicolor. *See* Tinea versicolor
Pityrosporum folliculitis, 99, 275
Pityrosporum orbiculare, in tinea versicolor, 312
Pityrosporum ovale, 90
in tinea versicolor, 312
Planar xanthomas, 543
Plantar warts, 104, 107, 107f, 108, 111, 283, 283f, 285, 286. *See also* Warts, nongenital
Plaquenil, for juvenile dermatomyositis, 177
Plaques, 4, 4f
pruritic urticarial papules and plaques of pregnancy, 513, 513f
Plateau (or late proliferative) phase, IH, 32
Plexiform neuromas, 179, 180f
Podofilox (Condylox), for HIV-associated molluscum contagiosum, 520
Podophyllin, for HIV-associated oral hairy leukoplakia, 529

Poikiloderma, 552, 552f
of Civatte, 379, 379f
Poison ivy, 9, 9f
Polycystic ovary syndrome (PCOS), hirsutism in, 336–337, 337f
Polyglactin 910 (Vicryl), for suturing, 582
Polyglycolic acid (Dexon), for suturing, 582
Poly-l-lactic acid (Sculptra®), for HIV-associated lipoatrophy, 533
Polyostotic fibrous dysplasia. *See* McCune–Albright syndrome
Polypropylene (Prolene), for suturing, 582
Pomade acne, 70
Port-wine stain (PWS), 29–31
basics of, 29
clinical manifestations of, 29
diagnosis of, 29
differential diagnosis, 29
on face, 29f
helpful hint on, 30
Klippel–Trenaunay syndrome (KTS), 31
on leg, 31f
location and associated syndrome of, 29t
management of, 30
pathogenesis, 29
Sturge–Weber syndrome (SWS), 30
on thigh, 31f
Postherpetic neuralgia (PHN), 295
Postinflammatory hyperpigmentation, 377, 377f
Postinflammatory hypopigmentation, 45, 372, 374–375, 374f
Potassium hydroxide, for superficial viral infections, 116
Potassium hydroxide (KOH) test, 572–574, 572f–574f
Povidone-iodine (Betadine), for impetigo, 272
PPGSS. *See* Papular-purpuric gloves and socks syndrome
Prednisolone, 35
Prednisone, 35. *See also* Corticosteroids
for hidradenitis suppurativa, 279
for oral lichen planus, 344
Pregnancy, 509–514
dermatoses of, 513–514
pemphigoid gestationis, 514, 514f
pruritic urticarial papules and plaques of pregnancy, 513, 513f
pruritus gravidarum, 513–514
recurrent cholestasis of pregnancy, 514
normal skin changes in, 510–512
connective tissue changes, 510, 510f
erythema multiforme, 511–512
erythema nodosum, 511, 512f
gums, 511
hair changes, 511
hyperpigmentation, 510, 510f
pyogenic granuloma, 511, 511f
vascular phenomena, 511, 511f
overview of, 509

pyogenic granuloma, 351
Pregnancy gingivitis, 512
Pretibial myxedema lesions, 541–542, 541f, 542f
Primary lesions, 2–5, 2f–5f. *See also* specific lesions
Procedures. *See* Diagnostic and therapeutic techniques; *specific techniques*
Progressive systemic sclerosis, 557–558, 557f–558f
Propionibacterium, 96
Propranolol, 34
Prostaglandins, for scleroderma, 558
Protopic ointment. *See* Tacrolimus (Protopic ointment)
Pruritic urticarial papules and plaques of pregnancy (PUPPP), 513, 513f
Pruritus, 382–387
aquagenic, 387
brachioradial pruritus, 387
delusions of parasitosis, 386
factitial dermatitis, 385, 385f
HIV-associated, 531
neurotic excoriations, 385, 385f
notalgia paresthetica, 387, 387f
overview of, 382
pruritus of unknown origin, 383–384, 383f
from systemic disease, 387
Pruritus gravidarum, 513–514
Pruritus of unknown origin, 383–384, 383f
Pseudofolliculitis barbae, 332–333, 332f–333f
Pseudomonas folliculitis, 274, 274f
Pseudomonas nail infection
green nail syndrome, 358, 358f
paronychia, 362
vs. onychomycosis, 308
Psoralen, for scleroderma, 558
Psoralen plus topical ultraviolet A (PUVA). *See also* UVA (ultraviolet light A)
for lichen planus, 268
for psoriasis of palms and soles, 253
for vitiligo vulgaris, 373
Psoriasis, 9f, 14, 14f, 43, 61f, 61t, 82, 91, 103, 235–258, 236f–237f, 361, 361f
acute guttate, 247, 247f
arthritis, 256, 256f
basics of, 236
clinical manifestations of, 237
clinical sequelae of, 237–238
course, 238
fissuring of plaques, 237
Köbner reaction (isomorphic response), 237, 237f–238f
pruritus, 237
psychosocial problems, 237–238
triggers, 238
diagnosis of, 238
differential diagnosis of, 238
exfoliative dermatitis, 257–258, 257f